P9-EEH-363

Oral Radiology

Principles and Interpretation

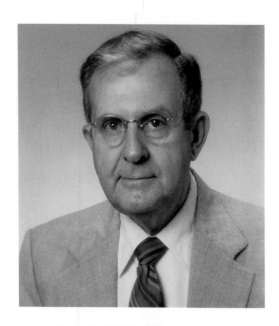

Dr. PAUL W. GOAZ
1922-1995

Shortly after publication of the previous release of this book,
Dr. Paul W. Goaz, lead author on the first three editions, passed away.
We remember him as a scholar with insatiable curiosity, as an author who
focused on clarity and thoroughness, as a teacher who loved his students,
and as a colleague and friend of great humor and patience.
We dedicate this edition to him.

Oral Radiology

Principles and Interpretation

STUART C. WHITE, DDS, PhD

Professor, Section of Oral and Maxillofacial Radiology
School of Dentistry
University of California, Los Angeles
Los Angeles, California

MICHAEL J. PHAROAH, DDS, MSc, FRCD(C)

Professor, Department of Radiology
Faculty of Dentistry
University of Toronto
Toronto, Ontario
Canada

Fourth Edition

with 1046 *illustrations*

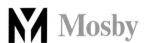

St. Louis Baltimore Boston Carlsbad Chicago Minneapolis New York Philadelphia Portland
London Milan Sydney Tokyo Toronto

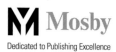

Publisher: John Schrefer
Editor: Penny Rudolph
Associate Developmental Editor: Kimberly Frare
Project Manager: Linda McKinley
Production Editor: Jennifer Furey
Designer: Renée Duenow
Cover Design: Elizabeth Rohne Rudder

FOURTH EDITION

Mosby, Inc.
A Harcourt Health Sciences Company
11830 Westline Industrial Drive
St. Louis, Missouri 63146

Printed in United States
Composition by Top Graphics
Lithography by Top Graphics
Printing/binding by Maple-Vail Book Manufacturing Group, Binghamton, New York

Library of Congress Cataloging in Publication Data

Oral radiology : principles and interpretation / [edited by] Stuart C.
  White, Michael J. Pharoah. — 4th ed.
    p. cm.
  Includes bibliographical references and index.
  ISBN 0-8151-9491-9
  1. Teeth—Radiography. 2. Jaws—Radiography. 3. Mouth—Radiography.
 I. White, Stuart C. II. Pharoah, M. J.
  [DNLM: 1. Radiography, Dental.   WN 230 G573o 1999]
RK309.07 1999
617.6′07572—dc21
DNLM/DLC
for Library of Congress   98-53444
                                     CIP

99 00 01 02 03 / 9 8 7 6 5 4 3 2 1

Contributors

KATHRYN A. ATCHISON, DDS, MPH
Professor,
University of California School of Dentistry,
Center for the Health Sciences,
Los Angeles, California

BYRON W. BENSON, DDS, MS
Professor,
Department of Diagnostic Sciences,
Baylor College of Dentistry,
Texas A&M University System,
Dallas, Texas

SHARON L. BROOKS, DDS, MS
Professor,
Department of Oral Medicine/Pathology/Oncology,
University of Michigan School of Dentistry;
Associate Professor,
Department of Radiology,
University of Michigan School of Medicine,
Ann Arbor, Michigan

NEIL L. FREDERIKSEN, DDS, PhD
Professor and Director, Oral and Maxillofacial Radiology,
Department of Diagnostic Sciences,
Baylor College of Dentistry,
Texas A&M University System,
Dallas, Texas

BARTON M. GRATT, DDS, PhD
Professor of Oral Radiology,
Department of Oral Medicine,
University of Washington,
Seattle, Washington

LINDA LEE, DDS, MSC, DIPL, ABOP, FRCD(C)
Assistant Professor,
Department of Radiology,
Faculty of Dentistry, University of Toronto;
Active Staff Dentist,
Department of Dentistry,
Ontario Cancer Institute,
Princess Margaret Hospital,
Toronto, Ontario,
Canada

STEPHEN R. MATTESON, DDS
Professor and Chairman,
Department of Dental Diagnostic Science,
University of Texas Health Science Center,
Dental School,
San Antonio, Texas

C. GRACE PETRIKOWSKI, DDS, MSC, DIP. ORAL RAD, FRCD(C)
Assistant Professor,
Department of Radiology,
Faculty of Dentistry, University of Toronto,
Toronto, Ontario,
Canada

AXEL RUPRECHT, DDS, MSCD, FRCD(C)
Professor and Director, Oral and Maxillofacial Radiology,
Department of Oral Pathology, Radiology, and Medicine,
College of Dentistry;
Professor,
Department of Radiology,
College of Medicine,
University of Iowa,
Iowa City, Iowa

VIVEK SHETTY, DDS, DR MED DENT
Associate Professor,
Department of Oral and Maxillofacial Surgery,
University of California School of Dentistry,
Los Angeles, California

ROBERT E. WOOD, DDS, MSC, PhD, FRCD(C)
Assistant Professor,
Radiology Department,
University of Toronto;
Active Staff Dentist,
Department of Dentistry,
Princess Margaret Hospital,
Toronto, Ontario,
Canada

To our wives and children

Liza
Heather and Kelly

Linda
Jayson, Edward, and Lian

"Man erblickt nur, was man shon weiss und versteht."

Johann Wolfgang von Goethe
Gespräche mit F.V. Müller
24.4.1819

One recognizes only what one already knows and understands.

Preface

As *we close* this century, we reflect on the changes and new opportunities in our lives, profession, and the world. This book inevitably reflects many of these changes. In the two decades since work on the first edition began, dentistry has experienced increasing awareness of the importance of infection control; the risks associated with exposure to ionizing radiation; the introduction of faster films; improved film/screen combinations; improved technology for complex motion tomography; rapid developments in new imaging modalities such as digital radiography, computed tomography (CT), and magnetic resonance imaging (MRI); and the development of new therapies, including osseous integrated implants. Our understanding of the molecular mechanisms and pathophysiology of diseases affecting the oral cavity is becoming increasingly sophisticated, as is our awareness of a growing range of radiographic manifestations, especially those contributed by new imaging modalities (e.g., CT, MRI) for oral disease. Because of these continuous changes, oral and maxillofacial radiology is an especially exciting field of study and practice. As we look to the future, we see only an acceleration of these trends. We can anticipate, for instance, that the field of digital imaging is in its infancy and will play an increasingly important role in image acquisition, display, and disease identification in the new millennium.

It is a particular pleasure for me (SCW) to welcome Michael J. Pharoah as a co-editor of this text. He has made significant contributions to this new edition, especially the chapters concerned with the interpretation of disease, and brings the benefit of knowledge acquired from teachers that included Drs. Harry Worth, Guy Poyton, and Douglas Stoneman.

In this edition of the book, as before, we seek to bring to the reader a clear presentation of the basic principles of oral and maxillofacial radiology. This text does not attempt to be an encyclopedia. We endeavor to convey the core body of knowledge required for dental students to be able to use imaging thoughtfully for the diagnosis and management of disease in the oral and maxillofacial region. Our intent is to describe the practical application of radiology as well as its underlying principles. This gives the student the knowledge to provide state-of-the-art care as well as the insight to evaluate the efficacy of future developments in this field.

Even as many aspects of oral and maxillofacial radiology change, others stay constant. We cannot overemphasize the importance of a sound knowledge of normal anatomy for radiographic interpretation. Only with a clear appreciation for the range of normal can abnormality be identified. Just as critical for effective radiographic interpretation is knowledge of the mechanisms of disease and the effects of pathologic processes on normal structures. By understanding the radiographic changes associated with disease processes, the clinician can classify lesions into general categories of disease, which results in a logical interpretation and treatment plan. With this edition we have made a special effort to standardize the presentation of the cardinal radiographic features of each condition considered, including its location, periphery, shape, internal structure, and effects on surrounding structures. As before, this information is placed in context with clinical features, differential diagnosis, and management.

Acknowledgments

This book is the product of the generous contributions of many. Twelve of the chapters of this edition are contributed in whole or part by colleagues. We thank them for sharing their expertise in this endeavor. We are also pleased to acknowledge the insightful comments of other colleagues, including Drs. Peter Hirschmann, Susan Kinder, Alan Lurie, Colin Price, and Donald Tyndall, who have reviewed parts of this work in draft form. Messrs. David Allen and Thomas Russell of Eastman Kodak Company made valuable suggestions regarding film and film processing. Also, Ms. Karen Strebel and Mr. Patrick Mason of the Media Department at UCLA made invaluable contributions to the quality of new illustrations. And, of course, our students are a helpful and continuing source of inspiration for better ways to present the material.

Stuart C. White
Michael J. Pharoah

Contents

Oral Radiology

Principles and Interpretation

The Physics of Ionizing Radiation

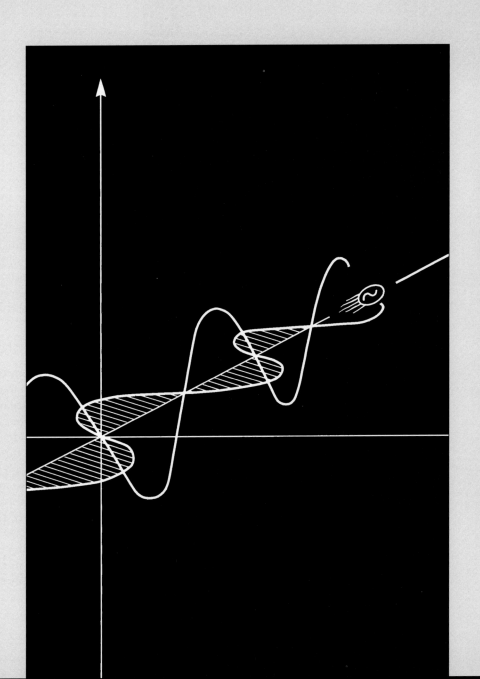

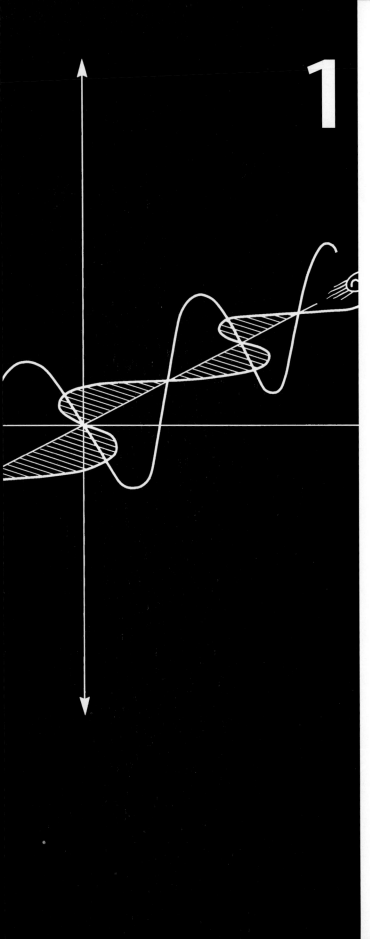

1

Radiation Physics

In collaboration with

ALBERT G. RICHARDS

Composition of Matter

All things are composed of matter. Matter is anything that occupies space and has inertia. It has mass and can exert force or be acted on by a force. It occurs in three states—solid, liquid, and gas—and may be divided into elements and compounds. Atoms, the fundamental units of elements, and cannot be subdivided by ordinary chemical methods but may be broken down into smaller (subatomic) particles by special high-energy techniques. More than 100 subatomic particles have been described; the so-called "fundamental" particles (electrons, protons, and neutrons) are of greatest interest in radiology because the generation, emission, and absorption of radiation occurs at the subatomic level.

ATOMIC STRUCTURE

Because the atom cannot be directly observed, various models are used to describe its structure, each of which is capable of explaining observable actions. The phenomena associated with radiology employ the quantum mechanical model proposed by Niels Bohr in 1913. Bohr conceived the atom as a miniature solar system, at the center of which is the nucleus, analogous to the sun. Electrons revolve around this nucleus at high speeds, analogous to the planets orbiting the sun. In all atoms except hydrogen, the nucleus consists of two primary subatomic particles: protons and neutrons. A single proton constitutes the nucleus of the hydrogen atom. Electrons orbit the nucleus of all atoms. All electrons are alike, as are all protons and neutrons.

Fig. 1-1, *A*, illustrates Bohr's model using a stylized rendering of three atoms. The paths of the electrons are drawn as sharply defined orbits to facilitate graphic representation of the generation of x-rays and their interaction with matter. In reality the orbit should be represented by broad parameters defining a space in which the electron is most likely to be found. The orbits, or shells, lie at defined distances from the nucleus and are identified by a letter (Fig. 1-1, *B*). The innermost shell is the K shell, and the next in order are the L, M, N, O, P, and Q shells. The shells also have numbers for identification: 1 for the K shell, 2 for the L shell, and so on. These are the principal quantum numbers, represented by the letter *n*. No known atom has more than seven shells. Only two electrons may occupy the K shell, with increasingly larger numbers of electrons occupying the outer shells. The maximal number of electrons in a given shell is $2(n^2)$, where *n* is the principal quantum number.

Electrons, protons, and neutrons have unique characteristics. The electron carries an electrical charge of -1, the proton a charge of $+1$, and the neutron no charge at all. The mass of an electron at rest is about 9.1×10^{-28} g. In contrast, the mass of a proton is 1.67×10^{-24} g, which is 1838 times the mass of an electron. The mass of a neutron is 1.68×10^{-24} g, making it 1841 times heavier than an electron and slightly heavier than a proton. Most of the mass of an atom consists of protons and neutrons concentrated in the nucleus. The nucleus contributes only a small fraction (about $\frac{1}{100,000}$) of the total size of an atom; most of the size of an atom is contributed by the cloud of electrons orbiting it.

The number of protons contained in the nucleus determines the positive charge. Because any atom in its ground state is electrically neutral, the total number of protons and electrons it carries must be the same. The number of protons in the nucleus also determines the identity of an element. This is its atomic number, which is designated by the symbol *Z*. Consequently, each of the more than 100 types of atoms (elements) has a definitive atomic number, a corresponding number of orbital electrons, and unique chemical and physical properties. Nearly the entire mass of the atom consists of the protons and neutrons in the nucleus. The total number of protons and neutrons in the nucleus of an atom is its atomic mass, designated by the symbol *A*.

The electrostatic attraction between a positively charged nucleus and its negatively charged electrons balances the centrifugal force of the rapidly revolving electrons and maintains them in their orbits. Consequently, the amount of energy required to remove an electron

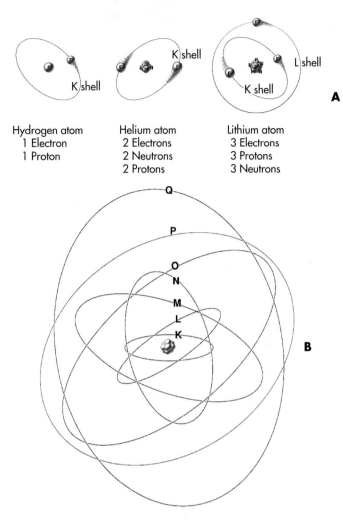

Hydrogen atom
1 Electron
1 Proton

Helium atom
2 Electrons
2 Neutrons
2 Protons

Lithium atom
3 Electrons
3 Protons
3 Neutrons

FIG. **1-1 A,** Atomic structures of hydrogen, helium, and lithium showing orbiting electrons surrounding neutrons and protons in the nucleus. **B,** Atom showing the structure and identification of electron shells around the nucleus.

from a given shell must exceed the electrostatic force of attraction between it and the nucleus. This is called the *binding energy* of the electron and is specific for each shell of each atom. Electrons in the K shell of a given atom have the greatest binding energy because they are closest to the nucleus. The binding energy of the electrons in each successive shell decreases. To move an electron from a specific orbit to another orbit farther from the nucleus, energy must be supplied in an amount equal to the difference in binding energies between the two orbits. In contrast, in moving an electron from an outer orbit to one closer to the nucleus, energy is lost and given up in the form of electromagnetic radiation. (See "Characteristic Radiation," p. 12.) The K-shell electrons or any other electrons of large (high-Z) atoms have greater binding energies than those in comparable shells of smaller (low-Z) atoms. This is because large atoms have more protons and thus bind the orbital electrons more tightly to the nucleus than do small atoms.

IONIZATION

If the number of orbiting electrons in an atom is equal to the number of protons in its nucleus, the atom is electrically neutral. If an electrically neutral atom loses an electron, it becomes a positive ion, and the free electron is a negative ion. This process of forming an ion pair is termed *ionization*. Heating or interactions (collisions) with high-energy x-rays or particles such as protons can remove electrons from an atom. Such ionization requires sufficient energy to overcome the electrostatic force binding the electrons to the nucleus. The electrons in the inner shells (K, L, and M) are so tightly bound to the nucleus that only x-rays, gamma rays, and high-energy particles can remove them. In contrast, the electrons in the outer shells have such low binding energies that they can be easily displaced by photons of lower energy (e.g., ultraviolet or visible light).

Nature of Radiation

Radiation is the transmission of energy through space and matter. It may occur in two forms: particulate and electromagnetic.

PARTICULATE RADIATION

Particulate radiation consists of atomic nuclei or subatomic particles moving at high velocity. Alpha rays, beta rays, and cathode rays are examples of particulate radiation. Alpha rays are high-speed doubly ionized helium nuclei consisting of two protons and two neutrons. They result from the decay of many radioactive elements. After acquiring two electrons, they become neutral helium atoms. Because of their double charge and heavy mass, they densely ionize matter through which they pass. Accordingly, they quickly give up their energy and penetrate only a few microns of body tissue. (An ordinary sheet of paper absorbs them.)

Beta and cathode rays are both high-speed electrons. Beta rays are emitted by radioactive nuclei, and cathode rays are produced by manufactured devices (e.g., x-ray tubes). The very high–speed beta particles are able to penetrate matter to a greater depth than alpha particles, to a maximum of 1.5 cm in tissue. This deeper penetration occurs because beta particles are smaller and

lighter and carry a single negative charge; therefore they have a much lower probability of interacting with matter than alpha particles. They ionize matter much less densely than alpha particles. Beta particles are used in radiation therapy for treatment of skin lesions.

The capacity of particulate radiation to ionize atoms depends on its kinetic energy, which equals $\frac{1}{2}$ (mass $\times$ velocity^2), and its charge. The rate of loss of energy from a particle as it moves along its track through matter (tissue) is its linear energy transfer (LET). A particle loses kinetic energy at each ionization; the greater its physical size and charge and the lower its velocity, the greater is its LET. For example, alpha particles (with their high charge and low velocity) have a high LET (are densely ionizing) and as a consequence lose kinetic energy rapidly and have short path lengths. Beta particles (which are much less densely ionizing because of their lighter mass and lower charge) have a lower LET than alpha particles and thus penetrate through tissue more readily.

ELECTROMAGNETIC RADIATION

Electromagnetic radiation is the movement of energy through space as a combination of electric and magnetic fields. It is generated when the velocity of an electrically charged particle is altered (Fig. 1-2). Gamma rays, x-rays, ultraviolet rays, visible light, infrared radiation (heat), microwaves, and radio waves are all exam-

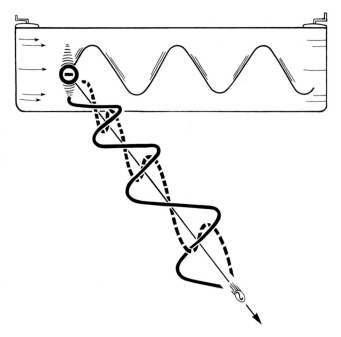

FIG. **1-2** A vibrating negatively charged particle generates electromagnetic radiation. Oscillations of the particle are traced on a strip recorder; they are equal in frequency to the electromagnetic waves produced.

ples of electromagnetic radiation (Fig. 1-3). Gamma rays are photons having the same energy range as x-rays, but they originate in the nuclei of radioactive atoms. X-rays, in contrast, originate from the interaction of electrons and nuclei in a manufactured device, an x-ray machine for example. The types of radiation in this spectrum are ionizing or nonionizing depending on their energy. If sufficient energy is associated with the radiation to remove orbital electrons from the atoms in the irradiated matter, the radiation is ionizing.

Some of the properties of electromagnetic radiation are best expressed by wave theory, whereas others are most successfully described by quantum theory. The wave theory of electromagnetic radiation maintains that radiation is propagated in the form of waves, not unlike the waves resulting from a disturbance in water. Such waves consist of electrical and magnetic fields oriented in planes at right angles to one another that oscillate perpendicular to the direction of motion (Fig. 1-4). They move forward much as a ripple moves over the surface of water. All electromagnetic waves travel at the velocity of light (3.0×10^8 m per sec; the velocity of light is represented by the letter c) in a vacuum. Waves of all kinds exhibit the properties of wavelength (λ) and fre-

Wavelength

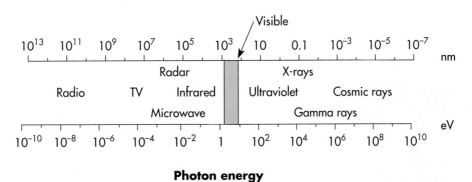

Photon energy

FIG. **1-3** Electromagnetic spectrum showing the relationship among wavelength, photon energy, and physical properties of various portions of the spectrum. Photons with shorter wavelengths have higher energy. Photons used in dental radiography have a wavelength of 0.1 to 0.001 nm.

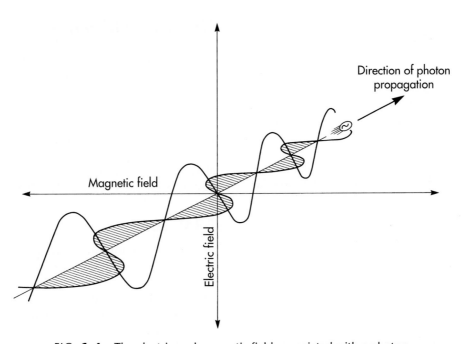

FIG. **1-4** The electric and magnetic fields associated with a photon.

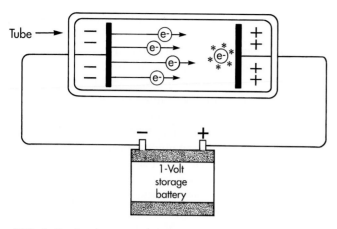

FIG. **1-5** An electron volt is the amount of energy acquired by one electron accelerating through a potential difference of 1 volt (1.602 × 10⁻¹⁹ joules).

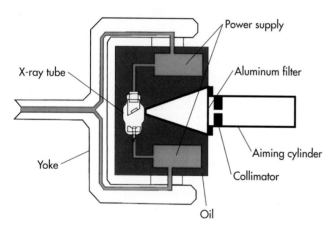

FIG. **1-6** Tube head (including the recessed x-ray tube), components of the power supply, and the oil that conducts heat away from the x-ray tube.

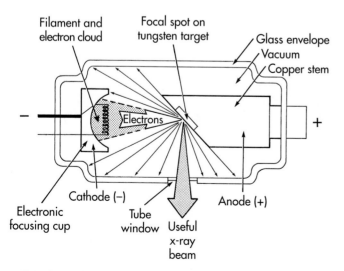

FIG. **1-7** X-ray tube with the major components labeled.

quency (v). Wavelength and frequency of electromagnetic radiation are related as follows:

$$\lambda \times v = c = 3 \times 10^8 \text{ m per sec}$$

where λ is in meters and v is in cycles per second (hertz). Wave theory is more useful for considering radiation in bulk when millions of quanta are being examined, as in experiments dealing with refraction, reflection, diffraction, interference, and polarization.

Quantum theory depicts electromagnetic radiation as small bundles of energy called *photons*. Each photon travels at the speed of light and contains a specific amount of energy. The unit of photon energy is the electron volt (eV) (Fig. 1-5). The relationship between wavelength and photon energy is as follows:

$$E = h \times (c/\lambda)$$

where E is energy in kiloelectron volts (keV), h is Planck's constant (6.25×10^{34} joule-seconds), c is the velocity of light, and λ is wavelength in nanometers. This expression may be simplified as follows:

$$E = 1.24/\lambda$$

The quantum theory of radiation has been successful in correlating experimental data on the interaction of radiation with atoms, the photoelectric effect, and the production of x-rays.

Typically, high-energy photons such as x-rays are characterized by their energy, whereas lower-energy photons (ultraviolet through radio waves) are characterized by their wavelength.

The X-Ray Machine

The heart of an x-ray machine is the x-ray tube and its power supply. The x-ray tube is positioned within the tube head along with some components of the power supply (Fig. 1-6). Often the tube is recessed within the tube head to improve the quality of the radiographic image. (See Chapter 5.) The tube head is supported by an arm that is usually mounted on a wall. A control panel allows the operator to adjust the time of exposure and often the energy and exposure rate of the x-ray beam.

X-RAY TUBE

The basic apparatus for generating x-rays, the x-ray tube, is composed of a cathode and an anode (Fig. 1-7). The cathode serves as a source of electrons to be directed at the anode. The cathode and anode lie within an evacuated glass envelope or tube. When electrons from the cathode strike the target in the anode, they produce x-rays. For the x-ray tube to function, a power supply is necessary to establish high-voltage potentials between the anode and cathode to accelerate the electrons (Fig. 1-8).

CATHODE

The cathode (see Fig. 1-7) of an x-ray tube consists of a filament and a focusing cup. The filament is the source of electrons within the x-ray tube. It is a coil of tungsten wire about 2 mm in diameter and 1 cm or less in length. It is mounted on two stiff wires that support it and carry the electric current. These two mounting wires lead through the glass envelope and connect to both the high- and low-voltage electrical sources. The filament is heated to incandescence by the flow of current from the low-voltage source and emits electrons at a rate proportional to the temperature of the filament.

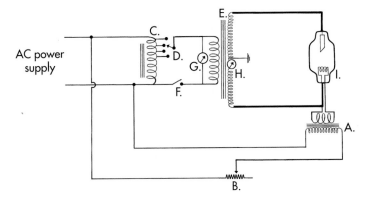

FIG. **1-8** Dental x-ray machine circuitry with the major components labeled. *A,* Filament step-down transformer; *B,* filament current control (mA switch); *C,* autotransformer; *D,* kVp selector dial (switch); *E,* high-voltage transformer; *F,* x-ray timer (switch); *G,* tube voltage indicator (volt-meter); *H,* tube current indicator (ammeter); *I,* x-ray tube.

The filament lies in a focusing cup (see Figs. 1-7 and 1-9, *A*), a negatively charged concave reflector made of molybdenum. The focusing cup electrostatically focuses the electrons emitted by the incandescent filament into a narrow beam directed at a small rectangular area on the anode called the *focal spot* (see Figs. 1-7 and 1-9, *B*). The electrons move in this direction because they are repelled by the negatively charged cathode and attracted to the positively charged anode. The x-ray tube is evacuated as completely as possible to prevent collision of the moving electrons with gas molecules, which would significantly reduce their speed. It also prevents oxidation and "burnout" of the filament.

ANODE

The anode consists of a tungsten target embedded in a copper stem (see Fig. 1-7). The purpose of the target in an x-ray tube is to convert the kinetic energy of the electrons generated from the filament into x-ray photons. The target is made of tungsten, a material that has many characteristics of an ideal target material. It has a high atomic number, high melting point, and low vapor pressure at the working temperatures of an x-ray tube. A target material with a high atomic number is best because it is most efficient for the production of x-rays. Only a small amount of the KE of electrons coming from the filament generates x-ray photons when the electrons strike the focal spot of the target. Because this is an inefficient process, with more than 99% of the electron kinetic energy converted to heat, the requirement for a high melting point is clear. Although the atomic number of tungsten (74) is lower than that of some other metals, its melting point is much higher. The low vapor pressure of tungsten at high temperatures also helps maintain the vacuum in the tube at high operating temperatures.

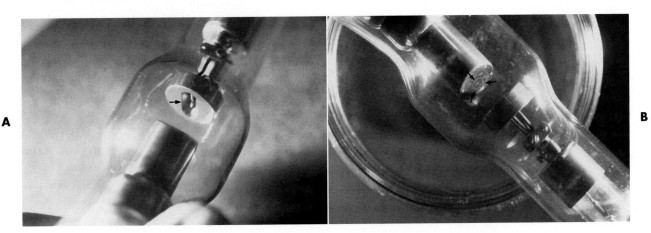

FIG. **1-9** **A,** Focusing cup *(arrow)* containing a filament in the cathode of the tube from a dental x-ray machine. **B,** Focal spot area *(arrows)* on the target of the tube. The size and shape of the focal area approximate those of the focusing cup.

Because the thermal conductivity of tungsten is relatively low, the tungsten target is typically embedded in a large block of copper. Copper, a good thermal conductor, dissipates heat from the tungsten, thus reducing the risk of target melting. In addition, an insulating oil may circulate between the glass envelope and the protective tube housing carrying away heat from the copper stem. This type of anode is a stationary anode.

The focal spot is the area on the target to which the focusing cup directs the electrons from the filament. The sharpness of the radiographic image increases as the size of the radiation source—the focal spot—decreases. (See Chapter 5.) The heat generated per unit target area, however, becomes greater as the focal spot decreases in size. To take advantage of the smaller focal spot while distributing the electrons over the surface of a larger target, the target is placed at an angle to the electron beam (Fig. 1-10). The projection of the focal spot perpendicular to the electron beam (the effective focal spot) is smaller than the actual size of the focal spot. Typically the target is inclined about 20 degrees to the central ray of the x-ray beam. This causes the effective focal spot to be almost 1×1 mm, as opposed to the actual focal spot, which is about 1×3 mm. The effect is a small apparent source of x-rays and an increase in sharpness of the image (see Fig. 5-2) with a larger actual focal spot for heat dissipation.

Another method of dissipating the heat from a small focal spot is to use a rotating anode. In this case the tungsten target is in the form of a beveled disk that rotates when the tube is in operation (Fig. 1-11). As a result, the electrons strike successive areas of the target, widening the focal spot by an amount corresponding to the circumference of the beveled disk and distribut-

ing the heat over this expanded area. As a consequence, small focal spots can be used with tube currents of 100 to 500 milliamperes (mA), 10 to 50 times that possible with stationary targets. The target and rotor (armature) of the motor lie within the x-ray tube, and the stator coils (which drive the rotor at about 3000 revolutions per minute) lie outside the tube. Such rotating anodes are not used in intraoral dental x-ray machines but may be used in cephalometric units and in medical x-ray machines requiring higher radiation output.

POWER SUPPLY

A brief review of some aspects of an electric circuit may be useful in understanding the power supply in an x-ray machine. An electric current is the movement of electrons in a conductor, for example, a wire. The rate of the current flow—the number of electrons moving past a point in a second—is measured in amperes. It depends on two factors: the pressure, or voltage, of the current measured in volts, and the resistance of the conductor to the flow of electricity, measured in ohms. These units are related by Ohm's law:

$$V = I \times R$$

where V is the electric potential in volts, I is the current flow in amperes, and R is the resistance of the conductor in ohms. Such an electric circuit is often compared to a simple water supply system in which the rate of water flow through a pipe (amperes) depends both on the wa-

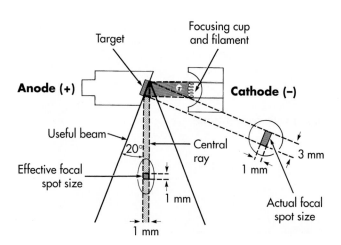

FIG. **1-10** The angle of the target to the central ray of the x-ray beam has a strong influence on the apparent size of the focal spot. The projected effective focal spot is much smaller than the actual focal spot size.

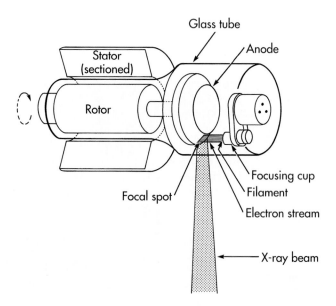

FIG. **1-11** X-ray tube with a rotating anode, which allows heat at the focal spot to spread out over a large surface area.

ter pressure (volts) and the pipe resistance or diameter (ohms).

The primary functions of the power supply of an x-ray machine are to (1) provide a low-voltage current to heat the x-ray tube filament by use of a step-down transformer and (2) generate a high potential difference between the anode and cathode by use of a high-voltage transformer. These transformers and the x-ray tube lie within an electrically grounded metal housing called the *head* of the x-ray machine. An electrical insulating material, usually oil, surrounds the transformers.

The filament step-down transformer (see Fig. 1-8, *A*) reduces the voltage of the incoming alternating current (AC) to about 10 volts. Its operation is regulated by the filament current control (mA switch) (see Fig. 1-8, *B*), which adjusts the resistance and thus the current flow through the low-voltage circuit, including the filament. This in turn regulates the temperature of the filament and thus the quantity of electrons emitted. The electrons emitted by the filament travel to the anode and constitute the tube current. The mA setting on the filament current control refers to the tube current, which is measured by the ammeter (see Fig. 1-8, *H*). The tube current is the flow of electrons from the filament to the anode and then back to the filament through the wiring of the power supply.

The output of the autotransformer (see Fig. 1-8, *C*) is regulated by the kilovolts peak (kVp) selector dial (see Fig. 1-8, *D*). The kVp dial selects varying voltages from different levels on the autotransformer and applies them across the primary winding of the high-voltage transformer. The kVp dial therefore controls the voltage between the anode and cathode of the x-ray tube. The high-voltage transformer (see Fig. 1-8, *E*) provides the high-voltage required by the x-ray tube to accelerate the electrons from the cathode to the anode and generate x-rays. It accomplishes this by boosting the peak voltage of the incoming line current to up to 60 to 100 kV and thus the peak energy of the electrons passing through the tube to up to 60 to 100 keV.

Because the line current is AC (60 cycles per second), the polarity of the x-ray tube alternates at the same frequency (Fig. 1-12, *A*). When the polarity of the voltage applied across the tube is such that the target anode is positive and the filament is negative, the electrons around the filament accelerate toward the positive target and current flows through the tube (Fig. 1-12, *B*). As the tube voltage is increased, the speed of the electrons toward the anode increases. Because the line voltage is variable, the voltage potential between the anode and cathode varies. The kVp selector dial setting controls the peak kilovoltage across the tube (see Fig. 1-8, *I*) during one cycle. When the electrons strike the focal spot of the target, some of their energy converts to x-ray photons. X-rays are produced at the target with greatest efficiency when the voltage applied across the tube is high. There-

fore the intensity of x-ray pulses tends to be sharply peaked at the center of each cycle (Fig. 1-12, *C*). During the following half (or negative half) of the cycle, the polarity of the AC reverses, and the filament becomes positive and the target negative (see Fig. 1-12, *B*). At these times the electrons stay in the vicinity of the filament and do not flow across the gap between the two elements of the tube. This half of the cycle is called *inverse voltage* or *reverse bias* (see Fig. 1-12, *B*). No x-rays are generated during this half of the voltage cycle (see Fig. 1-12, *C*). Therefore when an x-ray tube is powered with 60-cycle AC, 60 pulses of x-rays are generated each second, each having a duration of $\frac{1}{120}$ second. This type of power supply circuitry, in which the alternating high voltage is applied directly across the x-ray tube, limits x-ray production to half the AC cycle. It is called *self-rectified* or *half-wave rectified*. Almost all conventional dental x-ray machines are self-rectified.

A tube energized with a self-rectifying power supply must not be operated for extended periods. With overuse the target may get so hot that it emits electrons, and during the negative half cycle, the inverse voltage may drive electrons from the target to the filament, causing the filament to overheat and melt. The glass envelope also may be damaged if the electrons are driven in the wrong direction by the reverse bias on the tube.

Recently, some dental x-ray manufacturers have produced machines that replace the conventional 60-cycle AC high-voltage current of the x-ray tube with a high-frequency power supply. This effect is an essentially constant potential between the anode and cathode. The result is that the mean energy of the x-ray beam produced by these x-ray machines is higher than that from a conventional half-wave rectified machine operated at the same voltage. This is because the number of lower-energy (nondiagnostic) x-rays is reduced. These photons are produced as the voltage across the x-ray tube rises from zero to its peak and then decreases back again to zero during the voltage cycle in the half-wave rectified machine (see the "Production of X-Rays" section). For a given voltage setting and radiographic density, the images resulting from these constant-potential machines have a longer contrast scale and lower patient dose compared with conventional x-ray machines.

TIMER

A timer is built into the high-voltage circuit to control the duration of the x-ray exposure (see Fig. 1-8, *F*). The timer controls the time that high voltage is applied to the tube and therefore the time during which tube current flows and x-rays are produced. Before the high voltage is applied across the tube, however, the filament must be brought to operating temperature to ensure an adequate rate of electron emission. Subjecting the filament to con-

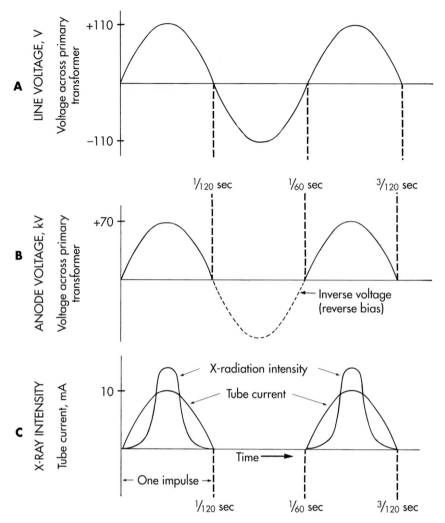

FIG. **1-12**   **A,** A 60-cycle AC line voltage at a primary transformer. **B,** Voltage at the anode varies up to the kVp setting (70 in this case). **C,** The intensity of radiation produced at the anode increases as the anode voltage increases. (Modified from Johns HE, Cunningham JR: *The physics of radiology,* ed 3, Springfield, Ill, 1969, Charles C Thomas.)

tinuous heating at normal operating current is not practical because maintaining the filament at a high temperature for a long period shortens its life. Failure of the filament is a common source of malfunction of x-ray tubes. To minimize filament burnout, the timing circuit first sends a current through the filament for about half a second to bring it to the proper operating temperature. After the filament is heated, the timer then applies power to the high-voltage circuit. In some circuit designs, a continuous low-level current passing through the filament maintains it at a safe low temperature. In this case the delay to preheat the filament before each exposure is even shorter. Accordingly, the machine should be left on continuously during working hours.

Some x-ray machine timers are calibrated in fractions and whole numbers of seconds. The time intervals on other timers are expressed as number of impulses per exposure (e.g., 3, 6, 9, 15). The number of impulses divided by 60 (the frequency of the power source) gives the exposure time in seconds. Therefore 30 impulses is equivalent to a half-second exposure.

TUBE RATING AND DUTY CYCLE

Each x-ray machine comes with tube rating specifications that describe the maximal exposure time that the tube can be energized without risk of damage to the target from overheating. These specifications describe in graph form the maximal safe intervals (seconds) that the tube can be used for a range of voltages (kVp) and filament current (mA) values. These tube ratings generally do not impose any restrictions on tube use for dental periapical radiography. If a dental x-ray unit is to be used for extraoral exposures, however, the tube rating chart should be mounted by the machine for easy reference.

The duty cycle relates to the frequency with which successive exposures can be made. The heat buildup at the anode is measured in heat units defined by the following equation: heat units (HU) = kVp × mA × sec (watt-sec), an actual measure of energy. The heat storage capacity for anodes of various diagnostic tubes ranges from 100,000 to 250,000 HU. Because of heat generated at the anode, the interval between successive exposures must be long enough for its dissipation. This characteristic is a function of the size of the anode and the method used to cool it. The cooling characteristics of anodes are described by the maximal number of heat units it can store without damage and the heat dissipation rate, which can be determined from the cooling curves provided by the manufacturer of each tube.

Production of X-Rays

Electrons traveling from the filament to the target convert some of their KE into x-ray photons by the formation of bremsstrahlung and characteristic radiation.

BREMSSTRAHLUNG RADIATION

Bremsstrahlung interactions, the primary source of x-ray photons from an x-ray tube, are produced by the sudden stopping or slowing of high-speed electrons at the target. When the electrons from the filament strike the tungsten target, x-ray photons are created if they either hit a target nucleus directly or their path takes them close to a nucleus. If a high-speed electron hits the nucleus of a target atom, all its kinetic energy is transformed into a single x-ray photon (Fig. 1-13, *A*). The energy of the resultant photon (in keV) is numerically equal to the energy of the electron. This in turn is equal to the kilovoltage applied across the x-ray tube at the instant of its passage.

Most high-speed electrons, however, have near or wide misses with atomic nuclei (Fig. 1-13, *B*). In these interactions, a negatively charged high-speed electron is attracted toward the positively charged nuclei and loses some of its velocity. This deceleration causes the electron to lose some kinetic energy, which is given off in the form of a photon. The closer the high-speed electron approaches the nuclei, the greater is the electrostatic attraction on the electron, the braking effect, and the energy of the resulting bremsstrahlung photon.

Bremsstrahlung interactions generate x-ray photons with a continuous spectrum of energy. The energy of an x-ray beam may be described by identifying the peak operating voltage (in kVp). A dental x-ray machine operating at a peak voltage of 70,000 volts (70 kVp) for ex-

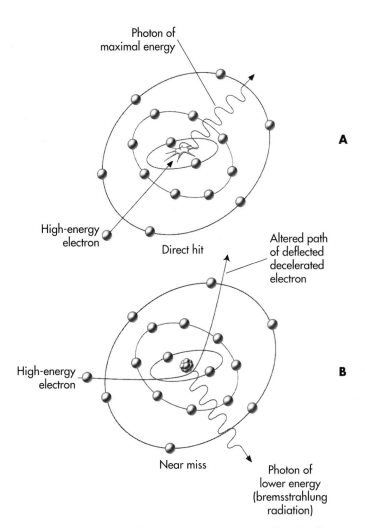

FIG. **1-13** Bremsstrahlung radiation is produced by the direct hit of electrons on the nucleus in the target **(A)** or by the passage of electrons near the nucleus, which results in electrons' being deflected and decelerated **(B)**.

ample, applies a fluctuating voltage of as much as 70 kVp across the tube. This tube therefore produces x-ray photons with energies ranging to a maximum of 70,000 eV (70 keV). Fig. 1-14 demonstrates the continuous spectrum of photon energies produced by an x-ray machine operating at 100 kVp. The reasons for this continuous spectrum are as follows:

1. The continuously varying voltage difference between the target and filament, which is characteristic of halfwave rectification, causes the electrons striking the target to have varying levels of kinetic energy.
2. Most electrons participate in many interactions before all their kinetic energy is expended. As a consequence, an electron carries differing amounts of energy at the time of each interaction with a tungsten atom that results in the generation of an x-ray photon.

3. The bombarding electrons pass at varying distances around tungsten nuclei and are thus deflected to varying extents. As a result, they give up varying amounts of energy in the form of bremsstrahlung photons.

CHARACTERISTIC RADIATION

Characteristic radiation occurs when an electron from the filament displaces an electron from a shell of a tungsten target atom, thereby ionizing the atom. When this happens, another electron in an outer shell of the tungsten atom is quickly attracted to the void in the deficient inner shell (Fig. 1-15). When the displaced electron is replaced by the outer-shell electron, a photon is emitted with an energy equivalent to the difference in the two orbital binding energies. Characteristic radiation from the K shell occurs only above 70 kVp with a tungsten target and occurs as discrete increments compared with bremsstrahlung radiation (see Fig. 1-14). The energies

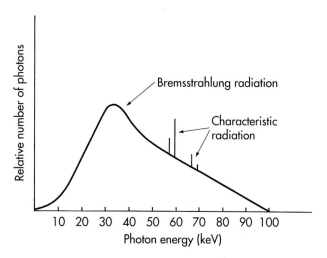

FIG. 1-14 Spectrum of photons emitted from an x-ray beam generated at 100 kVp. The vast preponderance of radiation is bremsstrahlung, with a minor addition of characteristic radiation.

of characteristic photons are a function of the energy levels of various electron orbital levels and hence are characteristic of the target atoms. Characteristic radiation is only a minor source of radiation from an x-ray tube.

Factors Controlling the X-Ray Beam

The x-ray beam emitted from an x-ray tube may be modified to suit the needs of the application by altering the beam exposure length (timer), exposure rate (mA), beam energy (kVp and filtration), beam shape (collimation), and target-patient distance.

EXPOSURE TIME

Figure 1-16 portrays the changes in the x-ray spectrum that result when the exposure time is increased while the tube current (mA) and voltage (kVp) remain constant. When the exposure time is doubled, the number of photons generated is doubled, but the range of photon energies is unchanged. Therefore changing the time simply controls the "quantity" of the exposure, the number of photons generated.

TUBE CURRENT (mA)

Fig. 1-17 illustrates the changes in the spectrum of photons that result from increasing tube current (mA) while maintaining constant tube voltage (kVp) and exposure time. As the mA setting is increased, more power is applied to the filament, which heats up and releases more electrons that collide with the target to produce radiation. Theoretically, a linear relationship exists between mA and radiation output. Therefore the quantity of radiation produced by an x-ray tube (i.e., the number of photons that reach the patient and film) is directly pro-

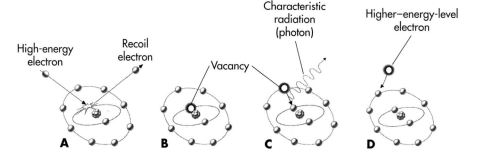

FIG. 1-15 Characteristic radiation. **A,** An incident electron in an inner orbit ejects a photoelectron, creating a vacancy. **B,** This vacancy is filled by an electron from an outer orbit. **C,** A photon is emitted with energy equal to the difference in energy levels between the two orbits. **D,** Electrons from various orbits may be involved, giving rise to other photons. The energies of the photons thus created are characteristic of the target atom.

portional to the tube current and the time the tube is operated. The quantity of radiation produced is expressed as the product of time and tube current. The quantity of radiation remains constant regardless of variations in mA and time as long as their product remains constant. For instance, a machine operating at 10 mA for 1 second (10 mAs) produces the same quantity of radiation when operated at 20 mA for 0.5 second (10 mAs). Although this is generally true, in practice some dental x-ray machines fall slightly short of this ideal.

TUBE VOLTAGE (kVp)

Fig. 1-18 shows the way the spectrum of photon energies in a x-ray beam increases through increases in tube voltage (kVp). Increasing the kVp increases the potential

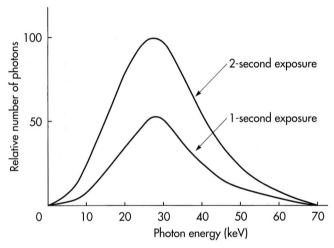

FIG. **1-16** Spectrum of photon energies showing that as exposure time increases, so does the total number of photons, but the mean energy and maximal energy of the beams are unchanged.

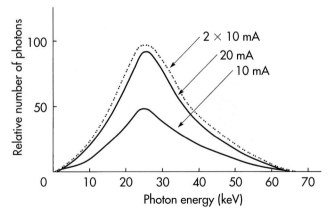

FIG. **1-17** Spectrum of photon energies showing that two 10-mA exposures result in slightly more radiation than one 20-mA exposure. The difference, however, is slight.

difference between the cathode and anode, thus increasing the energy of each electron when it strikes the target. This results in an increased efficiency of conversion of electron energy into x-ray photons, and thus an increase in (1) the number of photons generated, (2) their mean energy, and (3) their maximal energy. The increased number of high-energy photons produced per unit time by use of higher kVp results from the greater efficiency in the production of bremsstrahlung photons that occurs when increased numbers of higher-energy electrons interact with the target.

The ability of x-ray photons to penetrate matter depends on their energy. High-energy x-ray photons have a greater probability of penetrating matter, whereas relatively low-energy photons have a greater probability of being absorbed. Therefore the higher the kVp and mean energy of the x-ray beam, the greater the penetrability of the beam through matter. A useful way to characterize the penetrating quality of an x-ray beam is by its half-value layer (HVL). The HVL is the thickness of an absorber, such as aluminum, required to reduce by one half the number of x-ray photons passing through it. As the average energy of an x-ray beam increases, so does its HVL. The term *quality* refers to the mean energy of an x-ray beam.

FILTRATION

An x-ray beam consists of a spectrum of x-ray photons of different energies, but only photons with sufficient energy to penetrate through anatomic structures and reach the image receptor (usually film) are useful for diagnostic radiology. Those that are of low energy (long wavelength) contribute to patient exposure but do not have enough energy to reach the film. Consequently, to reduce patient dose, the less-penetrating photons should be removed. This can be accomplished by plac-

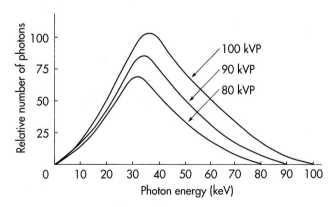

FIG. **1-18** Spectrum of photon energies showing that as the kVp is increased (with mA held constant), a corresponding increase occurs in the mean energy of the beam, the total number of photons emitted, and the maximal energy of the photons.

ing an aluminum filter in the path of the beam. Fig. 1-19 illustrates how the addition of an aluminum filter alters the energy distribution of the unfiltered beam. The aluminum preferentially removes many of the lower-energy photons with lesser effect on the higher-energy photons that are able to penetrate to the film.

In determinations of the amount of filtration required for a particular x-ray machine, kVp and inherent filtration of the tube and its housing must be considered. Inherent filtration consists of the materials that x-ray photons encounter as they travel from the focal spot on the target to form the usable beam outside the tube enclosure. These materials include the glass wall of the x-ray tube, the insulating oil that surrounds many dental tubes, and the barrier material that prevents the oil from

escaping through the x-ray port. The inherent filtration of most x-ray machines ranges from the equivalent of 0.5 to 2 mm of aluminum. Total filtration is the sum of the inherent filtration plus any added external filtration supplied in the form of aluminum disks placed over the port in the head of the x-ray machine. Governmental regulations require the total filtration in the path of a dental x-ray beam to be equal to the equivalent of 1.5 mm of aluminum to 70 kVp, and 2.5 mm of aluminum for all higher voltages. (See Chapter 3.)

COLLIMATION

A collimator is a metallic barrier with an aperture in the middle used to reduce the size of the x-ray beam (Fig. 1-20, *A, B*) and therefore the volume of irradiated tissue within the patient. Round and rectangular collimators are most frequently used in dentistry. Dental x-ray beams are usually collimated to a circle 2¾ inches (7 cm) in diameter. The round collimator (see Fig. 1-20, *A*) is a thick plate of radiopaque material (usually lead) with a circular opening centered over the port in the x-ray head through which the x-ray beam emerges. Typically, round collimators are built into open-ended aiming cylinders. Rectangular collimators (see Fig. 1-20, *B*) further limit the beam to a size just larger than that of the x-ray film. The size of the beam should be reduced to the size of the film being exposed to reduce further unnecessary patient exposure. Some types of film-holding instruments also provide rectangular collimation of the x-ray beam. (See Chapters 3 and 9.)

Use of collimation also improves image quality. When an x-ray beam is directed at a patient, about 90% of the x-ray photons are absorbed by the tissues and 10% of

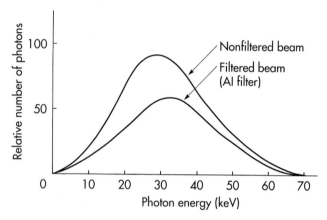

FIG. **1-19** Filtration of an x-ray beam with aluminum results in the preferential removal of low-energy photons, reducing the intensity of the beam but increasing its mean energy.

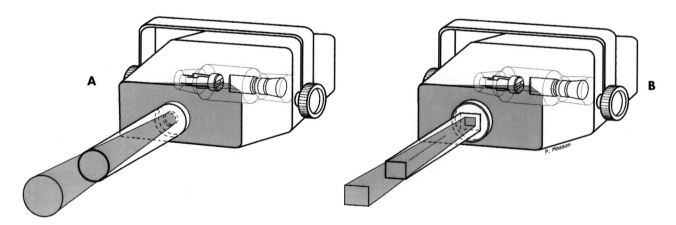

FIG. **1-20** Collimation of an x-ray beam *(dotted area)* is achieved by restricting its useful size. **A,** Circular collimator. **B,** Rectangular collimator restricts area of exposure to just larger than the detector size.

the photons pass through the patient and reach the film. Many of the absorbed photons generate scattered radiation within the exposed tissues by a process called *Compton scattering*. These scattered photons travel in all directions (Fig. 1-21). Many fog the film and thereby degrade image quality. The detrimental effect of scattered radiation on the images can be minimized by collimating the beam to reduce the number of scattered photons reaching the film.

INVERSE SQUARE LAW

The intensity of an x-ray beam at a given point (number of photons per cross-sectional area per unit exposure time) depends on the distance of the measuring device from the focal spot. For a given beam the intensity is inversely proportional to the square of the distance from the source (Fig. 1-22). The reason for this decrease in intensity is that the x-ray beam spreads out as it moves from the source. The relationship is as follows:

$$\frac{I_1}{I_2} = \frac{(D_2)^2}{(D_1)^2}$$

where *I* is intensity and *D* is distance. Therefore if a dose of 1 gray (Gy) is measured at a distance of 2 m, a dose of 4 Gy will be found at 1 m, and 0.25 Gy at 4 m.

Therefore changing the distance between the x-ray tube and patient has a marked effect on beam intensity. Such a change requires a corresponding modification of the kVp or mAs if the exposure of the film is to be kept constant.

Interactions of X-Rays with Matter

The intensity of an x-ray beam is reduced by interaction with the matter it encounters. This attenuation results from interactions of individual photons in the beam with atoms in the absorber. The x-ray photons are either absorbed or scattered out of the beam. In absorption, photons ionize absorber atoms and convert their energy into KE of the absorber electrons. In scattering, photons are ejected out of the primary beam as a result of interactions with the orbital electrons of absorber atoms. In the case of a dental x-ray beam, three mechanisms exist by which these interactions take place: (1) coherent scattering, (2) photoelectric absorption, and (3) Compton scattering. In addition, about 9% of the primary photons pass through the patient without interaction (Table 1-1).

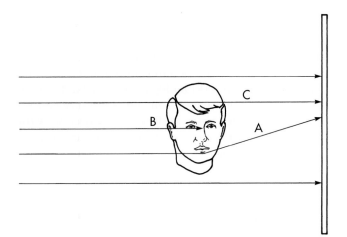

FIG. **1-21** Scattered radiation resulting from Compton interaction *(A)* may strike the film and degrade the radiographic image by causing film fog. Photons may also be absorbed *(B)* or pass through the object without interacting *(C)*.

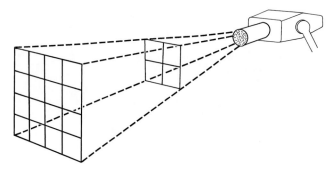

FIG. **1-22** The intensity of an x-ray beam is inversely proportional to the square of the distance between the source and the point of measure.

TABLE **1-1** *Fate of 2,000,000 Incident Photons in Bitewing Projections*			
INTERACTION	PRIMARY PHOTONS	SCATTERED PHOTONS*	TOTAL
Coherent scatterings	148,905	156,234	305,139
Photoelectric	536,208	522,082	1,058,290
Compton effect	1,131,878	1,098,720	2,230,598
Exit	183,009	758,701	941,710
	2,000,000	2,535,737	4,535,737

*Scattered photons result from primary, Compton, and coherent interactions.
From Gibbs SJ: Personal communication, 1986.

COHERENT SCATTERING

Coherent scattering (also known as *classical scattering*) may occur when a low-energy incident photon passes near an outer electron of an atom (which has a low binding energy). The photon may not be absorbed but scattered without a loss of energy (Fig. 1-23). The incident photon interacts with the electron by causing it to vibrate momentarily at the same frequency as the incoming photon. The incident photon then ceases to exist. The vibration causes the electron to radiate energy in the form of another x-ray photon with the same frequency and energy as in the incident beam. Usually the secondary photon is emitted at an angle to the path of the incident photon. In effect, the direction of the incident x-ray photon is altered. This interaction accounts for only about 8% of the total number of interactions (per exposure) in a dental examination (see Table 1-1). Coherent scattering contributes very little to film fog because the total quantity of scattered photons is small and its energy level is too low for much of it to reach the film.

PHOTOELECTRIC ABSORPTION

Photoelectric absorption occurs when an incident photon collides with a bound electron in an atom of the absorbing medium. At this point the incident photon ceases to exist. The electron is ejected from its shell and becomes a recoil electron (photoelectron) (Fig. 1-24). The kinetic energy imparted to the recoil electron is equal to the energy of the incident photon minus that used to overcome the binding energy of the electron. The absorbing atom is now ionized because it has lost an electron. In the case of atoms with low atomic numbers (e.g., those in most biologic molecules), the binding energy is small. As a result the recoil electron acquires most of the energy of the incident photon. Most photoelectric interactions occur in the K shell because the density of the electron cloud is greater in this region and a higher probability of interaction exists. About 30% of photons absorbed from a dental x-ray beam are absorbed by the photoelectric process.

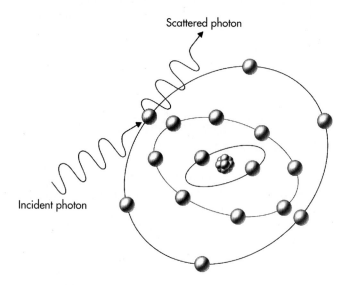

FIG. **1-23**   Coherent scattering resulting from the interaction of a low-energy incident photon with an outer electron, causing it to vibrate momentarily. After this, a scattered photon of the same energy is emitted at a different angle from the path of the incident photon.

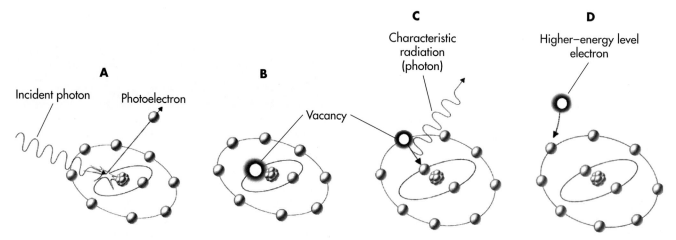

FIG. **1-24**   **A,** Photoelectric absorption occurs when an incident photon gives up all its energy to an inner electron ejected from the atom (a photoelectron). **B,** An electron vacancy in the inner orbit results in ionization of the atom. **C,** An electron from a higher energy level fills the vacancy and emits characteristic radiation. **D,** All orbits are subsequently filled, completing the energy exchange.

An atom that has participated in a photoelectric interaction is ionized. This electron deficiency (usually in the K shell) is instantly filled, usually by an L-shell electron, with the release of characteristic radiation (see Fig. 1-15). Whatever the orbit of the replacement electron, the characteristic photons generated are of such low energy that they are absorbed within the patient and do not fog the film.

The recoil electrons ejected during photoelectric absorptions travel only a short distance in the absorber before they give up their energy. As a consequence, all the energy of incident photons that undergo photoelectric interaction is deposited in the patient. This is beneficial in producing high-quality radiographs, because no scattered radiation fogs the film, but potentially deleterious for patients because of increased radiation absorption.

The frequency of photoelectric interaction varies directly with the third power of the atomic number of the absorber. For example, because the effective atomic number of compact bone (Z = 13.8) is greater than water (Z = 7.4), the probability that a photon will be absorbed by a photoelectric interaction in bone is approximately 6.5 times greater than in an equal distance of water. This difference is readily seen on dental radiographs. It is this difference in the absorption that makes the production of a radiographic image possible.

COMPTON SCATTERING

Compton scattering occurs when a photon interacts with an outer orbital electron (Fig. 1-25). In this interaction the incident photon collides with an outer electron, which receives kinetic energy and recoils from the point of impact. The incident photon is then deflected by its interaction and is scattered from the site of the collision. The energy of the scattered photon equals the energy of the incident photon minus the kinetic energy gained by the recoil electron plus its binding energy. As with photoelectric absorption, Compton scattering results in the loss of an electron and ionization of the absorbing atom.

Scattered photons travel in all directions. The higher the energy of the incident photon, however, the greater the probability that the angle of scatter of the secondary photon will be small and its direction will be forward. Approximately 30% of the scattered photons formed during a dental x-ray exposure (primarily from Compton scattering) exit the patient's head. This is advantageous to the patient because some of the energy of the

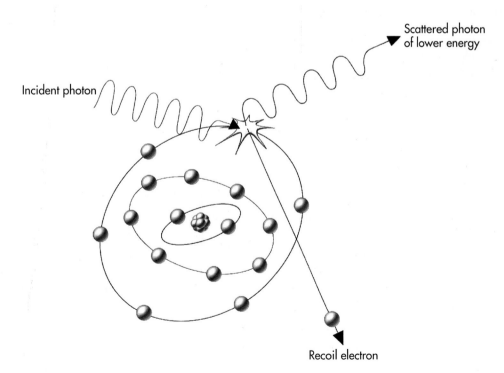

Incident photon

Scattered photon of lower energy

Recoil electron

FIG. 1-25 Compton absorption occurs when an incident photon interacts with an outer electron, producing a scattered photon of lower energy than the incident photon and a recoil electron ejected from the target atom.

incident x-ray beam escapes the tissue, but it is disadvantageous because it causes nonspecific film darkening. Scattered photons darken the film while carrying no useful information to it because their path is altered.

The probability of Compton scattering is directly proportional to the *electron density*. The number of electrons in bone (5.55×10^{23} per cc) is greater than in water (3.34×10^{23} per cc); therefore the probability of Compton scattering is correspondingly greater in bone than in tissue. In a dental x-ray beam, approximately 62% of the photons undergo Compton scattering.

The importance of photoelectric absorption and Compton scattering in diagnostic radiography relates to differences in the way photons are absorbed by various anatomic structures. The number of photoelectric and Compton interactions is greater in hard tissues than in soft tissues. As a consequence, more photons in the beam exit the patient after passing through soft tissue than through hard tissue. This allows a radiograph to provide a clear image of enamel, dentin, bone, and soft tissues.

SECONDARY ELECTRONS

In both photoelectric absorption and Compton scattering, electrons are ejected from their orbits in the absorbing material after interaction with x-ray photons. These secondary electrons give up their energy in the absorber by either of two processes: (1) collisional interaction with other electrons, resulting in ionization or excitation of the affected atom, and (2) radiative interactions, which produce bremsstrahlung radiation resulting in the emission of low-energy x-ray photons. Secondary electrons eventually dissipate all their energy, mostly as heat by collisional interactions, and come to rest.

BEAM ATTENUATION

As a dental x-ray beam travels through matter, individual photons are removed, primarily through photoelectric and Compton interactions. The reduction of beam intensity is predictable because it depends on physical characteristics of the beam and absorber. A monochromatic beam of photons, a beam in which all the photons have the same energy, provides a good example. When just the primary (not scattered) photons are considered, a constant fraction of the beam is attenuated as the beam moves through each unit thickness of an absorber. Therefore 1.5 cm of water may reduce a beam intensity by 50%, the next 1.5 cm by another 50% (to 25% of the original intensity), and so on. This is an exponential pattern of absorption (Fig. 1-26). The HVL described earlier in this chapter is a measure of beam energy describing the amount of an absorber that reduces the beam

intensity by half; in the preceding example, the HVL is 1.5 cm. The absorption of the beam depends primarily on the thickness and mass of the absorber and the energy of the beam.

The spectrum of photon energies (as illustrated by the kVp setting) in an x-ray beam is wide. In such a heterogeneous beam the probability of absorption of individual photons depends on their energy. Low-energy photons are much more likely than high-energy photons to be absorbed. As a consequence the superficial layers of an absorber tend to remove the low-energy photons and transmit the higher-energy photons. Therefore as an x-ray beam passes through matter, the intensity of the beam decreases but the mean energy of the resultant beam increases. In contrast to the absorption of a monochromatic beam, an x-ray beam is absorbed less and less by each succeeding unit of absorber thickness. For example, the first 1.5 cm of water might absorb about 40% of the photons in an x-ray beam with a mean energy of

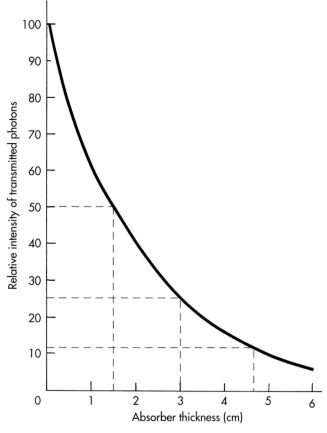

FIG. **1-26** Exponential decay of intensity in a homogeneous photon beam through the absorber, where the HVL is 1.5 cm of absorber. The curve for a heterogeneous x-ray beam does not drop quite as precipitously because of the preferential removal of low-energy photons and the increased mean energy of the resulting beam.

50 kVp. The mean energy of the remnant beam might increase 20% as a result of the loss of lower-energy photons. The next 1.5 cm of water removes only about 30% of the photons as the average energy of the beam increases another 10%. If the water test object is thick enough, the mean energy of the remnant beam approaches the peak voltage applied across the tube and absorption becomes similar to that of a monochromatic beam.

The attenuation of a beam depends on both the energy of the incident beam and the composition of the absorber. In general, as the energy of the beam increases, so does the transmission of the beam through the absorber. When the energy of the incident photon is raised to the binding energy of the K-shell electrons of the absorber, however, the probability of photoelectric absorption increases sharply and the number of transmitted photons is greatly decreased. This is called *K-edge absorption.* (The probability that a photon will interact with an orbital electron is greatest when the energy of the photon equals the binding energy of the electron; it decreases as the photon energy increases.) Photons with energy less than the binding energy of K-shell electrons interact photoelectrically only with electrons in the L shell and in shells even farther from the nucleus. Rare earth elements are sometimes used as filters because their K edges (50.2 keV for gadolinium) greatly increase the absorption of high-energy photons. This is desirable because these high-energy photons are not as likely to contribute to a radiographic image as mid-energy photons.

Dosimetry

Determining the quantity of radiation exposure or dose is termed *dosimetry.* The term *dose* is used to describe the amount of energy absorbed per unit mass at a site of interest. *Exposure* is a measure of radiation based on its ability to produce ionization in air under standard conditions of temperature and pressure (STP).

UNITS OF MEASUREMENT

Table 1-2 presents some of the more frequently used units for measuring quantities of radiation. In recent years a move has occurred to use a modernized version of the metric system called the SI system (Système International d'Unités). This book uses SI units.

Exposure

Exposure is a measure of radiation quantity, the capacity of radiation to ionize air. The roentgen (R) is the traditional unit of radiation exposure measured in air; 1 R is that amount of x-radiation or gamma radiation that produces 2.08×10^9 ion pairs in 1 cc of air (STP). It measures the intensity of radiation to which an object is exposed. No specific SI unit is equivalent to the R, but in terms of other SI units it is equal to coulombs per kilogram (C/kg); 1 R = 2.58×10^{-4} C/kg, and 1 C/kg equals 3.88×10^3 R. The roentgen applies only for x-rays and gamma rays. In recent years the roentgen has been replaced by air kerma, an acronym for *k*inetic *e*nergy *r*eleased in *m*atter. Kerma measures the KE transferred from photons to electrons ans is expressed in units of dose (Gy).

Absorbed Dose

Absorbed dose is a measure of the energy absorbed by any type of ionizing radiation per unit mass of any type of matter. The SI unit is the gray (Gy)—1 Gy equals 1 joule/kg. The traditional unit of absorbed dose is the rad (*rad*iation *a*bsorbed *d*ose), where 1 rad is equivalent to 100 ergs/g of absorber. One gray equals 100 rads.

Equivalent Dose

The equivalent dose (H_T) is used to compare the biologic effects of different types of radiation on a tissue or

---

TABLE **1-2**
Summary of Radiation Quantities and Units

QUANTITY	SI UNIT	TRADITIONAL UNIT	CONVERSION
Exposure	Coulomb per kilogram (C/kg)	Roentgen (R)	1 C/kg = 3876 R
			1 R = 2.58×10^{-4} C/kg
Kerma	Gray (Gy)	—	
Absorbed dose	Gray (Gy)	Rad	1 Gy = 100 rad
			1 rad = 0.01 Gy (1 cGy)
Equivalent dose	Sievert (Sv)	Rem	1 Sv = 100 rem
Effective dose (E)	Sievert (Sv)	—	1 rem = 0.01 Sv (1 cSv)
Radioactivity	Becquerel (Bq)	Curie (Ci)	1 Bq = 2.7×10^{-11} Ci
			1 Ci = 3.7×10^{10} Bq

organ. It is the sum of the products of the absorbed dose (D_T) averaged over a tissue or organ and the radiation weighting factor (W_R):

$$H_T = \Sigma\ W_R \times D_T$$

It is expressed as a sum to allow for the possibility that the tissue or organ has been exposed to more than one type of radiation. The radiation weighting factor is chosen for the type and energy of the radiation involved. Therefore high-LET radiations (which are more damaging to tissue than low-LET radiations) have a correspondingly higher W_R. For example, the W_R of photons is 1; of 5-keV neutrons and high-energy protons, 5; and of alpha particles, 20. The unit of equivalent dose is the sievert (Sv). For diagnostic x-ray examinations, 1 Sv equals 1 Gy. The traditional unit of equivalent dose is the rem (*r*oentgen *e*quivalent *m*an). One sievert equals 100 rem.

Effective Dose

The effective dose (E) is used to estimate the risk in humans. It is the sum of the products of the equivalent dose to each organ or tissue (H_T) and the tissue weighting factor (W_T):

$$E = \Sigma\ W_T \times H_T$$

The tissue weighting factors include gonads, 0.20; red bone marrow, 0.12; esophagus, 0.05; thyroid, 0.05; skin, 0.01; and bone surface, 0.01. The unit of effective dose is the sievert (Sv). The use of this term is described more fully in Chapter 3.

Radioactivity

The measurement of radioactivity (A) describes the decay rate of a sample of radioactive material. The SI unit is the becquerel (Bq); 1 Bq equals 1 disintegration/second. The traditional unit is the curie (Ci), which corresponds to the activity of 1 g of radium (3.7×10^{10} disintegrations/sec).

BIBLIOGRAPHY

Bushberg JT et al: *The essential physics of medical imaging*, Baltimore, 1994, Williams & Wilkins.

Bushong SC: *Radiologic science for technologists: physics, biology, and protection*, ed 5, St Louis, 1993, Mosby.

Curry TS, Dowdey JE, Murry RC: *Christensen's introduction to the physics of diagnostic radiology*, ed 4, Philadelphia, 1990, Lea & Febiger.

International Commission on Radiological Protection: *Radiation protection*, ICRP Publ. 60, Oxford, England, 1990, Author.

Biologic Effects of Radiation

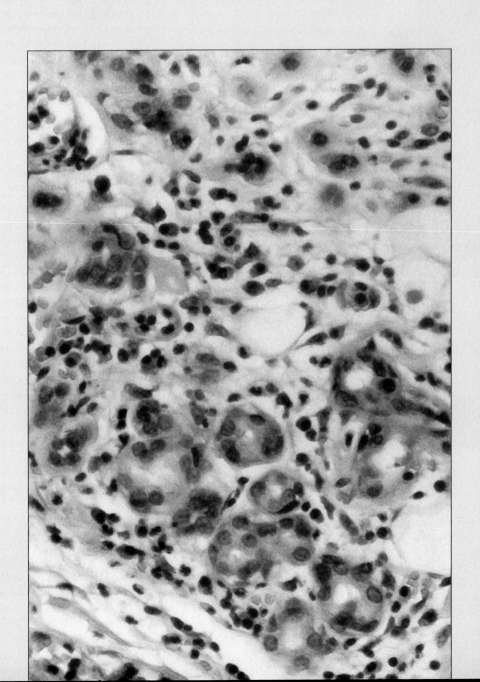

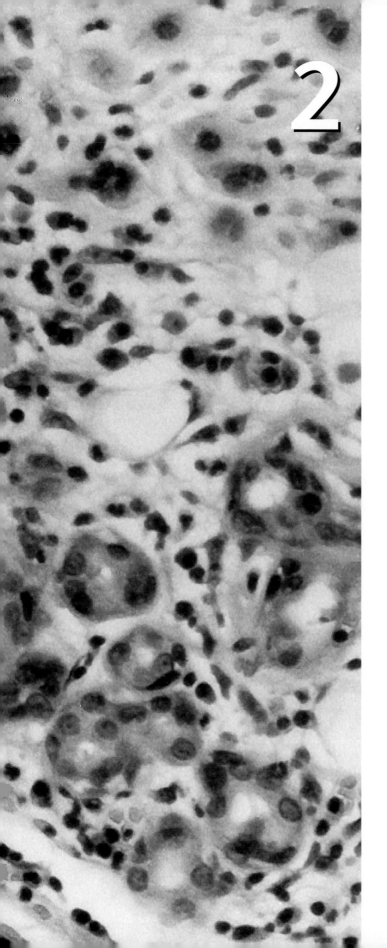

2 Radiation Biology

Radiation biology is the study of the effects of ionizing radiation on living systems. This discipline requires studying many levels of organization within biologic systems spanning broad ranges in size and temporal scale. The initial interaction between ionizing radiation and matter occurs at the level of the electron within the first 10^{-13} second after exposure. These changes result in modification of biologic molecules within the ensuing seconds to hours. In turn, the molecular changes may lead to alterations in cells and organisms that persist for hours, decades, and possibly even generations. They may result in injury or death of the cell or organism.

Biologic effects of ionizing radiation may be divided into two broad categories: deterministic effects and stochastic effects. *Deterministic effects* are those effects in which the severity of response is proportional to the dose. These effects occur in all people when the dose is large enough. Deterministic effects have a dose threshold below which the response is not seen. Examples of deterministic effects include oral changes after radiation therapy and radiation sickness after whole-body irradiation. By contrast, *stochastic effects* are those for which the probability of occurrence of the change, rather than its severity, is dose dependent. Stochastic effects are all-or-none: a person either has or does not have the condition. For example, radiation-induced cancer is a stochastic effect because greater exposure of a person or population to radiation increases the probability of cancer but not its severity. Stochastic effects are believed not to have dose thresholds.

Radiation Chemistry

Radiation acts on living systems through direct and indirect effects. When the energy of a photon or secondary electron ionizes biologic macromolecules, the effect is termed *direct*. Alternatively, the photon may be absorbed by water in an organism, ionizing the water molecules. The resulting ions form free radicals (radiolysis of water) that in turn interact with and produce changes in the biologic molecules. Because intermediate changes involving water molecules are required, this series of events is termed *indirect*.

DIRECT EFFECT

Direct alteration of biologic molecules (RH, where R is the molecule and H is a hydrogen atom) by ionizing radiation begins with absorption of energy by the biologic molecule and formation of unstable free radicals (atoms or molecules having an unpaired electron in the valence shell). They are extremely reactive and have very short lives, quickly reforming into stable configurations by dissociation (breaking apart) or cross-linking (joining of two molecules).

Free radical production:

$$RH + \text{x-radiation} \rightarrow R^{\bullet} + H^+ + e$$

Free radical fates:
Dissociation:

$$R^{\bullet} \rightarrow X + Y^{\bullet}$$

Cross-linking:

$$R^{\bullet} + S^{\bullet} \rightarrow RS$$

Because the altered molecules differ structurally and functionally from the original molecules, the consequence is a biologic change in the irradiated organism. *Approximately one third of the biologic effects of x-ray exposure result from direct effects.*

RADIOLYSIS OF WATER

A complex series of chemical changes occurs in water after exposure to ionizing radiation. Collectively these reactions result in the radiolysis of water. The first step is ionization of water resulting from the absorption of a photon or interaction with a photoelectron or Compton electron. Displacement of an electron from the water molecule results in an ion pair, a positively charged water molecule (H_2O^+) and the displaced electron:

$$\text{photon} + H_2O \rightarrow e^- + H_2O^+$$
$$\text{photoelectron } e^- + H_2O \rightarrow 2e^- + H_2O^+$$

The displaced electron is usually captured by a water molecule to form a negatively charged water molecule (H_2O^-):

$$e^- + H_2O \rightarrow H_2O^-$$

These molecules are not stable and dissociate rapidly to form a hydroxyl ion and hydrogen free radical:

$$H_2O^- \rightarrow OH^- + H^{\bullet}$$

The positively charged water molecule reacts with another water molecule to form a hydroxyl free radical:

$$H_2O^+ + H_2O \rightarrow H_3O^+ + OH^{\bullet}$$

Water may also be excited and dissociate directly into hydrogen and hydroxyl free radicals:

$$\text{Photon} + H_2O \rightarrow H_2O^* \rightarrow OH^{\bullet} + H^{\bullet}$$

Whereas the radiolysis of water is extremely complex, in balance water is largely converted to hydrogen and hydroxyl free radicals.

The generation of free radicals occurs in less than 10^{-10} second after the passage of a photon. These radicals play a dominant role in producing molecular changes in biologic molecules.

When dissolved molecular oxygen (O_2) is present in irradiated water, hydroperoxyl free radicals may also be formed:

$$H^{\bullet} + O_2 \rightarrow HO_2^{\bullet}$$

Hydroperoxyl free radicals also may contribute to the formation of hydrogen peroxide in tissues:

$$HO_2^{\bullet} + H^{\bullet} \rightarrow H_2O_2$$
$$HO_2^{\bullet} + HO_2^{\bullet} \rightarrow O_2 + H_2O_2$$

Both peroxyl radicals and hydrogen peroxide are oxidizing agents that can significantly alter biologic molecules and cause cell destruction. They are considered to be major toxins produced in the tissues by ionizing radiation.

INDIRECT EFFECTS

Because water is the predominant molecule in biologic systems (about 70% by weight), it frequently participates in the interactions between x-ray photons and the biologic molecules of an organism. About two thirds of radiation-induced biologic damage results from indirect effects. The interaction of hydrogen and hydroxyl free radicals with organic molecules can result in the formation of organic free radicals. Such reactions may involve the removal of hydrogen:

$$RH + OH^{\bullet} \rightarrow R^{\bullet} + H_2O$$
$$RH + H^{\bullet} \rightarrow R^{\bullet} + H_2$$

The OH⋅ free radical is more important in causing such damage.

Organic free radicals are unstable and transform into stable altered molecules as described in the earlier section in this chapter on direct effects (p. 23). These altered molecules have different chemical and biologic properties from the original molecules. The important role of water radiolysis and the indirect action of radiation may be seen by comparing the radiation dose required to inactivate enzymes when dry or in solution. The dose required to inactivate 37% of dry yeast invertase is 110 kGy but only 60 kGy when the enzyme is irradiated in solution.

CHANGES IN BIOLOGIC MOLECULES

Nucleic Acids

The last few decades have seen a growing appreciation for the crucial role of nucleic acids in determining cellular functions. It is clear that damage to the deoxyribonucleic acid (DNA) molecule is primarily responsible for cell death after radiation exposure. Radiation produces a number of different types of alterations in DNA, including the following:

1. Change or loss of a base
2. Disruption of hydrogen bonds between DNA strands
3. Breakage of one or both DNA strands
4. Cross-linking of DNA strands within the helix, to other DNA strands, or to proteins

The amount of radiation required to cause disruption of DNA molecules (e.g., an average of one single-strand break per molecule) is much higher than is required to cause cell death. Such evidence suggests that if DNA is the molecular target in a cell, relatively few biochemical lesions of the types just listed may be required to result in cell death. DNA sensitivity to radiation results from its complex replication mechanism in mitotically active cell populations.

Proteins

Irradiation of proteins in solution usually leads to changes in their secondary and tertiary structures through disruption of side chains or the breakage of hydrogen or disulfide bonds. Such changes lead to denaturation. The primary structure of the protein is usually not significantly altered. Irradiation may also induce intermolecular and intramolecular cross-linking. When an enzyme is irradiated, the biologic effect of the radiation may become amplified. For example, inactivation of an enzyme molecule results in its failure to convert many substrate molecules to their products. Thus many molecules become subsequently affected, although only a small number were initially damaged. The dose of radiation required to induce significant amounts of protein denaturation (or enzyme inactivation) is much higher than that required to induce gross cellular changes or cell death. Such data suggest that radiation-induced changes in protein structure and function are not the major cause of radiation effects after absorption of moderate doses (2 to 4 Gy) of radiation.

Radiation Effects at the Cellular Level

EFFECTS ON INTRACELLULAR STRUCTURES

The effects of radiation on intracellular structures result from radiation-induced changes in their macromolecules. Although the initial molecular changes are produced within a fraction of a second after exposure, cellular changes resulting from moderate exposures usually require a minimum of hours to become apparent. These changes are manifest initially as structural and functional changes in cellular organelles. Later, cell death may occur.

Nucleus

A wide variety of radiobiologic data indicate that the nucleus is more radiosensitive (in terms of lethality) than the cytoplasm, especially in dividing cells. *The sensitive site in the nucleus is the DNA within chromosomes.*

Chromosome Aberrations

Chromosomes serve as useful markers for radiation injury. They may be easily visualized and quantified, and the extent of their damage is related to cell survival. Chromosome aberrations are observed in irradiated cells at the time of mitosis when the DNA condenses to form chromosomes. The type of damage that may be observed depends on the stage of the cell in the cell cycle at the time of irradiation.

Fig. 2-1 shows the stages of the cell cycle. If radiation exposure occurs after DNA synthesis (i.e., in G_2 or mid and late S), only one arm of the affected chromosome is broken (chromatid aberration) (Fig. 2-2). If the radiation-induced break occurs before the DNA has replicated (i.e., in G_1 or early S), the damage manifests as a break in both arms (chromosome aberration) at the next mitosis. Most simple breaks are repaired by biologic processes and go unrecognized. Fig. 2-3 illustrates several common forms of chromosome aberrations resulting from incorrect repair. Such radiation-induced aberrations may result in unequal distribution of chromatin material to daughter cells or prevent completion of a subsequent mitosis. Chromosome aberrations have been

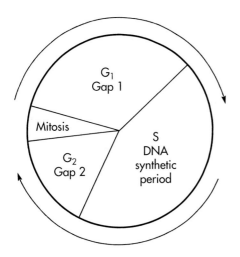

FIG. **2-1** *Cell cycle.* A proliferating cell moves in the cycle from mitosis to gap 1 *(G₁)* to the period of DNA synthesis *(S)* to gap 2 *(G₂)* to the next mitosis.

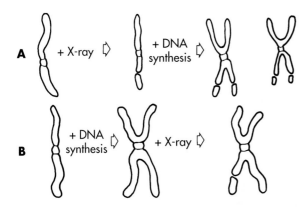

FIG. **2-2** *Chromosome aberrations.* **A,** Irradiation of the cell after DNA synthesis results in a single-arm chromatid aberration. **B,** Irradiation before DNA synthesis results in a double-arm aberration.

detected in peripheral blood lymphocytes of patients exposed to medical diagnostic procedures. Moreover, the survivors of the atom bombings of Hiroshima and Nagasaki have demonstrated chromosome aberrations in circulating lymphocytes more than two decades after the radiation exposure. The frequency of aberrations is generally proportional to the radiation dose received.

Cytoplasm

Radiation effects occur in cellular structures other than nuclei and chromosomes. After relatively large doses of radiation (30 to 50 Gy), mitochondria demonstrate increased permeability, swelling, and disorganization of the internal cristae. Such permeability and structural

changes probably play only a minor role in the cellular changes seen in rapidly dividing cells after exposure to moderate doses of radiation (2 to 4 Gy).

EFFECTS ON CELL KINETICS

The effects of radiation on the kinetics (turnover rate) of a cell population have been studied in rapidly dividing cell systems such as skin and intestinal mucosa and in cell culture systems. Irradiation of such cell populations will cause a reduction in size of the irradiated tissue as a result of mitotic delay (inhibition of progression of the cells through the cell cycle) and cell death (usually during mitosis).

Mitotic Delay

Mitotic delay occurs after irradiation of a population of dividing cells. Fig. 2-4 illustrates the effect of radiation on mitotic activity. A low dose of radiation induces mild mitotic delay in G₂ cells. The delayed cells subsequently pass through mitosis with other (nondelayed) cells, giving rise to an elevated mitotic index. A moderate dose results in a longer mitotic delay (G₂ block) and some cell death. The area under the curve of the following supranormal mitotic index is smaller than that of the preceding mitotic delay, indicating some cell death. Larger doses may cause a profound mitotic delay with incomplete recovery.

Cell Death

Mitosis-linked death in a cell population is loss of the capacity for mitotic division. Cell death results from damage to the nucleus that results in chromosome aberrations. This damage causes the cell to die, usually while attempting to complete the first few mitoses after irradiation. Reproductive death occurs in a dividing cell population after exposure to a moderate dose of radiation, which accounts for the radiosensitivity of tissues. When a population of nondividing cells is irradiated, much larger doses and longer time intervals are required for induction of interphase death.

Survival curves are used to study the response of replicating cells exposed in culture. Single cells grown in tissue culture are dispersed onto plates, where they form colonies. The plates are irradiated before colony growth, and the effect of the irradiation on the reproductivity of the cells is studied.

Fig. 2-5 shows typical survival curves for cells exposed to x-radiation in which the fraction of surviving cells is compared with the absorbed dose. The value *n* is the extrapolation number and measures the size of the shoulder. The shoulder in the survival curve represents either the accumulation of sublethal damage before cells die or a measure of the repair process active early in the period

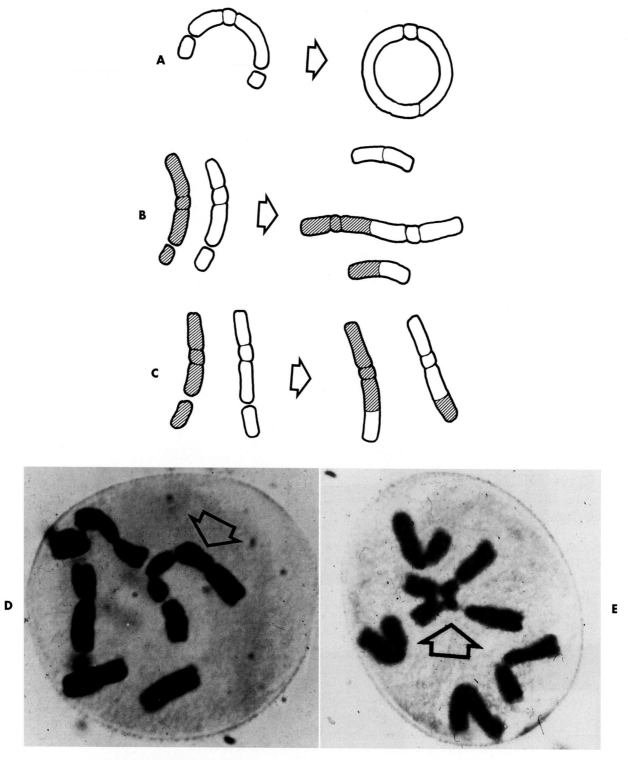

FIG. **2-3** *Chromosome aberrations.* **A,** Ring formation; **B,** dicentric formation; **C,** translocation. In **D** and **E** the arrows point to tetracentric exchange and chromatid exchange taking place in *Trandescantia,* an herb. (**D** and **E** courtesy Dr. M. Miller, Rochester, N.Y.)

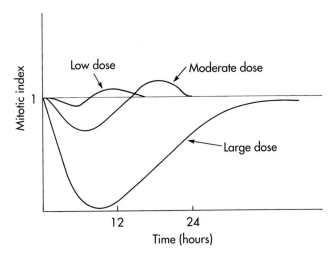

FIG. **2-4** *Radiation-induced mitotic delay.* The degree of delay in a replicating cell population depends on the amount of exposure. A large dose severely depresses mitosis and prolongs recovery.

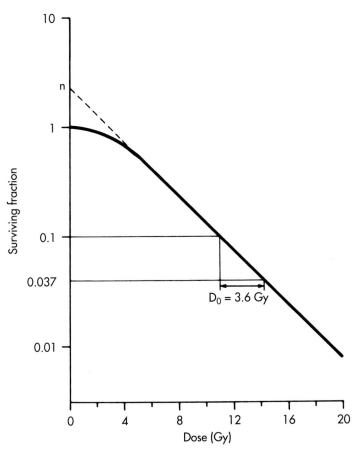

FIG. **2-5** *Survival curve for mammalian cells grown in culture after irradiation.* In this case the cells have an extrapolation number *(n)* of about 2 and a D_0 of about 3.6 Gy. The n value is a measure of the size of the shoulder; D_0 is the amount of radiation required to reduce the surviving population to 37% of its former size.

of irradiation. *D0* indicates the slope of the straight portion of the curve. It measures the amount of radiation required to reduce the number of colony-forming cells to 37% and thus is the dose required to deliver an average of one cell-killing event per cell. Survival curves have helped researchers understand the response of cells to irradiation under various conditions.

Recovery

Cell recovery involves enzymatic repair of single-strand breaks of DNA. Because of this repair, a higher total dose is required to achieve a given degree of cell killing when multiple fractions are used (e.g., in radiation therapy) than when the same total dose is given in a single brief exposure. Damage to both strands of DNA at the same site (usually caused by particulate radiation) is usually lethal to the cell.

RADIOSENSITIVITY AND CELL TYPE

Different cells from various organs of the same individual may respond to irradiation quite differently. This variation was recognized as early as 1906 by the French radiobiologists Bergonié and Tribondeau. They observed that the most radiosensitive cells are those that (1) have a high mitotic rate, (2) undergo many future mitoses, and (3) are most primitive in differentiation. These findings are still true except for lymphocytes and oocytes, which are very radiosensitive even though they are highly differentiated and nondividing.

Mammalian cells may be divided into five categories of radiosensitivity on the basis of histologic observations of early cell death:

1. *Vegetative intermitotic cells* are the most radiosensitive. They divide regularly, have long mitotic futures, and do not undergo differentiation between mitoses. These are stem cells that retain their primitive properties and whose function is to replace themselves. Examples include early precursor cells, such as those in the spermatogenic or erythroblastic series, and basal cells of the oral mucous membrane.
2. *Differentiating intermitotic cells* are somewhat less radio-sensitive than vegetative intermitotic cells because they divide less often. They divide regularly, although they undergo some differentiation between divisions. Examples of this class include intermediate dividing and replicating cells of the inner enamel epithelium of developing teeth, cells of the hematopoietic series that are in the intermediate stages of differentiation, spermatocytes, and oocytes.
3. *Multipotential connective tissue cells* have intermediate radiosensitivity. They divide irregularly, usually in re-

sponse to a demand for more cells, and are also capable of limited differentiation. Examples are vascular endothelial cells, fibroblasts, and mesenchymal cells.

4. *Reverting postmitotic cells* are generally radioresistant because they divide infrequently. They also are generally specialized in function. Examples include the acinar and ductal cells of the salivary glands and pancreas as well as parenchymal cells of the liver, kidney, and thyroid.

5. *Fixed postmitotic cells* are most resistant to the direct action of radiation. They are the most highly differentiated cells and, once mature, are incapable of division. Examples of these cells include neurons, striated muscle cells, squamous epithelial cells that have differentiated and are close to the surface of oral mucous membrane, and erythrocytes.

Radiation Effects at the Tissue and Organ Level

The radiosensitivity of a tissue or organ is measured by its response to irradiation. A fairly small number of lost cells results in no clinical effect. With an increased number of lost cells, all affected organisms display a clinical result. The severity of this change depends on the dose and thus the amount of cell loss. The following discussion pertains to the effect of irradiation of tissues and organs when the exposure is restricted to a small area. Moderate doses to a localized area may lead to repairable damage. Comparable doses to a whole organism may result in death from damage to the most sensitive systems in the body.

SHORT-TERM EFFECTS

The short-term effects of radiation on a tissue are determined primarily by the sensitivity of its parenchymal cells. If continuously proliferating tissues (e.g., bone marrow, oral mucous membranes) are irradiated with a moderate dose, cells are lost primarily by mitosis-linked death. The extent of cell loss depends on damage to the stem cell pools and the proliferative rate of the cell population. The effects of irradiation of such tissues become apparent relatively quickly as a reduction in the number of mature cells in the series. Tissues composed of cells that rarely or never divide (e.g., muscle) demonstrate little or no radiation-induced hypoplasia over the short term. The relative radiosensitivity of various tissues and organs is shown in Table 2-1.

TABLE **2-1** *Relative Radiosensitivity of Various Organs*		
HIGH	INTERMEDIATE	LOW
Lymphoid organs	Fine vasculature	Optic lens
Bone marrow	Growing cartilage	Mature erythrocytes
Testes	Growing bone	Muscle cells
Intestines	Salivary glands	Neurons
Mucous	Lungs	
membranes	Kidney	
	Liver	

LONG-TERM EFFECTS

The long-term deterministic effects of radiation on tissues and organs depend primarily on the extent of damage to the fine vasculature. The relative radiosensitivity of capillaries and connective tissue is intermediate between that of differentiating intermitotic cells and reverting postmitotic cells. Irradiation of capillaries causes swelling, degeneration, and necrosis. These changes increase capillary permeability and initiate a slow progressive fibrosis around the vessels. As a result, deposition of fibrous scar tissue is increased around the vessels, leading to premature narrowing and eventual obliteration of vascular lumens. This impairs the transport of oxygen, nutrients, and waste products and results in death of all cell types. The net result is progressive fibroatrophy of the irradiated tissue.

Such progressive atrophic changes lead to a loss of cell function and a reduced resistance of irradiated tissue to infection and trauma. These cellular changes are the basis for long-term radiation-induced atrophy of tissues and organs. Death of parenchymal cells after moderate exposure is thus the result of (1) mitotic-linked death of rapidly dividing cells in the short term and (2) the consequences of progressive fibroatrophy on all cell types over time.

MODIFYING FACTORS

The response of cells to irradiation depends on variations in exposure parameters and the environment of the cell.

Dose

The severity of deterministic damage seen in irradiated tissues or organs depends on the amount of radiation received. Very often a clinical threshold dose exists below which no adverse effects are seen. All individuals re-

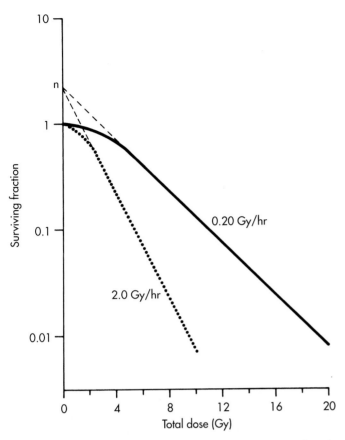

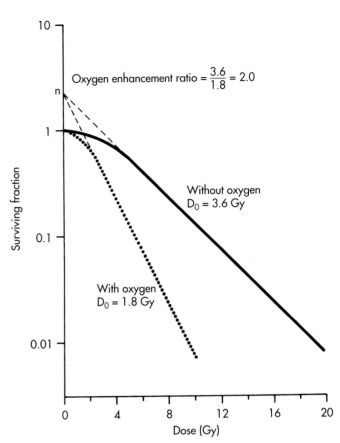

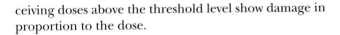

FIG. **2-6** *Survival curve for mammalian cells grown in culture after irradiation at low and high dose rates.* A high dose rate kills more cells because less time exists for repair of sublethal damage.

FIG. **2-7** *Survival curve for mammalian cells grown in culture after irradiation with and without oxygen.* The presence of oxygen increases the cells' sensitivity to radiation: the D_0 value is reduced from 3.6 Gy when irradiated without oxygen to 1.8 Gy in the presence of oxygen. The oxygen enhancement ratio measures the influence of oxygen.

ceiving doses above the threshold level show damage in proportion to the dose.

Dose Rate

The term *dose rate* indicates the rate of exposure. For example, a total dose of 5 Gy may be given at a high dose rate (5 Gy/min) or a low dose rate (5 mGy/min). Exposure of biologic systems to a given dose at a high dose rate causes more damage than exposure to the same total dose given at a lower dose rate. When organisms are exposed at lower dose rates, a greater opportunity exists for repair of damage, thereby resulting in less net damage. Fig. 2-6 illustrates the effects of dose rate schematically.

Oxygen

The radioresistance of many biologic systems increases by a factor of 2 or 3 when irradiation is conducted with reduced oxygen (hypoxia). The greater cell damage

sustained in the presence of oxygen is related to the increased amounts of hydrogen peroxide and hyperoxyl free radicals formed. The oxygen enhancement ratio measures the extent of this damage. It is the dose required to achieve a given endpoint (e.g., 50% survival of a cell population) under anoxic conditions divided by the dose required to produce the same endpoint under fully oxygenated conditions. Fig. 2-7 demonstrates oxygen's influence on cell survival curves.

Linear Energy Transfer

In general, the dose required to produce a certain biologic effect is reduced as the linear energy transfer (LET) of the radiation is increased. Thus higher-LET radiations (e.g., alpha particles) are more efficient in damaging biologic systems because their high ionization density is more likely than x-rays to induce double-strand breakage in DNA.

Radiation Effects on the Oral Cavity

RATIONALE OF RADIOTHERAPY

The oral cavity is irradiated during the course of treating radiosensitive oral malignant tumors, usually squamous cell carcinomas. The specific treatment of choice for a lesion depends on many tumor variables such as radiosensitivity, histology, size, location, invasion into adjacent structures, and duration of symptoms. Radiation therapy for malignant lesions in the oral cavity is usually indicated when the lesion is radiosensitive, advanced, or deeply invasive and cannot be approached surgically. Combined surgical and radiotherapeutic treatment often provides optimal treatment. Increasingly, chemotherapy is being combined with radiation therapy and surgery.

Fractionation of the total x-ray dose into multiple small doses provides greater tumor destruction than is possible with a large single dose. Fractionation characteristically also allows increased cellular repair of normal tissues, which are believed to have an inherently greater capacity for recovery than tumor cells. Fractionation also increases the mean oxygen tension in an irradiated tumor, rendering the tumor cells more radiosensitive. This results from rapid killing of tumor cells and shrinkage of the tumor mass after the first few fractions, reducing the distance that oxygen must diffuse through the tumor to reach the remaining viable tumor cells. The fractionation schedules currently in use have been established empirically.

RADIATION EFFECT ON ORAL TISSUES

The following sections describe the deterministic effects of a course of radiotherapy on the normal tissue of the oral cavity. This discussion assumes that 2 Gy is delivered daily, bilaterally through 8×10 cm fields over the oropharynx, for a weekly exposure of 10 Gy. This continues typically until a total of 50 Gy is administered.

Cobalt is often the source of gamma radiation; however, on occasion small implants containing radon or iodine-125 are placed directly in a tumor mass. Such implants deliver a high dose of radiation to a relatively small volume of tissue in a short time.

Oral Mucous Membrane

The oral mucous membrane contains a basal layer composed of radiosensitive vegetative and differentiating intermitotic cells. Near the end of the second week of therapy, as some of these cells die, the mucous membranes begin to show areas of redness and inflammation (mucositis). As the therapy continues, the irradiated mucous membrane begins to break down, with the for-

mation of a white to yellow pseudomembrane (the desquamated epithelial layer). At the end of therapy the mucositis is usually most severe, discomfort is at a maximum, and food intake is difficult. Good oral hygiene minimizes infection. Topical anesthetics may be required at mealtimes. Secondary yeast infection by *Candida albicans* is a common complication and may require treatment.

After irradiation is completed, the mucosa begins to heal rapidly. Healing is usually complete by about 2 months. At later intervals (months to years) the mucous membrane tends to become atrophic, thin, and relatively avascular. This long-term atrophy results from progressive obliteration of the fine vasculature and fibrosis of the underlying connective tissue. These atrophic changes complicate wearing of dentures because they may cause oral ulcerations of the compromised tissue. Ulcers can result from a denture sore, radiation necrosis, or tumor recurrence. A biopsy may be required to make the differentiation.

Taste Buds

Taste buds are sensitive to radiation. Doses in the therapeutic range cause extensive degeneration of the normal histologic architecture of taste buds. Patients often notice a loss of taste acuity during the second or third week of radiotherapy. Bitter and acid flavors are more severely affected when the posterior two thirds of the tongue is irradiated, and salt and sweet when the anterior third of the tongue is irradiated. Taste acuity usually decreases by a factor of 1000 to 10,000 during the course of radiotherapy. Alterations in the saliva may account partly for this reduction, which may proceed to a state of virtual insensitivity, with recovery to near-normal levels some 60 to 120 days after irradiation.

Salivary Glands

The major salivary glands are at times unavoidably exposed to 20 to 30 Gy during radiotherapy for cancer in the oral cavity or oropharynx. The parenchymal component of the salivary glands is rather radiosensitive (parotid glands more so than submandibular or sublingual glands). The first few weeks after initiation of radiotherapy usually sees a marked and progressive loss of salivary secretion. The extent of reduced flow is dose dependent and reaches essentially zero at 60 Gy. The mouth becomes dry (xerostomia) and tender, and swallowing is difficult and painful because the residual saliva also loses its normal lubricating properties.

Patients with irradiation of both parotid glands are more likely to complain of dry mouth than are those with unilateral irradiation. The small volume of viscous saliva that is secreted usually has a pH value 1 unit below normal (i.e., an average of 5.5 in irradiated patients compared with 6.5 in unexposed individuals). This pH is low enough to initiate decalcification of normal enamel. In addition, the buffering capacity of saliva falls as much as 44% during radiation therapy. If some portions of the major salivary glands have been spared, dryness of the mouth usually subsides in 6 to 12 months because of compensatory hypertrophy of residual salivary gland tissue. Reduced salivary flow that persists beyond a year is unlikely to show significant recovery.

Histologically an acute inflammatory response may occur soon after the initiation of therapy, particularly involving the serous acini. In the months after irradiation the inflammatory response becomes more chronic and the glands demonstrate progressive fibrosis, adiposis, loss of fine vasculature, and concomitant parenchymal degeneration (Fig. 2-8), thus accounting for the xerostomia.

Salivary changes have a profound influence on the oral microflora and secondarily on the dentition, often leading to radiation caries. After radiotherapy that includes the major salivary glands, the microflora undergo a pronounced change, rendering them acidogenic in the saliva and plaque. Patients receiving radiation therapy to oral structures have increases in *Streptococcus mutans*, *Lactobacillus*, and *Candida*. Because of their small volume of thick, viscous, acidic saliva, such patients are quite prone to radiation caries.

Teeth

Irradiation of teeth with therapeutic doses during their development severely retards their growth. Such irradiation may be for local disease (e.g., eosinophilic granuloma) or a generalized condition (leukemia being treated with whole-body irradiation followed by bone marrow transplantation). If it precedes calcification, it may destroy the tooth bud. Irradiation after calcification has begun may inhibit cellular differentiation, causing malformations and arresting general growth. Children receiving radiation therapy to the jaws may show defects in the permanent dentition such as retarded root development, dwarfed teeth, or failure to form one or more teeth (Fig. 2-9). Teeth irradiated during development may complete calcification and erupt prematurely. In general, the severity of the damage is dose dependent. Irradiation of teeth may retard or abort root formation, but the eruptive mechanism of teeth is relatively radiation resistant. Irradiated teeth with altered root formation still erupt.

Adult teeth are very resistant to the direct effects of radiation exposure. Pulpal tissue, which consists primarily of reverting and fixed postmitotic cells, demonstrates long-term fibroatrophy after irradiation. Radiation has no discernible effect on the crystalline structure of enamel, dentin, or cementum, and radiation does not increase their solubility.

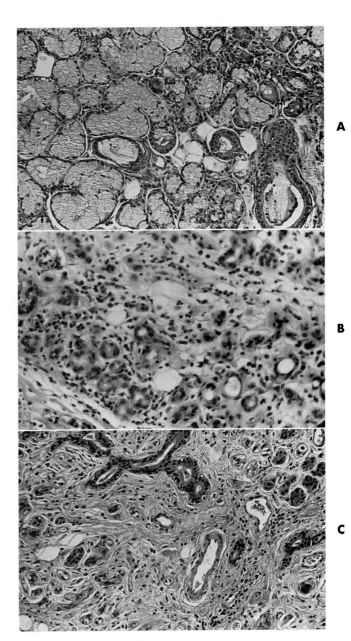

FIG. **2-8** *Radiation effects on human submandibular salivary glands.* **A,** Normal gland. **B,** A gland 6 months after exposure to radiotherapy. Note the loss of acini and presence of chronic inflammatory cells. **C,** A gland 1 year after exposure to radiotherapy. Note the loss of acini and extensive fibrosis.

Radiation Caries

Radiation caries is a rampant form of dental decay that may occur in individuals who receive a course of radiotherapy that includes exposure of the salivary glands. The carious lesions result from changes in the salivary glands and saliva, including reduced flow, decreased pH, reduced buffering capacity, and increased viscosity. Because of the reduced or absent cleansing action of normal

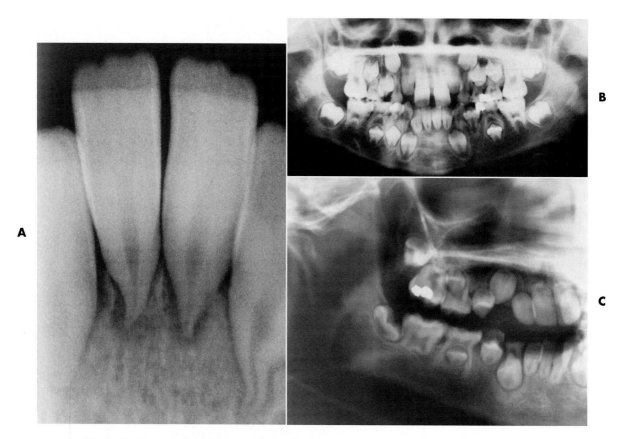

FIG. **2-9** *Dental abnormalities after radiotherapy in two patients.* The first, a 9-year-old girl who received 35 Gy at the age of 4 years because of Hodgkin's disease, had severe stunting of the incisor roots with premature closure of the apices at 8 years **(A)** and retarded development of the mandibular second premolar crowns with stunting of the mandibular incisor, canine, and premolar roots at 9 years **(B).** The other patient, **C,** a 10-year-old boy who received 41 Gy to the jaws at age 4 years, had severely stunted root development of all permanent teeth with a normal primary molar. (**A** and **B** courtesy Mr. P.N. Hirschmann, Leeds, England; **C** courtesy Dr. James Eischen, San Diego, Calif.)

saliva, debris accumulates quickly. Irradiation of the teeth by itself does not influence the course of radiation caries.

Clinically, three types of radiation caries exist. The most common is widespread superficial lesions attacking buccal, occlusal, incisal, and palatal surfaces. Another type involves primarily the cementum and dentin in the cervical region. These lesions may progress around the teeth circumferentially and result in loss of the crown. A final type appears as a dark pigmentation of the entire crown. The incisal edges may be markedly worn. Some patients develop combinations of all these lesions (Fig. 2-10). The histologic features of the lesions are similar to those of typical carious lesions. It is the rapid course and widespread attack that distinguish radiation caries.

The best method of reducing radiation caries is daily application for 5 minutes of a viscous topical 1% neutral

sodium fluoride gel in custom-made applicator trays. Use of topical fluoride causes a 6-month delay in the irradiation-induced elevation of *Streptococcus mutans.* Avoidance of dietary sucrose in addition to the use of a topical fluoride further reduces the concentrations of *S. mutans* and *Lactobacillus.* The best result comes from a combination of restorative dental procedures, excellent oral hygiene, and topical applications of sodium fluoride. Patient cooperation in maintaining oral hygiene is extremely important. Teeth with gross caries or periodontal involvement are often extracted before irradiation.

Bone

Treatment of cancers in the oral region often includes irradiation of the mandible. The primary damage to mature bone results from radiation-induced damage to the vasculature of the periosteum and cortical bone, which is

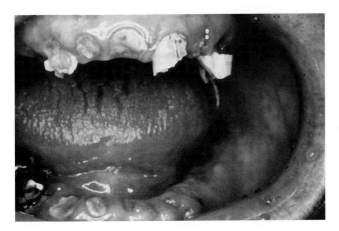

FIG. **2-10** *Radiation caries.* Note the extensive loss of tooth structure resulting from radiation-induced xerostomia.

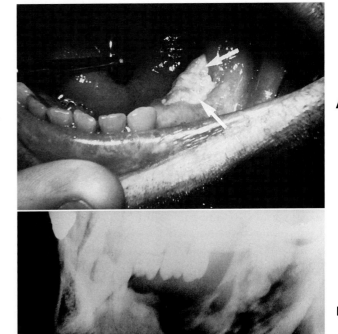

FIG. **2-11** *Osteoradionecrosis.* **A,** Area of exposed mandible after radiotherapy. Note the loss of oral mucosa. **B,** De-struction of irradiated bone resulting from the spread of infection.

normally already sparse. Radiation also acts by destroying osteoblasts and, to a lesser extent, osteoclasts. Subsequent to irradiation, normal marrow may be replaced with fatty marrow and fibrous connective tissue. The marrow tissue becomes hypovascular, hypoxic, and hypocellular. In addition, the endosteum becomes atrophic, showing a lack of osteoblastic and osteoclastic activity, and some lacunae of the compact bone are empty, an indication of necrosis. The degree of mineralization may be reduced, leading to brittleness, or little altered from normal bone. These changes are so severe that bone death results. The condition is termed *osteoradionecrosis.*

Osteoradionecrosis is the most serious clinical complication that occurs in bone after irradiation. The decreased vascularity of the mandible renders it easily infected by microorganisms from the oral cavity. This bone infection may result from radiation-induced breakdown of the oral mucous membrane, by mechanical damage to the weakened oral mucous membrane such as from a denture sore or tooth extraction, through a periodontal lesion, or from radiation caries. This infection may cause a nonhealing wound in irradiated bone that is difficult to treat (Fig. 2-11). It is more common in the mandible than in the maxilla, probably because of the richer vascular supply to the maxilla and the fact that the mandible is more frequently irradiated. The higher the radiation dose absorbed by the bone, the greater the risk of osteoradionecrosis.

Patients must be referred for dental care before undergoing a course of radiation therapy to reduce the severity of or prevent radiation caries and osteoradionecrosis. Radiation caries can be minimized by restoring all carious lesions before radiation therapy and initiating preventive techniques of good oral hygiene and daily topical fluoride. The risk of osteoradionecrosis and infection can be minimized by removing all poorly supported teeth, allowing sufficient time for the extraction wounds to heal before beginning radiation therapy, and adjusting dentures to minimize risk of denture sores. When teeth must be removed from irradiated jaws, the dentist should use atraumatic surgical technique to avoid elevating the periosteum, provide antibiotic coverage, and use low-concentration epinephrine-containing local anesthetics that do not contain lidocaine.

Often patients require a radiographic examination to supplement the clinical examination. These radiographs are especially important because untreated caries leading to periapical infection can be quite severe with the compromised vascular supply to bone. The amount of added radiation is negligible compared with the amount received during therapy and should not serve as a reason to defer radiographs. Whenever possible, however, it is desirable to avoid taking radiographs during the first 6 months after completion of radiotherapy to allow the mucosal membrane time to heal.

Effects of Whole-Body Irradiation

When the whole body is exposed to low or moderate doses of radiation, characteristic changes (called the *acute radiation syndrome*) develop. The clinical picture after whole-body exposure is quite different from that seen when a relatively small volume of tissue is exposed.

ACUTE RADIATION SYNDROME

The acute radiation syndrome is a collection of signs and symptoms experienced by persons after acute whole-body exposure to radiation. Information about this syndrome comes from animal experiments and human exposures in the course of medical radiotherapy, atom bomb blasts, and radiation accidents. Individually the clinical symptoms are not unique to radiation exposure, but taken as a whole, the pattern constitutes a distinct entity (Table 2-2). The following discussion pertains to whole-body exposure at a relatively high dose rate.

Prodromal Period

Within the first minutes to hours after exposure to whole-body irradiation of about 1.5 Gy, symptoms characteristic of gastrointestinal tract disturbances may occur. The individual may develop anorexia, nausea, vomiting, diarrhea, weakness, and fatigue. These early symptoms constitute the prodromal period of the acute radiation syndrome. Their cause is not clear but probably involves the autonomic nervous system. The severity and time of onset may be of significant prognostic value because they are dose related: the higher the dose, the more rapid the onset and the greater the severity of symptoms.

Latent Period

After this prodromal reaction comes a latent period of apparent well-being during which no signs or symptoms of radiation sickness occur. The extent of the latent period is also dose related. It extends from hours or days at supralethal exposures (greater than approximately 5 Gy) to a few weeks at sublethal exposures (less than 2 Gy). Symptoms follow the latent period when individuals are exposed in the lethal range (approximately 2 to 5 Gy) or supralethal range.

Hematopoietic Syndrome

Whole-body exposures of 2 to 7 Gy cause injury to the hematopoietic stem cells of the bone marrow and spleen. The high mitotic activity of these cells and the presence of many differentiating cells make the bone marrow a highly radiosensitive tissue. As a consequence, doses in this range cause a rapid and profound fall in the num-

TABLE **2-2** *Acute Radiation Syndrome*	
DOSE (GY)	MANIFESTATION
1 to 2	Prodromal symptoms
2 to 4	Mild hematopoietic symptoms
4 to 7	Severe hematopoietic symptoms
7 to 15	Gastrointestinal symptoms
50+	Cardiovascular and central nervous system symptoms

bers of circulating granulocytes and platelets, and finally erythrocytes. The mature circulating granulocytes, platelets, and erythrocytes themselves are very radioresistant, however, because they are nonreplicating cells. Their paucity in the peripheral blood after irradiation reflects the radiosensitivity of their precursors.

The differential changes in the blood count do not all appear at the same time (Fig. 2-12). Rather, the rate of fall in the circulating levels of a cell depends on the life span of that cell in the peripheral blood. Granulocytes, with short lives in circulation, fall off in a matter of days, whereas red blood cells, with their long lives in circulation, fall off only slowly.

The clinical consequences of the depression of these cellular elements become evident as the circulating levels decline. Hence, in the weeks after radiation injury, infection appears first, followed later by anemia. The clinical signs of the hematopoietic syndrome include infection (in part from the lymphopenia and granulocytopenia), hemorrhage (from the thrombocytopenia), and anemia (from the erythrocyte depletion). Individuals may survive exposure in this range if the bone marrow and spleen recover before the patient dies of one or more clinical complications. The probability of death is low after exposures at the low end of this range but much higher at the high end. When death results from the hematopoietic syndrome, it usually occurs 10 to 30 days after irradiation.

Because periodontitis results in a likely source of entry for microorganisms into the bloodstream, the role of the dentist is important in preventing infection in hematopoietic syndrome. After moderate injury, about 7 to 10 days pass before clinically significant leukopenia develops. During this time the dentist should remove all sites of infection from the mouth. The removal of sources of infection, the vigorous administration of antibiotics, and in some cases the transplantation of bone marrow have saved individuals suffering from the acute radiation syndrome.

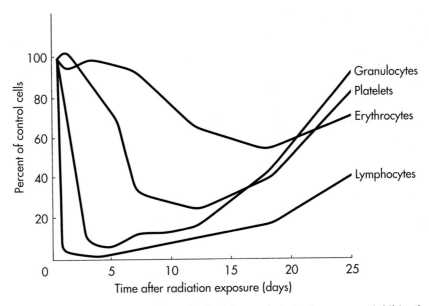

FIG. **2-12** *Radiation effects on blood cells.* When whole-body exposure inhibits the replacement of circulating cells by stem cell proliferation, the duration of the circulating cells' survival is largely determined by their life span.

Gastrointestinal Syndrome

Whole-body exposures in the range of 7 to 15 Gy cause extensive damage to the gastrointestinal system. This damage, in addition to the hematopoietic damage described previously, causes signs and symptoms called the *gastrointestinal syndrome.* Individuals exposed in this range may experience the prodromal stage within a few hours of exposure. Typically from the second through about the fifth day no symptoms are present (latent period) and the patient feels well. Such exposure, however, causes considerable injury to the rapidly proliferating basal epithelial cells of the intestinal villi and leads to a loss of the epithelial layer of the intestinal mucosa. The turnover time for cells lining the small intestine is normally 3 to 5 days. Because of the denuded mucosal surface, plasma and electrolytes are lost; efficient intestinal absorption cannot occur. Ulceration also occurs, with hemorrhaging of the intestines. All these changes are responsible for the diarrhea, dehydration, and loss of weight that are observed. Endogenous intestinal bacteria readily invade the denuded surface, producing septicemia.

The level of radiation required to produce the gastrointestinal syndrome (more than 7 Gy) is much greater than that causing sterilization of the blood-forming tissues. However, death (from destruction of the rapidly self-renewing cells in the intestines) occurs before the full effect of the radiation on hematopoietic systems can be evidenced. At about the time that developing damage to the gastrointestinal system reaches a maximum, the effect of bone marrow depression is just beginning to be manifested. By the end of 24 hours, the number of circulating lymphocytes falls to a very low level. This is followed by decreases in the number of granulocytes and then of platelets (see Fig. 2-12). The result is a marked lowering of the body's defense against bacterial infection and a decrease in effectiveness of the clotting mechanism. The combined effects on these stem cell systems cause death within 2 weeks from a combination of factors that include fluid and electrolyte loss, infection, and possibly nutritional impairment. Several of the firefighters at Chernobyl, in the former Soviet Socialist Republic Ukraine, died of the gastrointestinal syndrome.

Cardiovascular and Central Nervous System Syndrome

Exposures in excess of 50 Gy usually cause death in 1 to 2 days. The few human beings who have been exposed at this level showed collapse of the circulatory system with a precipitous fall in blood pressure in the hours preceding death. Autopsy revealed necrosis of cardiac muscle. Victims also may show intermittent stupor, incoordination, disorientation, and convulsions suggestive of extensive damage to the nervous system. Although the precise mechanism is not fully understood, these latter symptoms most likely result from radiation-induced damage to the neurons and fine vasculature of the brain.

The syndrome is irreversible, and the clinical course may run from only a few minutes to about 48 hours before death occurs. The cardiovascular and central nervous system syndromes have such a rapid course that the irradiated individual dies before the effects of damage to the bone marrow and gastrointestinal system can develop.

The initial clinical problems govern the management of different forms of the acute radiation syndrome. *Antibiotics* are indicated when infection threatens or the granulocyte count falls. *Fluid and electrolyte replacement* is used as necessary. *Whole blood transfusions* are used to treat anemia, and platelets may be administered to arrest thrombocytopenia. *Bone marrow grafts* are indicated between identical twins because there is no risk of graft-versus-host disease. Patients also receive such grafts when exposed to 8 to 10 Gy for treatment of leukemia.

RADIATION EFFECTS ON EMBRYOS AND FETUSES

Embryos and fetuses are considerably more radiosensitive than adults because most embryonic cells are relatively undifferentiated and rapidly mitotic. Prenatal irradiation may lead to death or specific developmental abnormalities depending on the stage of development at the time of irradiation. The description below of abnormalities resulting from embryo or fetal irradiation pertains to exposures far higher than those received during the course of dental radiography. The fetus of a patient exposed to dental radiography receives less than 0.25 µGy from a full-mouth examination when a leaded apron is used.

The effects of radiation on human embryos and fetuses have been studied in women exposed to diagnostic or therapeutic radiation during pregnancy and in women exposed to radiation from the atomic bombs dropped at Hiroshima and Nagasaki. These embryos received exposures of 0.5 to 3 Gy (well more than one million times the exposure from a dental examination). Exposures during the first few days after conception are thought to cause undetectable death of the conceptus.

The most sensitive period for inducing developmental abnormalities is during the period of organogenesis, between 18 and 45 days of gestation. These effects are deterministic in nature. The most common abnormality among the Japanese children exposed early in gestation was reduced growth and reduced head circumference (microcephaly), often associated with mental retardation. Other abnormalities included small birth size, cataracts, genital and skeletal malformations, and microphthalmia. The period of maximal sensitivity of the brain is 8 to 15 weeks postconception. The frequency of severe mental retardation after exposure to 1 Gy during this period is about 43%.

TABLE **2-3** *Comparative Risks during Pregnancy* *		
RISK FACTOR	RESULT	RATE OF RISK
Irradiation during gestation	Death from childhood leukemia	1 in 3333
10 mGy	Death from other childhood cancer	1 in 3571
10 mGy		
Maternal smoking		
1 pack or more per day	Infant death	1 in 3
Maternal alcohol consumption		
2 to 4 drinks per day	Signs of fetal alcohol syndrome	1 in 10
Major malformation at delivery		2.75%

*Adapted from Mettler and Moseley, 1985.

Irradiation during the fetal period (more than 50 days after conception) does not cause gross malformations. However, general retardation of growth persists through life. Evidence also exists for an increased risk of childhood cancer, both leukemia and solid tumors, after irradiation in utero. However, the risks to the embryo and fetus from exposure to radiation are less than from other sources. Table 2-3 shows that maternal smoking and alcohol consumption pose a greater risk than low-level radiation exposure.

Late Somatic Effects

Somatic effects are those seen in the irradiated individual. The most important are radiation-induced cancers. Such lesions are a stochastic effect of radiation in that the probability of an individual's getting cancer depends on the amount of radiation exposure but the severity of the disease is not related to the dose.

CARCINOGENESIS

Data on radiation-induced cancers come primarily from populations of people that have been exposed to high levels of radiation. By far, the group of individuals most intensively studied for estimating the cancer risk from radiation are the Japanese atomic bomb survivors. The cases of more than 120,000 individuals have been followed since 1950, of whom 91,000 were exposed. An estimated 5936 cases of cancer of all types have been observed in this group, most resulting from natural causes,

TABLE 2-4
Susceptibility of Different Tissues to Radiation-Induced Cancer

HIGH	MODERATE	LOW
Colon	Breast (women)	Bladder
Stomach	Esophagus	Liver
Lung		Thyroid
Bone marrow		Skin
(leukemia)		Bone surface
		Brain
		Salivary glands

with only 83 leukemias and 254 solid cancers attributed to radiation exposure.

British patients treated with spinal irradiation for anky-losing spondylitis have also demonstrated leukemia and other cancers. Several studies of patients receiving many fluoroscopic examinations in the course of treatment for tuberculosis, as well as women treated with radiation for postpartum mastitis, have helped researchers understand the risk of inducing breast cancer. The effects of thyroid gland exposure have also been studied in irradiated patients. Some Israeli children were irradiated to the scalp to aid in treatment for ringworm, whereas infants in Rochester, New York, received radiation treatments to reduce the size of their thymus glands. Many other studies on smaller groups of patients have provided useful information.

Estimation of the number of cancers induced by radiation is difficult. Most of the individuals in the studies mentioned above received exposure in excess of the diagnostic range. Thus the probability that a cancer will result from a small dose can be estimated only by interpolation from the rates observed after exposure to larger doses. Furthermore, radiation-induced cancers are not distinguishable from cancers produced by other causes. This means that the number of cancers can be estimated only as the number of excess cases found in exposed groups compared with the number in unexposed groups of people.

In the United States, cancer accounts for nearly 20% of all deaths. Accordingly, the estimated number of deaths attributable to low-level radiation exposure is a small fraction of the total number that occur spontaneously. Estimates indicate that a single, brief whole-body exposure of 100 mGy (about 30 times the average annual exposure) to 100,000 people would result in about 500 additional cancer deaths over the lifetime of the exposed individuals. This would be in addition to the

20,000 that would occur spontaneously. Such a calculation assumes a linear dose-response relationship and no threshold dose below which no risk exists.

These assumptions may be in error and, if so, most likely overestimate the actual risk. Tissues vary in their susceptibility to radiation-induced cancer (Table 2-4). Estimation of the risks associated with dental radiography are considered in Chapter 3, Health Physics.

The mechanism of induction of cancer by ionizing radiation is not well understood. Most likely the basis is radiation-induced gene mutation. Most investigators believe that radiation acts as an initiator, that is, it induces a change in the cell so that it no longer undergoes terminal differentiation. Evidence also exists that radiation acts as a promoter, stimulating cells to multiply. Finally, it may also convert premalignant cells into malignant ones.

The following brief discussion of somatic effects of exposure to radiation pertains primarily to those organs exposed in the course of dental radiography. All radiation-induced cancers, other than leukemia, generally show the following:

1. Most cancers appear approximately 10 years after exposure, and the elevated risk remains for as long as most exposed populations are followed, presumably for the lifetime of the exposed individuals.
2. The risk from exposure during childhood is estimated to be about twice as great as the risk during adulthood.
3. The number of excess cancers induced by radiation is considered to be a multiple of the spontaneous rate rather than independent of the spontaneous rate.

Thyroid Cancer

The incidence of thyroid carcinomas (arising from the follicular epithelium) increases in human beings after exposure. Only about 10% of individuals with such cancers die from their disease. The best-studied groups are Israeli children irradiated to the scalp for ringworm; children in Rochester, New York, irradiated to the thymus gland; and survivors of the atomic bomb in Japan. Susceptibility to radiation-induced thyroid cancer is greater early in childhood than at any time later in life and children are more susceptible than adults. Females are 2 to 3 times more susceptible than males to radiogenic and spontaneous thyroid cancers.

Esophageal Cancer

The data pertaining to esophageal cancer are relatively sparse. Excess cancers are found in the Japanese atomic bomb survivors and in patients treated with x-radiation for ankylosing spondylitis.

Brain and Nervous System Cancers

Patients exposed to diagnostic x-ray examinations in utero and to therapeutic doses in childhood or as adults (average midbrain dose of about 1 Gy) show excess numbers of malignant and benign brain tumors. Additionally, a case-control study has shown an association between intracranial meningiomas and previous medical or dental radiography. The strongest association was with a history of exposure to full-mouth dental radiographs when less than 20 years of age. Because of their age it is likely that these patients received substantially more exposure than is the case today with contemporary techniques.

Salivary Gland Cancer

The incidence of salivary gland tumors is increased in patients treated with irradiation for diseases of the head and neck, in Japanese atomic bomb survivors, and in persons exposed to diagnostic x-radiation. An association between tumors of the salivary glands and dental radiography has been shown, the risk being highest in persons receiving full-mouth examinations before the age of 20 years. Only individuals who received an estimated cumulative parotid dose of 500 mGy or more showed a significant correlation between dental radiography and salivary gland tumors.

Cancer of Other Organs

Other organs such as the skin, paranasal sinuses, and bone marrow (with respect to multiple myeloma) also show excess neoplasia after exposure. However, the mortality and morbidity rates expected after head and neck exposure are much lower than for the organs described previously.

Leukemia

The incidence of leukemia (other than chronic lymphocytic leukemia) rises after exposure of the bone marrow to radiation. Atomic bomb survivors and patients irradiated for ankylosing spondylitis show a wave of leukemias beginning soon after exposure, peaking at around 7 years, and nearly returning to baseline rates within 40 years. Leukemias appear sooner than solid tumors because of the higher rate of cell division and differentiation of hematopoietic stem cells compared with the other tissues. Persons younger than 20 years are more at risk than adults.

OTHER LATE SOMATIC EFFECTS

A number of late somatic effects other than carcinogenesis have been found in the survivors of the atomic bombing of Hiroshima and Nagasaki.

Growth and Development

Children exposed in the bombings showed impairment of growth and development. They have reduced height, weight, and skeletal development. The effects are more pronounced the younger the individual was at the time of exposure.

Mental Retardation

Studies of individuals exposed in utero have shown that the developing human brain is radiosensitive. An estimated 4% chance of mental retardation per 100 mSv exists at 8 to 15 weeks of gestational age, with less risk occurring from exposure at other gestational ages. During this period, rapid production of neurons and migration of these immature neurons to the cerebral cortex occur. The exposure to the embryo from a full set of dental radiographs, using a leaded apron, is less than 3 µSv.

Lenticular Opacities

The threshold for induction of opacities in the lens of the eye ranges from about 2 Gy when the dose is received in a single exposure to more than 5 Gy when the dose is received in multiple exposures over a period of weeks. These doses are far in excess of those received with contemporary dental radiographic techniques. Most affected individuals are unaware of their presence.

Radiation Genetics

GENE MUTATION

Radiation may induce damage in the genetic material of reproductive cells, and the offspring of irradiated parents may experience the effects of such damage. In his pioneering work in this field, Muller (1927) reported radiation-induced mutations in *Drosophila* (fruit flies). Intensive work in this field established a number of basic principles of radiation genetics. He found that radiation induces new mutations rather than simply increasing the frequency of spontaneous mutations. Furthermore, the frequency of mutations increases in direct proportion to the dose, even at very low doses, with no evidence of a threshold. The vast majority of mutations are deleterious to the organism.

Effects on Human Beings

Current knowledge of genetic effects (those effects seen in the progeny of irradiated persons) after radiation exposure come largely from the atomic bomb survivors. To date, no such radiation-related genetic damage has been demonstrated. No increase has occurred in adverse pregnancy outcome, leukemia or other cancers, or im-

TABLE 2-5
Estimated Genetic Effects of 10 mSv per Generation

DISORDER	CURRENT INCIDENCE/10^6 LIVEBORN	ADDITIONAL FIRST-GENERATION CASES/10^6 LIVEBORN
Autosomal dominant		
Severe	2500	5 to 20
Mild	7500	1 to 15
X-linked	400	<1
Recessive	2500	<1
Congenital abnormalities	20,000 to 30,000	10

Adapted from Committee on the Biological Effects of Ionizing Radiations: *Health effects of exposure to low levels of ionizing radiation, BEIR V,* Washington, DC, 1990, National Academy Press.

pairment of growth and development in the children of atomic bomb survivors. These findings do not exclude the possibility that such damage occurs but do show that it must be at a very low frequency.

Doubling Dose

One way to measure the risk from genetic exposure is by determining the doubling dose. This is the amount of radiation a population requires to produce in the next generation as many additional mutations as arise spontaneously. In human beings the genetic doubling dose for mutations resulting in death is approximately 2 Sv. Because the average person receives far less gonadal radiation, radiation contributes relatively little to genetic damage in populations.

For comparison, the gonadal dose to males from a full-mouth radiographic examination is very low; about 1 μSv or less. This exposure is contributed largely by the maxillary views, which are angled caudally. The dose to the ovaries is about 50 times less; in the range of 0.02 μSv. Table 2-5 shows the estimated genetic effects resulting from 10 mSv per generation.

BIBLIOGRAPHY

Hall E: *Radiobiology for the radiologist,* ed 3, Philadelphia, 1988, JB Lippincott.

Mettler F, Kelsey C, Ricks R: *Medical management of radiation accidents,* Boca Raton, Fla., 1990, CRC Press.

Mettler F, Moseley R: *Medical effects of ionizing radiation,* Orlando, Fla., 1985, Grune & Stratton.

Pizzarello D, Witcofski R: *Medical radiation biology,* ed 2, Philadelphia, 1982, Lea & Febiger.

Prasad K: *CRC handbook of radiobiology,* Boca Raton, Fla., 1984, CRC Press.

SUGGESTED READINGS

ODONTOGENESIS

Kimeldorf DJ: Radiation-induced alterations in odontogenesis and formed teeth. In Berdgis CC, editor: *Pathology of irradiation,* Baltimore, 1971, Williams & Wilkins.

OSTEORADIONECROSIS

Balogh JM, Sutherland SE: Osteoradionecrosis of the mandible: a review, *J Otolaryngol* 18:245, 1989.

Bras J, de Jonge HK, van Merkesteyn JP: Osteoradionecrosis of the mandible: pathogenesis, *Am J Otolaryngol* 11:244, 1990.

Jansma J et al: A survey of prevention and treatment regimens for oral sequelae resulting from head and neck radiotherapy used in Dutch radiotherapy institutes, *Int J Radiat Oncol Biol Phys* 24:359, 1992.

Marx RE, Johnson RP: Studies in the radiobiology of osteoradionecrosis and their clinical significance, *Oral Surg* 64:379, 1987.

Maxymiw WG, Rothney LM, Sutcliffe SB: Reduction in the incidence of postradiation dental complications in cancer patients by continuous quality improvement techniques, *Can J Oncol* 4:233, 1994.

Maxymiw WG, Wood RE: Postradiation dental extractions without hyperbaric oxygen, *Oral Surg Oral Med Oral Pathol* 72:270, 1991.

Mealey BL, Semba SE, Hallmon WW: The head and neck radiotherapy patient: part 2—management of oral complications, *Compendium* 15:442, 1994.

RADIATION CARIES

Jansmal J et al: The effect of x-ray irradiation on the demineralization of bovine dental enamel, *Caries Res* 22:199, 1988.

Joyston-Bechal S: The effect of x-radiation on the susceptibility of enamel to an artificial caries-like attack in vitro, *J Dent* 13:41, 1985.

Joyston-Bechal S: Management of oral complications following radiotherapy, *Dent Update* 19:232, 1992.

Ripa LW: Review of the anticaries effectiveness of professionally applied and self-applied topical fluoride gels, *J Public Health Dent* 49:297, 1989.

Semba SE, Mealey BL, Hallmon WW: The head and neck radiotherapy patient: part 1—oral manifestations of radiation therapy, *Compendium* 15:250, 1994.

SALIVA AND SALIVARY GLANDS

Atkinson JC, Wu AJ: Salivary gland dysfunction: causes, symptoms, treatment, *J Am Dent Assoc* 125:409, 1994.

Franzén L, Funegård U, Ericson T, Henriksson R: Parotid gland function during and following radiotherapy of malignancies in the head and neck. A consecutive study of salivary flow and patient discomfort, *Eur J Cancer* 28:457, 1992.

Greenspan D: Xerostomia: diagnosis and management, *Oncology (Huntingt)* 10 (3 suppl):7, 1996.

Karlsson G: The relative change in saliva secretion in relation to the exposed area of the salivary glands after radiotherapy of head and neck region, *Swed Dent J* 11:189, 1987.

Land CE et al: Incidence of salivary gland tumors among atomic bomb survivors, 1950-1987: evaluation of radiation-related risk, *Radiat Res* 146:28, 1996.

Liu RP et al: Salivary flow rates in patients with head and neck cancer 0.5 to 25 years after radiotherapy, *Oral Surg Oral Med Oral Pathol* 70:724, 1990.

Pogoda JM, Preston-Martin S: Comment on "Incidence of salivary gland tumors among atomic bomb survivors, 1950-1987. Evaluation of radiation-related risk" by Land et al. (Radiat. Res. 146, 28-36, 1996) [letter]. *Radiat Res* 146:356, 1996.

SOMATIC EFFECTS

Committee on the Biological Effects of Ionizing Radiations: *Health effects of exposure to low levels of ionizing radiation, BEIR V*, Washington, D.C., 1990, National Academy Press.

1990 Recommendations of the International Commission on Radiological Protection, ICRP Publ. 60, Annals of the ICRP 21, 1990.

Putnam FW: Hiroshima and Nagasaki revisited: the Atomic Bomb Casualty Commission and the Radiation Effects Research Foundation, *Perspect Biol Med* 37:515, 1994.

Schull WJ: *Effects of atomic radiation: a half-century of studies from Hiroshima and Nagasaki*, New York, 1995, Wiley-Liss.

United Nations Scientific Committee on the Effects of Atomic Radiation: *Sources and effects of ionizing radiation*, New York, 1996, UN.

TASTE

Conger AD: Loss and recovery of taste acuity in patients irradiated to the oral cavity, *Radiat Res* 53:338, 1973.

Mossman KL: Gustatory tissue injury in man: radiation dose response relationships and mechanisms of taste loss, *Br J Cancer* 7(suppl):9, 1986.

Radiation Safety and Protection

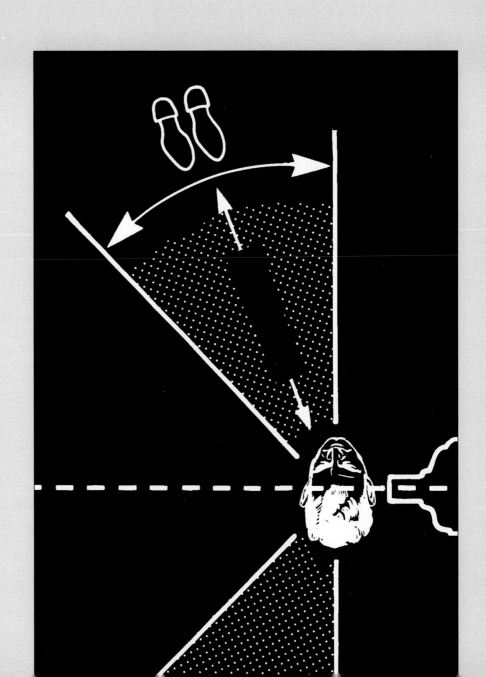

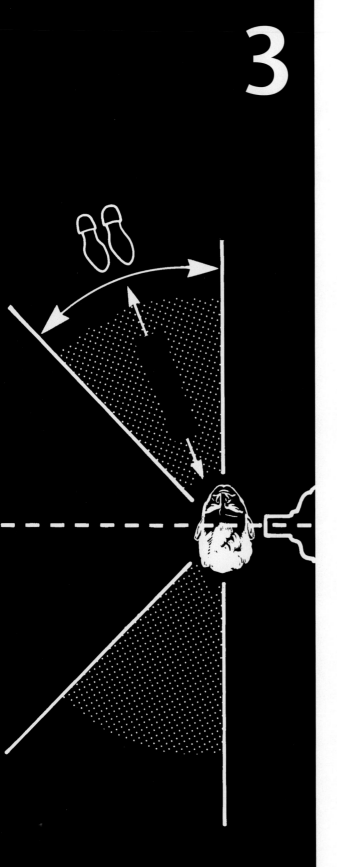

3 Health Physics

NEIL L. FREDERIKSEN

"Tests show radiation's bad effects!"
"Radiation cloud over medicine!"
"Single dose of 'safe' radiation found harmful!"
"Diagnostic x-rays deserve that negative reaction!"

These are headlines that have appeared in newspapers across the United States over the years. Before an appointment with the practitioner, the patient may read one of these articles and understandably form a negative opinion concerning the use of x-rays for diagnostic purposes. Practitioners must be prepared to discuss intelligently the benefits and possible hazards involved with the use of x-rays and describe the steps taken to reduce the hazard.

Practitioners who administer ionizing radiation must become familiar with the magnitude of radiation exposure encountered in medicine and dentistry, the possible risk that such exposure entails, and the methods used to affect exposure and reduce dose. This information provides the necessary background for explaining to concerned patients the benefits and possible hazards involved with the use of x-rays. This chapter is dedicated to the application of radiation protection principles, which are collectively known as *health physics*.

Sources of Radiation Exposure

A wide variety of conditions and circumstances, some that are controllable and others that are not, result in radiation exposure from a multitude of sources. Although the sources of radiation exposure are many and varied, they can be categorized as being derived from two sources: natural and artificial (Table 3-1). The radiation from these sources results in an average annual effective dose of 3.60 mSv to a person living in the United States.[69]

The effective dose, the dosimetric quantity used to relate radiation exposure to risk, is derived as follows: the equivalent dose (H_T), a quantity that expresses all kinds of radiation on a common scale, is defined as the sum of the products of the absorbed dose in grays (D) and the radiation weighting factor (w_R). The unit of equivalent dose is the sievert. The effective dose (E) is the sum of the equivalent doses to each tissue (H_T), multiplied by each tissue's weighting factor (w_T):

$$E = \Sigma \, H_T \times w_T$$

The tissue weighting factors are defined by the International Commission on Radiological Protection.[43] They allow practitioners to obtain a value for E that is estimated to be a measure of the somatic and genetic radiation-induced risks, even if the body is not uniformly exposed. The quantities of dose listed in Table 3-1 are an average for the total population. The contribution to the radiation exposure of an individual from each component may vary by one or more orders of magnitude depending on factors discussed later in this chapter.

NATURAL RADIATION

Natural or background radiation is by far the largest contributor (83%) to the radiation exposure of people living in the United States today[66,69,72] (see Table 3-1 and Fig. 3-1). Background radiation from external and internal sources yields an average annual E of about 3 mSv.

External

External exposure results from cosmic and terrestrial radiation, both of which originate from the environment. These sources contribute about 16% of the radiation exposure to the population.

Cosmic radiation. Cosmic radiation includes energetic subatomic particles, photons of extraterrestrial origin that reach the earth (primary cosmic radiation) and to a lesser extent the particles and photons (secondary cosmic radiation) generated by the interactions of primary cosmic radiation with atoms and molecules of the earth's atmosphere. In the lower atmosphere the E from cosmic radiation is primarily a function of altitude, almost doubling with each 2000-meter increase in eleva-

tion, because less atmosphere is present to attenuate the radiation. Therefore at sea level the exposure from cosmic radiation is about 0.24 mSv per year; at an elevation of 1600 m (approximately 1 mile, or the elevation of Denver, Colorado), it is about 0.50 mSv per year; and at an elevation of 3200 m (approximately 2 miles, or the elevation of Leadville, Colorado), it is about 1.25 mSv per year. Cosmic radiation is also greater at higher latitudes because of low-energy cosmic rays being deflected toward the poles by the earth's magnetic field. Considering the altitude and latitude distribution of the U.S. population and a 20% reduction in exposure because of structural shielding during time spent indoors, it can be calculated that the average cosmic radiation E rate is about 0.26 mSv per year.

Also included in this category is exposure resulting from airline travel. As more people travel frequently above the protection of the earth's atmosphere, cosmic radiation becomes a more significant contributor to exposure. Astronauts are an extreme example, being sub-

TABLE 3-1
Average Annual Effective Dose of Ionizing Radiation (mSv) to a Member of the U.S. Population

SOURCE	DOSE
Natural	
External	
Cosmic	0.27
Terrestrial	0.28
Internal	
Radon	2.00
Other	0.40
ROUNDED TOTAL	3.00
Artificial	
Medical	
X-ray diagnosis	0.39
Nuclear medicine	0.14
Consumer products	0.10
Other	
Occupational	<0.01
Nuclear fuel cycle	<0.01
Fallout	<0.01
Miscellaneous	<0.01
ROUNDED TOTAL	0.60
NATURAL PLUS ARTIFICIAL	3.60

From National Council on Radiation Protection and Measurements: NCRP Reports 93, 1987; 94, 1987; 95, 1987; 100, 1989.

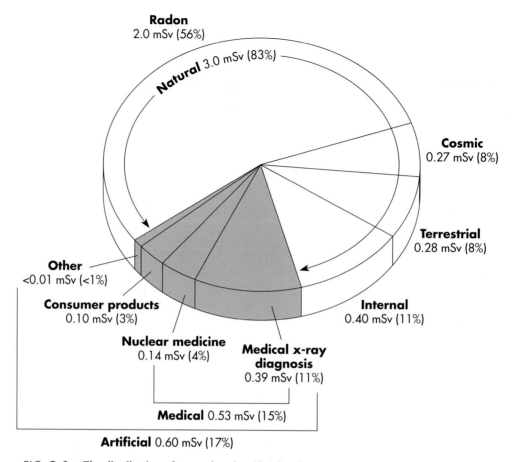

FIG. **3-1** *The distribution of natural and artificial radiation.* Natural radiation contributes more exposure than artificial radiation; x-ray diagnosis is the largest component of artificial radiation.

jected to whole-body dose equivalents of 1 to 10 mSv per mission. If these missions occurred during large solar particle events, it has been estimated that their exposure would be as much as 1 Sv.

More practical and relevant to the general population, an airline flight of 5 hours in the middle latitudes at an altitude of 12 km may result in a dose equivalent of about 25 µSv. With 340 million passengers in 1984 taking trips with an average duration of 1.5 hours, the average annual E is approximately 0.01 mSv. Thus in total, cosmic radiation, including that occurring in airline travel, contributes an exposure of 0.27 mSv, or about 8% of the average annual E to a member of the U.S. population.

Terrestrial radiation. Exposure from terrestrial sources varies with the type of soil and its content of the naturally occurring primordial radionuclides potassium-40 and the radioactive decay products of uranium-238 and thorium-232. Most of the gamma radiation from these sources comes from the top 20 cm of soil, with only a

small contribution by airborne radon and its decay products. Indoor exposure from primordial radionuclides is very close to that occurring outdoors. This results from a balance between the shielding provided by structural materials and the exposure from radioactive nuclides contained within these shielding materials.

Terrestrial radiation has been measured in air in more than 200 locations over a large portion of the United States. Dose rates vary from about 0.16 mSv per year on the Atlantic and Gulf coastal plains, to 0.63 mSv per year for a region on the eastern slopes of the Rocky Mountains, to about 0.30 mSv for the rest of the country. Combining this information with data on the geographic distribution of the U.S. population, it is estimated that the average terrestrial exposure rate is about 0.28 mSv per year, or approximately 8% of the average annual E to a person living in the United States. This quantity of radiation exposure appears minimal compared with that received by individuals living in certain towns and villages of Brazil and India, where the gamma radiation dose levels can be as high as 120 mSv per year. These unusually high terrestrial radiation levels are a result of the fact that these towns and villages were constructed on soil containing monazite, a mineral with a high content of thorium-232.[2]

Internal

The sources of internal radiation are radionuclides that are taken up from the external environment by inhalation and ingestion. Because an organism cannot discriminate between isotopes of a chemical element, all isotopes, radioactive or not, have an equal chance, modified by frequency of occurrence, of being incorporated into the body. This source, which results in about 67% (2.40 mSv) of the radiation exposure of the population, includes radon and its short-lived decay products.

Radon. Radon is estimated to be responsible for approximately 56% of the radiation exposure of the U.S. population. As such, it is the largest single contributor to natural radiation (2.00 mSv). Although the ubiquitous noble gas radon (radon-222) produced in the uranium-238 decay chain is transported in the water and atmosphere that enter our homes and buildings, its short-lived decay products (^{218}Po, ^{214}Po, ^{214}Pb, and ^{214}Bi) are of perhaps more concern. These products, produced during the decay of radon to stable lead-206, are attached primarily to aerosols that can deposit in the respiratory tract, contributing an average annual equivalent dose to the bronchial epithelium in the U.S. population of 24 mSv. It has recently been estimated[64] that exposure to this quantity of radiation may cause as many as 10,000 lung cancer deaths per year in the United States.

Other internal sources. The second largest source (11%) of natural radiation results from the ingestion of food and water that contain primordial radionuclides. Estimates place the average annual E because of the presence of uranium and thorium and their decay products (primarily potassium-40, but also rubidium-87, carbon-14, tritium, and a dozen or more extraterrestrially produced radionuclides) in the body at 0.40 mSv per year.

ARTIFICIAL RADIATION

Human beings, with all their technologic advances, have contributed a number of sources of radiation to the environment.[69,72,67] These may be categorized into three major groups—medical diagnosis and treatment, consumer and industrial products and sources, and other minor sources—which, in total, contribute an average annual E of about 0.60 mSv, or 17% of the annual radiation exposure to the U.S. population (see Table 3-1 and Fig. 3-1).

Medical Diagnosis and Treatment

In 1993 it was estimated that more than 1 billion medical x-ray examinations and 300 million dental examinations are performed annually worldwide.[115] Studies show that radiation used in the healing arts is the single largest component (0.53 mSv) of artificial radiation to which the U.S. population is exposed and second only to radon as a source. Although sources in this group include radiation therapy and diagnosis, diagnostic x-ray exposure is the largest contributor. It has been estimated that more than 330,000 x-ray units in the United States in 1981 were being used for medical and dental diagnoses, procedures that yield an average annual E of about 0.39 mSv.

The contribution made by oral radiography has been excluded from this calculated total because dental examinations are estimated[122] to be responsible for an average annual E of less than the negligible individual dose (0.01 mSv, Table 3-2). Dental x-ray examinations are responsible for only 2.5% of the average annual E resulting from x-ray diagnosis and 0.3% of the total average annual E. This is remarkable when the following facts are considered:

- In 1981 more than half (204,000) of the x-ray units in the United States were used by dentists.
- In 1982 it was estimated that 105 million x-ray examinations were performed using 380 million films.
- In that same year (1982), 456 x-ray examinations were performed per 1000 population.

Consumer and Industrial Products and Sources

Although only a minor contributor to the average annual E (3%), consumer and industrial products and sources contain some of the most interesting and unsuspected sources. In total, this group, which includes the domestic water supply (10 to 60 µSv), combustible fuels (1.0 to 6.0 µSv), dental porcelain (0.1 µSv), television receivers (less than 10 µSv), pocket watches (1.0 to 5.0×10^{-2} µSv), smoke alarms (less than 1.0×10^{-2} µSv), and airport inspection systems (less than 1.0×10^{-2} µSv), contributes about 0.10 mSv to the average annual E.

The contribution resulting from use of tobacco products is also included in this category. However, estimating the average annual E to the population from this source is impossible with current information. Nevertheless, by making several assumptions, an estimate of the E for the average smoker can be calculated. The annual average dose to a small area of the bronchial epithelium is estimated[17,53] to be 8.0 mGy as a result of the ^{210}Pb and ^{210}Po contained within tobacco. Applying a radiation quality factor (w_R) of 20 for alpha particles (^{210}Pb and ^{210}Po are alpha emitters) yields an annual equiva-

TABLE **3-2**
Recommendations on Annual Limits for Human Exposure to Ionizing Radiation*

RECOMMENDATION	NCRP	ICRP
Occupational Dose Limits		
Relative to stochastic effects	50 mSv annual effective dose limit and [10 mSv][age (yr)] cumulative effective dose limit	50 mSv annual effective dose limit and 100 mSv in 5 yr cumulative effective dose limit
Relative to deterministic effects	150 mSv annual equivalent dose limit to lens of eye and 500 mSv annual equivalent dose limit to skin and extremities	150 mSv equivalent dose limit to lens of eye and 500 mSv annual equivalent dose limit to skin and extremities
Nonoccupational (Public) Dose Limits		
Relative to stochastic effects	5 mSv annual effective dose limit for infrequent exposure and 1 mSv annual effective dose limit for continuous exposure	1 mSv annual effective dose limit and, if higher, not to exceed an annual average of 1 mSv over 5 yr
Relative to deterministic effects	50 mSv annual equivalent dose limit to lens of eye, skin, and extremities	15 mSv annual equivalent dose limit to lens of eye and 50 mSv annual equivalent dose limit to lens of eye, skin, and extremities
Embryo-fetus	0.5 mSv equivalent dose limit per month after pregnancy is known	2 mSv equivalent dose limit after the pregnancy has been declared
Negligible individual dose†	0.01 mSv annual effective dose	None established

*From National Council on Radiation Protection and Measurements: NCRP Report 116, 1993, and International Commission on Radiological Protection: Radiation protection, ICRP Publication 60, 1990.
†That dose below which any effort to reduce the radiation exposure cannot be justified.

lent dose (H_T) to the lungs of 160 mSv. Using a tissue weighting factor (w_T) of 0.08 for the portion of lungs exposed results in a calculation of an effective dose of approximately 13 mSv for the average smoker.

Other Artificial Sources

Because some primordial radionuclides have always existed in the environment, at least since the origin of humankind, they have always been in the body. Other artificial radionuclides are a product of modern times. After periods of nuclear weapons testing in the 1950s and early 1960s, the fission products cesium-137, strontium-90, and iodine-131 were discovered in the human body. Released into the environment by above-ground nuclear explosions, 90 of which occurred at the Nevada Test Site, they reached the body through normal food chains.

Of these, strontium-90 and iodine-131 are perhaps the most important. Because of its chemical similarity to calcium, strontium-90, a pure beta emitter, is readily assimilated in the bones and teeth of children and young adults. Concentration in these areas is a reason for justifiable concern because of its long half-life (28.8 years) and slow turnover rate (the effective half-life in bone is 17.5 years).[2] Iodine-131 accumulates in the thyroid

gland. It has been estimated that the average cumulative dose to the thyroid of approximately 160 million people in the United States resulting from the Nevada tests was 0.02 Gy, or about 21 times that delivered by a complete mouth survey (see "Thyroid Dose," p. 48).[75] The late effects of these exposures have yet to be determined. Currently, fallout is no longer considered a significant source of exposure to the public because of an almost worldwide ban on the atmospheric testing of nuclear weapons.

Of the sources in this category (which may contribute in total only about 0.01 mSv to the average annual E), nuclear power is of particular concern to the public. By 1979, 70 nuclear power reactors were licensed for operation in the United States[18]; by 1987, this figure had reached almost 100[69]; and as of 1990, 113 nuclear power plants were operating in the United States.[115] Additionally, in 1990, 75 nuclear reactors were being used for research and training, 70 were being operated at U.S. Department of Energy facilities, and at least 100 nuclear reactors were being used to power U.S. Navy ships and submarines. In spite of this number of nuclear power and support facilities, it is currently estimated that in normal operation these reactors add only about 0.6 µSv to the average annual *E*, a quantity up to 10 times less than that contributed by combustible fuels, coal, natural gas, and oil, which contain naturally occurring radionuclides that are released to the environment when burned.

In spite of this relatively low contribution to the average annual *E* made by nuclear power, accidents do happen that result in significant exposure to a segment of the population. Between 1945 and 1987, 284 nuclear reactor accidents, excluding Chernobyl, were reported in several countries, resulting in the exposure of more than 1300 people, with 33 fatalities.[55] In the majority of these accidents, the public was not directly affected. This was not the case, however, in the Three Mile Island incident in the United States and at Chernobyl in what was then the Ukrainian Soviet Socialist Republic. After the Three Mile Island nuclear plant incident in 1979, studies showed that the maximal individual dose was less than 1.0 mSv and individuals living within a 16-km radius of the plant received an average dose of only 0.08 mSv, an added exposure equal to some 2.7% of their natural background radiation exposure. From 1982 to 1984, a temporary increase occurred in the incidence of cancer among those living near the nuclear plant. This finding was not expected in view of the relatively long latent period for radiation-induced malignancy. Instead it is believed to be a result not of exposure to radiation, but of early detection as a result of increased surveillance of cancer prompted by postaccident concern.[40]

The nuclear accident at Chernobyl in 1986 made clear that the use of nuclear power facilities carries the real potential of causing considerable harm if not properly controlled. In that event, 29 persons in the immediate vicinity of the plant were reported to have died of acute radiation injury (see Chapter 2 for a discussion of the acute radiation syndrome) in the first months after exposure.[55] It has been estimated[19] that in the next 70 years at least 10,000 excess cancer deaths from leukemia and solid tumors of the thyroid gland and other organs will occur among the Ukrainian people. Although this large number of excess cancers should be considered a public health disaster, the projected excess among the Ukrainian people corresponds to less than 1% of the cancers expected to occur there spontaneously over the next 70 years.

Risk estimates to the United States population as a result of exposure to airborne debris from Chernobyl are considerably less:[12] three additional lung cancer deaths and an extra four deaths from cancer of the thyroid, breast, or bone marrow may be expected over the next 45 years in the United States because of this accident. (Compare this with the estimated 10,000 annual lung cancer deaths that may be caused by the presence of radon in the U.S. environment.)

Exposure and Dose in Radiography

The goal of health physics is to prevent the occurrence of deterministic effects and the likelihood of stochastic effects by minimizing the exposure of office personnel and patients during radiographic examinations. A *deterministic effect* is defined as any somatic effect that increases in severity as a function of radiation dose after a threshold has been reached.[70] These effects, resulting from relatively large doses of radiation not generally encountered in diagnostic radiology, may occur soon after exposure or months to years after exposure. Examples of deterministic effects include cataracts, skin erythema, fibrosis, and abnormal growth and development following exposure in utero. A *stochastic effect* is defined as one whose probability rather than severity is a function of radiation dose without a threshold. Stochastic effects represent an all-or-none response, modified by individual risk factors. These effects may occur after exposure to relatively low doses of radiation such as those that may be encountered in diagnostic radiology. Cancers and genetic effects are examples of stochastic effects.

DOSE LIMITS

Recognition of the harmful effects of radiation and the risks involved with its use led the National Council on Radiation Protection and Measurements (NCRP) and the International Commission on Radiological Protection (ICRP) to establish guidelines on limitations on the amount of radiation received by both occupationally exposed individuals and the public. Since their establishment in the 1930s, these dose limits have been revised downward several times. These revisions reflect the increased knowledge gained over the years concerning the harmful effects of radiation and the increased ability to use radiation more efficiently. The current occupational exposure limits have been established to ensure that the probability for stochastic effects is as low as reasonably and economically feasible (see Table 3-2).

Compliance with these limits should ensure that the risk of individual radiation workers being afflicted with fatal cancer as a result of their occupational exposure is no greater than that of fatal accidents in nonradiation occupations. Nonoccupational dose limits for members of the public have been established at 10% of that of occupationally exposed individuals. This lower dose limit was set because of uncertainties associated with risk estimates, the wider variation in mortality risks and levels of exposure to natural radiation, and the wider range of sensitivities to radiation found among the general public. The negligible individual dose, established by the

NCRP, is considered to be the dose below which any effort to reduce the radiation exposure may not be cost effective. In spite of the Council's endorsement of the nonthreshold hypothesis for purposes of radiation safety, it is believed that the impact on society of radiation exposure of this magnitude is negligible.

Although receiving 50 mSv of whole-body radiation exposure in 1 year as a result of performing one's occupation may be considered to present minimal risk, every effort should be made to keep the dose to all individuals as low as practical. All unnecessary radiation exposure should be avoided. This is a philosophy of radiation protection everyone should recognize. It is based on the principles of ALARA (*As Low As Reasonably Achievable*), which recognizes the possibility that no matter how small the dose, some stochastic effect may result.[43] The most current data available show that industrial workers in radiation industries are acting in accordance with this philosophy, insofar as their average annual individual effective dose was reported to be 1.56 mSv, 3% of the annual limit.[68] The dosage for individuals occupationally exposed in the operation of dental x-ray equipment was found to be even less, 0.20 mSv, or 0.4% of the allowable limit.

It is important to realize that these dose limits were formulated by the NCRP and ICRP, private nonprofit organizations, and as such have no force of law. Although the federal government and most state governments accept these recommendations, all those who administer ionizing radiation should consult with their state's bureau of radiation control or safety to obtain information on applicable and current laws. In addition, it is important to understand that these dose limits apply to exposure from manmade sources only and do not apply to either natural radiation or x-ray exposure that patients receive as a result of radiographic procedures in the course of dental and medical treatment.

PATIENT EXPOSURE AND DOSE

Patient dose from dental radiography is usually reported as the amount of radiation received by a target organ. One of the most common measurements is skin or surface exposure. The surface exposure, obtained by direct measurement, is the simplest way to record a patient's exposure to x-rays. Of little significance in itself, it is used in the calculation of doses received by organs that lie at or near the point of measurement. Other target organs commonly reported include the bone marrow, thyroid gland, and gonads. The mean active bone marrow dose is an important measurement because bone marrow is the target organ believed responsible for radiation-induced leukemia. Particular concern has been expressed over exposure of the thyroid because this gland has one of the highest radiation-induced cancer rates.[18] The gonad dose is important because of suspected genetic responses to diagnostic x-ray exposure.

Patient dose has also been reported as the *E*. This method of reporting resulted from an inability to make direct comparisons between radiographic techniques themselves and background radiation exposure in terms of dose because of the limited area of the body exposed during diagnostic radiology. It is only through the *E* that possible adverse effects from irradiation to a limited portion of the body can be compared with possible adverse effects from irradiation of the whole body.

Mean Active Bone Marrow Dose

The mean active bone marrow dose was derived as a specific tissue dose relevant to a particular stochastic effect, leukemia. The mean active bone marrow dose is that dose of radiation averaged over the entire active bone marrow.[14] The mean active bone marrow dose resulting from an intraoral full-mouth survey of 21 films exposed with round collimation has been reported to be 0.142 mSv; one exposed with rectangular collimation is only 0.06 mSv.[124] Panoramic radiography was found to contribute a mean active bone marrow dose of about 0.01 mSv per film. For comparison, the mean active bone marrow dose from one chest film is 0.03 mSv.[74]

Thyroid Dose

The proximity of the thyroid gland to the x-ray beam is of crucial importance in determining the magnitude of dose received. For example, a radiographic examination of the cervical spine may consist of four separate exposures that in total are responsible for a dose to the thyroid of about 5.5 mGy.[74] During this examination, the thyroid gland is almost directly in the center of the radiation field. On the other hand, a radiograph of the chest may result in a thyroid dose of only 0.01 mGy,[124] mainly from scatter radiation. Studies have reported that the dose to the thyroid from oral radiography is fairly low. A 21-film complete mouth examination results in a thyroid dose of 0.94 mGy. This value is one sixth that resulting from a radiographic examination of the cervical spine. Likewise, the thyroid dose from panoramic radiography has been reported as being about 74 μGy, 1% that from a cervical spinal examination.[36]

Gonad Dose

Radiographs that involve the abdomen result in the highest dose to the gonads; those involving the head, neck, and extremities result in the lowest. For example, a radiograph of the kidneys, ureters, and bladder (retrograde pyelogram) was reported to deliver a gonad dose of 1.07 mGy to women and 0.08 mGy to men, whereas a radiograph of the skull delivered a dose of less than 0.005 mGy to both sexes.[74] As a general category, dental x-ray examinations result in a genetically insignificant dose of only 1.0 µGy.[38] This contribution is only 0.003% of the average annual background exposure.

Effective Dose

It is tempting to make a direct comparison of the previously discussed values for purposes of risk estimation. However, the statement that a single dental periapical radiograph delivers more than 10 times the radiation of a chest film (in terms of surface exposure, i.e., 217 versus 16 mR[94,73]) is not entirely true because of differences in the exposed area and critical organs. These differences may be compensated for by a calculation of the E, which is an estimate of the uniform whole-body exposure carrying the same probability of radiation effect as a partial body exposure. By this method of calculation, a complete mouth survey of 20 films made by methods that were optimized for dose (i.e., E-speed film, rectangular collimation) has been found to deliver less than half the amount of radiation of a single chest film and less than 1% of the amount of a barium study of the intestines (Table 3-3).

ESTIMATES OF RISK

The degree of risk that may be associated with exposure to ionizing radiation may be expressed in two ways: days of equivalent natural exposure and probability of stochastic effects. Days of equivalent natural exposure is calculated as the product of the E resulting from a specific radiographic examination and the average daily E

TABLE 3-3
Effective Dose, Equivalent Natural Exposure, and Probability of Stochastic Effects from Diagnostic X-Ray Examinations

SURVEY	E (µSv)	DAYS OF EQUIVALENT NATURAL EXPOSURE	PROBABILITY OF STOCHASTIC EFFECTS ($\times 10^{-6}$)
Intraoral			
Round collimation, D-speed film*			
Periapical			
15 films	111	13.9	8.1
Interproximal			
4 films	38	4.8	2.8
Complete mouth survey			
19 films	150	18.8	11.0
Rectangular collimation, E-speed film†			
Complete mouth survey			
20 films	33	4.1	2.4
Extraoral			
Panoramic‡	26	3.3	1.9
Computed tomography			
Maxilla	104§ to 1202‖	13.0 to 150.3	7.6 to 87.7
Mandible	761§ to 3324‖	95.1 to 415.5	55.6 to 242.7
Lower gastrointestinal (GI)¶	4060	507.5	296.4
Upper GI¶	2440	305.0	178.1
Abdomen¶	560	70.0	40.9
Skull¶	220	27.5	16.1
Chest¶	80	10.0	5.8

*Avendanio B et al: Effective dose and risk assessment from detailed narrow beam radiography, *Oral Surg Oral Med Oral Pathol Oral Radiol Endod* 82:713, 1996.
†White SC: 1992 Assessment of radiation risks from dental radiography, *Dentomaxillofac Radiol* 21:118, 1992.
‡Frederiksen NL, Benson BW, Sokolowski TW: Effective dose and risk assessment from film tomography used for dental implant diagnostics, *Dentomaxillofac Radiol* 23:123, 1994.
§Frederiksen NL, Benson BW, Sokolowski TW: Effective dose and risk assessment from computed tomography of the maxillofacial complex, *Dentomaxillofac Radiol* 24:55, 1995.
‖Scaf G et al: Dosimetry and cost of imaging osseointegrated implants with film-based and computed tomography, *Oral Surg Oral Med Oral Pathol Oral Radiol Endod* 83:41, 1997.
¶National Council on Radiation Protection and Measurements: *Exposure of the U.S. population from diagnostic medical radiation*, NCRP Report 100, Bethesda, Md.,1989.

(8 µSv) delivered by natural sources (see Table 3-3). This expression of exposure may be used by the dentist to discuss potential risk with patients from a perspective that may be more easily understood. The dentist may point out to the patient that by optimizing the intraoral radiographic technique (E-speed film, rectangular collimation), the days of equivalent exposure may be reduced from about $2\frac{1}{2}$ weeks (18.8 days) to only about 4 days and that this quantity is significantly less when compared with almost $1\frac{1}{2}$ years (507.5 days), which is equivalent to that delivered by a barium examination of the lower intestinal tract. For another example, the dependence of physical location within the United States on exposure to natural radiation may be used. The E resulting from cosmic radiation in Denver is 0.24 mSv higher than the average of the United States because of its high elevation and reduced atmospheric protection. This means that a person living in an average location in the United States who had one complete mouth survey and one panoramic film made by optimized techniques every year (total E for these examinations = 59 µSv, see Table 3-3) would incur only one fourth the risk of a person living in Denver who was not exposed to dental radiography. Put another way, if a person living in an average location in the United States had four complete mouth surveys and panoramic films made by optimized techniques every year, they would incur only the same risk of a person living in Denver who was not exposed to dental radiography.

The significance of this method of comparison can be made even more dramatic by considering those locations in Brazil and India where the terrestrial gamma radiation levels can be as high as 0.12 Gy per year. This is equivalent to an annual excess exposure of about 40 years of average background radiation. Therefore if persons living in an average location in the United States were to receive at least one complete mouth survey and one panoramic examination every day for the rest of their lives, they would incur much less risk than individuals residing in these areas of Brazil or India who were not exposed to oral radiography.

The primary risk from dental radiography is radiation-induced cancer. The risk of cancer being induced in human beings as a result of exposure to low doses of radiation is difficult to estimate for a number of reasons. First, the number of known radiation-induced cases is small and the doses too high to allow for interpolation to low doses with any degree of certainty. Second, cancer is a prevalent disease. In 1997 approximately 1,382,400 new cases of invasive cancer (excluding basal and squamous cell carcinoma of the skin and carcinoma in situ of any site but the bladder) were diagnosed in the United States.[78] This makes the incidence resulting from radiation exposure difficult to detect. Third, radiation-induced cancer cannot be distinguished from cancer induced by other causes. Finally, the time between radiation exposure and the development of cancer may be years to decades, during which time individuals may be subjected to other carcinogens.

In spite of these difficulties, the ICRP has developed an estimate that includes the probability for the induction of both fatal and nonfatal cancer and hereditary effects in an exposed population.[43] The probability coefficient for these stochastic effects resulting from exposure to low doses of radiation is $7.3 \times 10^{-2} \text{Sv}^{-1}$. The product of this probability coefficient and the E resulting from a specific radiographic examination, which yields a probability of occurrence per million exposed people, is shown in Table 3-3. These data show that the risk of developing cancer or some heritable effect from radiation received as a result of intraoral radiography is estimated to be at most 11 per million examinations. If the contribution made by hereditary effects were ignored (assuming these 11 cases per million examinations to be cancers) and everyone in the United States (estimated population in 1997 was 266,449,000) were to have a complete mouth survey of intraoral radiographs made, this would increase the number of new cases of invasive cancer diagnosed by almost 3000 to approximately 1,385,326—an increase of only 0.2%.

Everyone is subject to risks in everyday life. Newspapers and news magazines occasionally publish articles dealing with the level of such risks. In consideration of the potential risk associated with dental radiography, it might be good to keep in mind that the average person's risk of choking to death is 13 per million and of dying in a boating accident, 4.6 per million. The risk from both of these events is greater than the risk from some intraoral radiographic procedures. On the other hand, it should be considered that the risk from these same radiographic procedures is greater than an individual's risk of dying as a result of an overseas terrorist attack (0.1 per million), being struck by falling airplane parts (0.1 per million), or being killed by a shark (0.003 per million).

Although the risk involved with dental radiography is certainly small in terms of many other risks that are a common part of everyday life, no statistical basis exists to assume that it is zero. Despite the fact that diagnostic radiation appears to be a weak carcinogen, the risk is increased because of the large number of people exposed. Practitioners must also conclude that it is their responsibility to ensure that patients avoid even the smallest unnecessary dose of radiation.

Methods of Exposure and Dose Reduction

The decision to use diagnostic radiography rests on professional judgment of its necessity for the benefit of the total health of the patient. This decision having been made, it then becomes the duty of the dental professional to produce a maximum yield of information per unit of x-ray exposure.[21]

Becoming aware of the potential risks associated with the use of ionizing radiation and its contribution to rising health care costs is the first step toward exposure and dose reduction in diagnostic radiography. After this awareness has been developed, the second step is to use techniques, materials, and equipment that optimize the radiologic process. Optimizing the radiologic process is the best way to ensure maximal patient benefit with a minimum of patient and operator exposure.[13]

In this section, methods of exposure and dose reduction are described that can be used in oral radiography. Each subsection begins with a recommendation of the American Dental Association (ADA) Council on Dental Materials, Instruments, and Equipment based on optimal use of the radiologic process. This is followed by a discussion of ways in which these recommendations can be satisfied. Included in the text are NCRP recommendations and federal regulations concerning the use of ionizing radiation.

In addition to federal regulations, states have their own laws dealing with ionizing radiation. Although most of them closely follow the recommendations of the ADA and the NCRP, all practitioners should consult with their state's bureau of radiation control or safety to obtain information on current and applicable state laws.

PATIENT SELECTION

Professional judgment should be used to determine the type, frequency, and extent of each radiographic examination (patient selection). Diagnostic radiography should be used only after clinical examination and consideration of both the dental and general health needs of the patient.[23]

No question exists about the diagnostic utility of radiographs. In one study of 490 patients, 44% of carious teeth were found only by radiographic examination.[125] In spite of their usefulness, the potential exists for misapplication resulting in increased patient exposure. It has been reported[4] that in three out of four cases, orthodontists were confident in their diagnosis before evaluating any existing radiographic evidence. In some instances, less than 1% of all radiographs made have any

influence in patient care.[127] These reports may cast some doubt on the reliability of "professional judgment" as the sole criterion for patient selection. Realization of this prompted two national conferences[77,104] to conclude that a need exists for the development and implementation of more specific radiographic selection criteria to guide the practitioner's professional judgment. Such criteria could serve as more definitive guidelines for patient selection, which in turn might reduce the number of unproductive radiographic examinations and patient exposure to x-rays.

Radiographic selection criteria, also known as *high-yield* or *referral criteria*, are clinical or historical findings that identify patients for whom a high probability exists that a radiographic examination will provide information affecting their treatment or prognosis. The Dental Patient Selection Criteria Panel, established by the Center for Devices and Radiological Health of the Food and Drug Administration, was assigned the responsibility of formulating selection criteria for oral radiography[118] (see Chapter 13).When used in ordering radiographs for caries detection, these guidelines have been found to result in 43% fewer radiographs being made while missing what was felt to be an insignificant number of lesions (3.3%).[125] Additionally, when these guidelines were used, the number of missed intraosseous and other dental conditions was considered inconsequential, given the range of variability among clinicians in diagnosis and treatment.[126] In spite of these findings, a survey reported that only 37% of dentists chose to prescribe selectively according to the patient's needs.[10]

CONDUCT OF THE EXAMINATION

When the decision has been made that a radiographic examination is justified (patient selection), the way in which the examination is conducted greatly influences patient exposure to x-radiation. The conduct of the examination may be divided into choice of equipment, choice of technique, operation of equipment, and processing and interpretation of the radiographic image.

Choice of Equipment
The choice of equipment includes selection of the image receptor, focal spot-to-film distance, x-ray beam collimation, filtration, and the type of leaded apron and collar.

Receptor Selection. The ADA has taken the following position[23]:

The basis for selecting films, film-intensifying screen combinations and other image receptors should be to obtain the maximum sensitivity (speed) consistent with the image quality required for the diagnostic task.

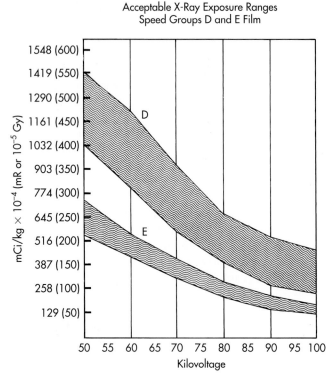

Acceptable X-Ray Exposure Ranges
Speed Groups D and E Film

FIG. 3-2 Relationship between surface exposures delivered to a patient by exposure of group D and group E intraoral films and diagnostic density at various kilovoltages. (From HHS Pub [FDA] 85-8245, 1985.)

Intraoral image receptors. In 1920, regular dental x-ray film was introduced by the Eastman Kodak Company. The images produced by this film were excellent for that time, but the speed was so slow that a radiograph of the maxillary molar area of an adult required 9 seconds of exposure.[89] Since that time, progressively faster films have been developed. Currently, intraoral dental x-ray film is available in two speed groups—D and E. Clinically, film of speed group E is almost twice as fast (sensitive) as film of group D and about 50 times as fast as regular dental x-ray film[91] (Fig. 3-2). In practice, this means that the 9-second exposure required for regular film in 1920 has been reduced to about 0.2 second with the use of E-speed film.

Faster films are desirable from the standpoint of exposure reduction. However, the possible decrease in image quality associated with increased speed, obtained in part by increasing the size or shape of silver halide crystals in the film's emulsion, must also be considered[27] (Table 3-4). If shorter exposure times are realized at the expense of image quality, it is not beneficial to use faster film. Shortly after the introduction of E-speed film (Ektaspeed, Eastman Kodak Company) in 1981,[97] studies were undertaken to compare film of speed group E with that of speed group D in terms of the diagnostic quality of the image. It was found that E-speed film had about the same useful density range, a greater latitude with slightly less contrast, and equal image quality as D-speed film if strict attention was paid to film handling and processing.[26,42,44,111] These and other studies of the compar-

TABLE **3-4**
Factors Affecting the Radiographic Quality of a Diagnostic Film

IMAGE FACTORS	CLARITY	IMAGE SIZE	SHAPE DISTORTION	FILM DENSITY	RADIOGRAPHIC CONTRAST
kVp*				X	X
mAs*	X			X	X
Collimation*		X		X	X
Filtration*				X	X
Focal spot size†	X	X			
Object-to-film distance†	X	X			
Focal spot-to-film distance†	X	X		X	
Motion	X	X			
Alignment‡			X		
Subject density§	X			X	X
Subject shape§	X			X	X
Film speed§	X			X	X
Developing time‖				X	X
Technique‡	X	X	X		
Screen speed§	X	X		X	X

*See Chapter 1
†See Chapter 5.
‡See Chapter 8.
§See Chapter 4.
‖See Chapter 6.

ative diagnostic value of D- and E-speed film suggested that the faster E film could be used in routine intraoral radiographic examinations without sacrifice of diagnostic information.*

In 1994 the Eastman Kodak Company introduced an improved E-speed film (Ektaspeed Plus), the emulsion of which was based on tabular grain technology similar to their T-Mat film. Ektaspeed Plus has been found to be faster and less sensitive to processing conditions, appear less grainy than Ektaspeed, and have a high contrast and exposure latitude similar to D-speed film.† Another speed group E film (M2 Comfort, Agfa-Gevaert, N.Y.) has been reported to be similar to Ektaspeed Plus for the detection of caries.[41] In spite of the reported benefits of using intraoral film of speed group E, 73% to 89% of dentists surveyed continue to use D-speed film.[9,63]

Patient dose reductions of 60% compared with E-speed film and 77% compared with D-speed film may be achieved using direct digital intraoral radiography. This significant reduction in patient dose must be balanced against the decreased image resolution associated with digital imaging. Radiographic film has the capability of resolving at least 20 line pairs per millimeter, whereas digital imaging at best can resolve only 11 (see Chapter 12, Digital Imaging).

Intensifying screens. Originally, intensifying screens used in extraoral radiography were made of crystals of calcium tungstate that emit blue light on interaction with x-rays (see Chapter 4). Calcium tungstate screens have been for the most part replaced by screens using the rare earth elements gadolinium and lanthanum. These rare earth phosphors emit green light on interaction with x-rays. When combined with green-sensitive films, these screens are as much as eight times more sensitive to x-rays than conventional intensifying screens using blue-sensitive film, without a significant loss of image quality.[39,52,107] The greater sensitivity or speed of the rare earth screen-film combinations results in a dramatic reduction in patient exposure. Compared with calcium tungstate screens, rare earth screens have been found to decrease patient exposure by as much as 55% in panoramic[39,98] and cephalometric[49] radiography.

A further reduction in patient exposure during extraoral radiography may be achieved with the use of T-grain film. Introduced as T-Mat by the Eastman Kodak Company in 1983, this film contains silver halide grains that are tabular or flat rather than pebblelike in shape. With their flat surface oriented toward the x-ray source, these grains present a greater cross section, which increases their ability to gather light from intensifying screens. T-grain film used with rare earth screens has been found to be twice as fast as calcium tungstate

screen-film combinations and one and a third times as fast as conventional rare earth screen-film combinations with no loss in image quality.[25,61,82,110]

Extraoral films have continued to be improved not only to decrease patient exposure but also to protect the environment. In 1990, Kodak introduced T-Mat/RA (Rapid Access) film, the emulsion of which was prehardened to allow for processing in chemistry that contains no hardener.[113] This improvement not only provided for processing times as short as 45 seconds but also made the processing chemistry environmentally safer by removing the glutaraldehyde hardener.

Extraoral films exposed by intensifying screens achieve a level of image resolution that is about half that of direct exposure intraoral film. One reason for image degradation in extraoral imaging systems is "crossover," which refers to the loss of image sharpness and resolution resulting from light emitted by one screen passing through the film to expose the emulsion on the opposite side of the double emulsion film.

The Ultra-Vision screen-film system (Du Pont) was designed to minimize this effect by using phosphors that emit ultraviolet light, which was found to be less able to pass through the film to expose the opposite emulsion. Results have shown that images produced by this system have higher resolution than corresponding rare earth screen-film systems. This allows for the use of a screen one speed class higher and a 50% reduction in patient exposure.[102] Kodak's recently introduced Ektavision system was also designed to prevent crossover, but its use has been reported to result in a slight increase in patient exposure compared with other, comparable rare earth screen-film combinations.[109]

Similar to digital intraoral imaging, digital panoramic imaging has been reported to result in an entry dose reduction of 70%. Image resolution with these systems appears to approach that obtained with rare earth regular-speed screens matched with T-Mat film (see Chapter 12, Digital Imaging).

Focal spot-to-film distance. The ADA states the following[22]:

> The combination of proper collimation and extended source-patient distance (focal spot-to-film distance) will reduce the amount of radiation to the patient.

Two standard focal spot–to-film distances (FSFDs) have evolved over the years for use in intraoral radiography, one 20 cm (8 inches) and the other 41 cm (16 inches). When the x-ray tube is operated above 50 kVp, each of these distances satisfies the federal regulation that the x-ray source–skin distance must not be less than 18 cm (7 inches) (assuming a 2.5-cm [1-inch] distance from the skin surface to the film).[16]

---

*References 33, 46, 51, 58, 128, 129.
†References 20, 54, 85, 108, 112.

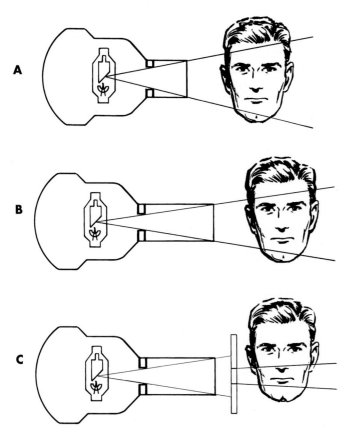

FIG. **3-3** *Effect of FSFD and collimation on the volume of tissue irradiated.* A larger volume of irradiated tissue results from **A** (with shorter FSFD) than from **B** (in which the longer FSFD produces a less divergent beam). In **C** the collimator between the round PID and the patient produces the effect of a rectangular PID on the tube housing or a rectangular collimating face shield on the film-holding instrument. This rectangular collimator (close to the patient in **C**) results in a smaller, less divergent beam and a smaller volume of tissue irradiated than in **A** or **B**.

Inasmuch as both distances comply with federal law, the decision as to which should be used may then be based on which FSFD results in less patient exposure and the best diagnostic image. One study of patient exposures from intraoral radiographic examinations[35] compared a 40-cm FSFD with a 20-cm FSFD in terms of organ doses. The results showed a 38% decrease in thyroid dose with the longer distance when 90 kVp x-rays were used and a 45% decrease with 70 kVp x-rays. These results occurred regardless of film speed used (i.e., D or E) and in spite of the fact that the intraoral examination using the 40-cm FSFD consisted of 21 films and the 20-cm FSFD examination consisted of only 18 films.

In addition to the decrease in thyroid dose obtained with the longer FSFD, use of the longer distance has been estimated to result in a 32% reduction in exposed tissue volume.[29] This is because at the greater distance, the x-ray beam is less divergent (Fig. 3-3). A reduction in

exposed tissue volume should be reflected in a reduction in the E. Recently a study reported a 30% decrease in the E resulting from the use of a 30-cm FSFD instead of a 20-cm FSFD for a simulated 19-film complete mouth survey using D-speed film.[15] The use of a longer FSFD also results in a smaller apparent focal spot size and thereby theoretically increases the resolution of the radiograph. (See Chapter 5.) The clinical significance of the effect of focal spot size on image resolution, however, has been questioned.[79]

Collimation. The ADA recommends the following[23]:

> The tissue area (and volume) exposed to the primary x-ray beam should not exceed the minimum coverage consistent with meeting diagnostic requirements and clinical feasibility. The collimation should comply with federal and state regulations. For periapical and bitewing radiography, restriction of the beam cross section to conform to the size of the image receptor (rectangular collimation) is recommended. Furthermore, shielded open-end position-indicating devices should be used.

The federal government requires[16] that the x-ray beam used in intraoral radiography be collimated so that the field of radiation at the patient's skin surface is "…containable in a circle having a diameter of no more than 7 cm (2¾ inches)…" when the x-ray tube is operated above 50 kVp. In view of the dimensions of no. 2 intraoral film (3.2 × 4.1 cm), a field size of this magnitude is almost three times that necessary to expose the film. Consequently, patient exposure may be significantly reduced by limiting the size of the x-ray beam even more than required by law. This results in not only decreased patient exposure but also increased image quality (see Table 3-4 and Fig. 3-3). Additionally, the amount of radiation scatter generated is proportional to the area exposed. If scatter radiation is decreased, film fog is decreased and image quality is increased.[130] Also, the reduction in beam size improves image definition (sharpness) by reducing the geometric phenomenon of penumbra. (See Chapter 5.)

Limitation of the size of the x-ray beam can be accomplished by one or a combination of several methods. First, a rectangular position-indicating device (PID) may be attached to the radiographic tube housing (Fig. 3-4). Use of a rectangular PID having an exit orifice of 3.5 × 4.4 cm (1.38 × 1.34 inches) reduces the area of the patient's skin surface exposed by 60% over that of a round (7 cm) PID (see Fig. 3-3, C). Depending on the FSFD, use of rectangular collimation may result in a 71% to 80% decrease in the E, a significant reduction.[15] This reduction in beam size, however, may make aiming the beam difficult. To avoid the possibility of unsatisfactory radiographs (cone cutting), a film-holding instrument that centers the beam over the film is recommended (Fig. 3-5).

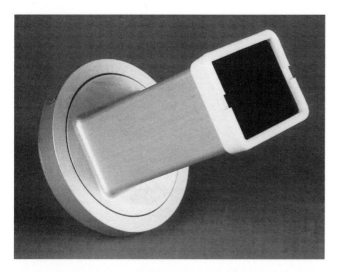

FIG. **3-4** A rectangular PID, which may be used to reduce the area of patient skin exposed. (Courtesy Dentsply/Rinn, Elgin, Ill.)

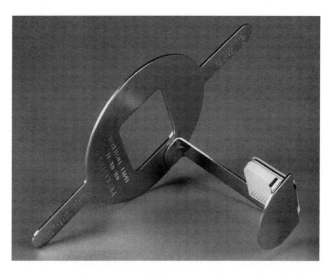

FIG. **3-6** *Precision film-holding instrument.* The face shield of the instrument absorbs radiation except for that required to expose the film. (Courtesy Masel Enterprises, Bristol, Penn.)

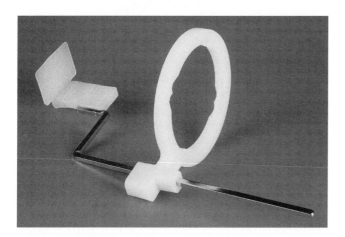

FIG. **3-5** Rinn XCP film-holding instrument. (Courtesy Dentsply/Rinn, Elgin, Ill.)

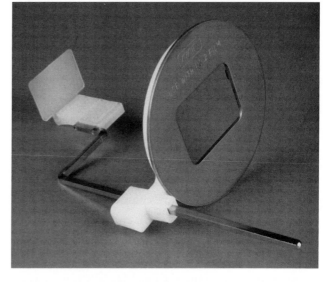

FIG. **3-7** *Rinn XCP instrument with a rectangular collimator clipped to the aiming ring.* As with the Precision instrument (Fig. 3-6), the collimator of this instrument absorbs radiation except for that required to expose the film. (Courtesy Dentsply/Rinn, Elgin, Ill.)

Second, film holders with rectangular collimators may be used with round PIDs (Fig. 3-6); they reduce patient exposure to the same degree as rectangular PIDs. In a study reviewing the *E* delivered during complete mouth examinations made with film holders using round and rectangular collimation,[124] rectangular collimation reduced the patient dose from intraoral examinations by about 60% (see Table 3-4). Both the Precision instrument (Masel Enterprises, Bristol, Penn.) and the XCP instrument (Dentsply/Rinn, Elgin, Ill.) with a rectangular collimator clipped to the aiming ring (Fig. 3-7) may be expected to produce similar results.

The benefits of rectangular collimation relative to image quality and patient exposure do not appear to be realized in clinical practice. Only 5% to 8% of dentists surveyed use rectangular collimation.[9,63]

Filtration. The ADA recommends the following[23]:

> Beam filtration should comply with federal and state regulations. The most judicious use of filtration involves selective filtration of excessively high-energy as well as excessively low-energy radiation.

The x-ray beam emitted from the radiographic tube consists of not only high-energy x-ray photons, but also many photons with relatively lower energy. (See Chapter 1.) Low-energy photons, which have little penetrating power, are absorbed mainly by the patient and contribute nothing to the information on the film. The purpose of conventional filtration is to remove these low-energy x-ray photons selectively from the x-ray beam. This results in decreased patient exposure with no loss of radiologic information (see Table 3-4).

The beneficial effect of filtration has been known for many years. When an x-ray beam is filtered with 3 mm of aluminum, the surface exposure is reduced to about 20% of that with no filtration.[114] In light of this and other information, the federal government has designated the specific amount of filtration required for dental x-ray machines operating at various kilovoltages. These quantities, expressed as beam quality (half-value layer [HVL]), are listed in Table 3-5. Compliance with these regulations by the dental profession was demonstrated in the results of the 1993 Nationwide Evaluation of X-Ray Trends (NEXT) study, which showed that the average calculated HVL was 2.3 mm aluminum, equivalent at an average kilovoltage of 73.[73]

Studies* have suggested that patient exposure may be reduced even further by removing both low- and high-energy x-ray photons from the beam, leaving the mid-range energy photons to expose the film. This suggestion resulted from the finding[90] that the x-ray energies most effective in producing the image are between 35 and 55 keV. Selective filtration of both low- and high-energy photons has been demonstrated with the rare earth elements samarium, erbium, yttrium, niobium, gadolinium, terbium-activated gadolinium oxysulfide (Lanex, Eastman Kodak), and thulium-activated lanthanum oxybromide (Quanta III, DuPont). The use of these materials in combination with aluminum filtration has reduced patient exposure by 20% to 80% compared with conventional aluminum filtration alone, which attenuates few high-energy photons. However, exposure reduction achieved with rare earth filtration is not without cost. Use of these filters requires a significant increase in exposure time (as much as 50%), increasing both x-ray tube loading and the possibility of patient movement during exposure. Additionally, depending on preference, image quality may suffer because of a decrease in contrast, sharpness, and resolution.[28,105,120,121]

Leaded aprons and collars. The ADA states the following[23]:

> Leaded aprons and collars should be used to minimize any unnecessary radiation.

The gonad dose resulting from oral radiography is minimal. (See "Gonad Dose," p. 48.) The philosophy of radiation protection currently in practice, however, is based on the principles of ALARA. This philosophy rec-

*References 33, 46, 51, 58, 128, 129.

TABLE **3-5** *Minumum Half-Value Layer*	
MEASURED X-RAY TUBE VOLTAGE	MINIMUM HALF-VALUE LAYER
(kVp)	(mm Al)
30 to 70	1.5
71	2.1
80	2.3
90	2.5
100	2.7

From Code of Federal Regulations 21, Subchapter J: *Radiological health, part 1000,* Washington, D.C., 1994, Office of the Federal Register, General Services Administration.

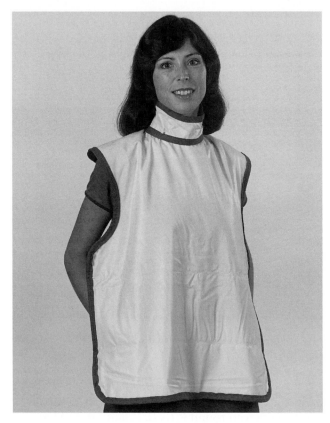

FIG. **3-8** Leaded apron with a thyroid collar attached. (Courtesy Ada Products, Milwaukee, Wisc.)

ognizes the possibility that, no matter how small the dose, some deleterious effect may result. Consequently, any dose that can be reduced without difficulty, great expense, or inconvenience should be reduced. Current data show that the mean exposure at skin entrance for a single dental periapical film is 217 mR. If the gonad dose is equal to $\frac{1}{10,000}$ of the total beam exposure,[88] the dose from one dental periapical film can be calculated to be 0.02 mR. No matter how small, this dose still represents a measurable quantity that is twice the negligible dose (see Table 3-2) and according to ALARA

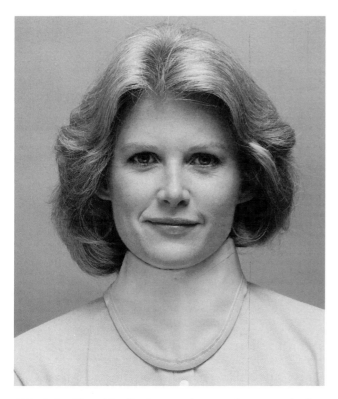

FIG. **3-9** Thyroid collar for use when one is not attached to the leaded apron. (Courtesy Ada Products, Milwaukee, Wisc.)

should be reduced if possible. A remedy for this is the use of a leaded apron, which may attenuate as much as 98% of the scatter radiation to the gonads.[7,45] Therefore with the use of either of these devices, the gonad dose from one dental periapical film can be calculated to be 0.4 μR. This quantity is more than 60 times less than the dose equivalent resulting from one airline flight. (See "Sources of Radiation Exposure," p. 43.)

Although these calculations and comparisons demonstrate that the gonad dose is quite small, no valid argument exists for not routinely using leaded aprons (Fig. 3-8). Indeed many states require their use in oral radiography. A similar argument can be made for thyroid shields, which have been found[96] to reduce the exposure of this gland by as much as 92% (Fig. 3-9). No difficulty, great expense, or inconvenience is encountered with their use; instead, using them demonstrates a real concern for the welfare of the patient.

This and other information regarding the dose to the fetus during oral radiographic procedures and NCRP recommendations concerning embryo-fetus exposure resulted in the decision by the Dental Patient Selection Criteria Panel to propose that oral radiographic examinations were not contraindicated because of pregnancy. However, the decision to use x-rays if the patient is pregnant is an individual one. The patient should be made aware of both the need for radiographs and the relative magnitude of exposure before any films are made.

CHOICE OF INTRAORAL TECHNIQUE

Practitioners should use receptor holders that position the image receptor to coincide with the collimation. They should not hold receptors in place for the patient.[23]

Currently no recommendations or regulations deal specifically with intraoral radiographic techniques. Consequently, the choice of technique (bisection of the angle or paralleling long cone) is left to the practitioner. Regardless of the technique chosen, a film holder should be used. A significant reduction in the number of unacceptable periapical films was found when film holders were used instead of patient manual support.[93]

The decision as to which technique is used should be based on the diagnostic quality of the resultant radiographs, the efficiency of using radiation, and the convenience of the technique (see Table 3-4). The more efficient the technique, the fewer radiograph retakes will be required, along with less patient exposure. A study of comparative efficiencies of the bisection and parallel techniques[6] found that the number of undiagnostic radiographs was reduced by more than half when intraoral complete mouth examinations were made with the parallel technique. If it is assumed that all undiagnostic radiographs are remade, use of the bisection technique leads to a significant increase in patient exposure. This study used the Rinn XCP instrument for parallel film placement (see Fig. 3-5), but similar reports on efficiency have appeared using the Precision instrument[123] (see Fig. 3-6). The Precision instrument with rectangular field collimation reduces patient exposure even more, although similar results might be obtained with the Rinn XCP instrument and a rectangular PID (see Figs. 3-4 and 3-5) or with a rectangular collimator clipped to the aiming ring (see Fig. 3-7). (See "Collimation," p. 54.)

Operating the Equipment
Operation of the x-ray generating equipment includes selection of the appropriate machine technique factors, kilovoltage, and milliampere-seconds.

Kilovoltage. The recommendation for selection of operating kilovoltage is stated in very general terms[23]:

A kilovoltage best suited to the diagnostic purpose should be used. Exposure should be established for optimal image quality.

This allows the practitioner to select either high (90) or low (70) kilovoltage, whichever is more suitable for the diagnostic purpose. Kilovoltage is the exposure factor that controls the energy of the x-ray beam. (See Chapter 1.) As the kilovoltage is decreased, the effective energy of the x-ray beam is decreased and radiographic image contrast increases (see Table 3-4). In theory, an image of high contrast should be better suited for visualizing large differences in density within an object such as caries or soft tissue calcifications.[99] However, the effect of kilovoltage on the accuracy of caries diagnosis has been reported to be negligible.[101] As the kilovoltage is increased, the effective energy of the x-ray beam is increased and radiographic image contrast decreases. An image of low contrast allows for the visualization of smaller differences in density within an object. This type of image contrast is more useful for periodontal diagnosis, where minute changes in bone must be detected.[29] High-kilovoltage techniques, which produce images of low contrast, also reduce the effective dose delivered per intraoral examination. It has been reported[35] that the effective dose resulting from the production of comparable-density radiographs was reduced by as much as 23% in one study, with an increase in kilovoltage from 70 to 90.

The introduction of a constant-potential (fully rectified) or high-frequency dental x-ray unit has made possible the production of diagnostic-quality radiographs with lower kilovoltage and at reduced levels of radiation.[100] The Intrex machine (Keystone X-Ray), which operated at 70 kVcp, was compared[60] with a conventional self-rectified x-ray unit also operating at 70 kVp. The surface exposure required to produce a comparable radiographic density was about 26% less for the constant-voltage Intrex unit. This finding results from the fact that the x-ray beam produced by the fully rectified Intrex machine has an equivalent photon energy approximately equal to that produced by a self-rectified unit operated at about 80 kVp.[32] Currently several other manu-facturers produce high-frequency dental x-ray units.

Milliampere-seconds. Of the three technical conditions (tube voltage, filtration, and exposure time), exposure time has been shown to be the most crucial factor in influencing diagnostic quality.[3] In terms of exposure, optimal image quality means that the radiograph is of diagnostic density, neither overexposed (too dark) nor underexposed (too light). Both overexposed and underexposed radiographs result in needless patient exposure. Image density is controlled by the quantity of x-rays produced, which in turn is best controlled by the combination of milliamperage and exposure time, termed *milliampere-seconds (mAs)* (see Table 3-4 and Chapter 1).

Diagnostic density is, for the most part, a matter of personal preference subject to certain guidelines. Patient exposure is directly related to mAs. Table 3-6 lists average mAs values needed to expose an intraoral film to proper density. In general a radiograph of correct density should demonstrate very faint soft tissue outlines.[29] This should correspond to an optical density of about 1.0 in enamel and dentin.[101] Such a degree of image density can be obtained by using values within the ranges listed, after considering the age and physical stature of the patient. For example, 2.2 mAs is suggested for an average adult when E-speed film and an operating kilovoltage of 90 are used. This value may be arrived at by using a milliamperage of 10 and an exposure time of 0.22 second (13 impulses). If the kilovoltage is increased to reduce image contrast, the mAs must be decreased or the radiograph will be overexposed.

Phototiming is routinely employed in some medical radiographic procedures.[14] This technique uses a phototimer to measure the quantity of radiation reaching the film and automatically terminates the exposure when enough radiation has reached the film to provide the required density. This technology is currently available with some panoramic machines; the availability of very small photodiodes has made feasible this type of automatic exposure control in intraoral radiography.[119]

PROCESSING THE FILM

A good darkroom and proper darkroom practices are important parts of performing diagnostic radiography.[24]

A major cause of unnecessary exposure of the patient to radiation is the deliberate overexposure of films. Overexposure is compensated for by underdevelopment of the film.[1] Not only does this procedure result in needless overexposure of the patient but it also (because of incomplete development) results in films that are of inferior diagnostic quality. On the other hand, a properly exposed radiograph is of no value if all its diagnostic information is lost as a result of poor processing procedures (see Table 3-4). A study by one dental insurance carrier[8] reported that some 6% of the dental radiographs it received were not readable because of improper processing. Another study of 500 panoramic radiographs[11] found that the average film contained at least one processing error. Time-temperature processing, in an adequately equipped and maintained darkroom, is the best way to ensure optimal film quality. (See Chapter 6.)

The use of machines to process dental x-ray film has become widespread. As many as 93% of dentists surveyed have reported using dental film processors.[9] Film processors, however, can actually increase patient exposure if not correctly maintained. One study[37] has shown that 30% of all retakes because of incorrect film density were directly related to processor variability. The introduction of a comprehensive maintenance program was found to reduce this retake rate significantly, resulting in a substantial savings in both patient exposure and operating costs.

TABLE 3-6

Milliampere-Seconds Required to Expose Speed Group D and E Intraoral Radiographic Film to Diagnostic Density at a Focal Spot to film Distance (FSFD) of 16 Inches

| OPERATING KILOVOLTAGE* | MILLIAMPERE-SECONDS† | | | | | |
| | D | | | E | | |
	LOW	HIGH	MEAN	LOW	HIGH	MEAN
70	6.7	10.9	8.8	3.6	4.8	4.2
90	3.1	6.0	4.6	1.7	2.6	2.2

*Using a half wave–rectified x-ray machine with minimal HVL, as shown in Table 3-5.
†For an 8-inch FSFD, divide by 4.

Interpretation of the Image

The maximal diagnostic information can be obtained from a radiograph only if it is viewed with even backlighting[23]:

> Radiographic images should be viewed under proper conditions with an illuminated viewer or transparent images to obtain maximum available information.

Radiographs are best viewed in a semidarkened room with light transmitted only through the films; all extraneous light should be eliminated. In addition, radiographs should be studied with the aid of a magnifying glass to detect even the smallest change in image density. A variable-intensity light source should also be available. This may compensate for overexposed or underexposed radiographs or radiographs with processing artifacts. Many radiographs can be "saved" in this way, precluding the necessity of remaking the film and subjecting the patient to additional radiation exposure.

At the beginning of this section it was stated that optimizing the radiologic process is the best way to ensure maximal patient benefit with minimal patient and operator exposure. Although the importance of this cannot be overemphasized, in spite of everything that can be done to optimize the radiologic process, the diagnostic accuracy of radiographic caries diagnosis is only 70%.[101] This fact should stimulate individuals to place a greater emphasis on accurate radiographic interpretation. Currently, failure to diagnose problems is an increasing source of liability claims.[62]

PROTECTION OF PERSONNEL

> Unless protective shielding is provided for the operator, the installation should be so arranged so that the operator can stand at least six feet from the patient during exposure.[23]

The methods of dose reduction discussed thus far have emphasized their effect on patient exposure. It should be apparent, however, that any procedure or technique that reduces radiation exposure to the patient also reduces the possibility of operator or office personnel exposure. In addition to those mentioned, several other steps can be taken to reduce the chance of occupational exposure.

Perhaps the single most effective way of limiting occupational exposure is the establishment of radiation safety procedures that are understood and followed by all personnel. Such written procedures are currently mandated by several states.[76,106] The procedures described below are based on a number of important facts concerning x-rays:

- They travel in straight lines from their source.
- The intensity of the radiation beam diminishes fairly rapidly as the distance from the source increases (inverse square law).
- They can be scattered or deflected in their path of travel.

First, every effort should be made so that the operator can leave the room or take a position behind a suitable barrier or wall during exposure of the film. Dental operatories should be designed and constructed to meet the minimal shielding requirement of the NCRP.[65] This recommendation states that walls must be of sufficient density or thickness that the exposure to nonoccupationally exposed individuals (e.g., someone occupying an adjacent office) is no greater than 10 mR per week. In most instances, it is not necessary to line the walls with lead to meet this requirement. Walls constructed of gypsum wallboard (drywall) have been found to be adequate for the average dental office.[56,87] The following factors are considered in calculating specific barrier thicknesses required: (1) workload, an expression of the amount of radiation emitted at a given kilovoltage in milliamperes per week; (2) use, the fraction of time an x-ray beam is directed toward the barrier; (3) occupancy,

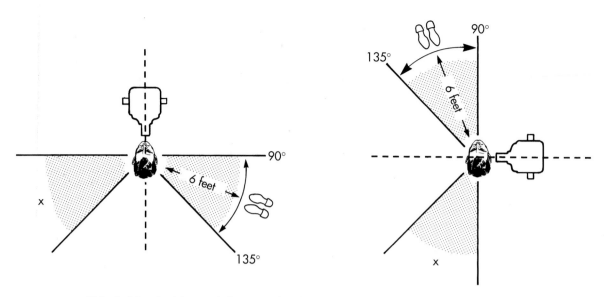

FIG. **3-10** *Position-and-distance rule.* If no barrier is available, the operator should stand at least 6 feet from the patient, at an angle of 90 to 135 degrees to the central ray of the x-ray beam when the exposure is made.

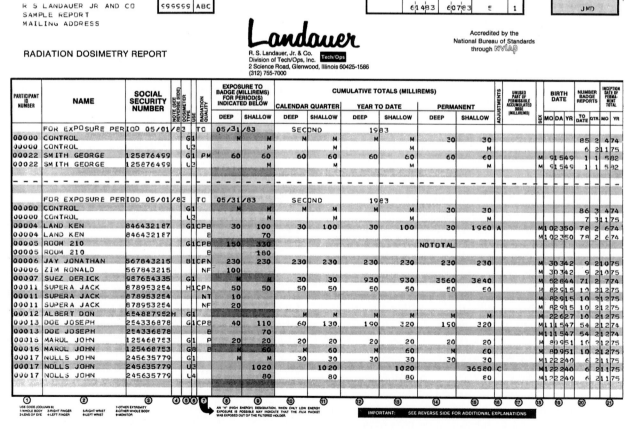

FIG. **3-11** Sample radiation dosimetry report showing that George Smith received an exposure of 0.60 mSv (60 mrem) during the month reported. The report also shows totals for the calendar quarter, year to date, and permanent or lifetime exposure. (Courtesy RS Landauer Jr & Co.)

an estimation of the amount of time the area behind the barrier is occupied; and (4) maximum permissible *E.* Examples of the way these parameters are used in calculating required barrier thickness can be found in NCRP Report 35.[65]

If leaving the room or making use of some other barrier is impossible, strict adherence to what has been termed the *position-and-distance rule* is required:[84] the operator should stand at least 6 feet from the patient, at an angle of 90 to 135 degrees to the central ray of the x-ray beam (Fig. 3-10). When applied, this rule not only takes advantage of the inverse square law to reduce x-ray intensity but also considers that in this position most scatter radiation is absorbed by the patient's head. All practitioners should check their state's regulations for use of ionizing radiation regarding operator position during x-ray exposures. At least one state (New Mexico) requires that the operator leave the room during the exposure.[76] Thus the position-and-distance rule is in violation of that state's regulations.

Second, the operator should never hold films in place.[65] Ideally, film-holding instruments should be used. (See "Collimation," p. 54.) If correct film placement and retention are still not possible, a parent or other individual responsible for the patient should be asked to hold the film in place and, of course, be afforded adequate protection with a leaded apron. Under no circumstances should this person be one of the office staff.

Third, the radiographic tube housing should never be stabilized by the operator or patient during the exposure.[65] Suspension arms should be adequately maintained to prevent housing movement and drift.

The best way to ensure that personnel are following office safety rules such as those described previously is with personnel-monitoring devices. Commonly referred to as *film badges,* they provide a useful record of occupational exposure. Their use is not only recommended but also required by law in certain states. Several companies in the United States offer a film badge service. For a reasonable charge, they provide badges that contain either a piece of sensitive film or a radiosensitive crystal (thermoluminescent dosimeter) and a printed report of accumulated exposure at regular intervals (Fig. 3-11). These reports indicate any undesirable change in work habits and help remove any apprehension office staff members may have about the possibility of exposure to x-rays.

QUALITY ASSURANCE

A quality assurance program should be established to ensure high-quality radiographic images.[23]

Quality assurance may be defined as "any systematic action to ensure that a dental office will produce consistently high-quality images with minimal exposure to pa-

tients and personnel."[57] Studies have indicated that dentists may be needlessly exposing their patients to compensate for improper exposure techniques, film processing practices, and darkroom procedures. One study reported that only 33% of panoramic radiographs that accompanied biopsy specimens were of acceptable diagnostic quality.[92] However, when demands are placed on dentists to improve their techniques, the number of unsatisfactory radiographs is significantly reduced. Two studies by a dental insurance carrier demonstrated that after claims were rejected for unsatisfactory radiographs and the dentist was made aware of the errors and ways in which they could be corrected, the number of satisfactory radiographs submitted doubled.[8] This suggests that when the dentist is presented with guidelines for quality assurance, along with proper motivation, patient exposure can be dramatically reduced.

Currently some states require dental offices to establish written guidelines for quality assurance and maintain written records of quality assurance tests.[76,106] Regardless, each dental office should establish maintenance and monitoring procedures as outlined in Box 3-1 according to the NCRP.[71] The frequency of

---

BOX 3-1
Guide for Establishing Maintenance and Quality Control Procedures

Following should be inspected at suitable intervals:
X-ray unit
  Leakage radiation
  Verification of FSFD
  Stability of radiographic tube housing
  X-ray beam
    Alignment
    Collimation
    Quality
  Timer accuracy
  Integrity of exposure switch
Darkroom
  Light leaks
  Adequacy of safe lighting
  Cleanliness
Ancillary equipment
  Leaded aprons and collars
  The brightness and color of view boxes
Procedures should be established for the following:
  Use of a reference film
  Proper handling and storage of film, cassettes, screens, grids, and chemicals
  X-ray exposure factors (posted by control console)
  Film processing techniques (posted in darkroom)
  Maintenance of processing systems

From National Council on Radiation Protection and Measurements: *NCRP Report 99*(1990), Washington, D.C., NCRP Publications.

these inspections varies according to state regulations and manufacturers' directions.

CONTINUING EDUCATION

Practitioners should stay informed of new developments in equipment, materials and techniques and adopt appropriate items to improve radiographic practices.[23]

Those who administer ionizing radiation must become familiar with the magnitude of exposure encountered in medicine, dentistry, and everyday life; the possible risks associated with such exposure; and the methods used to effect exposure and dose reduction. Although this chapter presents some of this information, acquiring knowledge and developing and maintaining skills is an ongoing process.

REFERENCES

1. Alcox RW: Biological effects and radiation protection in the dental office, *Dent Clin North Am* 22:517, 1978.
2. Arena V: *Ionizing radiation and life,* St Louis, 1971, Mosby.
3. Arnold LV: The radiographic detection of initial carious lesions on the proximal surfaces of teeth. I. The influence of exposure conditions, *Oral Surg* 64:221, 1987.
4. Atchison KA, Luke LS, White SC: Contribution of pretreatment radiographs to orthodontist's decision making, *Oral Surg* 71:238, 1991.
5. Avendanio B et al: Effective dose and risk assessment from detailed narrow beam radiography, *Oral Surg Oral Med Oral Pathol Oral Radiol Endod* 82:713, 1996.
6. Bean LR: Comparison of bisecting angle and paralleling methods of intraoral radiology, *J Dent Educ* 33:441, 1969.
7. Bean LR, Devore WD: The effect of protective aprons in dental roentgenography, *Oral Surg* 28:505, 1969.
8. Beideman RW, Pettigrew JC, Green PH: A follow-up study of a third-party radiographic evaluation system, *Oral Surg* 56:103, 1983.
9. Bohay RN, Kogon SL, Stephens RG: A survey of radiographic techniques and equipment used by a sample of general dental practitioners, *Oral Surg Oral Med Oral Pathol* 78:806, 1994.
10. Bohay RN, Stephens RG, Kogon SL: Survey of radiographic practices of general dentists for the dentate adult patient, *Oral Surg Oral Med Oral Pathol Oral Radiol Endod* 79:526, 1995.
11. Brezden NA, Brooks SL: Evaluation of panoramic dental radiographs taken in private practice, *Oral Surg* 63:617, 1987.
12. Broadway JA et al: Estimates of radiation dose and health risks to the United States population following the Chernobyl nuclear plant accident, *Health Phys* 55:533, 1988.
13. Brown RF, Shaver JW, Lamel DA: *The selection of patients for x-ray examinations,* DHEW Publ (FDA) 808104, 1980.
14. Bushong SC: *Radiologic science for technologists: physics, biology, and protection,* ed 5, St Louis, 1993, Mosby.
15. Cederberg RA et al: Effect of the geometry of the intraoral position-indicating device on effective dose, *Oral Surg Oral Med Oral Pathol Oral Radiol Endod* 84:101, 1997.
16. Code of Federal Regulations 21, Subchapter J: *Radiological health,* part 1000, Washington, D.C., 1994, Office of the Federal Register, General Services Administration.
17. Cohen BS, Eisenbud M, Harley NH: Measurement of the alpha-radioactivity on the mucosal surface of the human bronchial tree, *Health Phys* 39:619, 1980.
18. Committee on the Biological Effects of Ionizing Radiations: *The effects on populations of exposure to low levels of ionizing radiation,* Washington, D.C., 1980, National Academy Press.
19. Committee on the Biological Effects of Ionizing Radiations: *Health effects of exposure to low levels of ionizing radiation. BEIR V,* Washington, D.C., 1990, National Academy Press.
20. Conover GL, Hildebolt CF, Anthony D: Objective and subjective evaluations of Kodak Ektaspeed Plus dental x-ray film, *Oral Surg Oral Med Oral Pathol Oral Radiol Endod* 79:246, 1995.
21. Council on Dental Materials and Devices: Recommendations in radiographic practices: March 1978, *J Am Dent Assoc* 96:485, 1978.
22. Council on Dental Materials, Instruments, and Equipment: Recommendations on radiographic practices, 1984, *J Am Dent Assoc* 109:764, 1984.
23. Council on Dental Materials, Instruments, and Equipment: Recommendations on radiographic practices: an update, 1988, *J Am Dent Assoc* 118:115, 1989.
24. Council on Dental Materials, Instruments, and Equipment: Recommendations for radiographic darkrooms and darkroom practices, *J Am Dent Assoc* 104:886, 1982.
25. D'Ambrosio JA et al: Diagnostic quality versus patient exposure with five panoramic screen-film combinations, *Oral Surg* 61:409, 1986.
26. Diehl R, Gratt BM, Gould RG: Radiographic quality control measurements comparing D-speed film, E-speed film, and xeroradiography, *Oral Surg* 61:635, 1986.
27. Domon M, Yoshino N: Factors involved in the high radiographic sensitivity of E-speed films, *Oral Surg* 69:123, 1990.
28. Farman AG et al: Evaluation of aluminum-yttrium filtration for intraoral radiography, *Oral Surg* 67:244, 1989.
29. Frederiksen NL: The radiograph in the diagnosis of periodontal disease: a quality assurance program, *Technology Assessment Forum on Dental Radiology,* FDA/BRH 82:107, 1982.
30. Frederiksen NL, Benson BW, Sokolowski TW: Effective dose and risk assessment from computed tomography of the maxillofacial complex, *Dentomaxillofac Radiol* 24:55, 1995.
31. Frederiksen NL, Benson BW, Sokolowski TW: Effective dose and risk assessment from film tomography used for dental implant diagnostics, *Dentomaxillofac Radiol* 23:123, 1994.

32. Frederiksen NL, Goaz PW: Parameters affecting radiographic contrast, *Dentomaxillofac Radiol* 19:173, 1990.

33. Frommer HH, Jain RK: A comparative clinical study of group D and E dental film, *Oral Surg* 63:738, 1987.

34. Gelskey DE, Baker CG: Energy-selective filtration of dental x-ray beams, *Oral Surg* 52:565, 1981.

35. Gibbs SJ et al: Patient risk from intraoral dental radiography, *Dentomaxillofac Radiol* 17:15, 1988.

36. Gibbs SJ et al: Patient risk from rotational panoramic radiography, *Dentomaxillofac Radiol* 17:25, 1988.

37. Goldman L et al: Automatic processing quality assurance program: impact on a radiology department, *Radiology* 125:591, 1977.

38. *Gonad doses and genetically significant dose from diagnostic radiology: U.S., 1964 and 1970*, DHEW Publ (FDA) 76-8034, Washington, D.C., 1976.

39. Gratt BM et al: An evaluation of rare-earth imaging systems in panoramic radiography, *Oral Surg* 58:475, 1984.

40. Hatch MC et al: Cancer rates after the Three Mile Island nuclear accident and proximity of residence to the plant, *Am J Public Health* 81:719, 1991.

41. Hintze H, Christoffersen L, Wenzel A: In vitro comparison of Kodak Ultra-speed, Ektaspeed, and Ektaspeed Plus, and Agfa M2 Comfort dental x-ray films for the detection of caries, *Oral Surg Oral Med Oral Pathol Oral Radiol Endod* 81:240, 1996.

42. Horton PS et al: A clinical comparison of speed groups D and E dental x-ray films, *Oral Surg* 58:104, 1984.

43. International Commission on Radiological Protection: *Radiation protection*, ICRP Publ. 60, Oxford, England, 1990.

44. Kaffe I, Littner MM, Kuspet ME: Densitometric evaluation of intraoral x-ray films: Ektaspeed versus Ultraspeed, *Oral Surg* 57:338, 1984.

45. Kaffe I et al: Efficiency of the cervical lead shield during intraoral radiography, *Oral Surg* 62:732, 1986.

46. Kantor ML, Reisken AB, Lurie AG: A clinical comparison of x-ray films for detection of proximal surface caries, *J Am Dent Assoc* 111:967, 1985.

47. Kapa SF, Tyndall DA: A clinical comparison of image quality and patient exposure reduction in panoramic radiography with heavy metal filtration, *Oral Surg* 67:750, 1989.

48. Kapa SF, Tyndall DA, Ouellette TE: The application of added beam filtration to intra-oral radiography, *Dentomaxillofac Radiol* 19:67, 1990.

49. Kaugars GE, Fatouros P: Clinical comparison of conventional and rare-earth screen-film systems for cephalometric radiographs, *Oral Surg* 53:322, 1982.

50. Kircos LT, Staninec M, Chou L: Rare earth filters for intraoral radiography: exposure reduction as a function of kV(p) with comparisons of image quality, *J Am Dent Assoc* 118:605, 1989.

51. Kleier DJ, Hicks MJ, Flaitz CM: A comparison of Ultraspeed and Ektaspeed dental x-ray film: in vitro study of the radiographic appearance of interproximal lesions, *Oral Surg* 63:381, 1987.

52. *Kodak film screen combinations*, Publication M3-138, Rochester, N.Y., 1983, Eastman Kodak.

53. Little JB et al: Distribution of polonium 210 in pulmonary tissues of cigarette smokers, *N Engl J Med* 273:1343, 1965.

54. Ludlow JB, Platin E: Densitometric comparisons of Ultraspeed, Ektaspeed, and Ektaspeed Plus intraoral films for two processing conditions, *Oral Surg Oral Med Oral Pathol Oral Radiol Endod* 79:105, 1995.

55. Lushbaugh CC, Fry SA, Ricks RC: Medical and radiobiological basis of radiation accident management, *Br J Radiol* 60:1159, 1987.

56. MacDonald JCF, Reid JA, Berthoty D: Drywall construction as a dental radiation barrier, *Oral Surg* 55:319, 1983.

57. Manny EF et al: *An overview of dental radiology*, Washington, D.C., 1980, National Center for Health Care Technology (FDA/BRH).

58. Matteson SR et al: The effect of lesion size, restorative material, and film speed on the detection of recurrent caries, *Oral Surg* 68:232, 1989.

59. Mauriello SM et al: Clinical evaluation of a samarium/aluminum compound filter, *Oral Surg* 68:108, 1989.

60. McDavid WD et al: The Intrex: a constant-potential x-ray unit for periapical dental radiography, *Oral Surg* 53:433, 1982.

61. Miles DA, Van Dis ML, Peterson MGE: Information yield: a comparison of Kodak T-Mat G, Ortho L and RP X-Omat films, *Dentomaxillofac Radiol* 18:15, 1989.

62. Milgrom P, Getz T: Current therapy. Radiographic recommendations for transitional dentition, *Dental Claims and Insurance News* 9:1, 1995.

63. Nakfoor CA, Brooks SL: Compliance of Michigan dentists with radiographic safety recommendations, *Oral Surg Oral Med Oral Pathol* 73:510, 1992.

64. National Council on Radiation Protection and Measurements: *Control of radon in houses*, NCRP Report 103, 1989.

65. National Council on Radiation Protection and Measurements: *Dental x-ray protection*, NCRP Report 35, 1970.

66. National Council on Radiation Protection and Measurements: *Exposure of the population in the United States and Canada from natural background radiation*, NCRP Report 94, 1987.

67. National Council on Radiation Protection and Measurements: *Exposure of the U.S. population from diagnostic medical radiation*, NCRP Report 100, 1989.

68. National Council on Radiation Protection and Measurements: *Exposure of the U.S. population from occupational radiation*, NCRP Report 101, 1989.

69. National Council on Radiation Protection and Measurements: *Ionizing radiation exposure of the population of the United States*, NCRP Report 93, 1987.

70. National Council on Radiation Protection and Measurements: *Limitation of exposure to ionizing radiation*, NCRP Report 116, 1993.

71. National Council on Radiation Protection and Measurements: *Quality assurance for diagnostic imaging*, NCRP Report 99, 1990.

72. National Council on Radiation Protection and Measurements: *Radiation exposure of the U.S. population from consumer products and miscellaneous sources*, NCRP Report 95, 1987.

73. Nationwide Evaluation of X-Ray Trends (NEXT): *1993 Dental x-ray data*, HHS Publication (FDA), Washington, D.C., 1993.

74. Nationwide Evaluation of X-Ray Trends (NEXT): *Tabulations: representative sample data, January 1, 1983 to December 31, 1983*, HHS Publication (FDA), 1984.

75. *NCI releases results of nationwide study of radioactive fallout from nuclear tests*, press release, August 1, 1997. http://rex.nci.nih.gov.

76. New Mexico Health and Environment Department, Environmental Improvement Division: *Radiation protection regulations*, Santa Fe, 1989, The Department.

77. Nowak AJ et al: Summary of the Conference on Radiation Exposure in Pediatric Dentistry, *J Am Dent Assoc* 103:426, 1981.

78. Parker SL et al: Cancer statistics, 1997, *CA Cancer J Clin* 47:5, 1997.

79. Platin E, Mauriello S, Ludlow JB: Effects of focal spot size on caries diagnosis with D and E speed images, *Oral Surg Oral Med Oral Pathol Oral Radiol Endod* 81:235, 1996.

80. Ponce AZ, McDavid WD, Langland OE: The use of added erbium filtration in intraoral radiography, *Oral Surg* 66:513, 1988.

81. Ponce AZ et al: Adaptation of the Panorex II for use with rare earth screen-film combinations, *Oral Surg* 61:645, 1986.

82. Ponce AZ et al: Kodak T-Mat G film in rotational panoramic radiography, *Oral Surg* 61:649, 1986.

83. Ponce AZ et al: Use of E-speed film with added filtration, *Oral Surg* 61:297, 1986.

84. Preece JW, Morris CR: *The efficient and effective use of x-radiation in the dental office*. III. Office assessment GP Texas Acad Gen Dent Pub 6:1, 1980.

85. Price C: Sensitometric evaluation of a new E-speed dental radiographic film, *Dentomaxillofac Radiol* 24:30, 1995.

86. Price C, McDonnell D: Effects of niobium filtration and constant potential on the sensitometric responses of dental radiographic films, *Dentomaxillofac Radiol* 20:11, 1991.

87. Reid JA, MacDonald JDF: Use and workload factors in dental radiation: protection design, *Oral Surg* 57:219, 1984.

88. Richards AG: Roentgen-ray doses in dental radiography, *J Am Dent Assoc* 56:351, 1958.

89. Richards AG: Trends in dental radiography, *Oral Surg* 44:807, 1977.

90. Richards AG et al: Samarium filters for dental radiography, *Oral Surg* 29:704, 1970.

91. Richards AG, Colquitt WN: Reduction in dental x-ray exposures during the past 60 years, *J Am Dent Assoc* 103:713, 1981.

92. Rumberg H, Hollender L, Oda D: Assessing the quality of radiographs accompanying biopsy specimens, *J Am Dent Assoc* 127:363, 1996.

93. Rushton VE, Horner K: A comparative study of radiographic quality with five periapical techniques in general practice, *Dentomaxillofac Radiol* 23:37, 1994.

94. Ruter FG et al: Assessment of skin entrance KERMA in the United States: The Nationwide Evaluation of x-ray Trends (NEXT), *Radiation Protection Dosimetry* 43:71, 1992.

95. Scaf G et al: Dosimetry and cost of imaging osseointegrated implants with film-based and computed tomography, *Oral Surg Oral Med Oral Pathol Oral Radiol Endod* 83:41, 1997.

96. Sikorski PA, Taylor KW: The effectiveness of the thyroid shield in dental radiology, *Oral Surg* 58:225, 1984.

97. Silha RE: The new Kodak Ektaspeed dental x-ray film, *Dent Radiogr Photogr* 54:32, 1981.

98. Skoczylas LJ et al: Comparison of x-radiation doses between conventional and rare earth panoramic radiographic techniques, *Oral Surg* 68:776, 1989.

99. Svenson B et al: Accuracy of radiographic caries diagnosis at different kilovoltages and two film speeds, *Swed Dent J* 9:37, 1985.

100. Svenson B, Petersson A: Accuracy of radiographic caries diagnosis using different x-ray generators, *Dentomaxillofac Radiol* 18:68, 1989.

101. Svenson B et al: Exposure parameters and their effects on diagnostic accuracy, *Oral Surg Oral Med Oral Pathol* 78:544, 1994.

102. Sewerin I: Clinical testing of the Ultra-Vision screen-film system for maxillofacial radiography, *Oral Surg Oral Med Oral Pathol* 77:302, 1994.

103. Tanimoto K et al: A filter for use in lateral cephalography, *Oral Surg* 68:666, 1989.

104. Technology Assessment Forum on Dental Radiology, op. cit. reference 29.

105. Tetradis S et al: Niobium filtration of conventional and high-frequency x-ray generator beams for intraoral radiography. Effects on absorbed doses, image density and contrast, and photon spectra, *Oral Surg Oral Med Oral Pathol Oral Radiol Endod* 80:232, 1995.

106. Texas Department of Health, Division of Occupational Health and Radiation Control: *Texas regulations for control of radiation*, Austin, 1989, The Department.

107. Thunthy KH, Boozer CH, Weinberg R: Sensitometric evaluation of rare earth intensifying screen systems, *Oral Surg* 59:102, 1985.

108. Thunthy KH, Weinberg R: Effects of developer exhaustion on Kodak Ektaspeed Plus, Ektaspeed, and Ultra-speed dental films, *Oral Surg Oral Med Oral Pathol Oral Radiol Endod* 79:117, 1995.

109. Thunthy KH, Weinberg R: Film screen systems. Sensitometric comparison of Kodak Ektavision system to Kodak T-Maty/RA system, *Oral Surg Oral Med Oral Pathol Oral Radiol Endod* 83:288, 1997.

110. Thunthy KH, Weinberg R: Sensitometric and image analysis of T-grain film, *Oral Surg* 62:218, 1986.

111. Thunthy KH, Weinberg R: Sensitometric comparison of dental films of groups D and E, *Oral Surg* 54:250, 1982.

112. Thunthy KH, Weinberg R: Sensitometric comparison of Kodak Ektaspeed Plus, Ektaspeed, and Ultra-Speed dental films, *Oral Surg Oral Med Oral Pathol Oral Radiol Endod* 79:114, 1995.

113. Thunthy KH, Yeadon WR, Weinberg R: Sensitometric and archival evaluation of Kodak RA films in dental automatic processing, *Oral Surg Oral Med Oral Pathol* 77:427, 1994.

114. Trout ED, Kelley JP, Cathey GA: The use of filters to control radiation exposure to the patient in diagnostic radiology, *AJR* 67:946, 1952.

115. TSDR, *Case studies in environmental medicine. 34.* Ionizing radiation. Washington, D.C., 1993, U.S. Department of Health and Human Services, Public Health Service.

116. Tyndall DA: Spectroscopic analysis and dosimetry of diagnostic x-ray beams filtered by rare earth materials, *Oral Surg* 62:205, 1986.

117. Tyndall DA, Washburn DB: The effect of rare earth filtration on patient exposure, dose reduction, and image quality in oral panoramic radiology, *Health Phys* 52:1726, 1987.

118. U.S. Department of Health and Human Services, FDA: *Guidelines for prescribing dental radiographs*, Rockville, Md., 1987, HHS Publication FDA 88-8273.

119. van Lujik JA, Sanderink GCH: Application of a photodiode in dental radiology, *Oral Surg* 62:110, 1986.

120. Wakoh M et al: Diagnostic image quality and dose reduction using niobium filtration for cephalometric radiography, *Dentomaxillofac Radiol* 22:189, 1993.

121. Wakoh M et al: Quantitative assessment of image quality using niobium filtration for cephalometric radiography, *Dentomaxillofac Radiol* 23:73, 1994.

122. Wall BF, Kendall GM: Collective doses and risks from dental radiology in Great Britain, *Br J Radiol* 56:511, 1983.

123. Weissman DD, Longhurst GE: Clinical evaluation of a rectangular field collimating device for periapical radiography, *J Am Dent Assoc* 82:580, 1971.

124. White SC: 1992 Assessment of radiation risks from dental radiography, *Dentomaxillofac Radiol* 21:118, 1992.

125. White SC et al: Efficacy of FDA guidelines for ordering radiographs for caries detection, *Oral Surg Oral Med Oral Pathol* 77:531, 1994.

126. White SC et al: Efficacy of FDA guidelines for prescribing radiographs to detect dental and intraosseous conditions, *Oral Surg Oral Med Oral Pathol Oral Radiol Endod* 80:108, 1995.

127. White SC, Forsythe AB, Joseph LP: Patient-selection criteria for panoramic radiography, *Oral Surg* 57:681, 1984.

128. White SC, Hollender L, Gratt BM: Comparison of xeroradiographs and film for detection of calculus, *Dentomaxillofac Radiol* 13:39, 1984.

129. White SC, Hollender L, Gratt BM: Comparison of xeroradiographs and film for detection of proximal surface caries, *J Am Dent Assoc* 108:755, 1984.

130. Winkler KG: Influence of rectangular collimation on intraoral shielding of radiation dose in dental radiography, *J Am Dent Assoc* 77:95, 1968.

Imaging Principles and Techniques

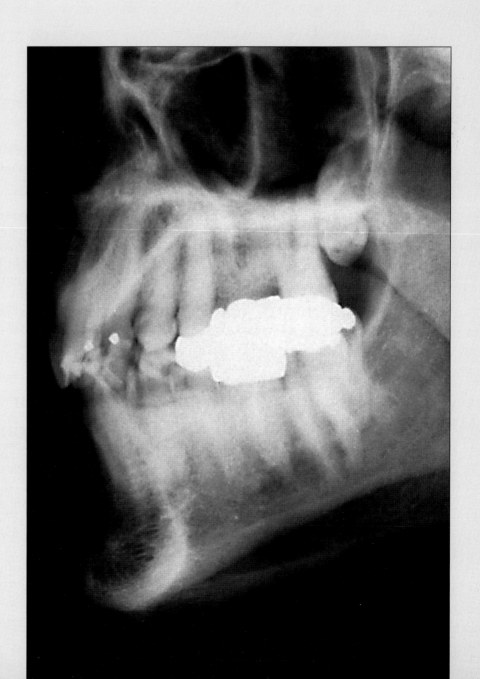

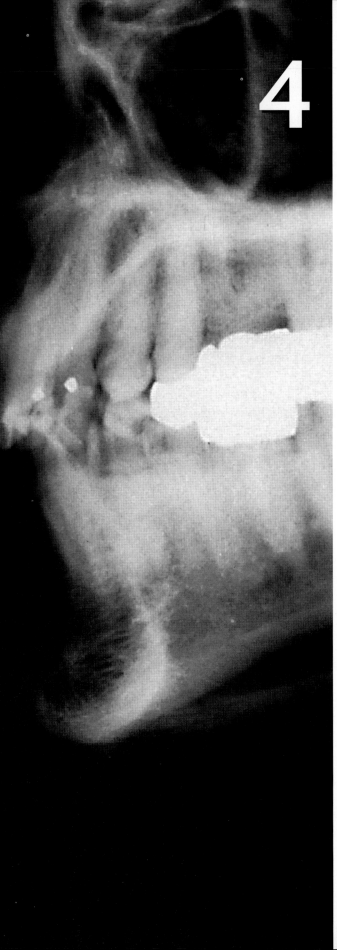

X-Ray Film, Intensifying Screens, and Grids

4

A ***beam of x-ray photons*** that passes through the dental arches is reduced in intensity (attenuated) by absorption and scattering of photons out of the primary beam. The pattern of the photons that exits the subject, the remnant beam, conveys information about the structure and composition of the absorber. For this information to be useful diagnostically, the remnant beam must be recorded on an image receptor. The image receptor most often used in dental radiography is x-ray film. This chapter describes x-ray film and its properties, as well as the use of intensifying screens and grids to modify radiographic images. Digital radiographic systems, which occasionally are used instead of film, are described in Chapter 12.

X-Ray Film

COMPOSITION

X-ray film has two principal components: emulsion and base. The emulsion, which is sensitive to x-rays and visible light, records the radiographic image. The base is a plastic supporting material onto which the emulsion is coated (Fig. 4-1).

Emulsion

The two principal components of emulsion are silver halide grains, which are sensitive to x-radiation and visi-

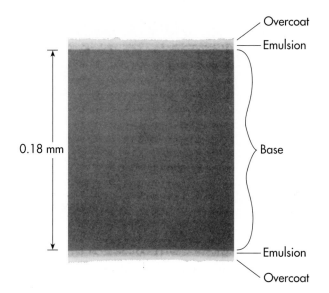

FIG. **4-1** *Scanning electron micrograph of Kodak Ultra-Speed dental x-ray film (300 ×).* Note the overcoat, emulsion, and base on this double-emulsion film. (Courtesy Eastman Kodak, Rochester, N.Y.)

TABLE **4-1** Coating Weight per Film Side (mg/cm²)					
FILM TYPE	SILVER	BROMIDE	IODIDE	EMULSION VEHICLE	OVERCOAT VEHICLE
Ultra-Speed	0.92	0.67	0.02	0.59	0.16
Ektaspeed Plus	0.92	0.66	0.03	0.75	0.08

Courtesy Eastman Kodak, Rochester, N.Y.

ble light, and a vehicle matrix in which the crystals are suspended. The *silver halide grains* are composed primarily of crystals of silver bromide and to a lesser extent silver iodide. The composition of a dental film emulsion is shown in Table 4-1. Iodide is added because its large-diameter crystals (compared to those of bromine) disrupt the regularity of the silver bromide crystal structure, thereby increasing its sensitivity to x-radiation. The photosensitivity of the silver halide crystals also depends on the presence of trace amounts of a sulfur-containing compound. In addition, trace amounts of gold are sometimes added to silver halide crystals to improve their sensitivity.

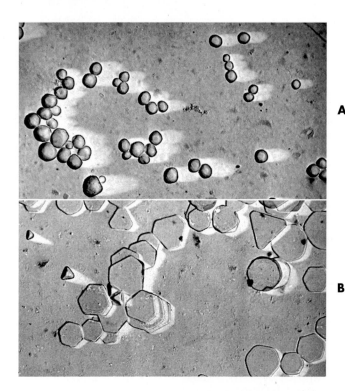

FIG. **4-2** Scanning electron micrographs of emulsion comparing globular silver halide crystals of Ultra-Speed film **(A)** and tabular silver halide crystals of Ektaspeed Plus film **(B)**. (Courtesy Eastman Kodak, Rochester, N.Y.)

The silver halide grains in Ektaspeed Plus film (an E-speed film) are flat, tabular crystals with a mean diameter of about 1.6 µm (Fig. 4-2). Ultra-Speed film (a D-speed film) is composed of globular crystals about 1 µm in diameter. The tabular grains of the E-speed film are oriented parallel with the film surface to offer a large cross-sectional area to the x-ray beam (Fig. 4-3).

In the manufacture of film, the silver halide grains are suspended in a surrounding *vehicle* that is applied to both sides of the supporting base. The vehicle, composed of gelatinous and nongelatinous materials, keeps the silver halide grains evenly dispersed. To ensure good adhesion of the emulsion to the film base, a thin layer of adhesive material is added to the base before the emulsion is applied. During film processing, the vehicle absorbs the processing solutions, allowing the chemicals to reach and react with the silver halide grains. An additional layer of vehicle is added to the film emulsion as an overcoat; this barrier helps protect the film from damage by scratching, contamination, or pressure from rollers when an automatic processor is used.

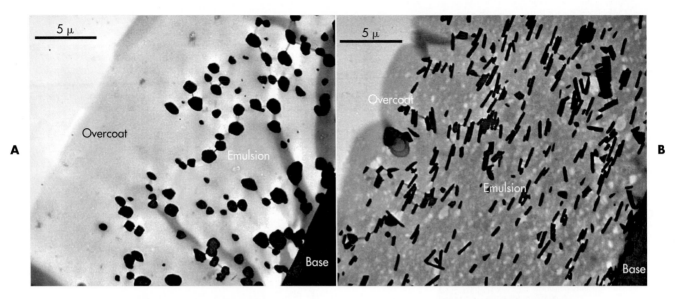

FIG. **4-3** Cross-sectional electron microscopic image of emulsion of Ultra-Speed film **(A)** and Ektaspeed Plus film **(B).** Note that the orientation of the tabular crystals in the Ektaspeed Plus film is essentially parallel to the film surface to increase the exposure surface area of the crystals to the x-ray beam. (Courtesy Eastman Kodak, Rochester N.Y.)

Film emulsions are made to be especially sensitive to either x-ray photons or visible light. Film intended to be exposed by x-rays is called *direct exposure* film. All intraoral dental film is direct exposure film. *Screen film,* which is most sensitive to visible light, is used with intensifying screens that emit visible light. Screen film and intensifying screens are used for extraoral projections such as panoramic and skull radiographs. Intensifying screens are described later in this chapter.

Base

The function of the film base is to support the emulsion. The base must have the proper degree of flexibility to allow easy handling of the film. The base for dental x-ray film is about 0.2 mm thick and is made of polyester polyethylene terephthalate. The film base is uniformly translucent and casts no pattern on the resultant radiograph. Some believe that a base with a slight blue tint improves viewing of diagnostic detail. The film base must also withstand exposure to processing solutions without becoming distorted.

INTRAORAL X-RAY FILM

A number of manufacturers around the world make intraoral dental x-ray film. In each case the film is made as a double-emulsion film, that is, *coated with an emulsion on each side of the base.* With a double layer of emulsion, less radiation can be used to produce an image. Direct exposure film is used for intraoral examinations because it provides higher-resolution images than screen-film

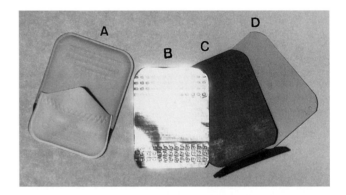

FIG. **4-4** Moisture- and light-proof packet *(A)* contains an opening tab on the side opposite the tube. Inside is a sheet of lead foil *(B)* and a black, light-proof, interleaf paper wrapper *(C)* that is folded around the film *(D).*

combinations. Some diagnostic tasks, such as detection of incipient caries or early periapical disease, require this higher resolution.

One corner of each dental film has a small, raised dot that is used for film orientation. When the film is placed in the patient's mouth, the side of the film with the raised dot is always positioned facing the x-ray tube. The side of the film with the depression thus is oriented toward the patient's tongue. After the film has been processed, the dot is used to identify the image as being the patient's right or left side (see Fig. 6-26).

Intraoral x-ray film packets contain either one or two sheets of film (Fig. 4-4). When double-film packs are

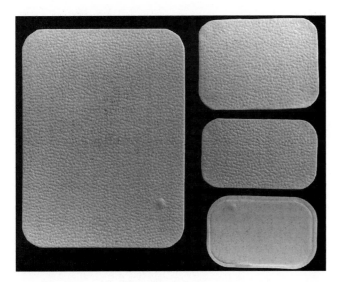

FIG. **4-5** Dental x-ray film is commonly supplied in various sizes. *Left,* Occlusal film; *top right,* adult posterior film; *middle right,* adult anterior film; *bottom right,* child-size film (in plastic wrapping).

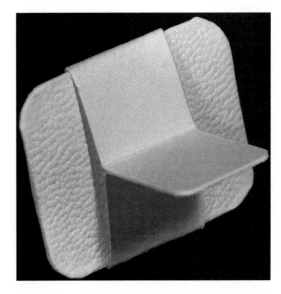

FIG. **4-6** Paper loop placed around a size 2 adult film to support the film when the patient bites on the tab for a bitewing projection. This projection reveals the tooth crowns and alveolar crests.

used, the second film serves as a duplicate record that can be sent to insurance companies or a colleague. The film is encased in a protective black paper wrapper and then in an outer white paper or plastic wrapping, which is resistant to moisture. The outer wrapping clearly indicates the location of the raised dot and which side of the film should be directed toward the x-ray tube.

Between the wrappers in the film packet is a thin lead foil backing with an embossed pattern. The foil is positioned in the film packet behind the film, away from the tube. This lead foil serves several purposes. It shields the film from backscatter (secondary) radiation, which fogs the film and reduces subject contrast (image quality). It also slightly reduces patient exposure by absorbing some of the residual x-ray beam. Most important, however, is the fact that if the film packet is placed backwards in the patient's mouth so that the tube side of the film is facing away from the x-ray machine, the lead foil is positioned between the subject and the film. Much of the radiation is absorbed by the lead foil, resulting in a light image showing the embossed pattern. This combination of a light film with the characteristic pattern indicates that the film packet was put in backwards and that the right side–left side designation indicated by the film dot was reversed.

Because intraoral direct exposure film packets have several uses, they are made in a variety of sizes. The composition of the film is identical.

Periapical View

Periapical views are used to record the crowns, roots, and surrounding bone. Film packs come in three sizes: 0

for small children (22×35 mm); 1, which is relatively narrow and used for views of the anterior teeth (24×40 mm); and 2, the standard film size used for adults (31×41 mm) (Fig. 4-5).

Bitewing View

Bitewing (interproximal) views are used to record the coronal portions of the maxillary and mandibular teeth in one image. They are useful for detecting interproximal caries and evaluating the height of alveolar bone. Size 2 film usually is used in adults; the smaller size 1 is preferred in children. In small children size 0 maybe used. A relatively long size 3 also is available.

Bitewing films often have a paper tab projecting from the middle of the film, on which the patient bites to support the film (Fig. 4-6). This tab is rarely visualized and does not interfere with the diagnostic quality of the image. Film-holding instruments for bitewing projections also are available.

Occlusal View

Occlusal film is more than three times larger than size 2 film (57×76 mm) (see Fig. 4-5). It is used to show larger areas of the maxilla or mandible than may be seen on a periapical film. These films also are used to obtain right-angle views to the usual periapical view. The name derives from the fact that the film usually is held in position by having the patient bite lightly on it to support it between the occlusal surfaces of the teeth (see Chapter 8).

SCREEN FILM

The extraoral projections used most frequently in dentistry are the panoramic, skull, and cephalometric views. For these projections and for virtually all other extraoral radiography, screen film is used with intensifying screens (described later in this chapter). Screen film is different from dental intraoral film in that it is designed to be particularly sensitive to visible light rather than to x-radiation because this film is placed between two intensifying screens when an exposure is made. The intensifying screens absorb x-rays and emit visible light, which exposes the screen film. Silver halide crystals are inherently sensitive to ultraviolet (UV) and blue light (300 to 500 nm) and thus are sensitive to screens that emit UV and blue light. When film is used with screens that emit green light, the silver halide crystals are coated with sensitizing dyes to increase absorption. Because the properties of intensifying screens vary, the dentist should use the appropriate screen-film combination recommended by the screen and film manufacturer so that the emission characteristics of the screen match the absorption characteristics of the film.

Several general types of screen film are suitable for extraoral radiography. Several manufacturers supply high-contrast, medium-speed film suitable for skull radiography. Other films are available that are faster (i.e., they require less radiation exposure), but these provide less image detail. Such films should be considered for panoramic radiography when fine image detail is not available because of movement of the x-ray tube head during the exposure.

Another type of film provides less contrast and a wider latitude. This type reveals a wide range of densities and is most suitable for cephalometric radiography, when both bony and soft tissue details are desired.

The design of screen films changes constantly to optimize imaging characteristics. Kodak, for example, has introduced T-Mat films, which have tabular-shaped (flat) grains of silver halide (Fig. 4-7). The tabular (T) grains are oriented with their relatively large, flat surfaces facing the radiation source, providing a larger cross-section (target) and resulting in increased speed without loss of sharpness. In addition, green-sensitizing dyes are added to the surface of the tabular grains, increasing their light-gathering capability and reducing the crossover of light from the phosphor layer on one side of the intensifying screen to the film emulsion on the other. Kodak's new Ektavision system also coats the film base with an absorbing dye to prevent crossover of light from one screen to the other emulsion. These properties increase both the speed of the film and the sharpness of the image. Sterling uses tabular grains in its Cronex 10T film, and Imation coats its XDA+ and XLA+ film base with an anticrossover agent as well.

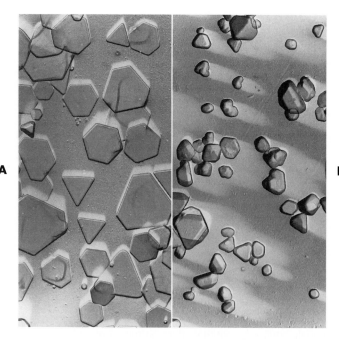

FIG. **4-7** T grains of silver halide in an emulsion of T-Mat film **(A)** are larger and flatter than the smaller, thicker crystals in an emulsion of conventional film **(B).** Note that the flat surfaces of the T grains are oriented parallel with the film surface, facing the radiation source. (Courtesy Eastman Kodak, Rochester, N.Y.)

Intensifying Screens

Early in the history of radiography, scientists discovered that various inorganic salts or phosphors *fluoresce* (emit visible light) when exposed to an x-ray beam. The intensity of this fluorescence is proportional to the intensity of the x-ray beam. These phosphors have been incorporated into intensifying screens for use with screen film. The sum of the effects of the x-rays and the visible light emitted by the screen phosphors exposes the screen film in an intensifying cassette.

FUNCTION

The presence of intensifying screens creates an image receptor system that is 10 to 60 times more sensitive to x-rays than the film alone. Consequently, use of intensifying screens means a substantial reduction in the dose of x-radiation to which the patient is exposed. Intensifying screens are used with films for virtually all *extraoral radiography*, including panoramic, cephalometric, and skull projections. The resolving power of screens is related to their speed: the slower the speed of the screen, the greater its resolving power and vice versa. Intensifying screens generally are not used intraorally with periapical or occlusal films because the resolution is not as great as with direct exposure film.

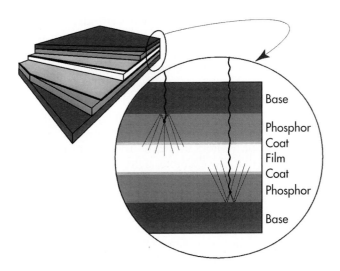

FIG. **4-8** The image on the left shows a schematic of two intensifying screens *(shades of gray)* enclosing a film *(white)*. The detailed view on the right shows x-ray photons entering at the top, traveling through the base, and striking phosphors in the base. The phosphors emit visible light, exposing the film. Some visible light photons may reflect off the reflecting layer of the base.

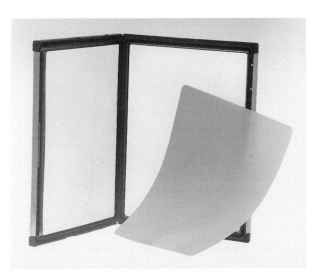

FIG. **4-9** *Cassette for 8 × 10 inch film.* When the cassette is closed, the film is supported between two intensifying screens.

TABLE **4-2**
Rare Earth Elements Used in Intensifying Screens

COMPANY	NAME	PHOSPHOR	EMISSION
Kodak	Lanex	Gadolinium oxysulfide, terbium activated	Green
Imation	Trimax	Gadolinium oxysulfide, terbium activated	Green
Sterling	Quanta	Yttrium tantalate, niobium activated	Blue and UV

COMPOSITION

Intensifying screens are made of a base supporting material, a phosphor layer, and a protective plastic coat (Fig. 4-8). Intensifying screens are used in pairs, one on each side of the film, and they are positioned inside a *cassette* (Fig. 4-9). The purpose of a cassette is to hold each intensifying screen in contact with the x-ray film to maximize the sharpness of the image. Most cassettes are rigid, but they may be flexible.

Base

The base material of most intensifying screens usually is some form of polyester plastic that is about 0.25 mm thick. The base provides mechanical support for the other layers. In some intensifying screens the base also is reflective; thus it reflects light emitted from the phosphor layer back toward the x-ray film. This has the effect of increasing the sensitivity of the intensifying screen. However, it also results in some image "unsharpness" because of the divergence of light rays reflected back to the film. Some fine detail intensifying screens omit the reflecting layer to improve image sharpness. In other intensifying screens the base is not reflective, and a separate coating of titanium dioxide is applied to the base material to serve as a *reflecting layer*.

Phosphor Layer

The phosphor layer is composed of radiation-sensitive phosphorescent crystals suspended in a plastic material. When the crystals are struck by photons, they fluoresce (see Fig. 4-8). The phosphor crystals are made of rare earth elements, most commonly lanthanum and gadolinium. Their fluorescence can be increased by the addition of small amounts of thulium, niobium, or terbium. Common phosphor combinations used in intensifying screens are shown in Table 4-2.

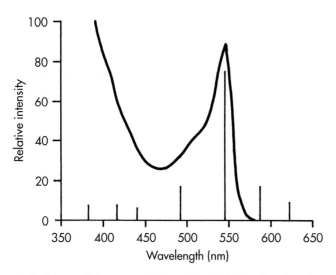

FIG. **4-10** Relative sensitivity of Kodak T-Mat film *(continuous line)* and emission of a Kodak Lanex regular screen (gadolinium oxysulfide, terbium activated). Intensifying screens emit light as a series of relatively narrow line emissions. The maximal emission of the screen at 545 nm corresponds well to a high-sensitivity region of the film. (Data courtesy Eastman Kodak, Rochester, N.Y.)

Rare earth elements are efficient phosphors. A pair of rare earth intensifying screens absorbs about 60% of the photons that reach the cassette after passing through a patient. These phosphors are about 18% efficient in converting this x-ray energy to visible light. Rare earth screens convert each absorbed x-ray photon into about 4000 lower-energy, visible light (green or blue) photons. These visible photons then expose the film.

Different phosphors fluoresce in different portions of the spectrum. For example, light emission from Kodak Lanex (Fig. 4-10) and Imation Trimax rare earth intensifying screens ranges from 375 to 600 nm and peaks sharply at 545 nm (green). This figure shows the spectral emission of a rare earth screen and the spectral sensitivity of an appropriate film. The Sterling Quanta Detail screen has a major peak at 350 nm (UV) and another at 450 nm (blue). It is important to match blue-emitting screens with blue-sensitive films and green-emitting screens with green-sensitive films.

Each screen-film combination has its own speed. Table 4-3 shows several contemporary screen and film combinations. Fast screens have large phosphor crystals and efficiently convert x-ray photons to visible light but produce

TABLE **4-3**
Speeds of Various Screen-Film Combinations

MANUFACTURER	SCREEN	FILM	SPEED
Eastman Kodak	Lanex (green)		
	Fine	T-Mat G, T-Mat L	100
	Medium	T-Mat G, T-Mat L	250
	Regular	T-Mat G, T-Mat L	400
	Ektavision	Ektavision	400
Imation	Trimax (green)		
	Fine	XLA+, XDA+	100
	Fast detail	XLA+, XDA+	300
	Medium	XLA+, XDA+	400
	Regular	XLA+, XDA+	600
Sterling	Quanta (blue)		
	Detail	Cronex 10T, 10TL	100
	Fast detail	Cronex 10T, 10TL	200
	Rapid	Cronex 10T, 10TL	400
	Super rapid	Cronex 10T, 10TL	800
	Ultra-Vision (ultraviolet)		
	Detail	Ultra-Vision G, L	100
	Fast detail	Ultra-Vision G, L	200
	Rapid	Ultra-Vision G, L	400
	Super rapid	Ultra-Vision G, L	800

T-Mat G, XDA+, 10T: Medium detail, medium speed, high contrast.
Ektavision, Ultra-Vision: High detail, high speed.
T-Mat L, XLA+, 10TL: Medium detail, medium speed, wide latitude.

images with low resolution. As the size of the crystals or the thickness of the screen decreases, the speed of the screen also declines, but image sharpness increases. In deciding on the combination to use, the practitioner must consider the resolution requirements of the task for which the image will be used. Most dental extraoral diagnostic tasks can be accomplished with screen-film combinations that have a speed of 250 or faster.

Coat

A protective coat of plastic (up to 8 μm thick) is placed over the phosphor layer to protect the phosphor and provide a surface that can be cleaned. The intensifying screens should be kept clean because any debris, spots, or scratches cause light spots on the resultant radiograph.

Image Characteristics

Processing an exposed x-ray film causes it to become dark in the exposed area. The degree and pattern of film darkening depend on numerous factors, including the energy and intensity of the x-ray beam, composition of the subject imaged, film emulsion used, and characteristics of film processing. This section describes the major imaging characteristics of x-ray film.

RADIOGRAPHIC DENSITY

When a film is exposed by an x-ray beam (or by light in the case of screen-film combinations) and then processed, the silver halide crystals in the emulsion that were stuck by the photons are converted to grains of metallic silver. These silver grains block the transmission of light from a viewbox and give the film its dark appearance. The overall degree of darkening of an exposed film is referred to as *radiographic density*. This density can be measured as the optical density of an area of an x-ray film where:

$$\text{Optical density} = \text{Log}_{10} \frac{I_o}{I_t}$$

where I_o is the intensity of incident light (e.g., from a viewbox) and I_t is the intensity of the light transmitted through the film. Thus the measurement of film density also is a measure of the opacity of the film. With an optical density of 0, 100% of the light is transmitted; with a density of 1, 10% of the light is transmitted; with a density of 2, 1% of the light is transmitted, and so on.

A plot of the relationship between film optical density and exposure is called a *characteristic curve* (Fig.

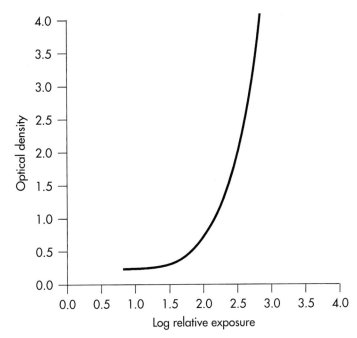

FIG. **4-11** Characteristic curve of direct exposure film. The contrast *(slope of the curve)* is greater in the high-density region than in the low-density region.

4-11). It usually is shown as the relation between the optical density of the film and the logarithm of the corresponding exposure. As exposure of the film increases, its optical density increases. A film is of greatest diagnostic value when the structures of interest are imaged on the relatively straight portion of the graph, between 0.6 and 3.0 optical density units. The characteristic curves of films reveal much information about film contrast, speed, and latitude.

An unexposed film, when processed, shows some density. This is caused by the inherent density of the base and added tint, as well as the development of unexposed silver halide crystals. This minimal density is called *gross fog*, or *base plus fog*. The optical density of gross fog typically is 0.2 to 0.3.

Radiographic density is influenced by exposure and the thickness and density of the subject.

Exposure

The overall film density depends on the number of photons absorbed by the film emulsion. Increasing the *milliamperage* (mA), *peak kilovoltage* (kVp), or *exposure time* increases the number of photons reaching the film and thus increases the density of the radiograph. Reducing the *distance* between the focal spot and film also increases film density.

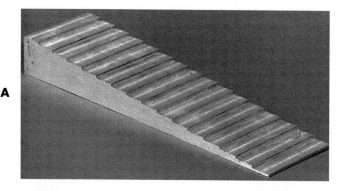

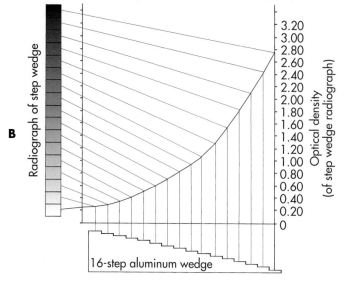

FIG. **4-12** **A,** Aluminum step wedge. **B,** Graph of the optical density of a radiograph made by exposing the step wedge. Note that as the thickness of the aluminum decreases, more photons are available to expose the film, and the image becomes progressively darker.

Subject Thickness

The thicker the subject, the more the beam is attenuated and the lighter the resultant image (Fig. 4-12). If exposure factors intended for adults are used on children or edentulous patients, the resultant films are dark because a smaller amount of absorbing tissue is in the path of the x-ray beam. The dentist should vary exposure (either kVp or time) according to the patient's size to produce radiographs of optimal density.

Subject Density

Variations in the density of the subject exert a profound influence on the image. The greater the density of a structure within the subject, the greater the attenuation of the x-ray beam directed through that subject

or area. In the oral cavity the relative densities of various natural structures, in order of decreasing density, are enamel, dentin and cementum, bone, muscle, fat, and air. Metallic objects (e.g., restorations) are far denser than enamel and hence better absorbers. Because an x-ray beam is differentially attenuated by these absorbers, the resultant beam carries information that is recorded on the radiographic film as light and dark areas. Dense objects (which are strong absorbers) cause the radiographic image to be light and are said to be *radiopaque.* Objects with low densities are weak absorbers. They allow most photons to pass through, and they cast a dark area on the film that corresponds to the *radiolucent* object.

RADIOGRAPHIC CONTRAST

Radiographic contrast is a general term that describes the range of densities on a radiograph. It is defined as the difference in densities between light and dark regions on a radiograph. Thus an image that shows both light areas and dark areas has *high contrast.* This also is referred to as a *short gray scale of contrast* because few shades of gray are present between the black and white images on the film. A radiographic image composed only of light gray and dark gray zones is *low contrast,* also referred to as having a *long gray scale of contrast* (Fig. 4-13). The radiographic contrast of an image is the result of the interplay of subject contrast, film contrast, and scattered radiation.

Subject Contrast

Subject contrast is the range of characteristics of the subject that influence radiographic contrast. It is influenced largely by the subject's thickness, density, and atomic number. The subject contrast of a patient's head and neck exposed in a lateral cephalometric view is high. The dense regions of the bone and teeth absorb most of the incident radiation, whereas the less dense soft tissue facial profile transmits most of the radiation.

Subject contrast also is influenced by beam energy and intensity. The energy of the x-ray beam, selected by the kVp, influences image contrast. Fig. 4-14 shows an aluminum step wedge exposed to x-ray beams of differing energies. Because increasing the kVp increases the overall density of the image, the exposure time has been adjusted so that the density of the middle step in each case is comparable. As the kVp of the x-ray beam increases, subject contrast decreases. Similarly, when relatively low kVp energies are used, subject contrast increases. Most clinicians select a kVp in the range of 70 to 80. At higher values the exposure time is reduced, but

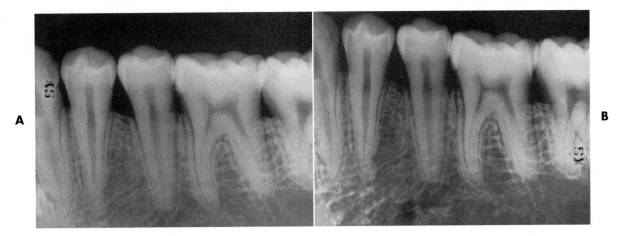

FIG. **4-13**   Radiograph of a dried mandible revealing low contrast **(A)** and high contrast **(B).**

the loss of contrast may be objectionable because subtle changes may be obscured.

Changing the time or mA of the exposure (and holding the kVp constant) also influences subject contrast. If the film is excessively light or dark, contrast of anatomic structures is diminished. Subtle changes in the mA may also slightly change subject contrast by changing the location of the radiographed structures on the characteristic curve, as described previously.

Film Contrast

The term *film contrast* describes the capacity of radiographic films to display differences in subject contrast, that is, variations in the intensity of the remnant beam. A high-contrast film reveals areas of small difference in subject contrast more clearly than does a low-contrast film. Film contrast usually is measured as the average gradient (slope) of the diagnostically useful portion of the characteristic curve (Fig. 4-15): the greater the average gradient of the curve in this region, the greater the film contrast. In this illustration, film *A* has a higher contrast than film *B*. When the average gradient of the curve in the useful range is greater than 1, the film exaggerates subject contrast. This desirable feature, which is found in most diagnostic film, allows visualization of structures that differ only slightly in density. Films used with intensifying screens typically have an average gradient in the range of 2 to 3.

As can be seen in Fig. 4-11, film contrast also depends on the density range being examined. With dental direct-exposure film the average gradient of the curve continually increases with increasing exposure. As a result, properly exposed films have more contrast than underexposed (light) films.

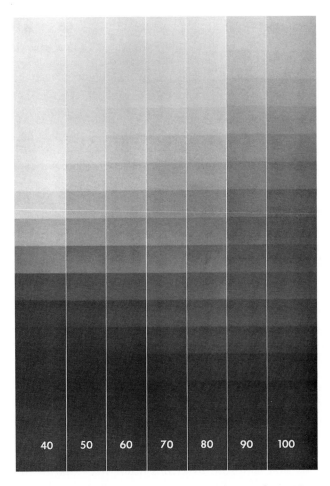

FIG. **4-14**   Radiographs of a step wedge made at 40 to 100 kVp. As the kVp increases, the mA is reduced to maintain the uniform middle-step density. Note the long gray scale (low contrast) with high kVp. (Courtesy Eastman Kodak, Rochester, N.Y.)

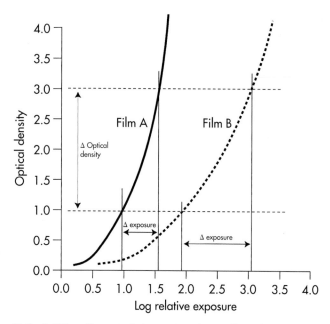

FIG. **4-15** Characteristic curves of two films demonstrating the greater inherent contrast of film *A* compared with film *B*. The slope of film *A* is greater than that of film *B*; film *A* therefore requires less change in exposure to increase its optical density from 1 to 3.

FILM SPEED GROUP	SPEED RANGE (RECIPROCAL ROENTGENS*)
C	6-12
D	12-24
E	24-48
F	48-96

TABLE **4-4**
Intraoral Film Speed Classification

American Dental Association, Council on Dental Materials and Devices: *Dentist's desk reference: materials, instruments, and equipment,* ed 2, 1983.
*Reciprocal roentgens are the reciprocal of the exposure in roentgens required to obtain a film with an optical density of 1.0 above base plus fog after processing.

Film processing is another factor that influences film contrast. Film contrast is maximized by optimal film processing conditions. Mishandling of the film through incomplete or excessive development results in diminished contrast of anatomic structures. Improper handling of film, such as storage at too high a temperature, exposure to excessively bright safelights, or light leaks in the darkroom, also degrades film contrast.

Fog on an x-ray film results in increased film density arising from causes other than exposure to the remnant beam. Film contrast is reduced by the addition of this undesirable density. Common causes of film fog are improper safelighting, storage of film at too high a temperature, and development of film at an excessive temperature or for a prolonged period. Film fog can be reduced by proper film processing and storage.

Scattered Radiation

Scattered radiation results from photons that have interacted with the subject by Compton or coherent interactions. These interactions cause the emission of photons that travel in directions other than that of the primary beam. The consequent scattered radiation causes fogging of a radiograph, an overall darkening of the image that results in loss of radiographic contrast. In most dental applications the best means of reducing scattered radiation are to (1) use a relatively low kVp, (2) collimate the beam to the size of the film to prevent

scatter from an area outside the region of the image, and (3) use grids in extraoral radiography.

RADIOGRAPHIC SPEED

Radiographic speed refers to the amount of radiation required to produce an image of a standard density. Film speed frequently is expressed as the reciprocal of the exposure (in roentgens) required to produce an optical density of 1 above gross fog. A fast film requires a relatively low exposure to produce a density of 1, whereas a slower film requires a longer exposure for the processed film to have the same density. Film speed is controlled largely by the size of the silver halide grains.

The speed of dental intraoral x-ray film is indicated by a letter designating a particular group (Table 4-4). The fastest dental film currently available has a speed rating of E. Only films with a D or E speed rating are appropriate for intraoral radiography. Currently the types of film used most often in the United States are Kodak Ultra-Speed (group D) and Kodak Ektaspeed Plus (group E). Ektaspeed Plus film is preferred because it requires only about half the exposure of Ultra-Speed film and offers comparable contrast and resolution. E-speed film is faster than the D-speed type because tabular crystal grains are used in the emulsion of E-speed film. The characteristic curves in Fig. 4-16 show that Ektaspeed Plus film (curve on the left) is faster than Ultra-Speed film (curve on the right) because less exposure is required to produce the same level of density even though the two films have similar contrast.

Film speed can be increased slightly by processing the film at a higher temperature, but this is achieved at the expense of increased film fog and graininess. Processing in depleted solutions can lower the effective speed. It is always preferable to use fresh processing solutions and follow the recommended processing time and temperature.

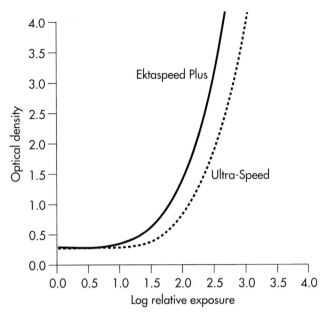

FIG. **4-16** *Characteristic curves for Ektaspeed Plus and Ultra-Speed film.* Ektaspeed Plus film is faster and has essentially the same contrast as Ultra-Speed film. (Courtesy Eastman Kodak, Rochester, N.Y.)

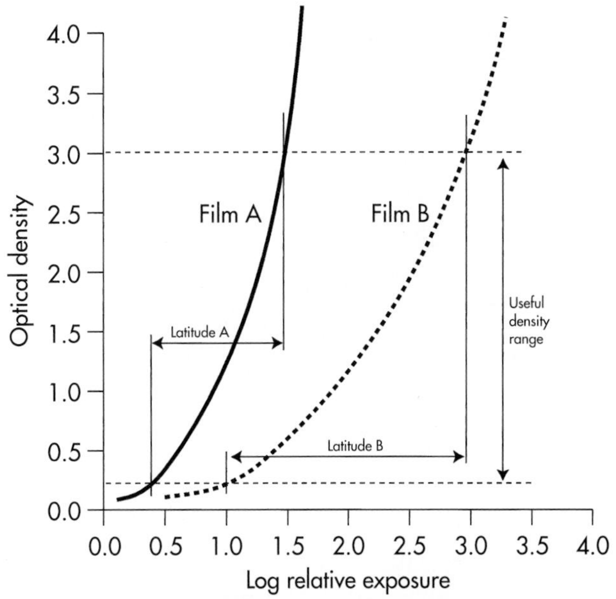

FIG. **4-17** Characteristic curves for two films demonstrating the greater inherent latitude of film *B* compared with film *A.* The slope of film *B* is less steep than that of film *A;* film *B* therefore records a greater range of exposures within the useful density range than does film *A.*

FILM LATITUDE

Film latitude is a measure of the range of exposures that can be recorded as distinguishable densities on a film. A film optimized to display a wide latitude can record a subject with a wide range of subject contrast. A film with a characteristic curve that has a long straight-line portion and a shallow slope has a wide latitude (Fig. 4-17). As a consequence, wide variations in the amount of radiation exiting the subject can be recorded. Films with a wide latitude have lower contrast (i.e., a long gray scale) than do films with a narrow latitude. Wide-latitude films are useful when both the osseous structures of the skull and the soft tissues of the facial region must be recorded.

To some extent the operator can modify the latitude of an image. A *high kVp* produces images with a wide latitude and low contrast. *Reduced exposure* produces a somewhat lighter image and shows a slightly wider range of anatomic structures with lower contrast. Wide-latitude film is recommended for imaging structures with a wide range of subject densities.

RADIOGRAPHIC NOISE

Radiographic noise is the appearance of *uneven density* of a uniformly exposed radiographic film. It is seen on a small area of film as localized variations in density. The primary causes of noise are radiographic mottle and ra-

diographic artifact. Radiographic mottle is uneven density resulting from the physical structure of the film or intensifying screens. Radiographic artifacts are defects caused by errors in film handling, such as fingerprints or bends in the film, or errors in film processing, such as splashing developer or fixer on a film or marks or scratches from rough handling.

On intraoral dental film, mottle may be seen as *film graininess,* which is caused by the visibility of silver grains in the film emulsion, especially when magnification is used to examine an image. Film graininess is most evident when high-temperature processing is used.

Radiographic mottle is also evident when the film is used with fast intensifying screens. Two important causes of the phenomenon are *quantum mottle* and *screen structure mottle.* Quantum mottle is caused by a fluctuation in the number of photons per unit of the beam cross-sectional area that are absorbed by the intensifying screen. Quantum mottle is most evident when fast film-screen combinations are used. Under these conditions the relative nonuniformity of the beam is highest. The longer exposures required by slower film-screen combinations tend to average out the beam pattern and thereby reduce quantum mottle. Screen structure mottle is graininess caused by screen phosphors. It is most evident when fast screens with large crystals are used.

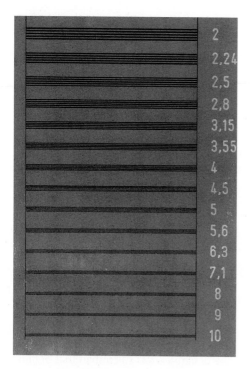

FIG. **4-18** Radiograph of a resolving power target consisting of groups of radiopaque lines and radiolucent spaces. Numbers at each group indicate the line pairs per millimeter represented by the group.

RADIOGRAPHIC BLURRING

Sharpness is the ability of a radiograph to *define an edge* precisely (e.g., the dentinoenamel junction, a thin trabecular plate). Resolution, or resolving power, is the ability of a radiograph to record *separate structures* that are close together. It usually is measured by radiographing an object made up of a series of thin lead strips with alternating radiolucent spaces of the same thickness. The groups of lines and spaces are arranged in the test target in order of increasing numbers of lines and spaces per millimeter (Fig. 4-18). The resolving power is measured as the highest number of line pairs (a line pair being the image of an absorber and the adjacent lucent space) per millimeter that can be distinguished on the resultant radiograph when examined with low-power magnification. Typically, panoramic film-screen combinations can resolve about five line pairs per millimeter; periapical film, which has better resolving power, can delineate clearly more than 10 line pairs per millimeter.

Radiographic blurring (unsharpness) is measured by the modulation transfer function (MTF). MTF measures the ability of a radiographic system (screens, film, and processing) to record information accurately. The higher the MTF, the greater the ability of the system to record

the signal. An MTF of 100% means that all the information in a signal is recorded. The MTF typically is high for gross information (e.g., one line pair per millimeter) and much lower for very fine detail (e.g., 10 line pairs per millimeter). Resolving power may be specified as the spatial frequency at which the MTF equals a certain value (e.g., 4%).

Radiographic blur is caused by image receptor (film and screen) blurring, motion blurring, and geometric blurring.

Image Receptor Blurring

With intraoral dental x-ray film, the *size of the silver grains* in the film emulsion determines image sharpness: the finer the grain size, the finer the sharpness. In general, slow-speed films have fine grains and faster films have larger grains.

Use of *intensifying screens* in extraoral radiography has an adverse effect on image sharpness. Some degree of sharpness is lost because visible light and ultraviolet radiation emitted by the screen spread out beyond the point of origin and expose a film area larger than the phosphor crystal (see Fig. 4-8). The spreading light causes a blurring of fine detail on the radiograph. Intensifying screens with large crystals are relatively fast, but image sharpness is diminished. Furthermore, fast intensifying screens have a relatively thick phosphor layer, which contributes to dispersion of light and loss of image sharpness. Diffusion of light from a screen can be minimized and image sharpness maximized by ensuring as close contact as possible between the intensifying screen and film.

The presence of an image on each side of a double-emulsion film also causes a loss of image sharpness through *parallax* (Fig. 4-19). Parallax results from the apparent change in position or size of a subject when it is viewed from different perspectives. Because dental film has a double coating of emulsion and the x-ray beam is divergent, the images recorded on each emulsion vary slightly in size. In intraoral images, the effect of parallax on image sharpness is unimportant but is most apparent when wet films are viewed. Under these conditions the emulsion is swollen with water and the loss of image sharpness caused by parallax is more evident. When intensifying screens are used, parallax distortion contributes to image unsharpness because light from one screen may cross the film base and reach the emulsion on the opposite side. This problem can be solved by incorporating dyes into the base that absorb the light emitted by the screens.

Motion Blurring

Image sharpness also can be lost through movement of the film, subject, or x-ray source during exposure. Movement of the x-ray source in effect enlarges the focal spot

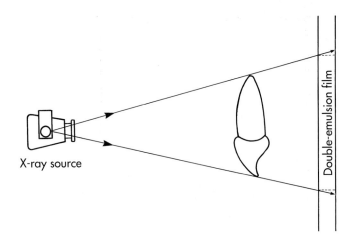

FIG. **4-19** Parallax unsharpness results when double-emulsion film is used because of the slightly greater magnification on the side of the film away from the x-ray source. Parallax unsharpness is a minor problem in clinical practice.

and diminishes image sharpness. Patient movement can be minimized by stabilizing the patient's head with the chair headrest during exposure. Using a higher mA and kVp and correspondingly shorter exposure times also helps resolve this problem.

Geometric Blurring

Several geometric factors influence image sharpness. Loss of image sharpness results in part because photons are not emitted from a point source (focal spot) on the target in the x-ray tube. The larger the focal spot, the greater the loss of image sharpness. Also, image sharpness is improved by increasing the distance between the focal spot and the object and reducing the distance between the object and the image receptor. Various means of optimizing projection geometry are discussed in Chapter 5.

IMAGE QUALITY

The term *image quality* describes the subjective judgment by the clinician of the overall appearance of a radiograph. It combines the features of density, contrast, latitude, sharpness, and resolution and perhaps other parameters. Various mathematic approaches have been used to evaluate these parameters further, but a thorough discussion of them is beyond the scope of this text. The detective quantum efficiency (DQE) is a basic measure of the efficiency of an imaging system. It encompasses image contrast, blur, speed, and noise. Often a system can be optimized for one of these parameters, but this usually is achieved at the expense of others. For instance, a fast system typically has a high level of noise.

Even with these and other sophisticated approaches, however, more information is needed for complete understanding of all the factors responsible for the subjective impression of image quality.

Grids

When an x-ray beam strikes a patient, many of the incident photons undergo Compton interactions and produce scattered photons. Typically the number of scattered photons in the remnant beam that reach the film is two to four times the number of primary photons that do not undergo absorption. The amount of scattered radiation increases with increasing subject thickness, field size, and kVp (energy of the x-ray beam). These scattered photons produce fog on the film and reduce the subject contrast.

FUNCTION

The function of a grid is to reduce the amount of scattered radiation exiting a subject that reaches the film. The grid, which is placed between the subject and the film, preferentially removes the scattered radiation and spares primary photons; this reduces nonimaging exposure and increases subject contrast.

COMPOSITION

A grid is composed of alternating strips of a radiopaque material (usually lead) and strips of radiolucent material (often plastic). The diagram in Fig. 4-20 shows the interaction between a grid and an x-ray beam. When secondary photons generated in the subject are scattered toward the film, they usually are absorbed by the radiopaque material in the grid. This occurs because the direction of the scattered photons deviates from that of the primary beam, and consequently they cannot pass through the parallel plates of the grid. *Focused grids* are used most often. In a focused grid the strips of radiopaque material are all directed toward a common point, the focal spot of the x-ray tube, some distance away. Because the lead strips are angled toward the focal spot, their direction coincides with the paths of diverging photons in the primary x-ray beam. The lead strips absorb the scattered photons as their paths diverge from those of the primary photons. A focused grid can be used only within a range of distances from the focal spot where the alignment of lead strips closely coincides with the path of the diverging x-ray beam. The range of distances is specified on the grid.

Grids are manufactured with a varying number of line pairs of absorbers and radiolucent spaces per inch.

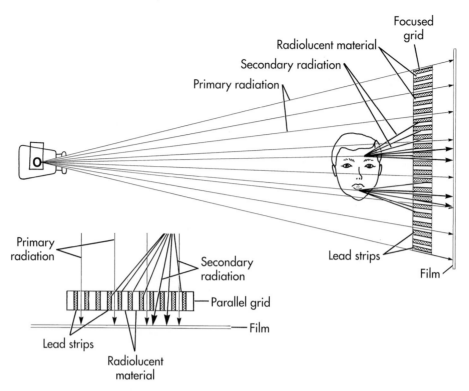

FIG. **4-20** An x-ray grid absorbs scattered x-ray photons from the primary beam and prevents them from fogging the film. In a focused grid the absorber plates are angled toward the anode; in a parallel grid the absorber plates are parallel.

Grids with 80 or more line pairs per inch do not show objectionable grid lines on the image. The ratio of grid thickness to the width of the radiolucent spacer is known as the *grid ratio*. The higher the grid ratio, the more effectively scattered radiation is removed from the x-ray beam. Grids with a ratio of 8 or 10 are preferred.

The image of the radiolucent grid lines on the film can be deleted by moving the grid perpendicular to the direction of the grid lines (but not moving the subject or the film) during exposure. This has the effect of blurring out the radiolucent lines and allowing a more uniform exposure. This movement does not interfere with the absorption of scattered photons. The apparatus for moving a grid is called a *Bucky*.

To compensate for the absorbing materials in the grid, the exposure required when a grid is used is approximately double that needed without a grid. Therefore grids should be used only when the improvement in diagnostic image quality is sufficient to justify the added exposure. For example, with lateral cephalometric examinations made for assessing the growth and development of the facial region (Chapter 11), use of a grid usually is not indicated because the improved contrast does not aid in identification of anatomic landmarks.

BIBLIOGRAPHY

Bushberg JT et al: *The essential physics of medical imaging*, Baltimore, 1994, Williams & Wilkins.

Bushong SC: *Radiological sciences for technologists: physics, biology, and protection*, ed 5, St Louis, 1993, Mosby.

Council on Dental Materials and Devices: Revised American Dental Association specification no. 22 for intraoral dental radiographic film adapted, *JADA* 80:1066, 1970.

Curry TS III et al: *Christensen's physics of diagnostic radiology*, ed 4, Philadelphia, 1990, Lea & Febiger.

Haus AG: The AAPM/RSNA physics tutorial for residents: measures of screen-film performance, *Radiographics* 16: 1165, 1996.

Ludlow JB et al: The efficacy of caries detection using three intraoral films under different processing conditions, *JADA* 128:1401, 1997.

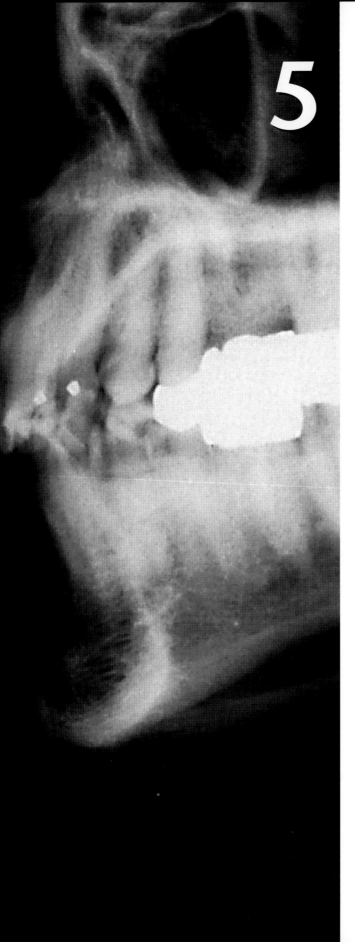

5

Projection Geometry

A *radiograph is a two-dimensional representation* of a three-dimensional object. To obtain the maximal value from a radiograph, a clinician must mentally reconstruct an accurate three-dimensional image of the anatomic structures of interest from one or more of these two-dimensional views. Using high-quality radiographs greatly facilitates this task. The principles of projection geometry describe the effect of focal spot size and position (relative to the object and the film) on image clarity, magnification, and distortion. The application of these imaging principles to clinical periapical radiography and object localization is described.

Image Sharpness and Resolution

Several geometric considerations contribute to image clarity, particularly image sharpness and resolution. *Sharpness* measures how well a boundary between two areas of differing radiodensity is revealed. Image *resolution* measures how well a radiograph is able to reveal small objects that are close together. Although sharpness and resolution are two distinct features, they are interdependent, being influenced by the same geometric variables. For clinical diagnosis it is desirable to optimize conditions that will result in images with high sharpness and resolution.

When x-rays are produced at the target in an x-ray tube, they originate from all points within the area of the focal spot. Because these rays originate from different points and travel in straight lines, their projections of a feature of an object do not occur at exactly the same location on a film. As a result, the image of the edge of an object is slightly blurred rather than sharp and distinct. Fig. 5-1 shows the path of photons that originate at the margins of the focal spot and provide an image of

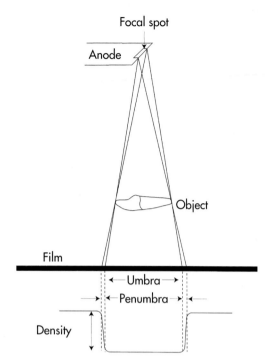

FIG. **5-1** Photons originating at different places on the focal spot result in a penumbra, or zone of unsharpness, on the radiograph. The density of the image changes from a high background value to a low value in the area of an edge of enamel, dentin, or bone.

the edges of an object. The resulting blurred zone on an image is called the *penumbra*. This blurring causes a loss in image clarity by reducing sharpness and resolution. The larger the focal spot area, the greater the loss of clarity.

Three methods exist for minimizing this loss of image clarity and improving the quality of radiographs:

1. *Using as small an effective focal spot as practical.* Dental x-ray machines should have a nominal focal spot size of 1.0 mm or less. Some tubes used in extraoral radiography have effective focal spots measuring 0.3 mm, which greatly adds to image clarity. X-ray tube manufacturers use as small an effective focal spot size as is consistent with the requirements for heat dissipation. As described in Chapter 1, the size of the effective focal spot is a function of the angle of the target with respect to the long axis of the electron beam. A large angle distributes the electron beam over a larger surface and decreases the heat generated per unit of target area, thus prolonging tube life. However, this results in a larger effective focal spot and loss of image clarity (Fig. 5-2). A small angle has a greater wearing effect on the target but results in a smaller effective focal spot, decreased penumbra, and increased image

FIG. **5-2** Decreasing the angle of the target perpendicular to the long axis of the electron beam decreases the actual focal spot size and decreases heat dissipation and thereby tube life. It also decreases the effective focal spot size and thus increases the sharpness of the image.

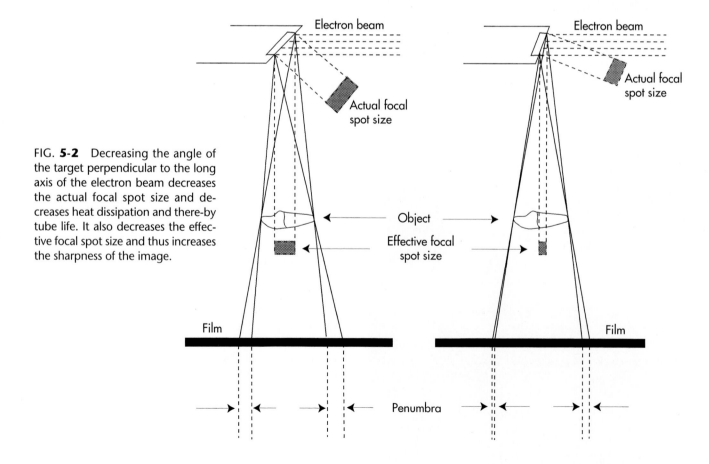

sharpness and resolution. This angle of the face of the target to the central x-ray beam is usually between 10 and 20 degrees.

2. *Increasing the distance between the focal spot and the object by using a long, open-ended cylinder.* Fig. 5-3 shows how increasing the focal spot–to-object distance reduces image blurring by reducing the divergence of the x-ray beam. The longer focal spot–to-object distance minimizes blurring by using photons whose paths are almost parallel. The benefits of using a long focal spot–to-object distance support the use of long, open-ended cylinders as aiming devices on dental x-ray machines.

3. *Decreasing the distance between the object and the film.* Fig. 5-4 shows that as the object-to-film distance is reduced, the penumbra decreases, resulting in enhanced image clarity. This is the result of minimizing the divergence of the x-ray photons.

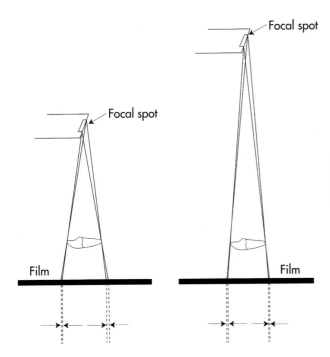

FIG. **5-3** Increasing the distance between the focal spot and the object results in an image with increased sharpness because the size of the penumbra is reduced. It also results in less magnification of the object.

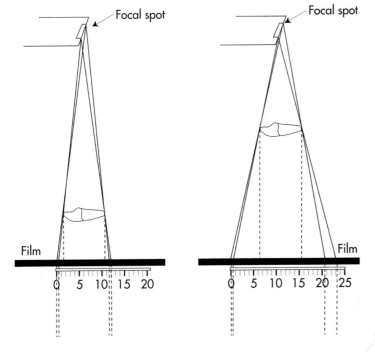

FIG. **5-4** Decreasing the distance between the object and the film increases the sharpness by decreasing the size of the penumbra. It also results in less magnification of the object.

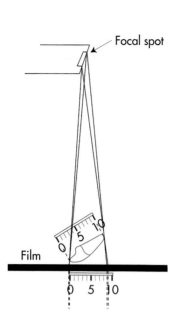

FIG. **5-5** Foreshortening of a radiographic image results when the central ray is perpendicular to the film but the object is not parallel with the film.

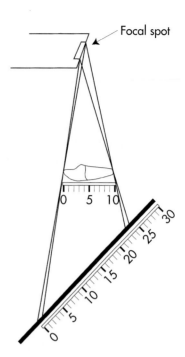

FIG. **5-6** Elongation of a radiographic image results when the central ray is perpendicular to the object but not the film.

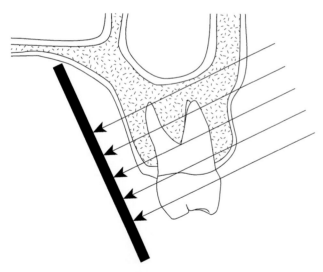

FIG. **5-7** The central ray should be perpendicular to the long axes of both the tooth and the film. When the direction of the x-ray beam is not at right angles to the long axis of the tooth, the appearance of the tooth is distorted, as seen by apparent elongation of the length of the palatal roots. Additionally, distortion of the relationship of the height of the alveolar crest relative to the cementoenamel junction (CEJ) occurs. In this case the buccal alveolar crest appears to lie superior to the palatal CEJ.

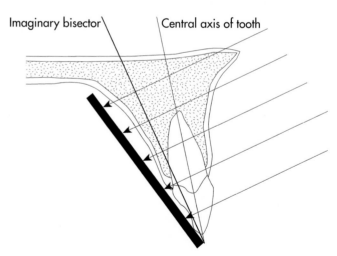

FIG. **5-8** In the bisecting-angle technique the central ray is directed at a right angle to the imaginary plane that bisects the angle formed by the film and the central axis of the object. This method results in an image that is the same length as the object.

Image Size Distortion

Image size distortion (magnification) is the increase in size of the image on the radiograph compared with the actual size of the object. The divergent paths of photons in an x-ray beam cause enlargement of the image on a radiograph. Image size distortion results from the relative distances of the focal spot–to-film and object-to-film (see Figs. 5-3 and 5-4). Accordingly, increasing the focal spot–to-film distance and decreasing the object-to-film distance minimizes image magnification. The use of a long, open-ended cylinder as an aiming device on an x-ray machine thus reduces the magnification of images on a periapical view. And, as mentioned above, this technique also improves image clarity by increasing the distance between the focal spot and object.

Image Shape Distortion

Image shape distortion is the result of unequal magnification of different parts of the same object. This situation arises when not all the parts of an object are at the same focal spot–to-object distance. The physical shape of the object may often prevent its optimal orientation, resulting in some shape distortion. Such a phenomenon is seen by the differences in appearance of the image on a radiograph compared with the true shape. To minimize shape distortion, the practitioner should make an effort to align the tube, object, and film carefully using the following guidelines:

1. *Position the film parallel to the long axis of the object.* Image shape distortion is minimized when the long axes of the film and tooth are parallel. Fig. 5-5 shows that the central ray of the x-ray beam is perpendicular to the film, but the object is not parallel to the film. The resultant image is distorted because of the unequal distances of the various parts of the object from the film. This type of shape distortion is called *foreshortening* because it causes the radiographic image to be shorter than the object. Fig. 5-6 shows the situation when the x-ray beam is oriented at right angles to the object but not the film. This results in *elongation,* with the object appearing longer on the film than its actual length.
2. *Orient the central ray perpendicular to the object and film.* Image shape distortion occurs if the object and film are parallel but the central ray is not directed at right angles to each. This is most evident on maxillary molar projections (Fig. 5-7). If the central ray is oriented with an excessive vertical angulation, the palatal roots appear disproportionately longer than the buccal roots.

The practitioner can prevent distortion errors by aligning the object and film parallel with each other and the central ray perpendicular to both.

Paralleling and Bisecting-Angle Techniques

From the earliest days of dental radiography, producing accurate images of dental structures that are normally visually obscured has been a clinical objective. One method for aligning the x-ray beam and film with the teeth and jaws that evolved early was the *bisecting-angle technique,* a term descriptive of the procedure (Fig. 5-8). In this method the film is placed as close to the teeth as possible without deforming it. However, when the film is in this position, it does not parallel the long axes of the teeth. This arrangement inherently causes distortion. Nevertheless, by directing the central ray perpendicular to an imaginary plane that bisects the angle between the teeth and the film, the practitioner can make the length of the tooth's image on the film correspond to the actual length of the tooth. This angle between a tooth and the film is especially apparent when radiographing teeth in the maxilla or anterior mandible. Even though the projected length of a tooth is correct, the image is still distorted because the film and object are not parallel and the x-ray beam is not directed at right angles to them. This distortion tends to increase along the image toward the apex.

When the central ray is not perpendicular to the bisector plane, the length of the image of a projected tooth changes. If the central ray is directed at an angle that is more positive than perpendicular to the bisector, the image of the tooth is *foreshortened.* Likewise, if it is inclined with more negative angulation to the bisector, the image is *elongated.* In recent years, the bisecting-angle technique has been used less frequently for general periapical radiography as use of the paralleling technique has increased.

The paralleling technique is the preferred method for making intraoral radiographs. It derives its name as the result of placing the film parallel with the long axis of the tooth (Fig. 5-9). This procedure minimizes image distortion and best incorporates the imaging principles described in the first three sections of this chapter.

To achieve this parallel orientation, the practitioner often must position the film toward the middle of the oral cavity, away from the teeth. Although this allows the teeth and film to be parallel, it results in some image magnification and loss of definition by increasing penumbra. As a consequence, the paralleling technique

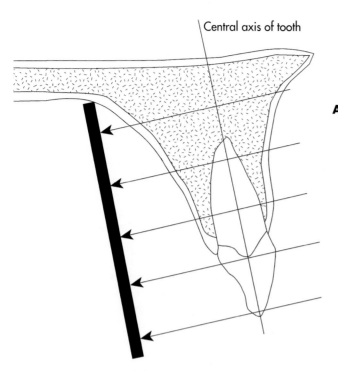

FIG. **5-9** In the paralleling technique the central ray is directed at a right angle to the central axes of the object and the film.

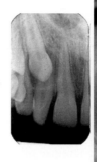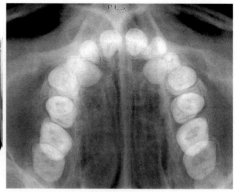

FIG. **5-10** **A,** The periapical radiograph shows impacted canine lying apical to roots of lateral incisor and first premolar. Note external root resorption of lateral incisor. **B,** The vertex occlusal view shows that the canine lies palatal to the roots of the lateral incisor and first premolar.

also uses a relatively long open-ended aiming cylinder ("cone") to increase the focal spot–to-object distance. This directs only the most central and parallel rays of the beam to the film and teeth and reduces image magnification while increasing image sharpness and resolution. The paralleling technique has benefited from the development of fast-speed film emulsions, which allow relatively short exposure times in spite of an increased target-to-object distance.

Because it is desirable to position the film near the middle of the oral cavity with the paralleling technique, film holders should be used to support the film in the patient's mouth. Chapter 8 discusses film-holding instruments and techniques for intraoral radiography using the paralleling technique.

Object Localization

In clinical practice, the dentist must often derive three-dimensional information concerning patients from a radiograph. The dentist may wish to use radiographs, for example, to determine the location of a foreign object or an impacted tooth within the jaw. Two methods are frequently used to obtain such three-dimensional information. The first is to examine two films projected at right angles to each other. The second method is to employ the so-called tube shift technique.

Fig. 5-10 shows the first method, in which *two projections taken at right angles to one another* localize an object in or about the maxilla in three dimensions. In clinical practice the position of an object on each radiograph is noted relative to the anatomic landmarks. This allows the observer to determine the position of the object or area of interest. For example, if a radiopacity is found near the apex of the first molar on a periapical radiograph, the dentist may take an occlusal projection to identify its mediolateral position. The occlusal film may reveal a calcification in the soft tissues located laterally or medially to the body of the mandible. This information is important in determining the treatment required. The right-angle (or cross-section) technique is best for the mandible. On a maxillary occlusal projection the superimposition of features in the anterior part of the skull may frequently obscure the area of interest.

The second method used to identify the spatial position of an object is the *tube shift technique.* Other names for this procedure are the *buccal object rule* and *Clark's rule* (Clark described it in 1910). The rationale for this procedure derives from the manner in which the relative positions of radiographic images of two separate objects change when the projection angle at which the images were made is changed.

Fig. 5-11 shows two radiographs of an object exposed at different angles. Compare the position of the object in question on each radiograph with the reference structures. If the tube is shifted and directed at the reference object (e.g., the apex of a tooth) from a more mesial angulation and the object in question also moves mesially with respect to the reference object, the object lies lingual to the reference object.

Alternatively, if the tube is shifted mesially and the object in question appears to move distally, it lies on the buccal aspect of the reference object (Fig. 5-12). These

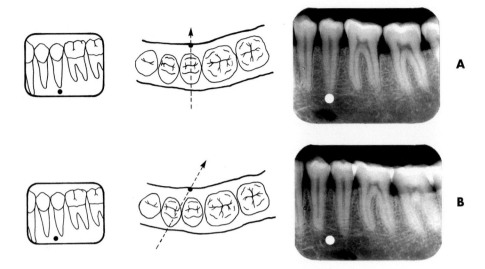

FIG. **5-11** The position of an object may be determined with respect to reference structures using the tube shift technique. In **A,** an object on the lingual surface of the mandible may appear apical to the second premolar. When another radiograph is made of this region angulated from the mesial, **B,** the object appears to have moved mesially with respect to the second premolar apex ("same lingual" in the acronym *SLOB*).

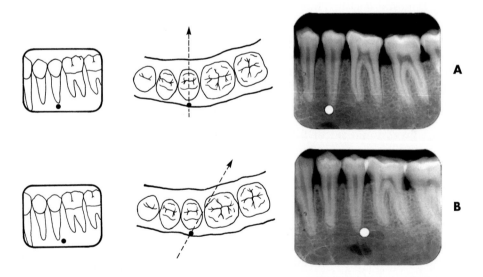

FIG. **5-12** The position of an object can be determined with respect to reference structures using the tube shift technique. In **A,** an object on the buccal surface of the mandible may appear apical to the second premolar. When another radiograph is made of this region angulated from the mesial, **B,** the object appears to have moved distally with respect to the second premolar apex ("opposite buccal" in the acronym *SLOB*).

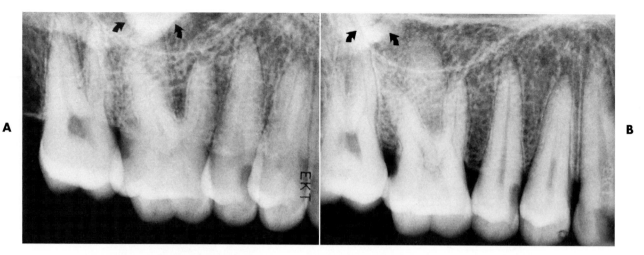

FIG. **5-13** The position of the maxillary zygomatic process in relation to the roots of the molars can help in identifying the orientation of projections. In **A** the inferior border of the process lies over the palatal root of the first molar, whereas in **B** it lies posterior to the palatal root of the first molar. This indicates that when **A** was made, the beam was oriented more from the posterior than when **B** was made. The same conclusion can be reached independently by examining the roots of the first molar. In **A** the palatal root lies behind the distobuccal root, but in **B** it lies between the two buccal roots.

relations can be easily remembered by the acronym *SLOB*: *S*ame *L*ingual, *O*pposite *B*uccal. Thus if the object in question appears to move in the same direction with respect to the reference structures as the x-ray tube, it is on the lingual aspect of the reference object; if it appears to move in the opposite direction as the x-ray tube, it is on the buccal aspect. If it does not move with respect to the reference object, it lies at the same depth (in the same vertical plane) as the reference object.

Examination of a conventional set of full-mouth films with this rule in mind demonstrates that the incisive foramen is indeed located lingual (palatal) to the roots of the central incisors and that the mental foramen lies buccal to the roots of the premolars. This technique assists in determining the position of impacted teeth, presence of foreign objects, and other abnormal conditions. It works just as well when the x-ray machine is moved in the vertical plane as in the horizontal plane.

As sometimes happens, the dentist may have two radiographs of a region of the dentition that were made at different angles, but no record exists of the orientation of the x-ray machine. Comparison of the anatomy displayed on the images helps distinguish changes in horizontal or vertical angulation. A more reliable method, however, is to compare the image fields (i.e., the changed positions of the bony anatomy with respect to the teeth).

In Fig. 5-13, *A*, the image of a lateral incisor on an incisor view is projected more from the mesial than the canine view. In Fig. 5-13, *B*, the relative positions of osseous landmarks—such as the inferior border of the

zygomatic process of the maxilla and the anterior border of the mandibular ramus—with respect to the teeth help identify changes in horizontal or vertical angulation. These two structures lie buccal to the teeth and appear to move mesially as the x-ray beam is oriented more from the distal. Similarly, as the angulation of the beam is increased vertically, the zygomatic process is projected occlusally over the teeth.

BIBLIOGRAPHY

Barr JH, Gron P: Palate contour as a limiting factor in intraoral x-ray technique, *Oral Surg* 12:459, 1959.

Clark CA: A method of ascertaining the relative position of unerupted teeth by means of film radiographs, *Proc R Soc Med Odontol Sect* 3:87, 1910.

Fitzgerald GM: Dental roentgenography. II. Vertical angulation, film placement and increased object-film distance, *J Am Dent Assoc* 34:160, 1947.

Fitzgerald GM: Dental roentgenography. III. The roentgenographic periapical survey of the upper molar region, *J Am Dent Assoc* 38:293, 1949.

Langlalis RA, Langland OE, Morris CR: Radiographic localization techniques, *Dent Radiogr Photogr* 52:69, 1979.

McCormack FW: Dental roentgenology: a technical procedure for furthering the advancement toward anatomical accuracy, *J S Calif Dent Assoc* 13:1, 1937.

McCormack FW: A plea for a standardized technique for oral radiography, with an illustrated classification of findings and their verified interpretation, *J Dent Res* 2:467, 1920.

Richards AG: The buccal object rule, *Dent Radiogr Photogr* 53:37, 1980.

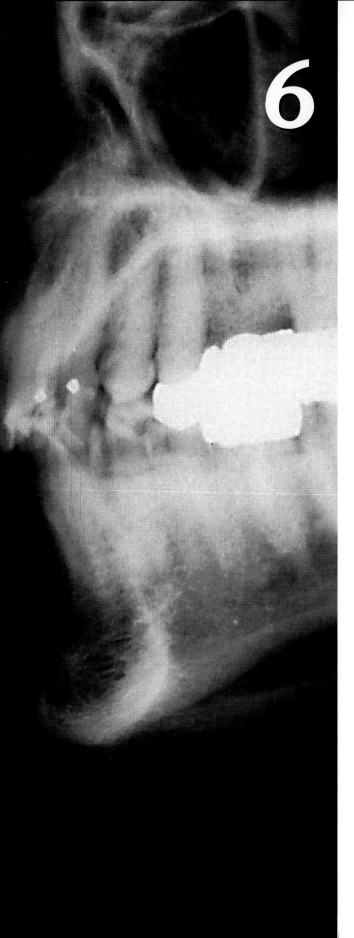

6 Processing X-Ray Film

The recording medium (image receptor) most frequently used in dental radiography is radiographic film. When a beam of photons exits an object and exposes an x-ray film, it chemically changes the photosensitive silver halide crystals in the film emulsion. These chemically altered silver bromide crystals constitute the latent (invisible) image on the film. The developing process converts the latent image into the visible radiographic image.

Formation of the Latent Image

Film emulsion consists of photosensitive crystals containing primarily silver bromide and small amounts of silver iodide suspended in a vehicle and layered on a thin sheet of transparent plastic base. These crystals contain a few free silver ions (interstitial silver ions) in the spaces between the crystalline lattice atoms (Figs. 6-1 and 6-2). Physical distortions occur in the regular array of the silver and bromide ions in the crystals when relatively large iodide ions are included (see Fig. 6-2, *A*). The silver halide crystals also may be chemically sensitized by the addition of trace amounts of sulfur compounds, which bind to the surface of the crystals. The sulfur compounds play a crucial role in image formation. Along with physical irregularities in the crystal produced by iodide ions, sulfur compounds create the sensitivity sites that contribute to latent image formation. The sensitivity sites begin the process of image formation by trapping the electrons generated when the emulsion is irradiated. Each crystal has many such sensitivity sites.

When the silver halide crystals are irradiated, x-ray photons interact primarily with the bromide ions by Compton and photoelectric interactions (see Fig. 6-2, *B*). These interactions result in the removal of an electron

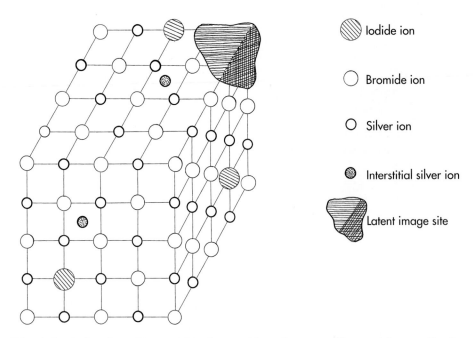

FIG. **6-1**   A silver bromide crystal in the emulsion of an x-ray film contains mostly silver and bromide ions with small amounts of iodide ions in a crystal lattice. Free interstitial silver ions and areas of trace chemicals serve as latent image sites.

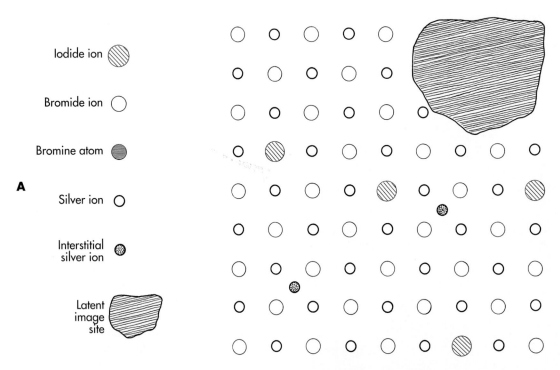

FIG. **6-2**   *Formation of the latent image.* **A,** A crystal contains silver, bromide, and iodide ions; before exposure it also has some interstitial silver ions and latent image sites.

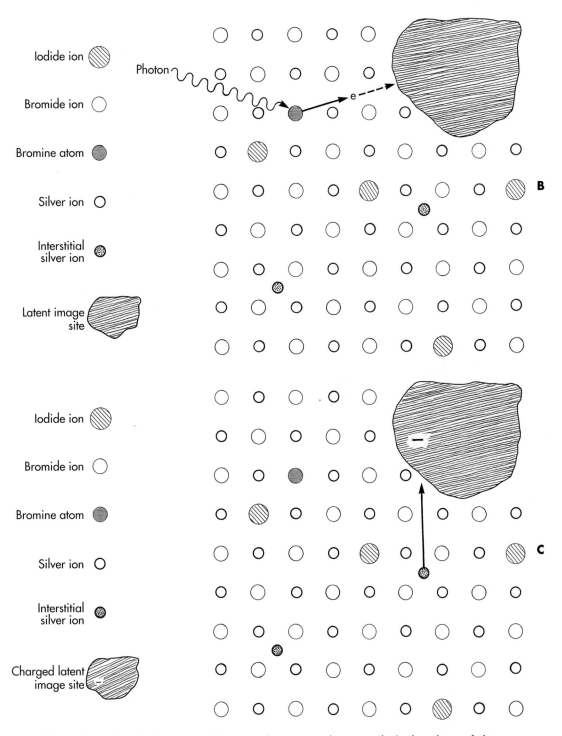

FIG. **6-2, cont'd   B,** Exposure of the crystal to an x-ray beam results in the release of electrons, usually by interaction with the bromide ions. Bromide ions are converted to bromine atoms, and the recoil electrons have sufficient kinetic energy to move about in the crystal. When they strike a latent image site, they impart a negative charge to this region. **C,** Free interstitial silver ions (with a positive charge) are attracted to the negatively charged latent image site.

Continued.

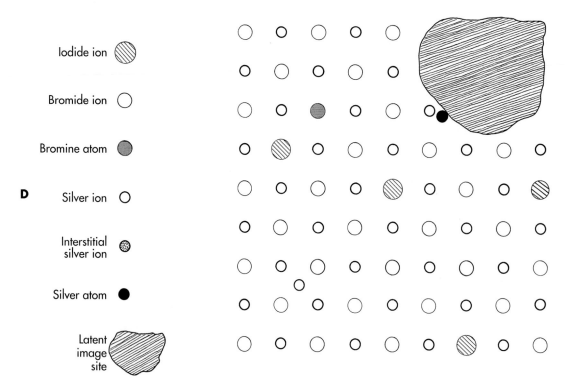

FIG. **6-2, cont'd** **D,** When the silver ions reach the site, they acquire an electron and become silver atoms; these silver atoms constitute the latent image. Developer causes the silver atoms to initiate the conversion of silver ions in the crystal into a grain of metallic silver.

from the bromide ions. By the loss of an electron a bromide ion is converted into a neutral bromine atom. The free electrons move through the crystal until they come across a sensitivity site, where they become trapped and impart a negative charge to the site. The negatively charged sensitivity site attracts positively charged free interstitial silver ions (see Fig. 6-2, *C*). When a silver ion reaches the negatively charged sensitivity site, it is reduced and forms a neutral atom of metallic silver (see Fig. 6-2, *D*). These neutral silver atoms form the latent image site. This process occurs many times at a single site within a crystal.

The metallic silver at each latent image site renders the crystals sensitive to development and image formation. The larger the aggregate of silver atoms, the more sensitive the crystal is to the effects of the developer. Most latent image sites that are capable of being developed in an optimally exposed film have four or five silver atoms. Developer converts crystals with metallic silver latent image sites into black, solid silver metallic grains that can be visualized. Fixer removes the unexposed, undeveloped silver halide crystals, leaving the film clear in unexposed areas.

Processing Solutions

Film processing involves the following procedures:

1. Exposed film is immersed in developer solution.
2. The film is rinsed in a running water bath.
3. The film is immersed in fixing solution.
4. The film is washed in a running water bath.
5. The film is dried and mounted for viewing.

This chapter describes the function of processing solutions. Procedures for each of these steps are described later.

DEVELOPER SOLUTION

The developer reduces all silver ions in the exposed crystals of silver halide (with a latent image) to flecks of black metallic silver (Fig. 6-3). To produce a diagnostic image, this reduction process must be restricted to crystals containing a latent image. Thus the reducing agents used as developers are those that are catalyzed by the metallic silver at the latent image sites. The metallic silver appears to act as a bridge by which electrons from the developing solution (reducing agents or chemical

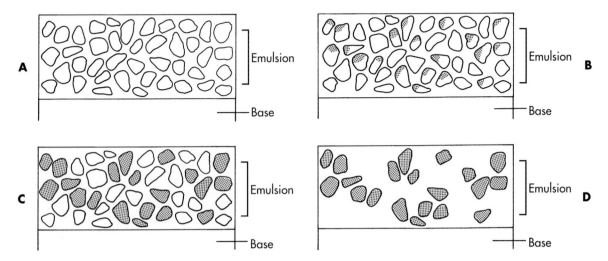

FIG. **6-3** *Emulsion changes during film processing.* **A,** Before exposure, many silver bromide crystals are present in the emulsion. **B,** After exposure, the exposed crystals containing silver particles at latent image sites constitute the latent image *(shaded areas in the crystals).* **C,** The developing solution converts the exposed crystals containing silver particles at the latent image sites into grains of metallic silver. **D,** The fixing solution and washing procedure dissolve and wash away the unexposed, undeveloped silver bromide crystals. (Courtesy C.L. Crabtree, DDS, Bureau of Radiological Health, Rockville, Md.)

electron donors) can reach silver ions in the crystal and convert them to metallic silver. Individual crystals are developed completely or not at all during the recommended developing times. Variations in density on the processed radiographs are the result of different ratios of developed (exposed) and undeveloped (unexposed) crystals. Areas with many exposed crystals are denser (blacker) because of their higher concentration of black metallic silver granules after development. If the developer remains too long in contact with silver bromide halide crystals that do not contain a latent image, it slowly reduces them also and thereby overdevelops the image.

When an exposed film is developed, the developer initially has no visible effect (Fig. 6-4). After this initial phase, the density increases, very rapidly at first and then more slowly. Eventually all the exposed crystals develop (become reduced to black metallic silver), and the developing agent starts to reduce the unexposed crystals. The development of unexposed crystals results in chemical fog on the film. The interval between maximal density and fogging explains why a properly exposed film does not become overdeveloped even though it may be in contact with the developer longer than the recommended interval. Thus dark films usually are the result of overexposure rather than overdevelopment. An overexposed film develops larger, more effective latent image sites, which explains why such a film develops acceptable density with a shorter developing time than

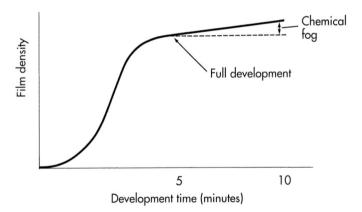

FIG. **6-4** Relationship between film density and development time. The density of film rises quickly initially and then levels off, increasing more slowly because of chemical fogging.

does a film that has been properly exposed. Unfortunately, this results in unnecessary overexposure of the patient.

The developing solution contains four components, all dissolved in water: (1) developer, (2) activator, (3) preservative, and (4) restrainer.

Developer

The primary function of the developing solution is to amplify the latent image by converting the exposed silver halide crystals into metallic silver grains. This process begins at the latent image sites, where electrons from the developing agents are conducted into the silver halide crystal and reduce the constituent silver ions (approximately 1 billion to 10 billion) to solid grains of metallic silver. Unexposed crystals, those without latent images, are unaffected during the time required for reduction of the exposed crystals. Two developing agents are used in dental radiology: a pyrazolidone-type compound, usually Phenidone (1-phenyl-3-pyrazolidone), and hydroquinone (paradihydroxy benzene). Pheni-done serves as the first electron donor that converts silver ions to metallic silver at the latent image site. This electron transfer generates the oxidized form of Pheni-done. Hydroquinone provides an electron to reduce the oxidized Phenidone back to its original active state so it can continue to reduce silver halide grains to metallic silver.

Activator

The developers are active only at alkaline pH values, usually around 10. This is achieved with the addition of alkali compounds (activators) such as sodium or potassium hydrozide. Buffers are used to maintain this condition—usually sodium carbonate, sodium hydroxide, or sodium metaborate or tetraborate. The activators also cause the gelatin to swell so that the developing agents can diffuse more rapidly into the emulsion and reach the suspended silver bromide crystals.

Preservative

The developing solution contains an antioxidant or preservative, usually sodium sulfite. The preservative protects the developers from oxidation by atmospheric oxygen and thus extends their useful life. The preservative also combines with the brown oxidized developer to produce a colorless soluble compound. If not removed, oxidation products interfere with the developing reaction and stain the film.

Restrainer

Bromide, usually as potassium or sodium bromide, is added to the developing solution to restrain development of unexposed silver halide crystals. Although bromide depresses the reduction of both exposed and unexposed crystals, it is much more effective in depressing the reduction of unexposed crystals. Consequently, the restrainer acts as an antifog agent.

DEVELOPER REPLENISHER

Developer becomes inactivated with use and by exposure to oxygen. Accordingly, the developing solution of both manual and automatic developers should be replenished with fresh solution each morning. The recommended amount to be added daily is 8 ounces of fresh developer (replenisher) per gallon of developing

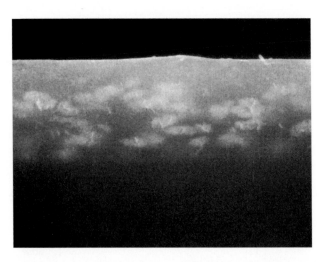

FIG. **6-5** Scanning electron micrograph of a processed emulsion of Kodak Ultra-Speed dental x-ray film (5000 ×). Note the white-appearing silver grains above the base. (Courtesy Eastman Kodak, Rochester, N.Y.)

solution. This assumes the development of an average of 30 periapical or five panoramic films per day. Some of the used solution may need to be removed to make room for the replenisher.

RINSING

After development the film emulsion swells and becomes saturated with developer. At this point the films are rinsed in water for 30 seconds with continuous, gentle agitation before they are placed in the fixer. Rinsing dilutes the developer, slowing the development process. It also removes the alkali activator, preventing neutralization of the acid fixer. This rinsing process is typical for manual processing but is not used with automatic processing.

FIXING SOLUTION

The primary function of fixing solution is to dissolve and remove the undeveloped silver halide crystals from the emulsion (see Fig. 6-3, *D*). The presence of unexposed crystals causes film to be opaque. If these crystals are not removed, the image on the resultant radiograph is dark and nondiagnostic. Fig. 6-5 is a photomicrograph of film emulsion showing the silver grains after fixer has removed the unexposed silver halide crystals. (Compare it with Fig. 4-2, *A*, which shows the unprocessed emulsion.) A second function of fixing solution is to harden and shrink the film emulsion. As with developer, fixer should be replenished daily at the rate of 8 ounces per gallon.

Fixing solution also contains four components, all dissolved in water: (1) clearing agent, (2) acidifier, (3) preservative, and (4) hardener.

Clearing Agent

After development the film emulsion must be cleared by dissolving and removing the unexposed silver halide. An aqueous solution of ammonium thiosulfate ("hypo") dissolves the silver halide grains. It forms stable, water-soluble complexes with silver ions, which then diffuse from the emulsion. The clearing agent does not have a rapid effect on the metallic silver grains in the film emulsion, but excessive fixation results in a gradual loss of film density because the grains of silver slowly dissolve in the acetic acid of the fixing solution.

Acidifier

The fixing solution contains an acetic acid buffer system (pH 4 to 4.5) to keep the fixer pH constant. The acidic pH is required to promote good diffusion of thiosulfate into the emulsion and of silver thiosulfate complex out of the emulsion. The acid fixing solution also inactivates any carryover developing agents in the film emulsion, blocking continued development of any unexposed crystals while the film is in the fixing tank.

Preservative

Sodium (or ammonium) sulfite is the preservative in the fixing solution, as it is in the developer. It prevents oxidation of the thiosulfate clearing agent, which is unstable in the acid environment of the fixing solution. It also binds with any colored oxidized developer carried over into the fixing solution and effectively removes it from the solution, which prevents oxidized developer from staining the film.

Hardener

The hardening agents most often used are aluminum salts. Aluminum complexes with the gelatin during fixing and prevents damage to the gelatin during subsequent handling. The hardeners also reduce swelling of the emulsion during the final wash. This lessens mechanical damage to the emulsion and limits water absorption, thus shortening drying time.

WASHING

After fixing, the processed film is washed in a sufficient flow of water for an adequate time to ensure removal of all thiosulfate ions and silver thiosulfate complexes. Washing efficiency declines rapidly when the water temperature falls below 60° F. Any silver compound or thiosulfate that remains because of improper washing discolors and causes stains, which are most apparent in the radiopaque (light) areas. This discoloration results from the thiosulfate reacting with silver to form brown silver sulfide, which can obscure diagnostic information.

Darkroom Equipment

The darkroom should be convenient to the x-ray machines and dental operatories and should be at least 4 × 5 feet (1.2 × 1.5 m) (Fig. 6-6). One of the most important requirements is that it be lightproof. To accomplish this, a light-tight door or doorless maze (if space permits) is used. The door should have a lock to prevent accidental opening, which might allow an unexpected flood of light that can ruin opened films. The room must be well ventilated for the comfort of those working in the area and to exhaust the heat from the dryer and moisture from the drying films. Also, a comfortable room temperature helps maintain optimal conditions for developing, fixing, and washing solutions. If supplies (including unexposed x-ray film) are to be stored in the darkroom, ventilation is doubly important because temperatures of 90° F or higher can cause a generalized increase in density (film fog) on the film.

SAFELIGHTING

Equipment

The processing room should have both white illumination and safelighting. Safelighting is low-intensity illumination of relatively long wavelength (red) that does not rapidly affect open film but permits one to see well enough to work in the area. It is best to place one safelight (Fig. 6-7) above the work area on the wall behind the processing tanks and somewhat to the right of the fixing tank. To minimize the fogging effect of prolonged exposure, the safelight should have a 15-watt bulb and should be mounted at least 4 feet above the surface where opened films are handled.

X-ray films are very sensitive to the blue-green region of the spectrum and less sensitive to yellow and red wavelengths. Accordingly, the red GBX-2 filter is recommended as a safelight in a darkroom where either intraoral or extraoral films are handled (Fig. 6-8). Film handling under a safelight should be limited to about 5 minutes because film emulsion shows some sensitivity to light from a safelight with prolonged exposure. The older ML-2 filters (yellow light) are not appropriate for fast intraoral dental film or extraoral panoramic or cephalometric film.

PROCESSING TANKS

All dental offices must have the capability to develop radiographs by tank processing. The tank must have hot and cold running water and a means of maintaining the temperature between 60° and 75° F. A practical size for a dental office is a master tank about 20 × 25 cm (8 × 10 inches) that can serve as a water jacket for two removable inserts that fit inside (Fig. 6-9). The insert tanks

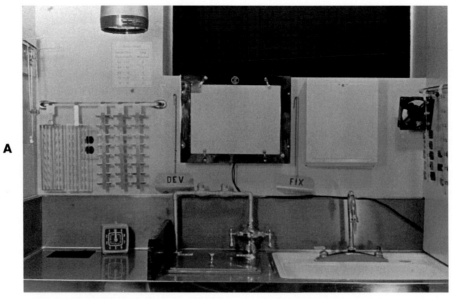

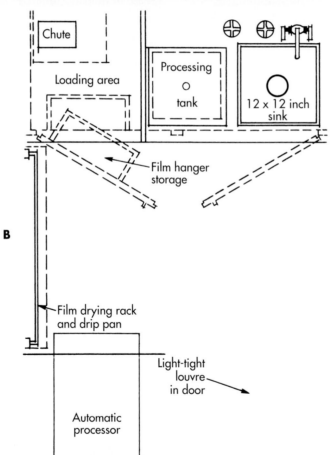

FIG. **6-6** **A,** Darkroom work area. *Left,* Film mounting area, timer, film racks, and safe-light above; *middle,* developing and fixing tanks below the viewbox and stirring paddles; *right,* sink and drying racks with fan. **B,** Floor plan. (**A,** Courtesy C.L. Crabtree, M.D., Bureau of Radiological Health, Rockville, Md; **B,** courtesy Eastman Kodak, Rochester, N.Y.)

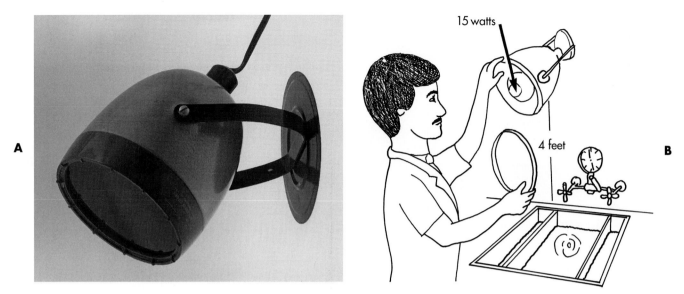

FIG. **6-7** **A,** A safelight may be mounted on the wall or ceiling in the darkroom and should be at least 4 feet from the work surface. **B,** The safelight uses a GBX-2 filter and 15-watt bulb.

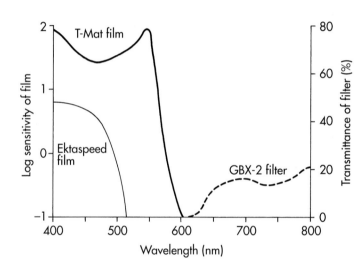

FIG. **6-8** Spectral sensitivities of T-Mat film *(heavy line)* and Ektaspeed film *(thin line)* shown with the transmission characteristics of a GBX-2 filter *(broken line)*. Note that the films are more sensitive in the blue-green portion of the spectrum (shorter than 600 nm); the GBX-2 filter transmits primarily red light (longer than 600 nm).

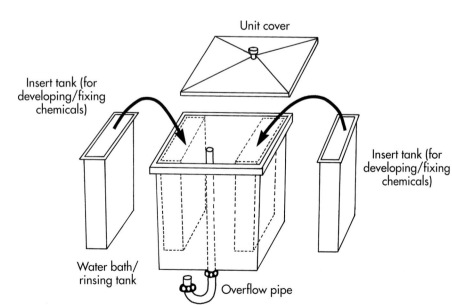

FIG. **6-9** *Processing tank.* The developing and fixing tanks are inserted into a bath of running water with an overflow drain.

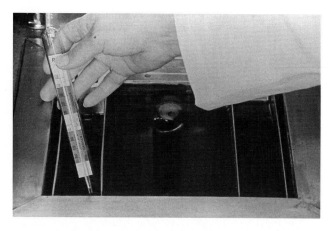

FIG. **6-10** A thermometer may float in the tank or may be attached to the tank wall. (Courtesy C.L. Crabtree, DDS, Bureau of Radiological Health, Rockville, Md.)

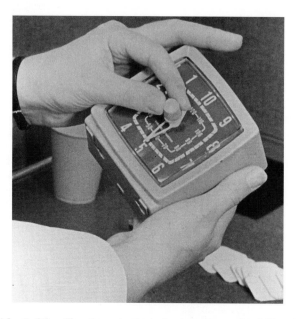

FIG. **6-11** The timer is started when the rack of films is placed in the developer. (Courtesy C.L. Crabtree, DDS, Bureau of Radiological Health, Rockville, Md.)

usually hold 3.8 L (1 gallon) of developer or fixer and are placed within the outer, larger master tank. The outer tank holds the running water for maintaining the temperature of the developer and fixer in the insert tanks and for washing films. The developer customarily is placed in the insert tank on the left side of the master tank and the fixer in the insert tank on the right. All three tanks should be made of stainless steel, which does not react with the processing solutions and is easy to clean. The master tank should have a cover to reduce oxidation of the processing solutions, protect the developing film from accidental exposure to light, and minimize evaporation of the processing solutions.

THERMOMETER

The temperature of the developing, fixing, and washing solutions should be closely controlled. A thermometer can be left in the water circulating through the master tank to monitor its temperature. The most desirable thermometers clip onto the side of the tank (Fig. 6-10). Thermometers should contain alcohol or metal but not mercury because they could break and contaminate the processor or solutions.

TIMER

The x-ray film must be exposed to the processing chemicals for specific intervals. An interval timer is indispensable for controlling development and fixation times (Fig. 6-11).

DRYING RACKS

Two or three drying racks can be mounted on a convenient wall for film hangers. Drip trays are placed underneath the racks to catch water that may run off the wet films. An electric fan can be used to circulate the air and speed the drying of films, but it should not be pointed directly at the films. Also, cabinet dryers are available that circulate warm air around the film and accelerate drying. Excessive heat must be avoided because it may damage the emulsion. If dryers are installed in the darkroom, they should be ventilated outside the darkroom to preclude high humidity and heat (which are detrimental to any unexposed film stored in the room).

Manual Processing Procedures

Manual processing of film requires the following eight steps:

1. *Replenish solutions*—The first step in manual tank processing is to replenish the developer and fixer. Eight ounces per gallon of fresh developer (replenisher) and fixer are added to maintain the proper strength of each solution. The levels of the solutions are checked to ensure that the developer and fixer cover the films on the top clips of the film hangers.
2. *Stir solutions*—Next, the developer and fixing solution are stirred to mix the chemicals and equalize the temperature throughout the tanks. To prevent cross-contamination, a separate paddle is used for each solution. It is best to label one paddle for the developer and the other for the fixer. Because proper developing time varies with the temperature of the solution, the temperature of the developer should be checked after stirring.

3. *Mount films on hangers*—Using only safelight illumination in the darkroom, the exposed film is removed from its lightproof packet or cassette. The films are held only by their edges to avoid damage to the film surface. Care must be taken that the film is not bent and the emulsion is not scratched or touched with wet fingers. The bare film is clipped onto a film hanger, one film to a clip (Fig. 6-12). To avoid any possible confusion later, the film racks are labeled with the patient's name and the exposure date.

4. *Set timer*—The temperature of the developer is checked, and the interval timer is set to the time indicated by the manufacturer for the solution temperature. For intraoral film processing in conventional solutions, the following development times are used:

TEMPERATURE	DEVELOPMENT TIME
68° F	5 minutes
70° F	4½ minutes
72° F	4 minutes
76° F	3 minutes
80° F	2½ minutes

Processing films at either higher or lower temperatures and for longer or shorter times than recommended by the manufacturer reduces the contrast of the processed film. Also, processing too long or at temperatures higher than those recommended can result in film fog, which may diminish film contrast and diagnostic information.

5. *Develop*—The timer mechanism is started, and the hanger and films are immersed immediately in the developer. The hanger is agitated mildly for 5 seconds to sweep air bubbles off the film. The films are left in the developer for the predetermined time without further agitation. When the films are removed, the excess developer is drained into the wash bath.

6. *Rinse*—After development, the film hanger is removed from the developer and placed in the running water bath for 30 seconds. The films are agitated continuously in the rinse water to remove excess developer and thus slow development and minimize contamination of the fixer.

7. *Fix*—The hanger and film are then placed in the fixer solution for 4 minutes and agitated for 5 seconds every 30 seconds. This eliminates bubbles and brings fresh fixer into contact with the emulsion. Excess fixation (several hours) removes some of the metallic silver grains, diminishing the density of the film. When the films are removed, the excess fixer is drained into the wash bath.

8. *Wash and dry*—After fixation of the films is complete, they are placed in running water for at least

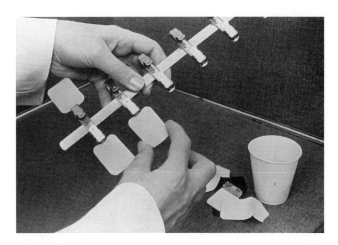

FIG. **6-12** Films are mounted securely on film clips. Film is always held by its edges to avoid fingerprints on the image. (Courtesy C.L. Crabtree, DDS, Bureau of Radiological Health, Rockville, Md.)

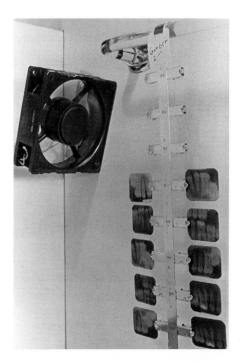

FIG. **6-13** Films dry in circulating air under a fan. (Courtesy C.L. Crabtree, DDS, Bureau of Radiological Health, Rockville, Md.)

10 minutes to remove residual processing solutions. After the films have been washed, surface moisture is removed by gently shaking excess water from the films and hanger. The films are dried in circulating, moderately warm air (Fig. 6-13). If the films dry rapidly with small drops of water clinging to their surface, the areas under the drops dry more slowly than the surrounding areas. This uneven drying causes distortion of the gelatin, leaving a drying artifact in some cases. The

result is spots that frequently are visible and detract from the usefulness of the finished radiograph. After drying, the films are ready to mount.

Rapid-Processing Chemicals

In recent years a number of manufacturers have produced rapid-processing solutions. These solutions typically develop films in 15 seconds and fix them in 15 seconds at room temperature. They have the same general formulation as conventional processing solutions but often are more concentrated. They are especially advantageous in endodontics and in emergency situations, when short processing time is essential. Although the resultant images may be satisfactory, they often do not achieve the same degree of contrast as films processed conventionally, and they may discolor over time. After viewing, rapidly processed films are placed in conventional fixing solution for 4 minutes and washed for 10 minutes. This improves the contrast and helps keep them stable in storage. Conventional solutions are preferred for most routine use.

Changing Solutions

All processing solutions deteriorate as a result of continued use and exposure to air. Although regular replenishment of the developer and fixer prolongs their useful life, the buildup of reaction products eventually causes these solutions to cease functioning properly. Exhaustion of the developer results from oxidation of the developing agents, depletion of the hydroquinone, and buildup of bromide. Use of exhausted developer results in films that show reduced density and contrast. When fixer becomes exhausted, silver thiosulfate complexes form and halide ions build up. The increased concentration of silver thiosulfate complexes slows the rate of diffusion of these complexes from the emulsion. The halide ions slow the rate of clearing of unexposed silver halide crystals. These changes result in films with incomplete clearing that turn brown with age. With regular replenishment, solutions may last 3 or 4 weeks before they must be changed. When the developer and fixer are replaced, the solutions must be prepared according to the directions on the containers.

A simple procedure can help in determining when solutions should be changed. A double film packet instead of a single film packet is exposed on one projection for the first patient radiographed after new solutions have been prepared. One film is placed in the patient's chart, and the other is mounted on a corner of a viewbox in the darkroom. As successive films are processed, they are compared with this reference film. Loss of image contrast and density become evident as the solutions deteriorate, indicating when the time has come to change them. The fixer is changed when the developer is changed.

Automatic Film Processing

Equipment is available that automates all processing steps (Fig. 6-14). Although automatic processing has a number of advantages, the most important is the time saved. Depending on the equipment and the temperature of operation, an automatic processor requires only 4 to 6 minutes to develop, fix, wash, and dry a film. Many dental automatic processors have a light-shielded (daylight loading) compartment in which the operator can unwrap films and feed them into the machine without working in a darkroom. This is desirable because the individual doing the developing does not have to work in the dark. However, special care must be taken to maintain infection control when using these daylight loading compartments (see Chapter 7).

When extraoral films are processed, the light-shielded compartment is removed to provide room for feeding the larger film into the processor. Another attractive feature of the automatic system is that the density and contrast of the radiographs tend to be consistent. However, because of the higher temperature of the developer and the artifacts caused by rollers, the quality of films processed automatically often is not as high as that of those carefully developed manually. With automatically processed films, more grain usually is evident in the final image.

Whether automatic processing equipment is appropriate for a specific practice depends on the dentist and the nature and volume of the practice. The equipment is expensive and must be cleaned frequently. Also, the automated equipment may break down, and conventional darkroom equipment may be needed as a backup system.

MECHANISM

Automatic processors have an in-line arrangement. Typically, this consists of a transport mechanism that picks up the unwrapped film and passes it through the developing, fixing, washing, and drying sections (Fig. 6-15). The transport system most often used is a series of rollers driven by a constant-speed motor that operates through gears, belts, or chains. The rollers often consist of independent assemblies of multiple rollers in a rack, with one rack for each step in the operation. Although these assemblies are designed and positioned so that the film crosses over from one roller to the next, the opera-

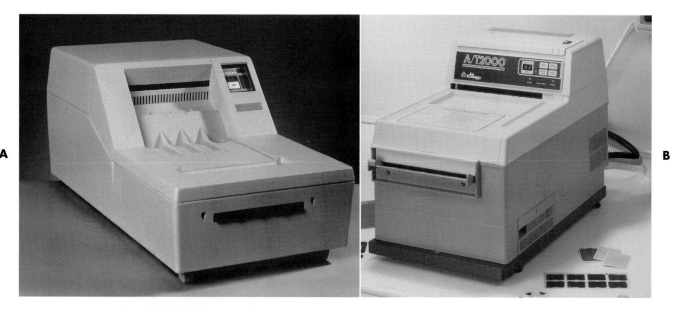

FIG. **6-14** *Automatic film processors.* **A,** Dent-X 9800. **B,** A/T 2000XR. (**A,** Courtesy Dent-X, Elmsford, N.Y.; **B,** courtesy Air Techniques, Inc., Hicksville, N.Y.)

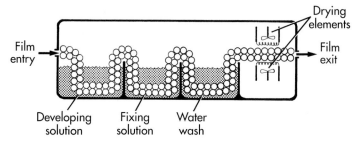

FIG. **6-15** Automatic film processors generally consist of a roller assembly that transports the film between the rollers through developing, fixing, washing, and drying stations.

tor may remove them independently for soaking, cleaning, and repairing.

The primary function of the rollers is to move the film through the developing solutions, but they also serve at least three other purposes. First, their motion helps keep the solutions agitated, which contributes to the uniformity of processing. Second, in the developer, fixer, and water tanks the rollers press on the film emulsion, forcing some solution out of the emulsion. The emulsions rapidly fill again with solution, thus promoting solution exchange. Finally, the top rollers at the crossover point between the developer and fixer tanks remove developing solution, minimizing carryover of developer into the fixer tank. This feature helps maintain the uniformity of processing chemicals.

The chemical compositions of the developer and fixer are modified to operate at higher temperatures than those used for manual processing and to meet the more rapid development, fixing, washing, and drying requirements of automatic processing. The fixer has an additional hardener that helps the emulsion withstand the rigors of the transport system.

REPLENISHMENT

It is important to maintain the constituents of the developer and fixer carefully to preserve the optimal sensitometric and physical properties of the film emulsion within the narrow limits imposed by the speed and temperature of automatic processing. As the activity of the developing and fixing solutions lessens, its effect on the film diminishes. To compensate for this loss of activity, some automatic processors include an automatic replenishment system, which adds fresh developer to the developer tank and fresh fixer to the fixer tank. As with manual processing, 8 ounces of fresh developer and fixer should be added per gallon of solution per day. This assumes an average workload of 30 intraoral or five extraoral films per day. Insufficient replenishment of the developer results in a loss of image contrast. Exhaustion of the fixing solution causes poor clearing of the film, insufficient hardening of the emulsion, and unreliable transport from the fixer assembly through the drying operation.

Management of Radiographic Wastes

To prevent environmental damage, many communities and states have passed laws governing the disposal of wastes. Such laws often derive from the federal Resource Conservation and Recovery Act of 1976. Although dental radiographic waste constitutes only a small potential hazard, it should be discarded properly. The primary ingredient of concern in processing solutions is the dissolved silver found in used fixer. Another material of concern is the lead foil found in film packets.

Several means are available for properly disposing of the silver and lead. Silver may be recovered from the fixer by using either metallic replacement or electroplating methods. Metallic replacement uses cartridges through which waste solutions are poured. In this process, iron goes into the solution and the silver precipitates as a sludge. In the electroplating method, the waste solutions come in contact with two electrodes, through which a current passes. The cathode captures the silver. In either case, the scrap silver can be sold to silver refiners and buyers.

The lead foil is separated from the packet and collected until enough has been accumulated to sell to a scrap metal dealer. Dental offices also should consider using companies licensed to pick up waste materials. The names of such companies can be found in the telephone directory or obtained from the state hazardous waste management agency.

Common Causes of Faulty Radiographs

Although film processing can produce radiographs of excellent quality, inattention to detail may lead to many problems and images that are diagnostically suboptimal. Poor radiographs contribute to a loss of diagnostic information and loss of professional and patient time. Box 6-1 presents a list of common causes of faulty radiographs. The steps necessary for correction are self-evident.

BOX **6-1**
Common Problems in Film Development

Light Radiographs (Fig. 6-16)
- Processing errors
  Underdevelopment (temperature too low; time too short; thermometer inaccurate)
  Depleted developer solution
  Diluted or contaminated developer
  Excessive fixation

- Underexposure
  Insufficient milliamperage
  Insufficient peak kilovoltage
  Insufficient time
  Film-source distance too great
  Film packet reversed in mouth (Fig. 6-17)

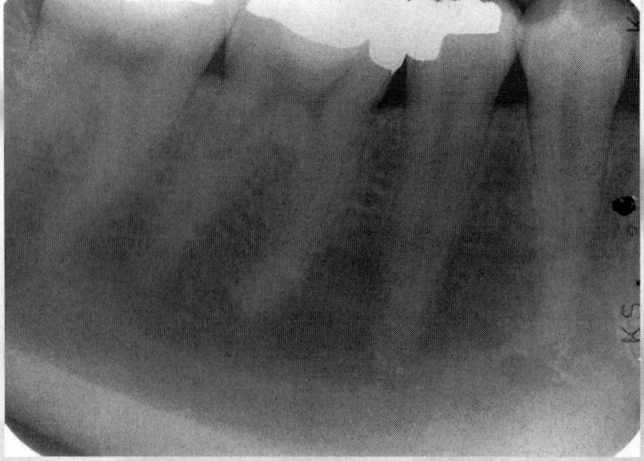

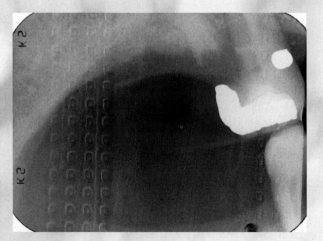

FIG. **6-16** A radiograph that is too light because of inadequate processing or insufficient exposure.

FIG. **6-17** A radiograph that is too light because the film packet was placed backward in the patient's mouth. Note the characteristic markings caused by exposure through the lead foil.

BOX **6-1**
Common Problems in Film Development—cont'd

Dark Radiographs (Fig. 6-18)

- Processing errors
  Overdevelopment (temperature too high; time too long)
  Developer concentration too high
  Inadequate fixation
  Accidental exposure to light
  Improper safelighting
- Overexposure
  Excessive milliamperage
  Excessive peak kilovoltage
  Excessive time
  Film-source distance too short

Insufficient Contrast (Fig. 6-19)

- Underdevelopment
- Underexposure
- Excessive peak kilovoltage
- Excessive film fog

Film Fog (Fig. 6-20)

- Improper safelighting (improper filter; excessive bulb wattage; inadequate distance between safelight and work surface; prolonged exposure to safelight)

- Light leaks (cracked safelight filter; light from doors, vents, or other sources)
- Overdevelopment
- Contaminated solutions
- Deteriorated film (stored at high temperature; stored at high humidity; exposed to radiation; outdated)

Dark Spots or Lines (Fig. 6-21)

- Fingerprint contamination
- Black wrapping paper sticking to film surface
- Film in contact with tank or another film during fixation
- Film contaminated with developer before processing
- Excessive bending of film
- Static discharge to film before processing
- Excessive roller pressure during automatic processing
- Dirty rollers in automatic processing

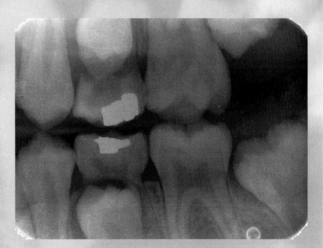

FIG. **6-19** A radiograph with insufficient contrast, showing gray enamel and gray pulp chambers.

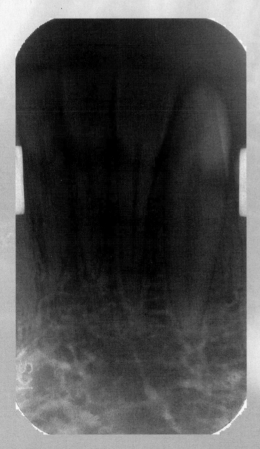

FIG. **6-18** A radiograph that is too dark because of overdevelopment or overexposure.

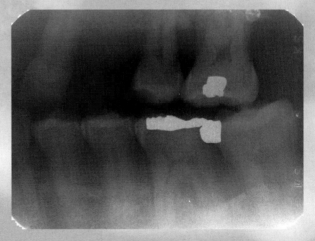

FIG. **6-20** Fogged radiograph marked by lack of image detail.

Continued.

BOX **6-1**

Common Problems in Film Development—cont'd

Light Spots (Fig. 6-22)
- Film contaminated with fixer before processing
- Film in contact with tank or another film during development
- Excessive bending of film

Yellow or Brown Stains
- Depleted developer
- Depleted fixer
- Insufficient washing
- Contaminated solurions

Blurring (Fig. 6-23)
- Movement of patient
- Movement of x-ray tube head
- Double exposure

Partial Images (Fig. 6-24)
- Top of film not immersed in developing solution
- Misalignment of x-ray tube head ("cone cut")

Emulsion Peel
- Abrasion of image during processing
- Excessive time in wash water

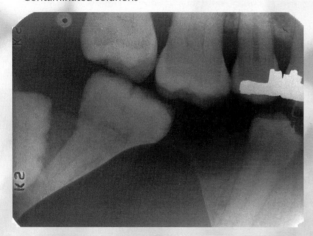

FIG. **6-21** Dark spot on an x-ray film caused by film contact with the tank wall during fixation.

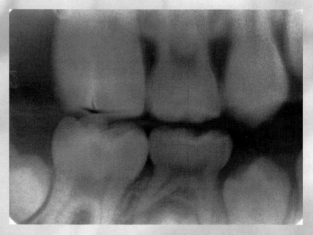

FIG. **6-23** Blurred radiograph caused by movement of the patient during exposure.

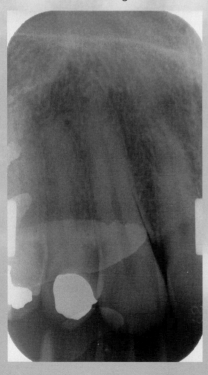

FIG. **6-22** Light spots on an x-ray film caused by film contact with drops of fixer before processing.

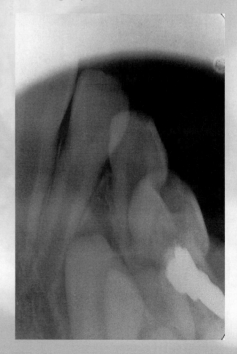

FIG. **6-24** Partial image caused by poor alignment of the tube head with the film.

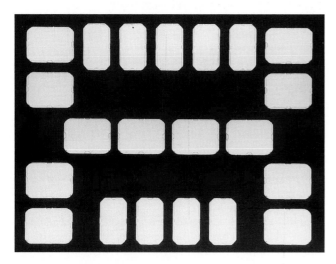

FIG. **6-25** Film mount for holding nine narrow anterior periapical views, eight posterior periapical view, and four bitewing views.

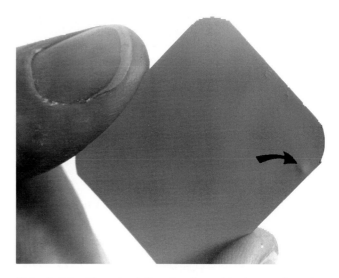

FIG. **6-26** The raised film dot *(arrow)* indicates the tube side of the film and identifies the patient's right and left sides.

Mounting Radiographs

Radiographs must be preserved and maintained in the most satisfactory and useful condition. Periapical, interproximal, and occlusal films are best handled and stored in a film mount (Fig. 6-25). The operator can handle them with greater ease and there is less chance of damaging the emulsion. Mounts are made of plastic or cardboard and may have a clear plastic window that covers and protects the film. However, the window may have scratches or imperfections that interfere with radiographic interpretation. The operator can arrange several films from the same individual in a film mount in the proper anatomic relationship. This facilitates correlation of the clinical and radiographic examinations. Opaque mounts are best because they prevent stray light from the viewbox from reaching the viewer's eyes.

The preferred method of positioning periapical and occlusal films in the film mount is to arrange them so that the images of the teeth are in the anatomic position and have the same relationship to the viewer as when the viewer faces the patient. The radiographs of the teeth in the right quadrants should be placed in the left side of the mount and those of the left quadrants in the right side. This system, advocated by the American Dental Association, allows the examiner's gaze to shift from radiograph to tooth without crossing the midline. The alternative arrangement, with the images of the right quadrants on the right side of the mount and those of the left quadrant on the left, is not recommended.

Identification Dot

A round impression in a corner of each film, the "dot," allows rapid and proper film orientation (Fig. 6-26). The manufacturer orients the film in the packet so that the convex side of the dot is toward the front of the packet and faces the source of radiation. Consequently, to mount the films with the images of the teeth in the anatomic position as described above, each film is first oriented with the convex side of the dot toward the viewer. Then, on the basis of the features of the teeth and anatomic landmarks in the adjacent bone, the films are placed in their normal sequential relationship in the mount.

DUPLICATING RADIOGRAPHS

Occasionally radiographs must be duplicated; this is best accomplished with duplicating film. The film to be duplicated is placed against the emulsion side of the duplicating film, and the two films are held in position by a glass-topped cassette or photographic printing frame. The films are exposed to light, which passes through the clear areas of the original radiograph and exposes the duplicating film. The duplicating film is then processed in conventional x-ray processing solutions.

Unlike conventional x-ray film, duplicating film gives a positive image. Thus areas exposed to light come out clear, as on the original radiograph. Duplication typically results in images with less resolution and more contrast than the original radiograph. The best images are obtained when a circular, ultraviolet light source is used. In contrast to the usual negative film, images on duplicating film that are too dark or too light are underexposed or overexposed, respectively.

BIBLIOGRAPHY

Curry TS et al: *Christensen's introduction to the physics of diagnostic radiology,* ed 3, Philadelphia, 1984, Lea & Febiger.

Fitterman AS et al: *Processing chemistry for medical imaging,* Technical and Scientific Monograph No 5, N-327, Rochester, N.Y., 1995, Eastman Kodak.

Fletcher JC: A comparison of Ektaspeed and Ultra-Speed films using manual and automatic processing solutions, *Oral Surg* 63:94, 1987.

Fredholm U, Julin P: Rapid developing of Ektaspeed dental film by increase of temperature, *Swed Dent J* 11:121, 1987.

Haist G: *Modern photographic processing,* vol 1, New York, 1979, Wiley & Sons.

Hashimoto K et al: Automatic processing: effects of temperature and time changes on sensitometric properties of Ultra-Speed and Ektaspeed films, *Oral Surg* 71:120, 1991.

Hedin M: Developing solutions for dental x-ray processors, *Swed Dent J* 13:261, 1989.

Kitts EL: The AAPM/RSNA physics tutorial for residents: physics and chemistry of film and processing, *Radiographics* 16:1467, 1996.

Mees DEK, James TH: *The theory of the photographic process,* New York, 1977, Macmillan.

Sturge JM, editor: *Neblette's handbook of photography and reprography: materials, processes, and systems,* New York, 1977, Van Nostrand Reinhold.

Thunthy KH et al: Automatic processing: effects of temperature and time changes on the sensitometric properties of light-sensitive films, *Oral Surg* 72:112, 1991.

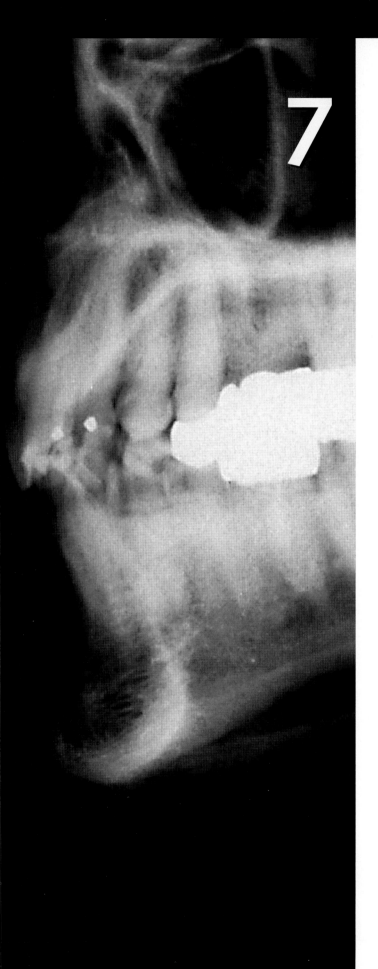

7

Radiographic Quality Assurance and Infection Control

Proper practice of dental radiology requires careful attention to detail, both in making and interpreting radiographs. This chapter focuses on the means of making radiographs and includes *quality assurance*, the methods used to ensure consistent high-quality radiographic processing conditions, and *infection control*, the methods used to avoid cross-contamination among patients and between patients and operators.

Quality Assurance

Because radiographs are indispensable for patient diagnosis, the dentist must ensure that optimal processing conditions are maintained. Quality assurance uses a plan of action to ensure radiographs of consistently high quality. This plan includes several routine assessments of x-ray systems and suggests corrective actions when necessary. The assessments include evaluation of the performance of x-ray machines, manual and automatic processing procedures, image receptors, and viewing conditions. Optimization of these conditions results in the most accurate diagnostic images and the lowest possible exposure for patients. Most of these steps are quickly accomplished, yet can have a significant influence on radiographic quality (Box 7-1). Further quality assurance is accomplished by keeping records of all test results.

BOX 7-1
Schedule of Radiographic Quality Assurance Procedures

Daily
Compare radiographs to reference film
Enter findings in a retake log
Replenish processing solutions
Check temperature of processing solutions for proper time-temperature processing
Make step-wedge test of processing system

Weekly
Replace processing solutions weekly or on alternate weeks
Clean manual and automatic processing equipment
Check and clean viewboxes
Review retake log and implement corrective actions

Monthly
Check darkroom safelight and check for light leaks using penny test
Check and clean all intensifying screens
Check that exposure charts are posted by each x-ray machine

Yearly
Calibrate x-ray machine

X-ray machine: brand name
Location: room
mA: 15
kVp: 70
E-speed film: brand name

Projection	Exposure time Seconds	Exposure time Impulses
Adult periapicals		
Incisors	0.25	15
Premolars	0.30	18
Molars	0.35	21
Occlusal	0.40	24
Adult bitewings		
Premolar	0.30	18
Molar	0.35	21
Edentulous periapicals		
Incisors	0.20	12
Premolars	0.25	15
Molars	0.30	18
Occlusal	0.35	21
Children		
Anterior periapicals	0.25	15
Posterior periapicals	0.25	15
Bitewing	0.25	15
Occlusal	0.30	18

FIG. 7-1 Sample wall chart showing identification information for x-ray machine, film type used, mA and kVp settings, and appropriate exposure times for various anatomic locations and patient sizes. The optimal exposure times must be determined empirically in each office because they vary with the machine settings used, source-to-skin distance, and other factors.

IMAGE RECEPTORS

Dental x-ray film is quite stable when properly handled. Store it in a cool, dry facility away from a radiation source. Rotate stock when new film is received so that old film does not accumulate in storage. Always use the oldest film first but never after its expiration date has passed.

Monthly cleaning of intensifying screens in panoramic and cephalometric film cassettes is important. The presence of scratches or debris results in recurring light areas on the resultant images. The foam supporting the screens must be intact and capable of holding the screens closely against the film. If close contact between the film and screens is not maintained, the image loses sharpness.

EXPOSURE TABLES

Exposure tables listing the proper peak kilovoltage (kVp), milliamperes (mA), and exposure times for making radiographs of each region of the oral cavity should be posted by each x-ray machine (Fig. 7-1). These help ensure that all operators use the appropriate exposure factors. Typically the mA is fixed at its highest setting;

the kVp is fixed, usually at 70 kVp; and the exposure time is varied to account for patient size and location of the area of interest in the mouth. Exposure times are initially determined empirically. Careful time-temperature processing (described in Chapter 6) must be used with fresh solutions during this initial determination.

MANUAL AND AUTOMATIC FILM PROCESSING

Quality control of manual and automatic film processing is important because deficiencies in this process are the most common cause of faulty radiographs. Several steps, followed carefully, greatly increase the likelihood of producing radiographs of consistently high quality.

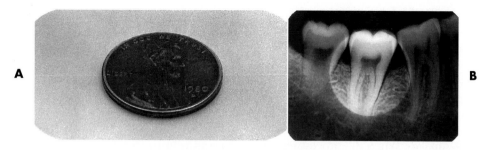

FIG. **7-2** *Penny test for unsafe illumination.* **A,** Leave a penny on the exposed duplicate film from the double-film pack on the working surface during the time that any film would be opened (usually about 5 minutes). **B,** If the processed radiograph shows an outline of the penny, the film is being fogged by inappropriate safelighting conditions.

Replenish Solutions Daily

At the beginning of the workday, check the levels of the processing solutions and replenish if necessary. The developer should be replenished with fresh developer or preferably with developer replenisher. The fixer should be replenished with fixer.

Check Solution Temperature

At the beginning of the workday, check the temperature of the processing solutions. The solutions must reach the optimal temperature before use—68° F (20° C) for manual processing and 82° F (28° C) for heated automatic processors. The instructions accompanying the film and processor verify the optimal temperature. Unheated automatic processors should be located away from windows or heaters that may cause their temperature to vary during the day. Proper temperature regulation is required for accurate time-temperature processing.

Clean Regularly

Regular cleaning of the processing equipment is necessary for optimal operation. The solution tanks of manual and automatic processing equipment should be cleaned when the solutions are changed. The rollers of automatic film processors should be cleaned weekly according to the manufacturers' instructions. Rinsing the tanks and rollers well after contact with cleaning solution prevents the cleaner from interfering with the action of the processing solutions.

Replace Solutions Regularly

The replacement frequency of processing solutions depends primarily on the rate of use of the solutions but also on the size of tanks, whether a cover is used, and the temperature of the solutions. In most offices the solutions should be changed every second week.

Avoid Light Leaks

Inspect the darkroom monthly to assess the integrity of the safelights (preferably GBX-2 filters with 15-watt bulbs). The glass filter should be intact, with no cracks. Turn off all lights, allow your vision to accommodate to the dark, and check for light leaks, especially around doors and vents. Mark light leaks with chalk or masking tape. Weather stripping is useful for sealing light leaks under doors.

Film may become fogged in the darkroom from inappropriate safelight filters, excessive exposure to safelights, and stray light from other sources. Such films are dark, show low contrast, and have a muddy gray appearance. The following simple penny test can be used monthly to evaluate for fogging caused by inappropriate safelighting conditions (Fig. 7-2):

1. Open the packet of an exposed film and place the test film in the area where the films are usually unwrapped and clipped on the film hanger.
2. Place a penny on the film and leave it in this position for the approximate time required to unwrap and mount a full-mouth set of films, usually about 5 minutes.
3. Develop the test film as usual. If the image is visible on the resultant film, the room is not light safe for the particular film tested. Each type of film used in the office should be tested to measure the integrity of the darkroom, sources of light leaks can be detected by standing in the darkroom for 5 minutes to allow the eyes to accommodate.

Reference Film

A simple and effective means for constant monitoring of the quality of images produced in an office is to check daily films against a reference film. Soon after film-processing solutions are replaced, mount a patient film that has been properly exposed and processed with exact time-temperature technique on a corner of the viewbox. This image, with optimal density and contrast, serves as a reference for the radiographs made in the following days and weeks (Fig. 7-3). All subsequent images should be compared with this reference film.

Comparison of daily images with the reference film may reveal problems before they interfere with the diagnostic quality of the images. When the processing solutions become depleted, the resultant radiographs are light and have reduced contrast. Both developer and fixer should be changed when degradation of the image quality is evident. Light images may also result from cold solutions or insufficient developing time. Dark images may be caused by excessive developing time, developer that is too warm, or light leaks.

Step-Wedge Test

In addition to the use of a reference film described above, a step-wedge test can provide accurate monitoring of day-to-day processing conditions. It measures the speed of the imaging system and image contrast. Both are sensitive measures of the processing environment.

A step wedge is readily made with the lead foil from film packets. Stack five sheets together and staple at one end (Fig. 7-4). Cut off $\frac{4}{5}$ of the top layer, $\frac{3}{5}$ of the second layer, $\frac{2}{5}$ of the third layer, and $\frac{1}{5}$ of the fourth layer. This creates a five-step wedge. Lay the wedge on top of a film packet and expose using the usual setting for an adult bitewing view. The resultant image should show five steps from dark to light.

Processing efficacy and consistency are measured by monitoring an index of speed. The density of the image is a measure of the speed. When film processing solutions are depleted or too cold, the resultant image becomes light. Solutions that are excessively warm cause a dark image. The speed index should be monitored at the beginning of each day to ensure that the processing system is operational for patient care.

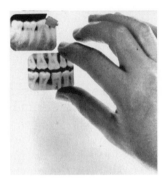

FIG. **7-3** Check radiographs daily against a reference film made with fresh solutions. As processing solutions become exhausted, the daily images become increasingly light and lose contrast. When these changes are clear, change both the developer and the fixer. (Courtesy C.L. Crabtree, DDS, Bureau of Radiological Health, Rockville, Md.)

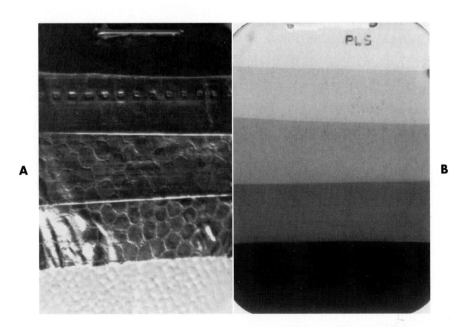

FIG. **7-4** **A,** Step wedge made of strips of lead foil from film packets. This step wedge is positioned over a film, and an exposure is made. **B,** Processed radiograph showing each step. Such an image should be made daily after replenishing processing solutions and compared with an image made with fresh solutions. When the step wedge has become one full step lighter, it is time to change both the developer and the fixer.

The best way to monitor the speed index in an office is to expose a series of films at one time. Soon after processing solutions are replaced, expose 21 films with the step wedge using posterior adult bitewing factors. Process one image and place it on the viewbox. Store the other 20 films in a cool, dry place. A refrigerator is best. At the beginning of each day, after the processing solutions are at the optimal temperature, process one of the exposed films. Compare this image to the reference image. When the resultant image has become one full step lighter, the solutions have become depleted and should be changed.

VIEWING CONDITIONS

Viewboxes should be cleaned weekly to remove any particles or defects that may interfere with proper film interpretation.

RETAKE LOG

Another simple and effective means of reducing the number of faulty radiographs is to keep a retake log. Record in this log the errors of all films that must be re-exposed. Review this record weekly and identify any recurring problems with film processing conditions or operator technique. This information assists in implementing corrective actions.

X-RAY MACHINE TESTS

X-ray machines are generally quite stable and only rarely cause poor radiographs. Accordingly, they need to be calibrated only annually unless a specific problem is identified or substantive repair is necessary that may affect their operation. Usually dental service companies or health physicists should make these machine measurements because of the specialized equipment required. The following parameters should be measured:

1. *X-ray output*—A radiation dosimeter is used to measure the intensity and reproducibility of radiation output, usually measured in milliroentgens (Fig. 7-5). Acceptable values are shown in Fig. 3-2.
2. *Collimation and beam alignment*—The field diameter for dental intraoral x-ray machines should be no greater than 2¾ inches. The tip of the position-indicating device (PID, aiming cylinder) should be closely aligned with the x-ray beam. This may be evaluated by making a star pattern with dental films, marking them with pinholes, and centering the aiming cylinder over the pattern (Fig. 7-6). Expose the films using usual bitewing values, process the films, and reconstitute the star pattern. The size and alignment of the beam can then be determined.

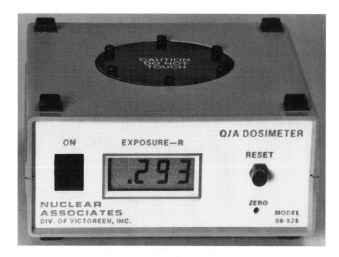

FIG. **7-5** *Device for measuring exposure output of an x-ray machine.* The aiming cylinder of the x-ray machine is positioned on the center of the top and an exposure made. The display on the front gives the output in roentgens.

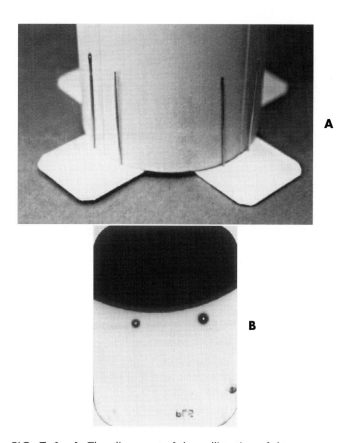

FIG. **7-6** **A,** The alignment of the collimation of the x-ray beam and the end of the aiming cylinder can be checked by making a cross pattern of film, centering the aiming cylinder, marking the periphery with needles, and making an exposure. **B,** One of the processed radiographs showing the dark exposed area just inside the holes. If this pattern is seen on all films, then good alignment is demonstrated.

For panoramic machines the beam exiting the patient should not be larger than the film slit holding the film cassette. This may be tested by taping dental films in front of and behind the slit. A pin stick should be made through both films to allow subsequent realignment. Expose, process, and realign both films. The exposure to the film in front of the slit should be comparable in size to the film exposure behind the slit. Service is required if the front film exposure is larger or not well oriented with the film exposure behind the slit.

3. *Beam energy*—The kVp or half-value layer (HVL) of the beam should be measured to ensure that the beam has sufficient energy for film exposure without excessive soft tissue dosage. Measurement of kVp requires specialized equipment. It should be accurate within 5 kVp. Measurement of HVL requires a dosimeter. The HVL should be at least 1.5 mm aluminum (Al) at 70 kVp and 2.5 mm Al at 90 kVp.

4. *Timer*—Electric pulse counters count the number of pulses generated by an x-ray machine during a preset time interval. The timer should be accurate and reproducible. This test can also be performed by using a spinning top with a notch on the edge (Fig. 7-7). Place the top over an occlusal film, give it a twist to start it spinning, and make an exposure. The number of images of the notch on the resultant image will reveal the number of pulses generated by the x-ray machine during the preset time interval (Fig. 7-8).

5. *mA*—The linearity of the mA control should be verified with a dosimeter. It also may be measured with the step wedge described previously. If two or more mA settings are available on the machine, the higher value is used routinely. Make an exposure using the usual adult bitewing setting. Then reduce the mA to the lower value and select another exposure time, ensuring that the product of the mA and time in seconds (impulses) is the same as for the adult bitewing. For example, if the machine has 10- and 15-mA settings, and 15 mA and 24 impulses are used for adult bitewings, select 10 mA and 36 impulses (15 × 24 = 10 × 36). Expose another image at 10 mA and 36 impulses, and process both films. The densities at each step should be the same. A discrepancy implies nonlinearity in the mA control or a fault in the timer.

6. *Tube head stability*—The tube head should be stable when placed around the patient's head and not drift during the exposure. When it is not stable, service is necessary to adjust the suspension mechanism.

7. *Focal spot size*—The size of the focal spot should be measured because it may become enlarged with excessive heat buildup within an x-ray machine. An enlarged focal spot contributes to geometric fuzziness in the resultant image. A specialized piece of equipment is required for this test.

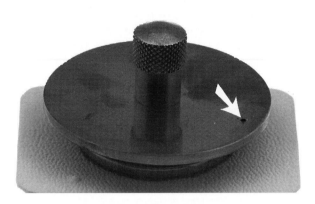

FIG. **7-7** Spinning top with hole *(arrow)* positioned over film packet. In use, the top is set spinning and exposed from above.

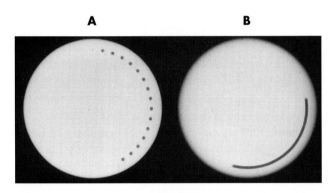

FIG. **7-8** *Radiograph made with spinning top.* **A,** Exposure of 15 impulses made with self-rectified dental x-ray machine. As each pulse of radiation is emitted, it is recorded on the film through the hole in the edge of the spinning top. **B,** Exposure with GEX unit having essentially continuous radiation output.

Infection Control

Dental personnel and patients are at increased risk of acquiring tuberculosis, herpes viruses, upper respiratory infections, and hepatitis strains A through E. After the recognition of acquired immunodeficiency syndrome (AIDS) in the 1980s, rigorous hygienic procedures were introduced in dental offices. The American Dental Association and the Centers for Disease Control and Prevention stress the use of universal precautions (hygiene procedures followed for all patients) because many patients are unaware that they are carriers of infectious disease or choose not to reveal this information. Under universal precautions, all human blood and saliva are treated as if known to be infectious for human immunodeficiency virus (HIV) and hepatitis B virus. The goal is to block the transmission of infectious agents between patients and dental personnel or other patients.

Radiographic infection control procedures are now an integral part of the dental practice. This chapter focuses on the use of universal precautions in dental radiography, including preparation of the radiographic areas and equipment, conduct of the examination, and film processing. Although radiographic procedures are not invasive, saliva is a potentially infectious medium because of its frequent contamination with blood. Furthermore, oral radiographic procedures are likely performed in the same dental units that are used for all different types of procedures, including invasive procedures. Because a medical history and clinical examination do not guarantee identification of patients with HIV infection or other serious infectious diseases, such as hepatitis, it is wise to treat all patients as potentially infectious. One set of procedures is used for all patients, regardless of their presumed status.

OVERVIEW

The primary goal of infection-control procedures is to prevent cross-contamination between patients as well as between patients and health care providers. In dental radiography the potential for cross-contamination is great. An operator's hands may become contaminated by contact with a patient's mouth and saliva-contaminated films and film holders. The operator then must adjust the x-ray tube head and PID as well as the x-ray machine control panel to make the exposure.

Cross-contamination also may occur when operators open film packets to process the films in the darkroom. The procedures described in the following sections minimize or eliminate cross-contamination. Each dental practice should have a written policy describing its infection control practices. It is best if one individual in a practice, usually the dentist, assumes responsibility for implementing these procedures. This person also educates other members of the practice.

In radiographic practice the goal of preventing cross-contamination is addressed by using surface disinfectants on all surfaces and by using barriers to isolate equipment from direct contact. Most items that accumulate on working surfaces in the operatory should be stored in a central preparation (cleaning and sterilizing) room and brought as necessary to the treatment area on trays. This eliminates the probability of touching items and surfaces that have not been properly prepared and defeating all the precautions that have been observed. Although barriers greatly aid infection control, they do not replace the need for effective surface cleaning and disinfection. Experience has demonstrated that, during the daily activity of treatment, failure of mechanical barriers is not uncommon. It is advantageous and reassuring to the operator to know that whenever this happens the surfaces that may become accidentally exposed are clean and disinfected.

INFECTION-CONTROL PROCEDURES

The following techniques facilitate infection control during radiography. They are presented in the order in which they should be performed. The sequence of the steps in the following guidelines is important because adherence to this order contributes significantly to their effectiveness in preventing disease transmission. The preparation and cleanup work described here necessitate wearing disinfected, thick, general-purpose utility gloves. After use, wash the gloves with soap and water; then rinse and dry them and apply a disinfectant. Discard the utility gloves weekly. All individuals who participate in disinfection routines should have their own gloves.

The infection-control sequence for radiography is as follows:

1. Prepackage x-ray film and sterilize film-holding instruments.
2. Disinfect and cover PID, x-ray head and support, working surfaces, chair, and apron.
3. Expose radiographs.
4. Process contaminated x-ray films.
5. Remove all barriers and spray or wipe all working surfaces and apron with disinfectant.
6. Disinfect panoramic machine and cephalostat.

Prepackage X-Ray Film and Sterilize Film-Holding Instruments

To prevent contamination of bulk supplies of film, dispense them in procedure quantities. Prepackage the required number of films for a full-mouth or interproximal series in coin envelopes or paper cups in the central preparation room. Dispense these envelopes of films with the film-holding instruments. If Kodak ClinAsept Dental Barrier protective plastic envelopes are used, the films may be inserted into these envelopes at the time they are packaged in the coin envelopes (Fig. 7-9). For unanticipated occasions in which an unusual number of films is required, a small container of films can be on hand in the central preparation and sterilizing room. No one wearing contaminated gloves should retrieve a film from this supply. Films should be dispensed only by a staff member with clean hands or wearing clean gloves.

The film-holding instruments described in Chapter 8, the Precision and the XCP, can both be sterilized with steam under pressure (autoclaved) or with exposure to ethylene oxide gas. The Precision instrument can also be dry-heat sterilized, but the plastic XCP instruments cannot. Both should be mechanically cleaned in soapy water and well rinsed to remove saliva before sterilizing. The instruments may now be placed in sterilization bags. The bite blocks used with the Precision instruments are disposable and should be discarded after use.

After sterilization, keep the instruments in bags for storage and subsequent transport to the radiography

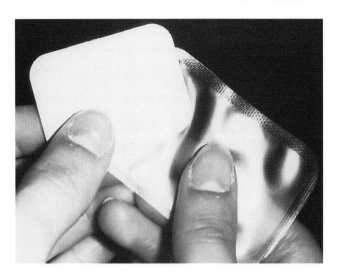

FIG. **7-9** Place films in plastic barrier envelopes in the stockroom before the radiographic examination.

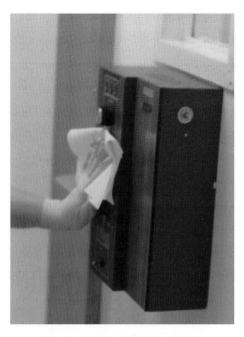

FIG. **7-10** Vigorously wipe the front of the console and the exposure switch with a folded double paper towel moistened with disinfectant. Wear utility gloves to protect hands.

storage and subsequent transport to the radiography area. When the instruments are taken to the radiography area, it is good technique to use them out of the bag immediately before use. After use, replace instruments in the bag to reinforce cleanliness in the area. Use the same sterilization bag to transport the contaminated instruments back to the cleaning and sterilizing room.

Disinfect and Cover PID, X-Ray Head and Support, Working Surfaces, Chair, and Apron
Any surface that may be contaminated should be surface disinfected. This includes the x-ray machine control panel, tube head, and beam alignment device, dental chair and headrest, surfaces on which film is placed, leaded apron and thyroid collar, and doorknob of operatory. Operators should avoid touching walls and other surfaces with contaminated gloves. Good surface disinfectants include iodophors, chlorines, and synthetic phenolic compounds. The iodophors are generally less expensive than the phenolic compounds because they can be diluted with more water. They are also less corrosive then hypochlorite, the least expensive of all, but perhaps the least pleasant to use.

Although the American Dental Association does not recommend specific chemical disinfectants and sterilants, it does suggest that when dentists use a chemical agent for disinfection or sterilization, it should carry Environmental Protection Agency (EPA) registration. It should also be tuberculocidal—an effective killer of tuberculosis—and capable of preventing other infectious diseases, including hepatitis B and HIV.

To clean surfaces, a spray-wipe-spray technique is recommended. First, liberally spray all exposed surfaces with a disinfecting solution. Then wipe the surfaces dry to clean them. Then spray the surfaces again and allow the solution to dry. This disinfects the surfaces. This practice should be observed daily unless a surface becomes contaminated.

Surfaces with electronic controls need special attention. Spray the top and sides of the x-ray control console with disinfectant, but do not spray the front because contact with liquid may damage the switches, dials, and meters. Wipe the front of the console and the exposure switch vigorously with a folded double paper towel that has been well moistened with disinfectant (Fig. 7-10). Similarly, if the positioning of the chair is electrically controlled, wipe the switches with a folded double towel liberally moistened with disinfectant.

Use barriers to cover working surfaces that were previously cleaned and disinfected. Barriers protect the underlying surface from becoming contaminated. An effective barrier for the countertops and x-ray control console is plastic wrap, which can be obtained in 1200-foot rolls that are 18 inches wide. This plastic may be conveniently stored in a butcher's paper dispenser mounted on a wall out of heavy traffic patterns to preclude it being repeatedly brushed by passing patients and staff (Fig. 7-11). These sheets may be secured to the countertops quite effectively (by electrostatic attraction) if they are pulled tight, lapped over the edges, and rubbed down. When

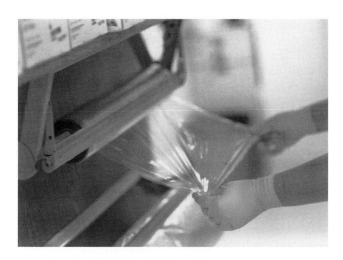

FIG. **7-11** Obtain plastic wrap from dispenser to cover countertops and x-ray machine console.

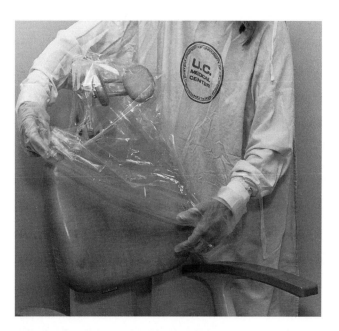

FIG. **7-13** Place a new garment bag over chair and headrest for each patient.

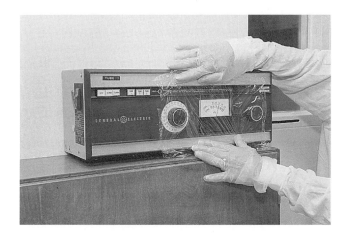

FIG. **7-12** Cover console with plastic wrap on parts that are touched during the radiographic examination.

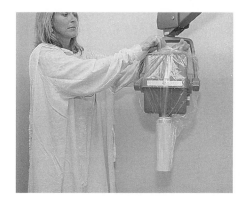

FIG. **7-14** Slip a plastic garment bag over x-ray tube head. Place a large rubber band just proximal to the swivel or tie ends as shown here. Pull the plastic tight over the PID and secure with a light rubber band slipped over the PID and placed next to the head.

exposure switch and the exposure time control if they are integral parts of the unit (Fig. 7-12). The application of plastic wrap over the kVp meter may cause electrostatic deflection of the meter needle and result in an erroneous voltage reading. Experiment with your equipment to determine whether the application of plastic wrap influences the meter reading. Cover an x-ray exposure switch that is independent of the console with a sandwich bag or food storage bag, or wrap it with plastic wrap.

The dental chair headrest, headrest adjustments, and chair back may be easily covered with a plastic bag (Fig. 7-13). Cover the x-ray tube head, PID, and yoke while they are still wet with disinfectant with a barrier to stop any dripping (Fig. 7-14). A commercially available, dis-

posable plastic sleeve made to cover the x-ray head and cone can be used. Slide the barrier over the PID and head and as far proximally onto the support arm as the bag permits. Secure it by tying a knot in the open end or by placing a heavy rubber band over the head just proximal to the swivel.

Also clean, disinfect, and cover the leaded apron between patients because it is frequently contaminated with saliva as the result of handling (readjusting its position) during a radiographic procedure. Suspend the apron on a heavy coat hanger to permit turning front to back. Spray it with detergent containing disinfec-

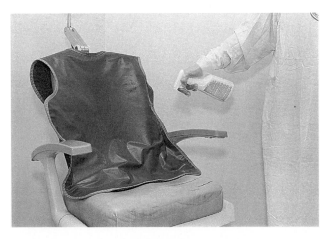

FIG. **7-15**　Spray hanging apron with disinfectant, then dry and cover with a garment bag.

tant, then wipe, and cover with the same type of plastic garment bag used for the x-ray head and chair back (Fig. 7-15). The operatory is now prepared for radiography.

Expose Radiographs

After seating the patient, wash your hands and put on disposable gloves in sight of the patient if the operatory arrangement permits. Some authorities recommend having the patients rinse their mouths before the examination with an antimicrobial mouthrinse, either 0.12% chlorhexidine gluconate or a phenolic product. Because dental radiography does not produce an aerosol, it is usually not necessary to use a face mask or protective eyewear unless splatter is anticipated. All objects that are touched from this point on have been disinfected or sterilized. Keep charts away from sources of contamination and do not handle them during the radiographic examination. Make chair adjustments in advance, or make adjustments on control surfaces that are covered, such as the headrest control.

Film should be obtained in advance from a central source. If an additional film is needed, a co-worker should supply it, or operators should remove their gloves while obtaining a film from the central supply. Film packets are exposed to saliva and possibly blood during exposure in the patient's mouth. To prevent saliva from seeping into a paper film packet, place a paper towel beside the container for exposed films. Use this towel to wipe each film as you remove it from the patient's mouth and before placing it with the other exposed films. This problem may also be avoided by using film packaged in plastic. If a digital radiographic system is used, cover the receptor with a barrier when placing it in the patient's mouth. No film processing concerns are involved with these systems.

Process Contaminated X-Ray Films

After making all exposures, remove your gloves and take the container of contaminated films to the darkroom. The goal in the darkroom is to break the infection chain so that only clean films are placed into processing solutions. Lay out two towels on the darkroom working surface. Place the container of contaminated films on one of these towels. After removing the exposed film from its packet, place it on the second towel. The film packaging is discarded on the first towel with the container.

Removing film from a packet without touching (contaminating) it is a relatively easy procedure if specific steps are observed, steps based on knowing the way the film is wrapped within the packet (see Fig. 4-4). Fig. 7-16 illustrates the method for opening a contaminated film packet while wearing contaminated gloves without touching the film. Put a pair of gloves back on, pick up the film packet by the color-coded end, and grasp the tab. Pull the tab upward and away from the packet to reveal the black paper tab wrapped over the end of the film. Now, holding the film over the second towel, carefully grasp the black paper tab that wraps the film and pull the film from the packet. When the film is pulled from the packet, it will fall from the paper wrapping onto the clean towel. The paper wrapper may need to be shaken lightly to cause the film to fall free. Place the packaging materials on the first paper towel. After opening all films, gather the contaminated packaging and container and discard them along with the contaminated gloves. Process the clean films in the usual manner. It is not necessary to wear gloves when handling processed films, film mounts, or patient charts.

A recent commercial development has simplified the handling of contaminated exposed films. Eastman Kodak has introduced intraoral D- and E-speed films sealed in a plastic envelope (Kodak dental film with ClinAsept barrier) (Fig. 7-17). This plastic barrier protects the film from contact with saliva and blood during exposure. These protected films are relatively expensive, but the empty polyester envelopes (ClinAsept barriers) may be purchased separately and used to seal and protect conventional film. Although the barrier envelopes are large enough to accommodate no. 2 film, a no. 1 can be placed in the envelope and the excess plastic folded over the film. Both sizes of barrier-protected film fit in the Precision and XCP film-holding instruments (Fig. 7-18). An attractive feature of the protective envelopes is the ease with which they may be opened and the film extracted. For best results, immerse the packet in a disinfectant after they have been exposed in the patient's mouth. Then dry the packets and open, allowing the film to drop out. The barrier envelopes can be conveniently opened in a lighted area, the film dropped onto

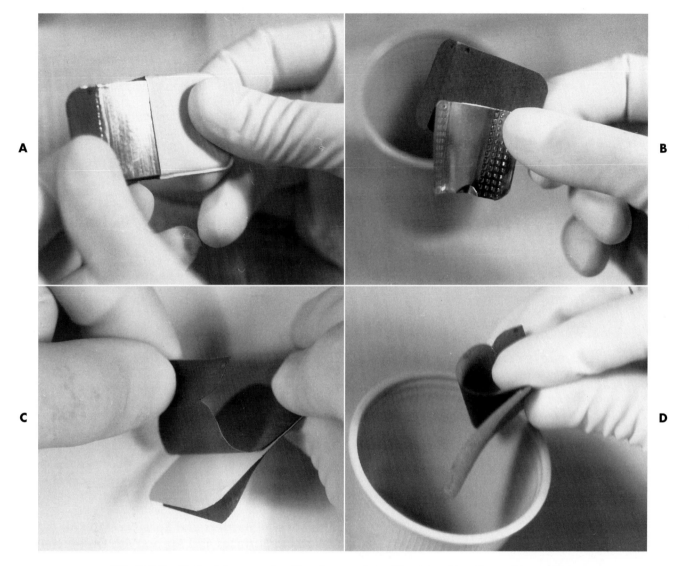

FIG. **7-16** *Method for removing films from packet without touching them with contaminated gloves.* **A,** Open packet tab and slide lead foil and black interleaf paper from wrapping. **B,** Rotate foil away from black paper and discard. **C,** Open paper wrapping. **D,** Allow film to fall into a clean cup.

a clean work area or into a clean paper or plastic cup, and the film transferred to the daylight loader or darkroom for processing. Use of these envelopes provides the best method of using a daylight loader and maintaining the integrity of an infection control procedure.

An alternate procedure when exposing films in plastic packaging is to place the exposed film, still in the protective plastic envelope, in an approved disinfecting solution when it is removed from the mouth and after wiping it with a paper towel. It should remain in the disinfectant after the exposure of the last film for the recommended time. Immersion for 30 seconds in a 5.25% solution of sodium hypochlorite is effective.

To increase the time available for the action of the disinfectant on the film packets, clean and disinfect the radiography area before proceeding with film processing. The envelope containing the film can then be dried with a clean paper towel, opened in the light or in the dark, and the film removed and processed without gloves and without transferring infectious material to the daylight loader or darkroom equipment.

Daylight loaders offer a special problem because of the risk of contaminating the sleeves with contaminated gloves or film packets. One approach is to clean the films by immersion in a disinfectant, with or without a plastic envelope, as described above. With this method

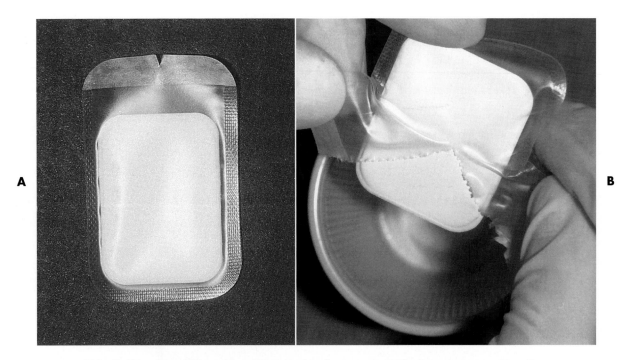

FIG. **7-17**   *Dental film with a ClinAsept barrier to protect film from contact with saliva.* **A,** Note notch on side of plastic envelope for opening. **B,** During opening, the plastic is removed and the clean film allowed to drop into a container.

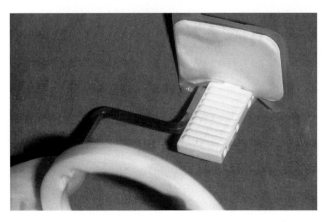

FIG. **7-18**   Film-holding instrument with barrier envelope protecting film from saliva.

the operator cleans the films, puts on clean gloves, and then takes only cleaned film packets into the daylight loader.

An alternate approach is to open the top of the loader, place a clean barrier on the bottom, and insert the cup of exposed film packets and a clean cup. The operator then closes the top, puts on clean gloves, pushes his or her hands through the sleeve, and opens the film packets, allowing the film to drop into the clean

cup. After all film packets have been opened, remove the contaminated gloves, load the films into the developer, and remove hands. Then the top of the loader may be removed and the contaminated materials removed.

Remove All Barriers and Spray or Wipe All Working Surfaces and Apron With Disinfectant

After completing the patient exposures, remove the barriers, spray contaminated working surfaces (including those in the darkroom) and the apron with disinfectant, and wipe them as described previously. Then replace the barriers in preparation for the next patient.

Disinfect Panoramic Machine and Cephalostat

The panoramic machine should receive the same maintenance for decontamination and disinfection as other equipment. However, in the use of the panoramic machine, fewer areas are contacted and contaminated by the patient, the patient's saliva, or the operator. Clean the bite blocks, chin rest, and patient handgrips with detergent-iodine disinfectant. Cover the chin rest and bite blocks with a plastic bag. Carefully wipe the head-positioning guides, control panel, and exposure switch with a paper towel that is well moistened with disinfectant. The radiographer should wear disposable gloves while positioning and exposing the patient. Remove the gloves before removing the cassette from the machine for processing because the cassette and film remain extraoral and should not be handled while wearing contaminated disposable gloves.

Clean and disinfect cephalostat ear posts, ear post brackets, and forehead support or nasion pointer by vigorous wiping with a paper towel generously moistened with the iodine-detergent disinfectant. These may then also be covered in plastic.

BIBLIOGRAPHY

QUALITY ASSURANCE

American Academy of Dental Radiology Quality Assurance Committee: Recommendations for quality assurance in dental radiography, *Oral Surg Oral Med Oral Pathol* 55:421, 1983.

Quality assurance for dental facilities, X-Ray Inspection Service, Ministry of Health, Ontario, Canada, May 1990.

Quality assurance in dental radiography, Kodak Dental Radiography series, N-416, Rochester, N.Y., 1995, Eastman Kodak.

Valachovic RW, Reiskin AB, Kirshof ST: A quality assurance program in dental radiology, *Pediatr Dent* 3:26, 1981.

INFECTION CONTROL

American Academy of Oral and Maxillofacial Radiology infection control guidelines for dental radiographic procedures, *Oral Surg Oral Med Oral Pathol* 73:248, 1992.

American Dental Association: Infection control recommendations for the dental office and dental laboratory, *JADA* 127:672, 1996.

American Dental Association Council on Scientific Affairs and American Dental Association Council on Dental Practice: Infection control recommendations for the dental office and the dental laboratory, *JADA* 127:672, 1996.

Bachman CE et al: Bacterial adherence and contamination during radiographic processing, *Oral Surg Oral Med Oral Pathol* 70:669, 1990.

Centers for Disease Control and Prevention: Recommended infection-control practices for dentistry, *MMWR* 42(RR-8):1, 1993.

Ciola B: A readily adaptable, cost-effective method of infection control for dental radiography, *JADA* 117:349, 1988.

Cottone JA, Terezhalmy GT, Molinari JA: *Practical infection control in dentistry,* Baltimore, 1996, Williams & Wilkins.

Glass BJ: Infection control in dental radiology, *N Y State Dent J* 60:42, 1994.

Hovius M: Disinfection and sterilization: duties and responsibilities of dentists and dental hygienists, *Int Dent J* 42:241, 1992.

Hubar JS, Oeschger MP, Reiter LT: Effectiveness of radiographic film barrier envelopes, *Gen Dent* 42:406, 1994.

Jefferies D, Morris J, White V: kVp meter errors induced by plastic wrap, *J Dent Hygiene* 65:91, 1991.

Katz JO et al: Infection control protocol for dental radiology, *Gen Dent* 38:261, 1990.

Miller CH: Sterilization and disinfection: what every dentist needs to know, *JADA* 123:46, 1992.

Miller CH, Palenik CJ: *Infection control and management of hazardous materials for the dental team,* ed 2, St Louis, 1998, Mosby.

Neaverth EJ, Pantera EA: Chairside disinfection of radiographs, *Oral Surg Oral Med Oral Pathol* 71:116, 1991.

Puttaiah R et al: Infection control in dental radiology, *CDA J* 23:21, 1995.

Stanczyk DA, Paunovich ED: Microbiologic contamination during dental radiographic film processing, *Oral Surg Oral Med Oral Pathol* 76:112, 1993.

Thomas LP, Abramovitch K: Aseptic techniques for dental radiography, *J Greater Houston Dent Soc* 63:21, 1992.

U.S. Department of Labor, Occupational Safety and Health Administration: *Occupational exposure to bloodborne pathogens, final rule,* Federal Register 1991;56(235):64004.

Wolfgang L: Analysis of a new barrier infection control system for dental radiographic film, *Compend Cont Ed Dent* 13:68, 1993.

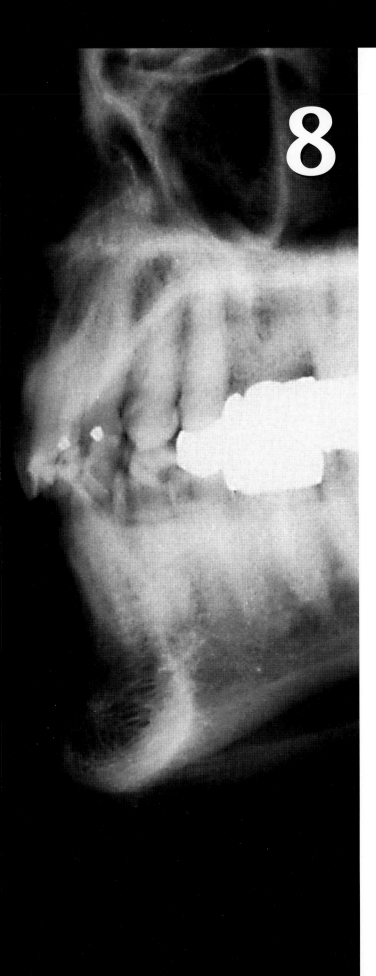

8 Intraoral Radiographic Examinations

Intraoral examinations are the backbone of dental radiography. Intraoral radiographs can be divided into three categories: periapical projections, bitewing projections, and occlusal projections. Periapical radiographs should show all of a tooth, including the surrounding bone. Bitewing radiographs show only the crowns of teeth and the adjacent alveolar crests. Occlusal radiographs show an area of teeth and bone larger than periapical films. The term *film* is used in this chapter because most intraoral radiographs are made with radiographic film. When intraoral digital image receptors are used, the radiographic principles are the same as those for radiographic film.

A full-mouth set of radiographs consists of periapical and bitewing projections (Fig. 8-1). These projections, when well exposed and properly processed, can provide considerable diagnostic information to complement the clinical examination. As with any clinical procedure, the operator must clearly understand the goals of dental radiography and the criteria for evaluating the quality of performance. The operator who demonstrates the skill and pride required to expose a good full-mouth set of radiographs is amply rewarded when the time arrives for radiographic interpretation.

Radiographs should be made only when a clear diagnostic need exists for the information the radiograph may provide. Accordingly, the frequency of such examinations varies with the individual circumstances of each patient (see Chapter 13).

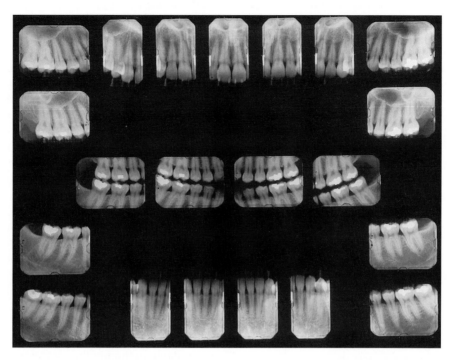

FIG. **8-1** Mounted full-mouth set of radiographs consisting of 17 periapical views and four bitewing views.

Criteria of Quality

Every radiographic examination should produce radiographs of optimal diagnostic quality, incorporating the following features:

- The radiographs should record the complete areas of interest on the image. In the case of intraoral periapical radiographs, the full length of the roots and at least 2 mm of the periapical bone must be visible. If evidence of a pathologic condition is present, the area of the entire lesion plus some surrounding normal bone should show on one radiograph. Sometimes, however, this is difficult to achieve on a periapical radiograph; in such an instance an occlusal projection may be required as well as an extraoral projection. Bitewing examinations should demonstrate each proximal surface at least once.
- The radiographs should have the least possible amount of distortion. Most distortion is caused by improper angulation of the x-ray beam rather than by curvature of the structures being examined or inap-

propriate positioning of the film. Close attention to proper positioning of the film and x-ray tube results in diagnostically useful images.
- The radiographs should have optimal density and contrast, which are essential for interpretation. Although tube current in milliamperes (mA), peak kilovoltage (kVp), and exposure time are crucial parameters influencing density and contrast, film processing also makes an important contribution to the quality of the radiograph. Faulty processing can adversely affect the quality of a properly exposed radiograph.

When evaluating radiographs and considering whether to retake a view, the practitioner should consider the initial reason for making the image. When a full-mouth set is indicated, it is not necessary to retake a view that fails to open a contact or show a periapical region if the missing information is available on another view. If few views or only one view is needed, they should be repeated only if they fail to reveal the desired information.

Periapical Radiography

Two intraoral projection techniques may be used for periapical radiography: the paralleling technique and the bisecting-angle technique. Although each has evolved as the result of efforts to minimize image distortion, most clinicians prefer the paralleling technique because it provides a less distorted view of the dentition. However, morphologic variations from mouth to mouth and even within the same oral cavity pose a variety of geometric problems that repeatedly emphasize that each technique has disadvantages and advantages and must be continually modified to accommodate the immediate circumstances. The following discussion describes the principles and uses of the paralleling technique to obtain a full-mouth set of radiographs. When anatomic configuration (e.g., palate, floor of the mouth) precludes strict adherence to the paralleling concept, slight modifications may have to be made. If the anatomic constraints are extreme, some of the principles of the bisecting-angle technique may be used to accomplish the required film placement and determine the vertical angulation of the tube. The bisecting-angle technique is described later in the chapter.

GENERAL STEPS FOR MAKING AN EXPOSURE

Greet and seat the patient—Position the patient upright in the chair with the back and head well supported and briefly describe the procedures that are to be performed. Do not comment on any discomfort the patient may experience during the procedure. The more apologetic the operator is, the more apprehensive most patients become. If it seems necessary to apologize for any discomfort, do it after the examination. Also, if the patient is experiencing considerable discomfort, the film-holding device is probably not being manipulated correctly. Position the dental chair low for maxillary projections and elevated for mandibular projections. Ask the patient to remove eyeglasses and all removable appliances. Drape the patient with a lead apron whether a single film or a full series is to be made. Occasionally the supine position is used in intraoral radiography instead of an upright posture. This may most easily be accomplished using reclining dental chairs, although an x-ray table may be used. Use of the supine position does not affect the frequency and distribution of technique errors compared with use of paralleling instruments in the upright position. In addition, patients, especially apprehensive ones, generally react favorably to the supine position.

Adjust the x-ray unit setting—Set the x-ray machine for the proper kVp, mA, and exposure time according to the recommendations of the film manufacturer or guidelines that experience has demonstrated produce the highest-quality films with the least radiation exposure to the patient.

Position the tube head—Bring the tube head to the side to be examined so that it is readily available after the film has been positioned.

Wash hands thoroughly—Wash your hands with soap and water, preferably in front of the patient or at least in an area where the patient can observe or be aware of the washing. Put on disposable gloves.

Examine the oral cavity—Before placing the film in the mouth, examine the teeth to estimate their axial inclination, which influences the placement of the film. Also note tori or other obstructions that modify film placement.

Position the film—Remove the film from the film dispenser, insert it into the film-holding device, and position the film in the region of the patient's mouth to be examined. Leading with the apical end of the film, rotate the film into the oral cavity. Place the film as far from the teeth as possible. This contradicts the principle that a short object-to-film distance reduces penumbra and increases sharpness and resolution. However, this compromise provides the maximal space available in the midline of the palate and the greatest depth toward the center of the floor of the mouth. The added space allows the film to be oriented parallel with the long axis of the teeth. Make an effort to avoid contact with the very sensitive attached gingiva covering the alveolar processes when placing a film for a mandibular anterior or posterior projection. Ask the patient to close, gently, holding the instrument and film in place.

When placing films intraorally, first rest the film gently on the palate or floor of the mouth. Next, rotate the instrument either up or down until the bite-block rests on the teeth to be radiographed. Then ask the patient to close. If the bite-block is not on the teeth when the patient closes, the film moves into the palate or floor of the mouth and may cause discomfort. For mandibular anterior projections, place the film gently on the floor of the mouth in front of the tip of the tongue near the second premolar. Ask the patient to close the mouth slowly. As the patient is closing, tip the instrument upward, and the film should move into the floor of the mouth with ease. Do not allow the film packet to contact the very sensitive attached gingiva on the lingual surface of the mandible.

To position the anterior Precision instrument, center the landmark on the support bar. Do not center on the bite-block because it is slightly displaced to one side or the other. When using the XCP anterior instrument, center the landmark on the bite-block.

Place a cotton roll between the bite-block and the teeth opposite those being radiographed. Hold it in place with an orthodontic elastic. This helps stabilize the instrument and in many cases contributes to the patient's comfort.

Position the x-ray tube—Adjust the vertical and horizontal angulation of the tube head to correspond to the beam-guiding instrument. The end of the aiming cylinder of the x-ray machine must be flush or parallel with the face shield of the Precision instrument or the guide ring of the XCP instrument. The aiming cylinder does not have to be centered on the face shield. Alignment is satisfactory when the aiming cylinder covers the port and is within the limits of the face shield. When a beam-guiding instrument is not used, aim the central ray at the appropriate entry point on the skin (identified later in this chapter). Caution the patient not to move.

Make the exposure—After exposure, remove the film from the patient's mouth, dry it with a paper towel, and place it in an appropriate receptacle outside the exposure area.

Projections

A typical full-mouth set of radiographs consists of 21 films (see Fig. 8-1):

Anterior periapical (use no. 1 film)
    Maxillary central incisors: one projection
    Maxillary lateral incisors: two projections
    Maxillary canines: two projections
    Mandibular centrolateral incisors: two projections
    Mandibular canines: two projections
Posterior periapical (use no. 2 film)
    Maxillary premolars: two projections
    Maxillary molars: two projections
    Maxillary distomolar (as needed): two projections
    Mandibular premolars: two projections
    Mandibular molars: two projections
    Mandibular distomolar (as needed): two projections
Bitewing (use no. 2 film)
    Premolars: two projections
    Molars: two projections

Establish a regular sequence when making exposures to avoid overlooking individual projections. Make the anterior projections before the posterior projections because the former cause less discomfort for the patient. The following description of procedures pertains to the paralleling technique. When using that technique, use film-holding instruments that also guide the position of the x-ray tube. Position each film-holding instrument to locate the film in the position described. Using a film-holding device with an external guide for film positioning automatically establishes the point of entry. However, if a great discrepancy seems apparent between the

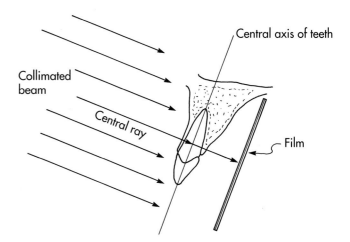

FIG. 8-2 Paralleling technique illustrates the parallelism between the long axis of the tooth and the film. The central ray is directed perpendicular to each.

point of entry indicated by the device and the point described below, check the placement of the film-holding instrument and the position of the film.

PARALLELING TECHNIQUE

The essence of the paralleling technique (also called the *right-angle* or *long cone technique*) is that the x-ray film is supported parallel to the long axis of the teeth and the central ray of the x-ray beam is directed at right angles to the teeth and film (Fig. 8-2). This orientation of the film, teeth, and central ray minimizes geometric distortion. To reduce geometric distortion further, the x-ray source should be located relatively distant from the teeth. In addition, the use of a long source-to-object distance reduces the size of the apparent focal spot. These factors result in images with less magnification and increased definition.

Film-Holding Instruments

Use film-holding instruments to position the film properly in the patient's mouth and maintain the film in position. To position the film parallel to the teeth and project the periapical areas onto the film, position the film away from the teeth and toward the center of the mouth to use the maximal height of the palate. The long source-to-object distance used in the paralleling technique minimizes the disadvantages imposed by the increased object-to-film distance. For maxillary projections, the superior border of the film generally rests at the height of the palatal vault in the midline. Similarly, for mandibular projections, use the film to displace the tongue lingually to allow the inferior border of the film to rest on the floor of the mouth away from the mucosa on the lingual surface of the mandible.

A number of available commercial devices can hold the film parallel and at varying distances from the teeth:

1. The XCP (extension cone paralleling) instruments (Fig. 8-3, *A*)
2. The Precision rectangular collimating instruments, which restrict the beam size at the patient's face to the size of the radiograph (Fig. 8-3, *B*)
3. The Stabe disposable film holder (Fig. 8-3, *C*)
4. The Snap-A-Ray intraoral film holder (Fig. 8-3, *D*)
5. A hemostat inserted through a flattened rubber bite-block, which serves in much the same manner as the Snap-A-Ray film holder (Fig. 8-3, *E*)

The Precision instrument (Isaac Masel, Philadelphia, Penn.) and the XCP instrument used with a rectangular aiming device (Rinn Corp., Elgin, Ill.) are recommended because they significantly reduce patient exposure by limiting the field of exposure to the size of the film.

Angulation of the Tube Head

Adjust the position of the x-ray machine's tube head in the vertical and horizontal planes. Control the third dimension by bringing the end of the aiming cylinder up to the film-holding instrument or within 2 cm of the patient's face. When using the paralleling technique with

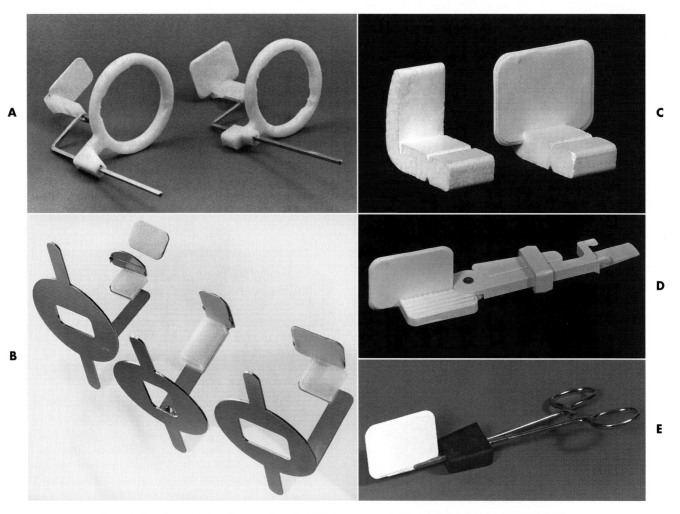

FIG. **8-3** *Film-holding instruments.* **A,** XCP instruments: *left,* instrument for anterior views; *right,* instrument for posterior views. During use, the aiming cylinder on the x-ray tube head is positioned against the localizing ring. **B,** Precision x-ray film holders show instruments for posterior projections *(left and right)* and anterior projections *(middle).* During use, the cylinder on the x-ray tube head is positioned against the face shield. **C,** Stabe bite-blocks. **D,** Snap-A-Ray intraoral film holder. **E,** Hemostat and rubber bite-block. (**A, C,** and **D,** Courtesy Rinn Corp., Elgin, Ill.)

an instrument that provides an external guide for positioning the aiming cylinder (such as the Precision instrument), the practitioner must place the end of the open-ended cylinder flush with the guide. This arrangement helps eliminate most shield cuts and ensures that the central ray is oriented at right angles to the film. A shield cut is an artifact that appears as a clear, unexposed area on a film. It is the result of a beam that is misdirected so that the radiation does not completely cover the film.

Positioning the tube head to direct the beam downward from the horizontal, in the vertical plane, is termed *positive vertical angulation*; directing the beam upward is *negative vertical angulation*. Vertical angulation usually is described in positive or negative degrees, established by the dial on the side of the tube head. The horizontal direction of the beam primarily influences the degree of overlapping of the images of the crowns at the interproximal spaces (Fig. 8-4).

BISECTING-ANGLE TECHNIQUE

The bisecting-angle technique is based on a simple geometric theorem, Cieszynski's rule of isometry, which states that two triangles are equal when they share one complete side and have two equal angles. (In addition, their corresponding sides are equal.) Dental radiography applies the theorem as follows: Position the film as close as possible to the lingual surface of the teeth, resting in the palate or in the floor of the mouth (Fig. 8-5). The plane of the film and the long axis of the teeth form an angle with its apex at the point where the film is in contact with the teeth. When an imaginary plane bisects this angle, it forms two congruent angles, with a common side (the imaginary bisector). A line, representing the central ray of the x-ray beam, completes the third side of the two triangles when it is directed through the apices of the teeth perpendicular to the bisecting plane; the two triangles are right-angle triangles and congruent, with the corresponding sides equal. Two of the cor-

Text continued on p. 150.

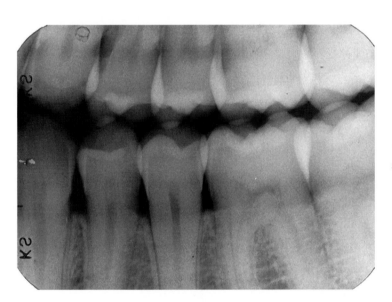

FIG. **8-4** Horizontal overlapping of crowns is the result of misdirection of the central ray.

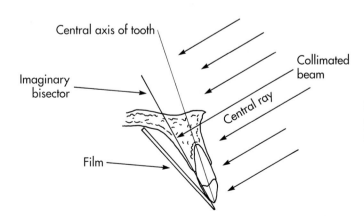

FIG. **8-5** Bisecting-angle technique shows the central ray directed at a right angle to the plane that bisects the angle between the long axis of the tooth and the film.

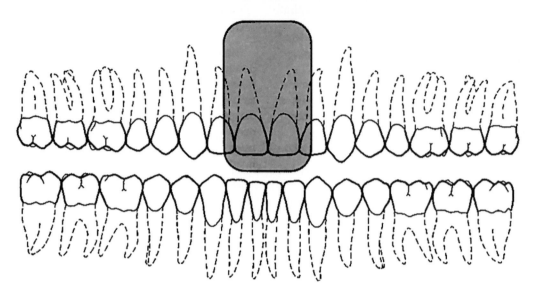

Image field. The field of view on these radiographs *(shaded area)* should include both central incisors and their periapical areas.

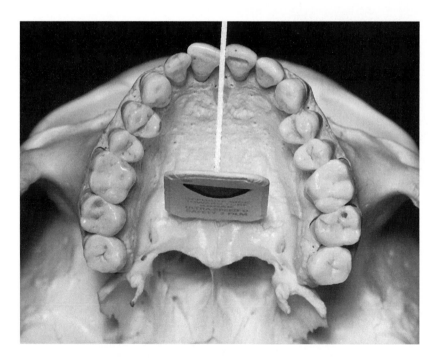

Film placement. Place a no. 1 film at about the level of the second premolars or first molars to take advantage of the maximal palatal height so that the entire length of the teeth can be projected on it. Have the film resting on the palate with its midline centered with the midline of the arch. Position the packet's long axis parallel to the long axis of the maxillary central incisors

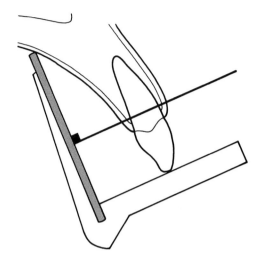

Projection of central ray. Direct the central ray through the contact point of the central incisors and perpendicular to the plane of the films and roots of the teeth. Because the axial inclination of the maxillary incisors is about 15 to 20 degrees, the vertical angulation of the tube should be at the same positive angle. The tube should have 0 horizontal angulation.

---

*Projection of the central ray and point of entry are described in the discussion of the paralleling technique for instances when using a film-holding device without a tube-alignment ring or face-shield. When using a film-holding device with a tube-aligning ring or face-shield, position the device in the mouth to give the appropriate horizontal and vertical angulation.

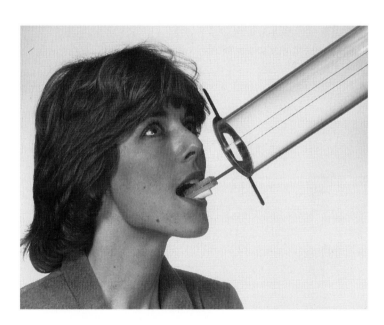

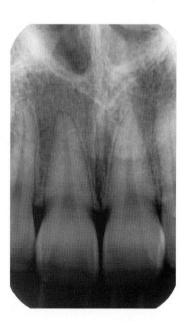

Point of entry. Direct the point of entry of the central ray high on the lip, in the midline, just below the septum of the nostril. If the palatal vault is unusually low or a palatal torus is present, it may be necessary to tilt the film holder positively and compromise a completely parallel relationship between the film and the teeth to ensure that the periapical region is included on the image.

PARALLELING TECHNIQUE
Maxillary Lateral Projection

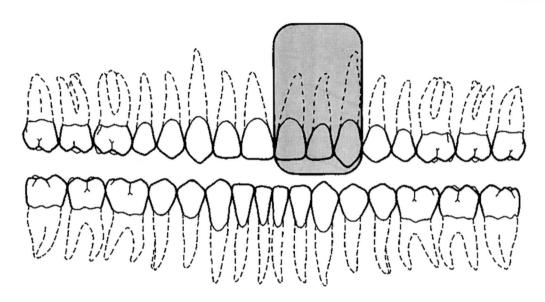

Image field.   This projection should show the lateral incisor and its periapical field centered on the radiograph. Include the mesial interproximal area with the distal aspect of the central incisor on the radiograph so that no overlap is evident.

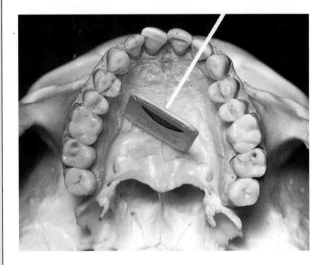

Film placement.   Place a no. 1 film deep in the oral cavity parallel with the long axis and the mesiodistal plane of the maxillary lateral incisor.

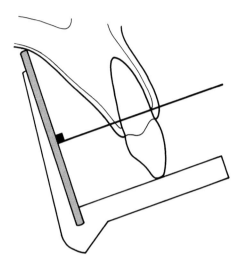

Projection of central ray. Direct the central ray through the middle of the lateral incisor, with no overlapping of the margins of the crowns at the interproximal space on its mesial aspect. Do not attempt to visualize the distal contact with the canine.

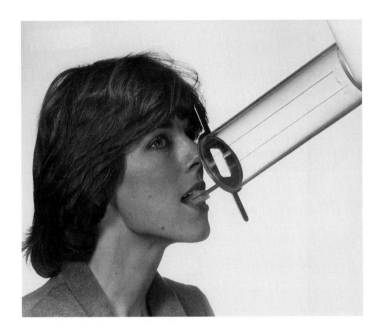

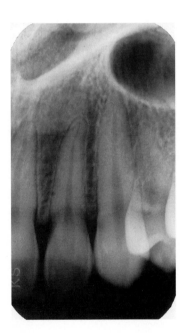

Point of entry. Orient the central ray to enter high on the lip about 1 cm from the midline.

PARALLELING TECHNIQUE
Maxillary Canine Projection

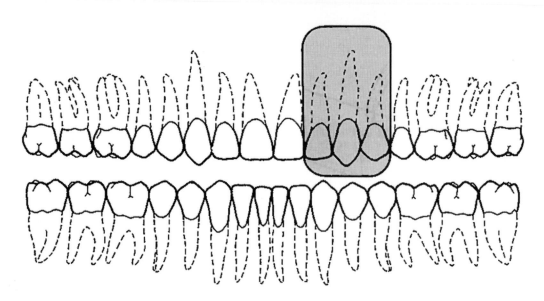

Image field.   This projection should demonstrate the entire canine, with its periapical area, in the midline of the radiograph. Open the mesial contact area. Ignore the distal contact because it will be visualized on other projections.

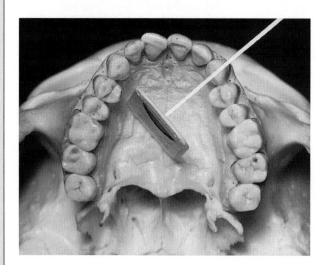

Film placement.   Place a no. 1 film against the palate, well away from the palatal surface of the teeth. Orient the film packet with its anterior edge at about the middle of the lateral incisor and its long axis parallel with the long axis of the canine.

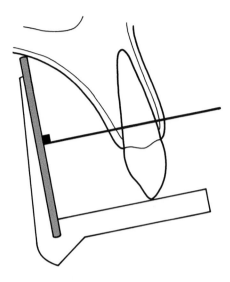

Projection of central ray. Position the holding instrument so that it directs the beam through the mesial contact of the canine. Do not attempt to open the distal contact.

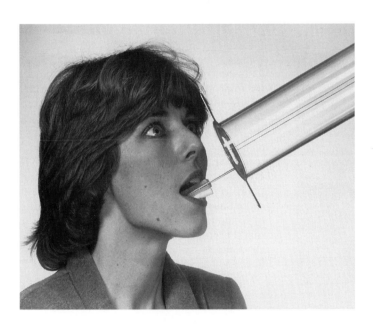

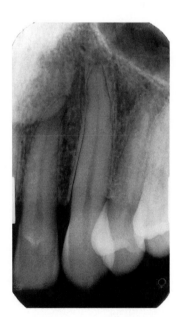

Point of entry. Direct the central ray through the canine eminence. The point of entry will be at about the intersection of the distal and inferior borders of the ala of the nose.

PARALLELING TECHNIQUE
Maxillary Premolar Projection

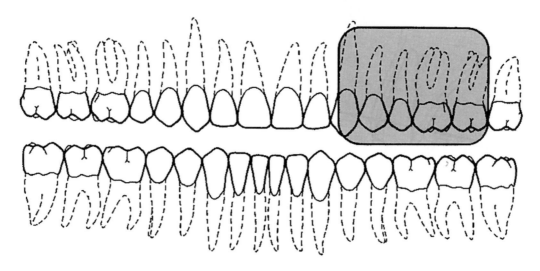

Image field. The radiograph of this region should include the images of the distal half of the canine and the premolars, with room for at least the first molar.

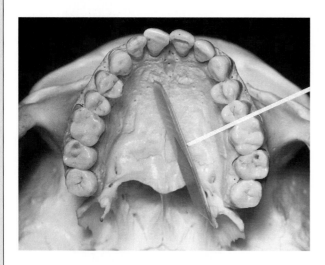

Film placement. Place a no. 2 film in the mouth with the long dimension parallel with the occlusal plane and in the midline. The packet should cover the distal half of the canine, the premolars, and the first molar; it probably will reach to the mesial portion of the second molar. Orient the Precision posterior instrument so that the tip of the canine is in the anterior groove of the bite-block. This ensures that the image includes the distal half of the canine. The exact position of the canine tip in this groove depends on the size of the mouth. The plane of the film should be nearly vertical to correspond with the long axis of the premolar teeth. Position the film-holding device so that the long axis of the film is parallel with the mean buccal plane of the premolars. This establishes the proper horizontal angulation.

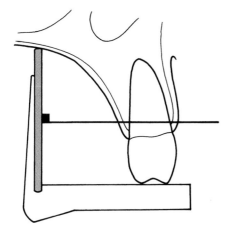

Projection of central ray. Direct the central ray perpendicular to the film. The horizontal angulation of the holding instrument should be adjusted to permit the beam to pass through the interproximal area between the first and second premolars.

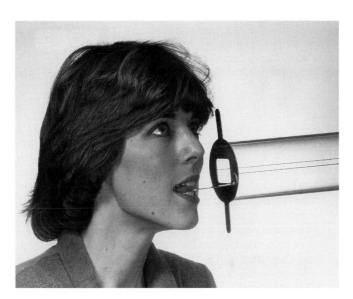

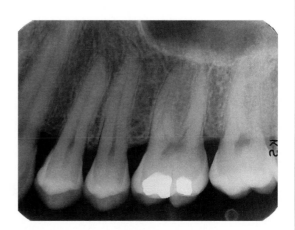

Point of entry. Place the holding instrument so that the central ray passes through the center of the second premolar root. This point usually is below the pupil of the eye.

PARALLELING TECHNIQUE
Maxillary Molar Projection

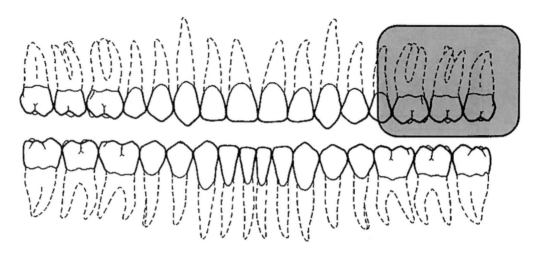

Image field.   The radiograph of this region should show the images of the distal half of the second premolar, the three maxillary permanent molars, and some of the tuberosity. Include the same area on the film even if some or all molars are missing. If the third molar is impacted in an area other than the region of the tuberosity, a distal oblique or extraoral projection (e.g., panoramic or oblique lateral jaw view) may be required.

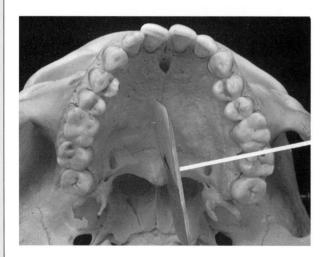

Film placement.   When placing the no. 2 film for this projection, position the wide dimension of the film nearly horizontal to minimize brushing the palate and dorsum of the tongue. When the film is in the region to be examined, rotate it into position with a firm and definite motion. This maneuver is important in avoiding the gag reflex, and resolute action by the operator enhances the patient's confidence. Place the film far enough posterior to cover the first, second, and third molar areas and some of the tuberosity. The anterior border should just cover the distal aspect of the second premolar. To cover the molars from crown to apices, place the film at the midline of the palate. In this position room should be available to orient the film parallel with the molar teeth. The mesial or distal rotation of the film-holding device should ensure that the long axis of the film is parallel with the mean buccal plane of the molars (to establish the proper horizontal angulation). A shallow palate may require slight tipping of the holding instrument to avoid bending the film.

NOTE: In some cases the size of the mouth (length of the arch) does not allow positioning of the film (holding device) as far posterior as recommended for the molar projection. However, by placing the film-holding device so that half the tube alignment ring or face shield is behind the outer canthus of the eye, the molars and part of the tuberosity usually can be included in the image of the molar projection.

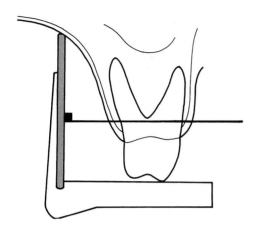

Projection of central ray. Direct the central ray perpendicular to the film. Adjust the horizontal angulation of the film-holding instrument to direct the beam at right angles to the buccal surfaces of the molar teeth. Orient the horizontal angulation of the Precision instrument so that the lateral groove on the bite-block is parallel with the mean buccal plane of the molars.

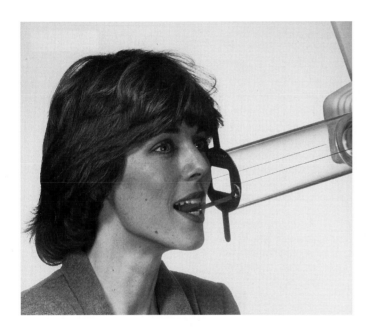

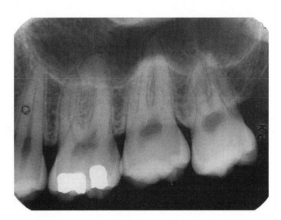

Point of entry. The point of entry of the central ray should be on the cheek below the outer canthus of the eye and the zygoma at the position of the maxillary second molar.

PARALLELING TECHNIQUE
Maxillary Distal Oblique Molar Projection

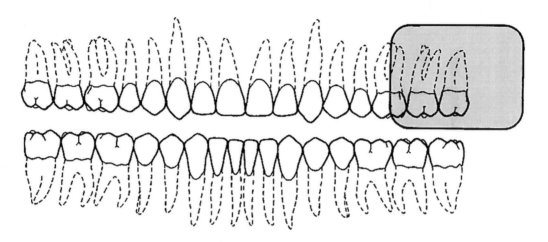

Image field. This projection provides a view of the maxillary tuberosity region more posterior than usually is seen in the molar projection. It allows detection or evaluation of impacted teeth or pathologic conditions in the bone of this area.

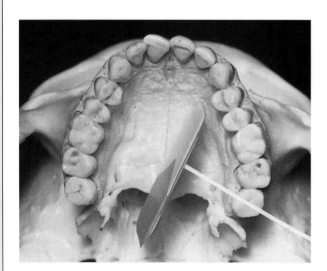

Film placement. Position the holding device with a no. 2 film in the molar region of the maxilla and rotate distally, angling the film across the midline so that the posterior border is away from the teeth of interest and the anterior border is near the molars on the side being radiographed. Position this film with a definite movement to minimize patient discomfort.

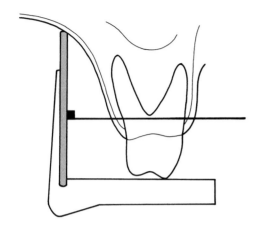

Projection of central ray. Direct the central ray from the posterior aspect through the third molar region and perpendicular to the angled film, projecting the more posterior objects anteriorly onto the film.

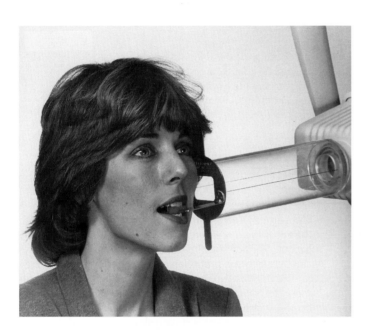

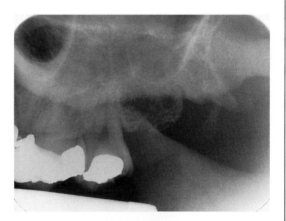

Point of entry. The central ray enters the maxillary third molar region just below the middle of the zygomatic arch, distal to the lateral canthus of the eye.

NOTE: Occasionally a hypersensitive patient gags when a film is placed for the usual maxillary molar projection. However, if a modified distal oblique projection is used, moving the posterior border of the film more medially frequently is less irritating to the patient, and the image is obtained with comfort. The patient's reaction of relief indicates when a sufficient rotation has been achieved. Although this maneuver may result in some overlapping of the molar contact areas, these surfaces will be apparent on the bitewing projection. Slight overlapping of contact areas is preferable to no radiograph of the region.

PARALLELING TECHNIQUE
Mandibular Centrolateral Projection

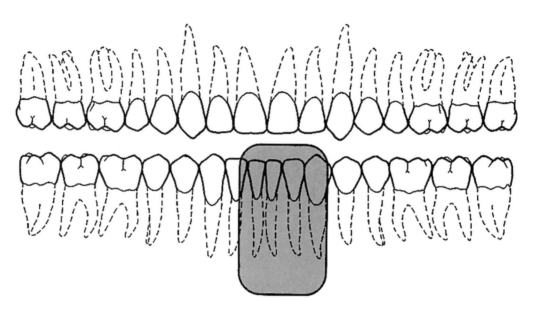

Image field.   Center the image of the mandibular central and lateral incisors and their periapical areas on the film. Because the space in this area frequently is restricted, use two of the narrower anterior periapical films for the incisors to provide good coverage with minimal discomfort. In addition, the incisor contact areas are better visualized on two narrower anterior films because the angulation of the central ray can be adjusted for the contact area on each side.

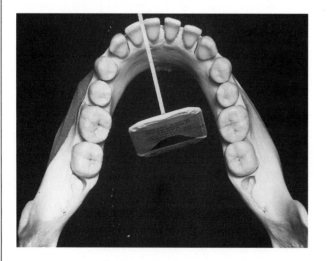

Film placement.   Place the long dimension of the no. 1 film vertically behind the central and lateral incisors with the contact area centered and the lower border below the tongue. Position the film posteriorly as far as possible, usually between the premolars. With the film resting gently on the floor of the mouth as the fulcrum, tip the instrument downward until the film-holder bite-block is resting on the incisors. Instruct the patient to close the mouth slowly. As the patient is closing slowly and the floor of the mouth is relaxing, rotate the instrument with the teeth as the fulcrum to align the film to be more parallel with the teeth.

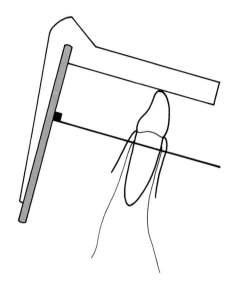

Projection of central ray. Orient the central ray through the interproximal space between the central and lateral incisors.

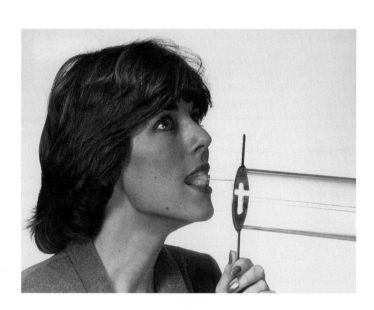

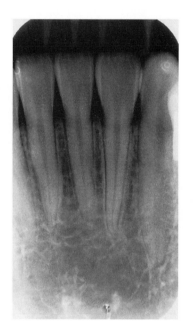

Point of entry. The central ray enters below the lower lip and about 1 cm lateral to the midline.

PARALLELING TECHNIQUE
Mandibular Canine Projection

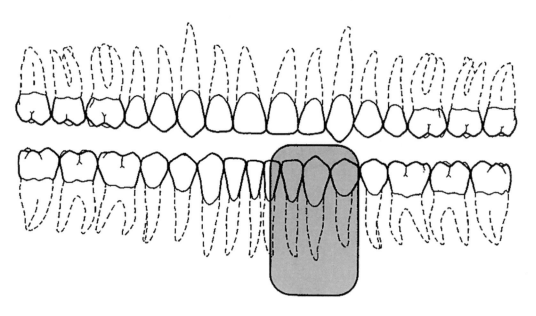

Image field. This image should show the entire mandibular canine and its periapical area. Open its mesial contact area. The distal contact is included on other projections.

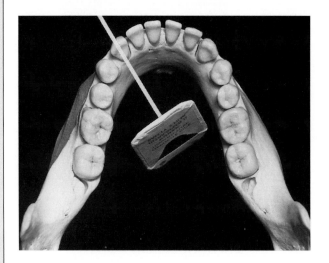

Film placement. Place a no. 1 film packet in the mouth with its long dimension vertical and the canine in the midline of the film. Position it as far lingual as the tongue and contralateral alveolar process permit, with its long axis parallel and in line with the canine. The instrument must be tipped with the bite-block on the canine before the patient is asked to close.

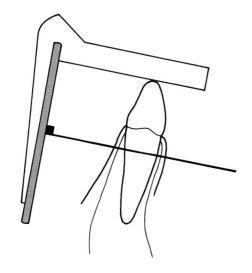

Projection of central ray. Direct the central ray through the mesial contact of the canine without regard to the distal contact.

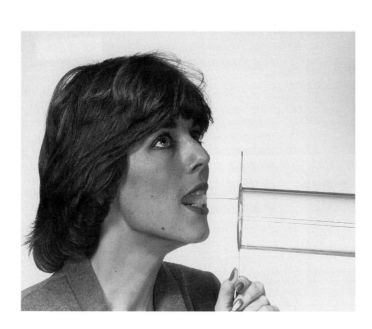

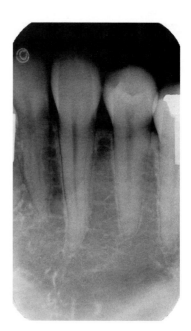

Point of entry. The point of entry is nearly perpendicular to the ala of the nose, over the position of the canine, and about 3 cm above the inferior border of the mandible.

PARALLELING TECHNIQUE
Mandibular Premolar Projection

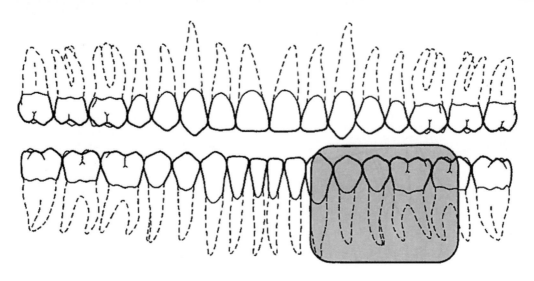

Image field. The radiograph of this area should show the distal half of the canine, the two premolars, and the first molar.

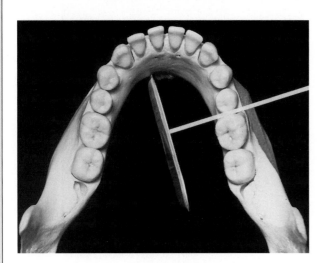

Film placement. Bring the no. 2 film into the mouth with its plane nearly horizontal. Rotate the lead edge to the floor of the mouth between the tongue and the teeth with the anterior border near the midline of the canine. Place the film away from the teeth to position it in the deeper portion of the mouth. Placing the film toward the midline also provides more room for the anterior border of the film in the curvature of the jaw as it sweeps anteriorly. Prevent the anterior border from contacting the very sensitive attached gingiva on the lingual surface of the mandible.

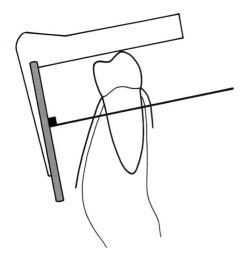

Projection of central ray. Position the film-holding instrument to project the central ray through the second premolar-molar area. The vertical angulation should be small, nearly parallel with the occlusal plane, to keep the film as nearly parallel with the long axis of the teeth as possible. Adjust the horizontal angulation and the placement of the film-holding device to direct the beam through the premolar contact points.

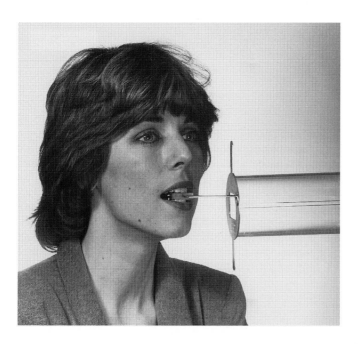

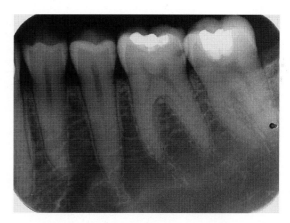

Point of entry. The point of entry of the central ray is below the pupil of the eye and about 3 cm above the inferior border of the mandible.

PARALLELING TECHNIQUE
Mandibular Molar Projection

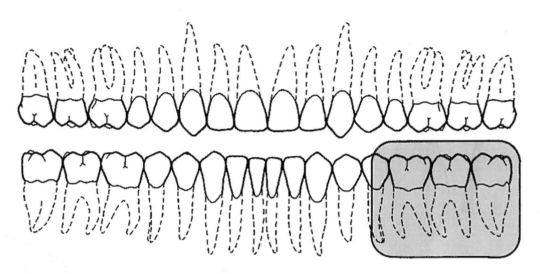

Image field. The radiograph of this region should include the distal half of the second premolar and the three mandibular permanent molars. In the case of an impacted third molar or a pathologic condition distal to the third molar, a distal oblique molar projection or even additional extraoral projections (panoramic or lateral ramus) may be required to demonstrate the area adequately. If the molar area is edentulous, place the film far enough posterior to include the retromolar area in the examination.

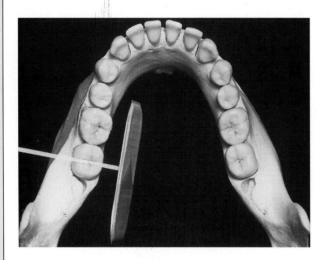

Film placement. Place the no. 2 film in the mouth with its plane nearly horizontal. Rotate the inferior edge downward beneath the lateral border of the tongue, displacing it medially. The anterior edge of the film should be at about the middle of the second premolar. Orient the lateral groove of the bite-block used with the Precision instrument parallel with the mean plane of the molars' buccal surfaces. In most cases the tongue forces the film near the alveolar process and molars, aligning it parallel with the long axis of the teeth and the line of occlusion.

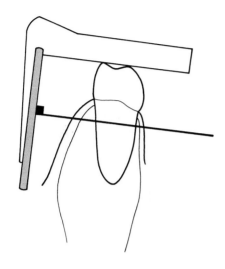

Projection of central ray. Proper placement of the holding instrument directs the central ray through the second molar. Adjust the horizontal angulation to project the beam through the contact areas. Because of the slight lingual inclination of the molars, the central ray may have some slight positive angulation (approximately 8 degrees).

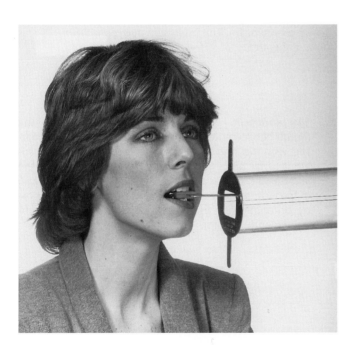

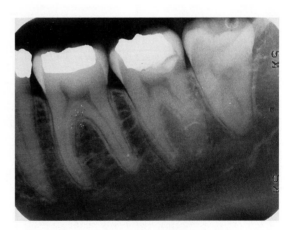

Point of entry. Direct the point of entry of the central ray below the outer canthus of the eye about 3 cm above the inferior border of the mandible.

PARALLELING TECHNIQUE
Mandibular Distal Oblique Molar Projection

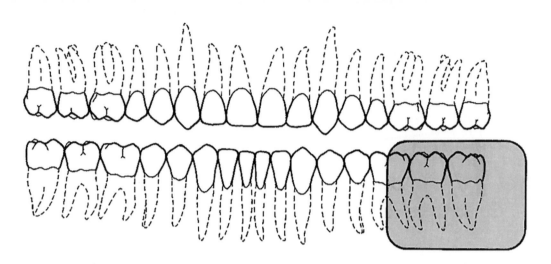

Image field.   The distal oblique projection provides a view of the third molar and the retromolar area of the mandible that usually is not included in the molar radiograph. It is intended primarily for detection or examination of impacted teeth and pathologic conditions in the bone in this area rather than for the teeth themselves; the images of the teeth are distorted and overlap because of the oblique path of the x-ray beam. This projection may eliminate the requirement for an extraoral radiograph of the area.

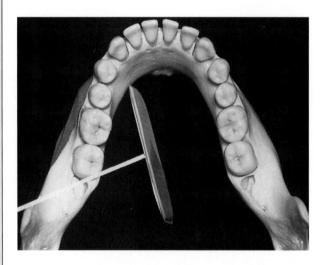

Film placement.   Place the film holder in the floor of the mouth between the tongue and alveolar process and parallel with the long axis of the molars. Position the instrument as far posteriorly as possible and then rotate the film-holding device distally, moving the posterior margin of the film toward the midline. The beam is directed posteroanteriorly, and more distal objects are projected anteriorly onto the film.

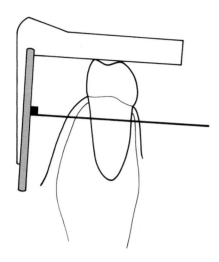

Projection of central ray. The position of the holding instrument projects the central ray from a more posterior aspect through the third molar area to the film.

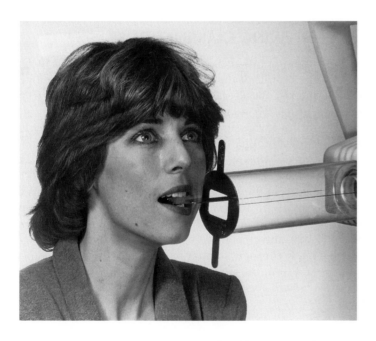

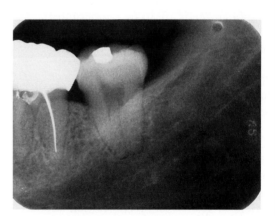

Point of entry. Orient the point of entry about 3 cm above the antegonial notch on the inferior border of the mandible, in line with the anterior border of the ramus.

responding sides, the hypotenuses of each imaginary congruent triangle, are represented by the long axis of the tooth and the long axis of the film. Consequently, when these conditions are satisfied, the images cast on the film theoretically are the same length as the projected object. To reproduce the length of each root of a multirooted tooth accurately, the central beam must be angled differently for each root.

Film-Holding Instruments

Several methods can be used to support films intraorally for bisecting-angle projections. The preferred method is to use a film-holding instrument (e.g., the Snap-A-Ray) or bisecting-angle instruments. Both provide an external device for localizing the x-ray beam. The bisecting-angle instrument uses a fixed average bisecting angle. The method most often used is to use the patient's forefinger to support the film from the lingual surface. However, this method has several drawbacks. Patients often use excessive force and bend the film, causing distortion of the image. Also, the film might slip without the operator's expertise, resulting in an improper image field. Finally, without an external guide to the position of the film, the x-ray beam may miss part of the film, resulting in a partial image ("cone cut").

Positioning of the Patient

To radiograph the maxillary arch, the patient's head should be positioned upright with the sagittal plane vertical and the occlusal plane horizontal. When the mandibular teeth are to be radiographed, the head is tilted back slightly to compensate for the changed occlusal plane when the mouth is opened.

Film Placement

The projections described for the paralleling technique are also used for the bisecting-angle technique. Often the anterior region is covered by using a no. 2 film behind the central incisors in the midline and one lingual to each canine. The film is positioned behind the area of interest, with the apical end against the mucosa on the lingual or palatal surface. The occlusal or incisal edge is oriented against the, teeth with an edge of the film extending just beyond the teeth. If necessary for the patient's comfort, the anterior corner of the film can be softened by bending it before it is placed against the mucosa. Care must be taken not to bend the film excessively because this may result in considerable image distortion and pressure defects in the emulsion that are apparent on the processed film.

Angulation of the Tube Head

Horizontal angulation. When a film-holding device with a beam-localizing ring is used, the instrument is positioned horizontally so that when the tube is aligned with the ring, the central ray is directed through the contacts in the region being examined. If the film-holding device does not have a beam-localizing feature, the tube is pointed so as to direct the central ray through the contacts. In this situation the radiation beam is also centered on the film. This angulation usually is at right angles (in the horizontal projection) to the buccal or facial surfaces of the teeth in each region.

Vertical angulation. In practice, the clinician's goal is to aim the central ray of the x-ray beam at right angles to a plane bisecting the angle between the film and the long axis of the tooth. This principle works well with flat, two-dimensional structures, but teeth that have depth or are multirooted show evidence of distortion. Excessive vertical angulation results in foreshortening of the image, whereas insufficient vertical angulation results in image elongation. The angle that directs the central ray perpendicular to the bisecting plane varies with the individual's anatomy. Several measurements can be used as a general guide when the occlusal plane is oriented parallel with the floor.

BITEWING EXAMINATIONS

Bitewing (also called *interproximal*) radiographs include the crowns of the maxillary and mandibular teeth and the alveolar crest on the same film. Bitewing films are particularly valuable for detecting interproximal caries in the early stages of development before it becomes clinically apparent. Because of the horizontal angle of the x-ray beam, these radiographs also may reveal secondary caries below restorations that may escape recognition in the periapical views. Bitewing projections are also useful for evaluating the periodontal condition. They provide a good perspective of the alveolar bone crest, and changes in bone height can be assessed accurately through comparison with the adjacent teeth. In addition, because of the angle of projection directly through the interproximal spaces, the bitewing film is

Angulation Guidelines for Bisecting-Angle Projections*		
Projection	**Maxilla**	**Mandible**
Incisors	+ 40 degrees	−15 degrees
Canine	+ 45 degrees	−20 degrees
Premolar	+ 30 degrees	−10 degrees
Molar	+ 20 degrees	−5 degrees

*When the occlusal plane is oriented parallel with the floor.

especially effective and useful for detecting calculus deposits in interproximal areas. (Because of its relatively low radiodensity, calculus is better visualized on radiographs made with reduced exposure.) Bitewing films usually are oriented horizontally but may be oriented vertically.

Horizontal Bitewing Films

To obtain the desirable characteristics of the bitewing examination described above, the beam is carefully aligned between the teeth and parallel with the occlusal plane. As the film or film-holding instrument is placed in the mouth, the portion of the mandibular quadrant that is being radiographed is in view. The position of the teeth in this segment of the mandibular quadrant is evaluated, and the beam is directed through the contacts. Some difference may exist in the curvature of the mandibular and maxillary arches. However, when the x-ray beam is accurately directed through the mandibular premolar contacts, overlapping is minimal or absent in the maxillary premolar segment. A few degrees of tolerance are available in the horizontal angulation before overlapping becomes critical. The contact between the maxillary first and second molars often is angled a few degrees more anteriorly than between the mandibular first and second molars. The aiming cylinder is positioned about +10 degrees to project the beam parallel with the occlusal plane (occlusal dentinoenamel junction [DEJ]). This minimizes overlapping of the opposing cusps onto the occlusal surface and thus improves the probability of detecting early occlusal lesions at the DEJ.

The XCP bitewing instrument has an external guide ring for positioning the tube head. This reduces the pos-sibility of cone cutting the film (Fig. 8-6). To position the XCP instrument properly, the guide bar is placed parallel with the direction of the beam that opens the contacts of the dentition being examined.

A film fitted with a bitewing tab or loop may be used instead of a holding device (Fig. 8-7). The film is placed in a comfortable position lingual to the teeth to be examined. The aiming cylinder is oriented in the predetermined direction that passes the x-ray beam through the interproximal spaces. To help prevent cone cutting, the central ray is directed toward the center of the bitewing tab, which protrudes to the buccal side. The beam is angulated +7 to +10 degrees vertically to preclude overlap of the cusps onto the occlusal surface.

Two posterior bitewing views, a premolar and a molar, are recommended for each quadrant. However, for children 12 years old or younger, one bitewing film (no. 2 film) usually suffices. The premolar projection should include the distal half of the canines and the crowns of the premolars. Because the mandibular canines usually are more mesial than the maxillary canines, the mandibular canine is used as the guide for placement of the premolar bitewing film. The molar bitewing film is placed 1 or 2 mm beyond the most distally erupted molar (maxillary or mandibular).

Vertical Bitewing Films

Vertical bitewing films usually are used when the patient has moderate to extensive alveolar bone loss. Orienting the length of the film vertically increases the likelihood that the residual alveolar crests in the maxilla and the mandible will be recorded on the radiograph (Fig. 8-8). The principles for positioning the film and orienting the

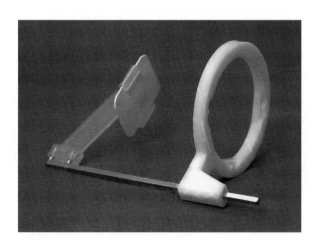

FIG. **8-6** Film-holding device for bitewing radiographs. Note the external localizing ring, which is used to position the aiming tube of the x-ray machine to ensure that the entire film is in the x-ray beam.

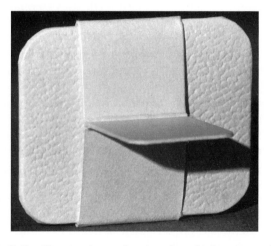

FIG. **8-7** Bitewing loop, showing the tab that the patient bites on to support the film during exposure.

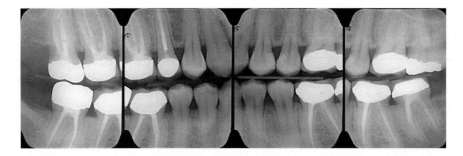

FIG. **8-8** *A set of vertical bitewings.* Orienting the length of the film vertically increases the likelihood that even in patients with extensive alveolar bone loss the residual alveolar crests in the maxilla and the mandible will be recorded on the radiograph.

x-ray beam are otherwise the same as for horizontal bitewing projections.

Occlusal Radiography

An occlusal radiograph displays a relatively large segment of a dental arch. It may include the palate or floor of the mouth and a reasonable extent of the contiguous lateral structures. Occlusal radiographs also are useful when patients are unable to open wide enough for periapical radiographs or for other reasons cannot accept periapical radiography. Because occlusal radiographs are exposed at a steep angulation, they may be used with conventional periapical radiographs to determine the location of objects in all three dimensions. Typically, the occlusal radiograph is especially useful in the following cases:

- To precisely locate roots and supernumerary, unerupted, and impacted teeth (this technique is especially useful for impacted canines and third molars)
- To localize foreign bodies in the jaws and stones in the ducts of sublingual and submandibular glands
- To demonstrate and evaluate the integrity of the anterior, medial, and lateral outlines of the maxillary sinus
- To aid in the examination of patients with trismus, who can open their mouths only a few millimeters; this condition precludes intraoral radiography, which may be impossible or at least extremely painful for the patient
- To obtain information about the location, nature, extent, and displacement of fractures of the mandible and maxilla
- To determine the medial and lateral extent of disease (e.g., cysts, osteomyelitis, malignancies) and detect disease in the palate or floor of the mouth

To make an occlusal radiograph, a relatively large film (7.7 × 5.8 cm [3 × 2.3 inches]) is inserted between the occlusal surfaces of the teeth. As its name implies, the film lies in the plane of occlusion. The "tube" side of this film is positioned toward the jaw to be examined, and the x-ray beam is directed through the jaw to the film. Because of its size, the film allows examination of relatively large portions of the jaw. Standardized projections are used, which stipulate a desired relationship between the central ray, film, and region being examined. However, the clinician should feel free to modify these relationships to meet a specific clinical requirement.

Radiographic Examination of Children

Concern about radiation protection is most important for children because of their greater sensitivity to irradiation. The best way to reduce unnecessary exposure is for the dentist to make the minimal number of films required for the individual patient. These judgments are based on a careful clinical examination and consideration of the patient's age, medical history, growth considerations, and general oral health, as well as whether caries is present and the time elapsed since previous examinations. No simple formulas have been devised for determining the frequency and extent of optimal radiographic examinations. Prudence suggests making bitewing examinations for caries assessment at periodic intervals after the patient's contacts have closed. The frequency should be determined partly by the patient's caries rate. A periapical survey often is recommended for children early in the mixed dentition stage. Special attention should be paid to procedures that reduce exposure (see Chapter 3). These include, in particular, use of fast film, proper processing, beam-limiting devices, and leaded aprons and thyroid shields.

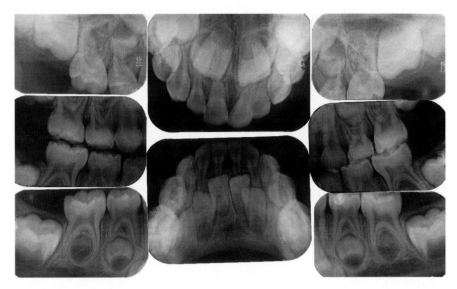

FIG. **8-9** Radiographic examination of primary dentition consists of two anterior occlusal views, four posterior periapical views, and two bitewing views.

Radiography in a child can be an interesting and challenging experience. Although the principles of periapical radiography for children are the same as for adults, in practice children present special considerations because of their small anatomic structures and possible behavioral problems. The smaller size of the arches and dentition requires the use of smaller periapical film. The relatively shallow palate and floor of the mouth may require further modification of film placement. Special radiographic examinations using occlusal film for extraoral projections have been suggested.

PATIENT MANAGEMENT

Children often are apprehensive about the radiographic examination, much as they are about many other types of dental procedures. The radiographic examination usually is the first manipulative procedure performed on a young patient. If this examination is nonthreatening and comfortable, subsequent dental experiences usually are accepted with little or no apprehension. This apprehension is best allayed by familiarizing children with the procedure, which is done by explaining it in a manner they can comprehend. It often is wise to describe the x-ray machine as a camera used to take pictures of teeth. The child can become more comfortable with the film and x-ray machine by touching them before the examination. The operator should carry on a conversation with children to distract them and gain their confidence. It may be advantageous for the child to watch an older brother or sister being radiographed or to have the parent or dental assistant serve as a model. For children who experience a gagging sensation, the clinician can have them breathe through their nose, curl their toes, make a fist, or follow other such devices to distract their attention from the radiographic procedure. However, if the procedure is postponed until the next appointment, the gag reflex may not be encountered or often is much easier for the patient to control. It is especially important to explain to the patient that it will be much easier the next time—plant the positive thought. In any case, if the dentist is adamant about completing the examination, the problem is likely to become chronic and even progressive.

EXAMINATION COVERAGE

When a complete radiographic survey is necessary, it should show the periapical region of all teeth, the proximal surfaces of all posterior teeth, and the crypts of the developing permanent teeth. The number of projections required depends on the child's size. Also, an exposure appropriate to the child's size should be used. For example, a 50% reduction in the mA used for the usual young adult gives the proper density for patients under 10 years of age. Exposure is reduced about 25% for those between 10 and 15 years of age.

Primary Dentition (3 to 6 Years)

A combination of projections can be used to provide adequate coverage for the pedodontic patient. This examination may consist of two anterior occlusal films, two posterior bitewing films, and up to four posterior periapical films as indicated (Fig. 8-9). For the maxil-

Text continued on p. 164.

Premolar Bitewing Projection

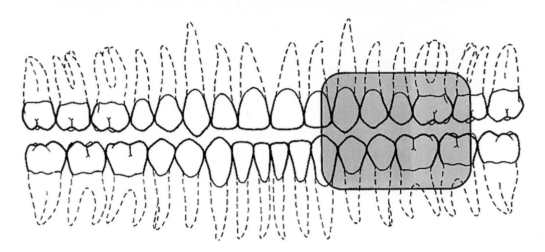

Image field. This projection should cover the distal portion of the mandibular canine anteriorly and show equally the crowns of the maxillary and mandibular premolar teeth.

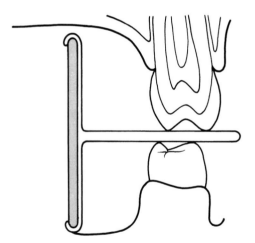

Film placement. Place the film between the tongue and the teeth, far enough from the lingual surface of the teeth to prevent interference by the palate on closing and parallel to the long axes of the teeth. The anterior border of the film should extend beyond the contact area between the mandibular canine and first premolar. Hold the film in place until the patient's mouth is completely closed. Holding the film while closing prevents it from being displaced distally.

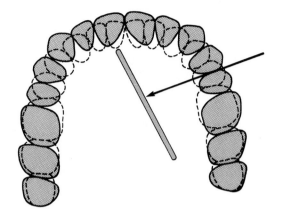

Projection of central ray. Adjust the horizontal angulation of the cone to project the central ray to the center of the film through the premolar contact areas. To compensate for the slight inclination of the film against the palatal mucosa, the vertical angulation should be about +5 degrees. (In the drawing, the mandibular teeth are in *dashed lines*.)

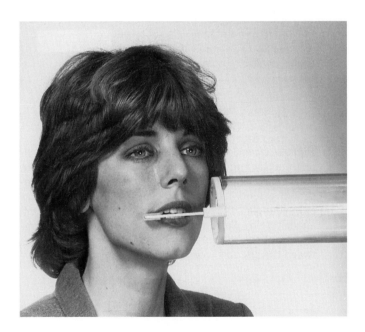

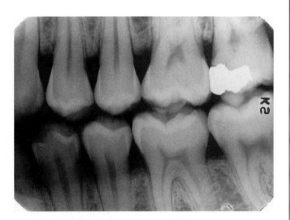

Point of entry. Identify the point of entry by retracting the cheek and determining that the central ray will enter the line of occlusion at the point of contact between the second premolar and first molar.

Molar Bitewing Projection

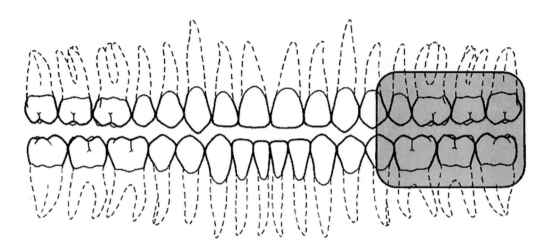

Image field. This projection should show the distal surface of the most posterior erupted molar and equally the crowns of the maxillary and mandibular molars. Because the maxillary and mandibular molar contact areas may not be open from the same horizontal angulation, they may not be visible on one film. In this case it may be desirable to open the maxillary molar contacts because the mandibular molar contacts usually are open on the periapical films.

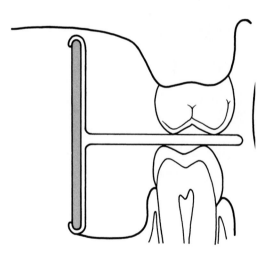

Film placement. Place the film between the tongue and teeth, as far lingual as practical to avoid contacting the sensitive attached gingiva. The distal margin of the film should extend 1 to 2 mm beyond the most posterior erupted molar. When using the XCP, adjust the horizontal angulation by placing the guide bar parallel with the direction of the central ray to open the contact area between the first and second molars.

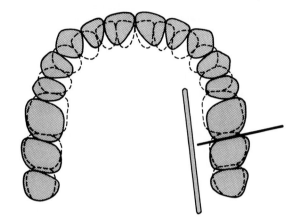

Projection of central ray. Project the central ray to the center of the film and through the contact of the first and second maxillary molars. Angle the central ray slightly from the anterior because the molar contacts usually are not oriented at right angles to the buccal surfaces of these teeth. A vertical angulation of +10 degrees is recommended. (In the drawing, the mandibular teeth are in *dashed lines*.)

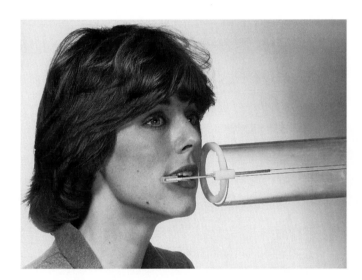

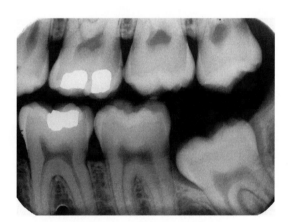

Point of entry. The central ray should enter the cheek below the lateral canthus of the eye at the level of the occlusal plane.

Anterior Maxillary Occlusal Projection

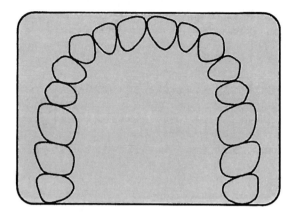

Image field. The primary field of this projection includes the anterior maxilla and its dentition, as well as the anterior floor of the nasal fossa and teeth from canine to canine.

Film placement. Adjust the patient's head so that the sagittal plane is perpendicular and the occlusal plane is horizontal to the floor. Place the film in the mouth with the exposure side toward the maxilla, the posterior border touching the rami, and the long dimension of the film perpendicular to the sagittal plane. The patient stabilizes the film by gently closing the mouth or using gentle bilateral thumb pressure.

Projection of central ray. Orient the central ray through the tip of the nose toward the middle of the film with approximately +45 degrees vertical angulation and 0 degrees horizontal angulation.

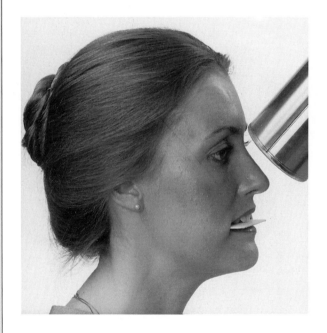

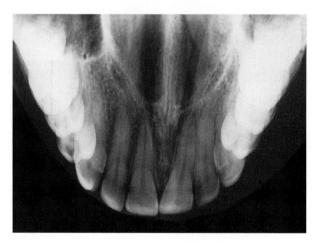

Point of entry. The central ray enters the patient's face approximately through the tip of the nose.

Cross-Sectional Maxillary Occlusal Projection

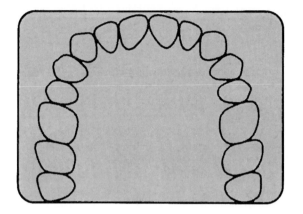

Image field. This projection shows the palate, zygomatic processes of the maxilla, anteroinferior aspects of each antrum, nasolacrimal canals, teeth from second molar to second molar, and nasal septum.

Film placement. Seat the patient upright with the sagittal plane perpendicular to the floor and the occlusal plane horizontal. Place the film, with its long dimension perpendicular to the sagittal plane, crosswise in the mouth. Gently push the film in backward until it contacts the anterior border of the mandibular rami. The patient stabilizes the film by gently closing the mouth.

Projection of central ray. Direct the central ray at a vertical angulation of +65 degrees and a horizontal angulation of 0 degrees, to the bridge of the nose just below the nasion, toward the middle of the film.

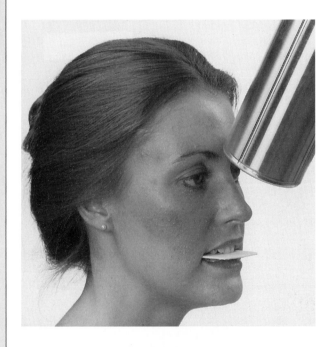

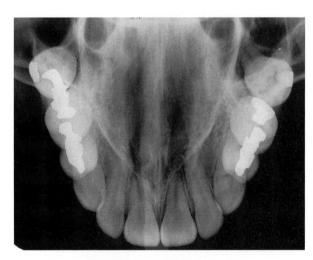

Point of entry. Generally, the central ray enters the patient's face through the bridge of the nose.

Lateral Maxillary Occlusal Projection

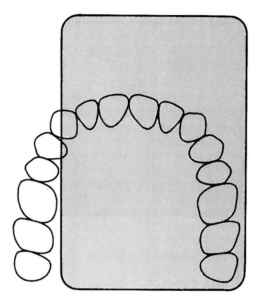

Image field. This projection shows a quadrant of the alveolar ridge of the maxilla, inferolateral aspect of the antrum, tuberosity, and teeth from the lateral incisor to the contralateral third molar. In addition, the zygomatic process of the maxilla superimposes over the roots of the molar teeth.

Film placement. Place the film with its long axis parallel with the sagittal plane and on the side of interest, with the tube side toward the side of the maxilla in question. Push the film posteriorly until it touches the ramus. Position the lateral border parallel with the buccal surfaces of the posterior teeth, extending laterally approximately 1 cm past the buccal cusps. Ask the patient to close gently to hold the film in position.

Projection of central ray. Orient the central ray with a vertical angulation of +60 degrees, to a point 2 cm below the lateral canthus of the eye, directed toward the center of the film.

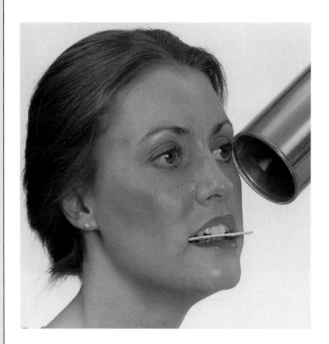

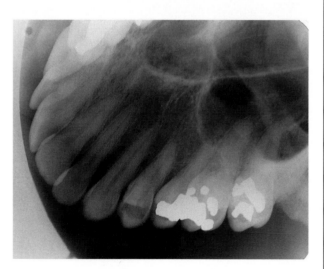

Point of entry. The central ray enters at a point approximately 2 cm below the lateral canthus of the eye.

Anterior Mandibular Occlusal Projection

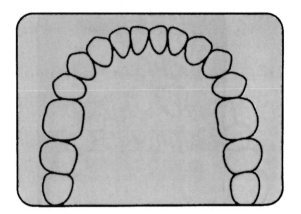

Image field. This projection includes the anterior portion of the mandible, dentition from canine to canine, and inferior cortical border of the mandible.

Film placement. Seat the patient tilted back so that the occlusal plane is 45 degrees above horizontal. Place the film in the mouth with the long axis perpendicular to the sagittal plane and push it posteriorly until it touches the rami. Center the film with the pebbled side (tube side) down and ask the patient to bite lightly to hold the film in position.

Projection of central ray. Orient the central ray with −10 degrees angulation through the point of the chin toward the middle of the film; this gives the ray −55 degrees of angulation to the plane of the film.

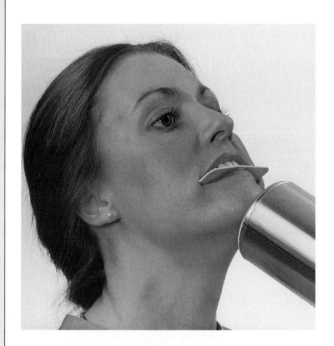

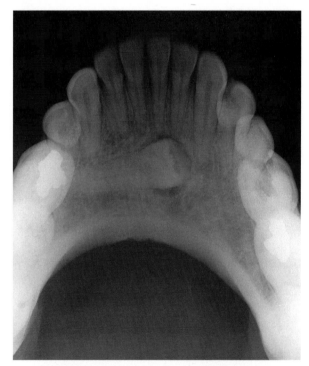

Point of entry. The point of entry of the central ray is in the midline and through the tip of the chin.

Cross-Sectional Mandibular Occlusal Projection

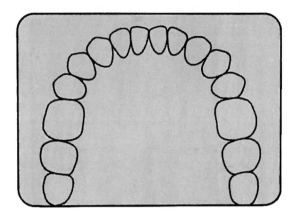

Image field. This projection includes the soft tissue of the floor of the mouth and reveals the lingual and buccal plates of the mandible from second molar to second molar. When this view is made to examine the floor of the mouth (e.g., for sialoliths), the exposure time should be reduced to one half the time used to create an image of the mandible.

Film placement. Seat the patient in a semireclining position with the head tilted back so that the ala-tragus line is almost perpendicular to the floor. Place the film in the mouth with its long axis perpendicular to the sagittal plane and with the tube side toward the mandible. The anterior border of the film should be approximately 1 cm beyond the mandibular central incisors. Ask the patient to bite gently on the film to hold it in position.

Projection of central ray. Direct the central ray at the midline through the floor of the mouth approximately 3 cm below the chin, at right angles to the center of the film.

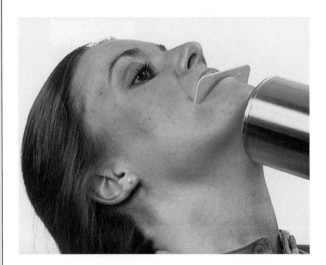

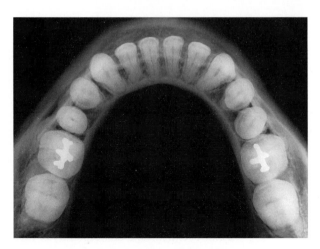

Point of entry. The point of entry of the central ray is in the midline through the floor of the mouth approximately 3 cm below the chin.

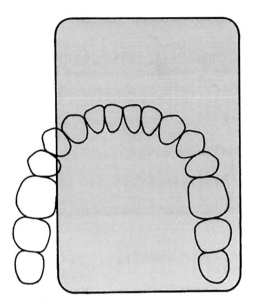

Image field. This projection covers the soft tissue of half the floor of the mouth, the buccal and lingual cortical plates of half of the mandible, and the teeth from the lateral incisor to the contralateral third molar. When this view is used to provide an image of the floor of the mouth, the exposure time should be reduced to one half that used to provide an image of the mandible.

Film placement. Seat the patient in a semireclining position with the head tilted back so that the alatragus line is almost perpendicular to the floor. Place the film in the mouth with its long axis initially parallel with the sagittal plane and with the pebbled side down toward the mandible. Place the film as far posterior as possible, then shift the long axis buccally (right or left) so that the lateral border of the film is parallel with the buccal surfaces of the posterior teeth and extends laterally approximately 1 cm.

Projection of central ray. Direct the central ray perpendicular to the center of the film through a point beneath the chin, approximately 3 cm posterior to the point of the chin and 3 cm lateral to the midline.

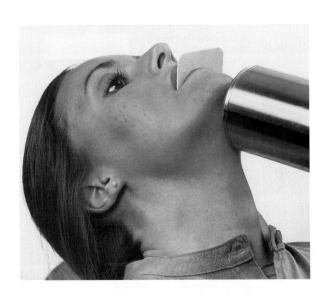

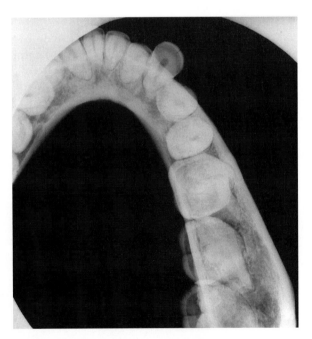

Point of entry. The point of entry of the central ray is beneath the chin, approximately 3 cm posterior to the chin and approximately 3 cm lateral to the midline.

lary and interproximal projections, the child is seated upright with the sagittal plane perpendicular to and the occlusal plane parallel with the floor (horizontal plane). For mandibular projections, except the occlusal, the child is seated upright with the sagittal plane perpendicular. The tragus corner of the mouth line is oriented parallel to the floor. Some find that a panoramic film, rather than the four periapical films, is more informative and results in less exposure to the child (see Chapter 3).

Maxillary anterior occlusal projection. Place a no. 2 film in the mouth with its long axis perpendicular to the sagittal plane and the pebbled surface toward the maxillary teeth. Center the film on the midline with the anterior border extending just beyond the incisal edges of the anterior teeth. Direct the central ray at a vertical angulation of +60 degrees through the tip of the nose toward the center of the film.

Mandibular anterior occlusal projection. Seat the child with the head tipped back so that the occlusal plane is about 25 degrees above the plane of the floor. Place a no. 2 film with the long axis perpendicular to the sagittal plane and the pebbled surface toward the mandibular teeth. Orient the central ray at −30 degrees vertical angulation and through the tip of the chin toward the film.

Bitewing projection. Use a no. 0 film with a paper loop film holder. Place the film in the child's mouth as in the adult premolar bitewing projection. The image field should include the distal half of the canine and the de-

ciduous molars. Use a positive vertical angulation of +5 to +10 degrees. Orient the horizontal angle to direct the beam through the interproximal spaces.

Deciduous maxillary molar periapical projection. Use a no. 0 film in a modified XCP or BAI bite-block, either with or without the aiming ring and indicator bar. Position the film in the midline of the palate with the anterior border extending to the maxillary primary canine. The image field of this projection should include the distal half of the primary canine and both primary molars.

Deciduous mandibular molar projection. Position a no. 0 film in a modified XCP or BAI bite-block, with or without the aiming ring and indicator bar, between the posterior teeth and tongue. The exposed radiograph should show the distal half of the mandibular primary canine and the primary molar teeth.

Mixed Dentition (7 to 12 Years)

A complete examination of the mixed dentition, if indicated, consists of two incisor periapical films, four canine periapical films, four posterior periapical films, and two or four posterior bitewing films (Fig. 8-10). For the maxillary and interproximal projections, seat the child upright with the sagittal plane perpendicular and the occlusal plane parallel to the floor. For the mandibular projections, seat the child upright with the sagittal plane perpendicular and the alatragus line parallel to the floor. Use the Precision Pedodontic or XCP instruments for larger children. The BAI bite-blocks may be more comfortable for smaller individuals.

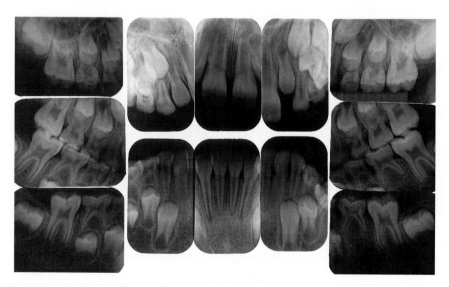

FIG. **8-10** Radiographic examination of mixed dentition consists of two incisor views, four canine views, four posterior views, and two bitewing views.

Maxillary anterior periapical projection. Center a no. 1 film on the embrasure between the central incisors in the mouth behind the maxillary central and lateral incisors. Center the film on the midline.

Mandibular anterior periapical projection. Position a no. 1 film behind the mandibular central and lateral incisors.

Canine periapical projection. Position a no. 1 film behind each of the canines.

Deciduous and permanent molar periapical projection. Position a no. 1 or no. 2 film (if the child is large enough) with the anterior edge behind the canine.

Posterior bitewing projection. Expose bitewing projections in the premolar region with no. 1 or no. 2 film as previously described, using either bitewing tabs or the Rinn bitewing instrument. Expose four bitewing projections when the second permanent molars have erupted.

Special Considerations

The radiographic procedures that have been described in this chapter are for the "well" patient. These procedures may need to be modified for patients who have unusual difficulties. Specific modifications depend on the patient's physical and emotional characteristics. As with any dental procedure, however, the dental assistant begins the examination by showing appreciation of the patient's condition and sympathy for any problems that might occur for either of them. If the assistant is kind but firm, the patient's confidence increases, which helps the patient relax and cooperate. Following are a few conditions and circumstances that may be encountered, with some recommendations and suggestions that may help the clinician achieve an adequate radiographic examination.

INFECTION

Infection in the orofacial structures may result in edema and lead to trismus of some of the muscles of mastication. As a result, intraoral radiography may be painful to the patient and difficult for both the patient and radiologist. Under such circumstances extraoral or occlusal techniques may offer the only possibility of an examination. The choice of a specific extraoral projection depends on the condition and the areas to be examined. Although the resulting radiograph may not be ideal in many respects, it usually provides more useful information than the diagnostician would have without it. In the case of edema in an area to be examined, increased exposure is required to compensate for the tissue swelling. Such an increase can be accomplished by increasing the kVp, mA, or duration of exposure. With dental x-ray machines, exposure time usually is the easiest and most convenient variable that provides the most consistent results (except with patients who have difficulty remaining motionless for a few seconds).

Often patients with communicable diseases such as acquired immunodeficiency syndrome (AIDS), tuberculosis, herpes, hepatitis, and syphilis require a dental radiographic examination. Strict observance of infection control procedures prevents the dentist from acquiring the disease or passing the infection to other patients. Chapter 7 discusses these infection control procedures in detail.

TRAUMA

A patient who has suffered trauma and may have a fracture of the facial skeleton may be bedridden because of involvement of several other areas of the skeleton. Consequently, an extraoral radiographic examination with the patient in the supine position is necessary. However, the circumstances need not compromise the techniques, and satisfactory radiographs can be produced if the proper relative positions of the tube, patient, and film are observed.

Often intraoral periapical radiographs are not large enough to delineate the size and extent of oral neoplasms. In these cases occlusal and extraoral projections must be used because these examinations have a greater chance of revealing all such lesions. When examining such conditions, it is always desirable to have all the borders of the lesion recorded on a single film.

MENTALLY DISABLED PATIENTS

Patients with mental disabilities may cause some difficulty for the radiologist who is attempting an examination. The difficulty usually is the result of the patient's lack of coordination or inability to comprehend what is expected. However, by performing the radiographic examination speedily, unpredictable moves by the patient can be avoided. Using a higher kVp or mA or fast film and intensifying screens reduces exposure time and the possibility that involuntary movement by the patient will make the film unusable. If coordination is a major difficulty, sedation may be required. If heavy sedation is used, the radiographic examination is performed with the patient in the supine position. When an intraoral radiographic examination is performed with the patient supine, film-holding and beam-aiming devices are used to ensure proper film placement and tube angulation.

PHYSICALLY DISABLED PATIENTS

Patients with physical disabilities (e.g., loss of vision, loss of hearing, loss of the use of any or all extremities, congenital defects such as cleft palate) may require special handling during a radiographic examination. These patients usually are cooperative and eager to assist. They may well have or have had so much discomfort and inconvenience that their tolerance level is high, and they are not challenged by the relatively slight irritation represented by the x-ray procedures. Generally, intraoral and extraoral radiographic examinations may be performed for these patients if a good rapport between the patient and radiology technician is established and maintained. Members of the patient's family often are very helpful in assisting the patient into and out of the examination chair and in film positioning and holding, inasmuch as they usually are familiar with the patient's condition and accustomed to coping with it.

GAG REFLEX

Occasionally, patients who need a radiographic examination manifest a gag reflex at the slightest provocation. These patients usually are very apprehensive and frightened by unknown procedures; others simply seem to have very sensitive tissue that precipitates a gag reflex when stimulated. This sensitivity is manifested when the film is placed in the oral cavity. To overcome this disability, the radiologist should make an effort to relax and reassure the patient. The radiologist can describe and explain the procedures. Often gagging can be controlled if the operator bolsters the patient's confidence by demonstrating technical competence and showing authority tempered with compassion. The gag reflex often is worse when a patient is tired; therefore it is advisable to perform the examination in the morning, when the individual is well rested, especially in the case of children.

Stimulating the posterior dorsum of the tongue or the soft palate usually initiates the gag reflex. Consequently, during the placement of the film, the tongue should be very relaxed and positioned well to the floor of the mouth. This can be accomplished by asking the patient to swallow deeply just before opening the mouth for placement of the film. (The dentist should never mention the tongue, nor ask patients to relax the tongue; this usually makes them more conscious of it and precipitates involuntary movements.) The film is carried into the mouth parallel to the occlusal plane. When the desired area is reached, the film is rotated with a decisive motion, bringing it into contact with the palate or the floor of the mouth. Sliding it along the palate or tongue is likely to stimulate the gag reflex. Also, the dentist must keep in mind that the longer the

film stays in the mouth, the greater the possibility that the patient will start to gag. The patient should be advised to breathe rapidly through the nose because mouth breathing usually aggravates this condition.

Any little exercise that can be devised that does not interfere with the x-ray examination but shifts the patient's attention from the film and the mouth is likely to relieve the gag reaction. Such a distraction often can be created by asking patients to hold their breath or to keep a foot or arm suspended during film placement and exposure. In extreme cases, topical anesthetic agents in mouthwashes or spray can be administered to produce temporary numbness of the tongue and palate to reduce gagging. However, in our experience this procedure gives limited results. The most effective approach is to reduce apprehension, minimize tissue irritation, and encourage rapid breathing through the nose. If all measures fail, an extraoral examination may be the only means, short of administering general anesthesia, to examine the patient radiographically.

RADIOGRAPHIC TECHNIQUES FOR ENDODONTICS

Radiographs are essential to the practice of endodontics. Not only are they indispensable for determining the diagnosis and prognosis of pulp treatment, they also are the most reliable method of managing endodontic treatment. The presence of a rubber dam, rubber dam clamp, and root canal instruments may complicate an intraoral periapical examination by impairing proper film positioning and aiming cylinder angulation. Despite these obstacles, certain requirements must be observed:

1. The tooth being treated must be centered in the image.
2. The film must be positioned as far from the tooth and apex as the region permits to ensure that the apex of the tooth and some periapical bone are apparent on the radiograph.

Projection Technique

For maxillary projections, the patient is seated so that the sagittal plane is perpendicular and the occlusal plane is parallel to the floor. For mandibular projections, the patient is seated upright with the sagittal plane perpendicular and the tragus corner of the mouth line parallel to the floor. A hemostat is used as a film holder because it occupies minimal space and is easy for the operator and patient to manage (see Fig. 8-3, *E*); specially designed instruments for endodontic use also may be used (Fig. 8-11).

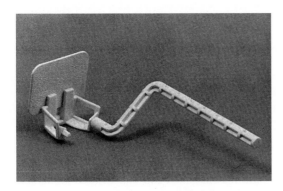

FIG. **8-11** Endo-Ray film holder used for endodontic radiographs. (Courtesy Demac, Ltd., St. Charles, Ill.)

A no. 2 periapical film is used for all projections. For anterior projections, the film is grasped along the edge of the short dimension of the film. For posterior projections, the long side of the film is engaged. The film in the hemostat is inserted into the mouth with the film parallel to the occlusal plane. The film is placed in the proper position by rotating the hemostat and film into a position as near parallel as possible to the long axis of the tooth to be radiographed.

The aiming cylinder is aligned so as to direct the central ray perpendicular to the center of the film. The plane of the end of the aiming cylinder should be parallel with the hemostat handle. After the film is positioned, the patient's hand is guided, with instructions, to hold and stabilize the hemostat against the teeth in the same arch during exposure. As an alternative, the hemostat can be inserted through a bite-block onto which the patient can bite, providing stabilization of the instrument and film.

Often a single radiograph of a multirooted tooth made at the normal vertical and horizontal projection does not display all the roots. In these cases, when it is prudent to separate the roots on multirooted teeth, a second projection may be made. The horizontal angulation is altered 20 degrees mesially to the hemostat handle for the maxillary premolars, 20 degrees mesially or distally for the maxillary molars, or 20 degrees distally for an oblique projection of the mandibular molar roots.

If a sinus tract is encountered, its course is tracked by threading a no. 40 gutta-percha cone through the tract before the radiograph is made. It also is possible to localize and determine the depth of periodontal defects with this gutta-percha tracking technique.

A final radiograph of the treated tooth is made to demonstrate the quality of the root canal filling and the condition of the periapical tissues after removal of the clamp and rubber dam. An oblique projection is used if a possibility of superimposing any of the canals exists.

PREGNANCY

Although a fetus is sensitive to ionizing radiation, the amount of exposure received by an embryo or fetus during dental radiography is extremely low. No incidences have been reported of damage to a fetus from dental radiography. Prudence suggests that such radiographic examinations be kept to a minimum consistent with the mother's dental needs. As with any patient, radiographic examination is limited during pregnancy to cases with a specific diagnostic indication. With the low patient dose afforded by use of optimal radiation safety techniques (see Chapter 3), an intraoral or extraoral examination can be performed whenever a reasonable diagnostic requirement exists.

EDENTULOUS PATIENTS

Radiographic examination of edentulous patients is important, whether the area is one tooth in extent or an entire arch. These areas may contain roots, residual infection, impacted teeth, cysts, or other pathologic entities that may adversely affect the usefulness of prosthetic appliances or the patient's health. After a determination has been made that these entities are not present, repeated examinations to detect them are not warranted. Edentulous patients typically represent an older age group, and their potential for developing malignant tumors is higher. However, the low probability of developing a malignancy does not constitute a continuing indication for periodic radiographic examination in the absence of other clinical signs or symptoms. After a determination has been made that the jaws are free of disease, periodic radiographs are not warranted in the absence of symptoms.

Radiographic Techniques for Edentulous Patients

If available, a panoramic examination of the edentulous jaws is most convenient. If abnormalities of the alveolar ridges are identified, the higher resolution of periapical film is used to make intraoral projections to supplement the panoramic examination.

In a completely or partly edentulous patient, a film-holding device is used for intraoral radiography of the alveolar ridges. Placement of the film-holding instrument may be complicated by its tipping into the voids normally occupied by the crowns of the missing teeth. To manage this difficulty, cotton rolls are placed between the ridge and the film holder, supporting the holder in a horizontal position. An orthodontic elastic to hold cotton rolls to the bite-block on the film holder often is useful when several such projections must be exposed. With elastics, it is simple to maneuver the cotton rolls into the areas that require support. The patient may steady the film-holding instrument with a hand or an opposing denture.

If panoramic equipment is not available, an examination consisting of 14 intraoral films provides an excellent survey. The exposure required for an edentulous ridge is approximately 25% less than that for a dentulous ridge. This examination consists of seven projections in each jaw (adult no. 2 film) as follows:

Central incisors (midline)	1 projection
Lateral-canine	2 projections
Premolar	2 projections
Molar	2 projections

BIBLIOGRAPHY

Bean LR: Comparison of bisecting angle and paralleling methods of intraoral radiology, *J Dent Educ* 33:441, 1969.

Jones PE, Warner B: A teaching method for the paralleling technique, *Oral Surg* 42:126, 1976.

Manson-Hing LR: On the evaluation of radiographic techniques, *Oral Surg* 27:631, 1969.

Medwedeff FM, Elcan PD: A precision technique to minimize radiation, *Dent Surv* 43:45, 1967.

Scandrett FR et al: Radiographic examination of the edentulous patient. 1. Review of the literature and preliminary report comparing three methods, *Oral Surg* 35:266, 1973.

Shawkat AH et al: Evaluation of the utilization of the supine position in intraoral radiology, *Oral Surg* 43:963, 1977.

Silha RE: Paralleling technique with a disposable film holder, *Dent Radiogr Photogr* 48:27, 1975.

Updegrave WJ: Simplified and standardized intraoral radiography with reduced tissue irradiation, *JADA* 85:861, 1972.

van der Stelt PF et al: In vitro study into the influence of x-ray beam angulation on the detection of artificial defects on bitewing radiographs, *Caries Res* 23:334, 1989.

Walton RE: Endodontic radiographic techniques, *Dent Radiogr Photogr* 46:51, 1973.

Weissman DD, Longhurst GE: Clinical evaluation of a rectangular field collimating device for periapical radiography, *JADA* 82:580, 1971.

Weissman DD, Sobkowski FJ: Comparative thermoluminescent dosimetry of intraoral periapical radiography, *Oral Surg* 29:376, 1970.

Wuehrmann AH, Manson-Hing LR: *Dental radiology*, ed 4, St Louis, 1977, Mosby.

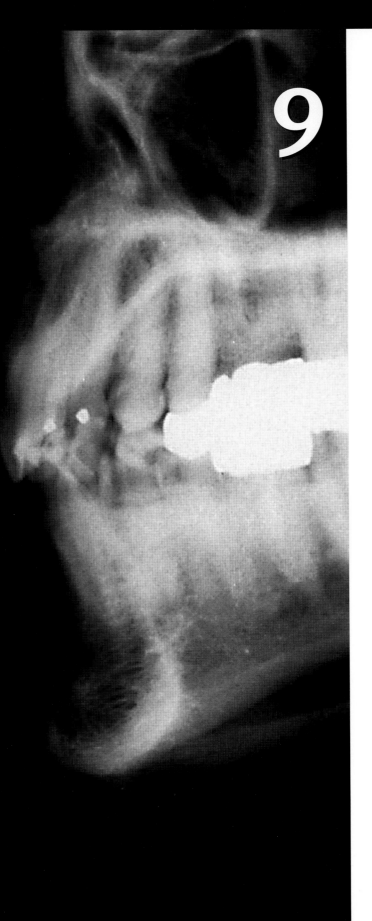

Normal Radiographic Anatomy

The radiographic recognition of disease requires a sound knowledge of the radiographic appearance of normal structures. Intelligent diagnosis mandates an appreciation of the wide range of variation in the appearance of normal anatomic structures. Similarly, most patients demonstrate many of the normal radiographic landmarks, but it is a rare patient who shows them all. Accordingly, the absence of one or even several such landmarks in any individual should not necessarily be considered abnormal.

Teeth

Teeth are composed primarily of dentin, with an enamel cap over the coronal portion and a thin layer of cementum over the root surface (Fig. 9-1). The enamel cap characteristically appears more radiopaque than the other tissues because it is the most dense naturally occurring substance in the body. Being 90% mineral, it causes the greatest attenuation of x-ray photons. The dentin is about 75% mineralized, and because of its lower mineral content its radiographic appearance is roughly comparable to that of bone. Dentin is smooth and homogeneous on radiographs because of its uniform morphology. The enamelodentinal junction, between enamel and dentin, appears as a distinct interface that separates these two structures. The thin layer of cementum on the root surface has a mineral content (50%) comparable to that of dentin. Cementum is not usually apparent radiographically because the contrast between it and dentin is so low and the cementum layer is so thin.

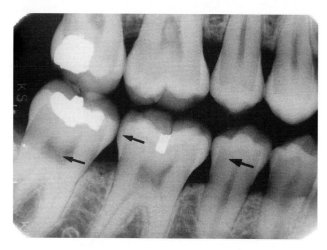

FIG. **9-1** Teeth are composed of pulp (*arrow* on the second molar), enamel (*arrow* on the first molar), dentin (*arrow* on the second premolar), and cementum (usually not visible radiographically).

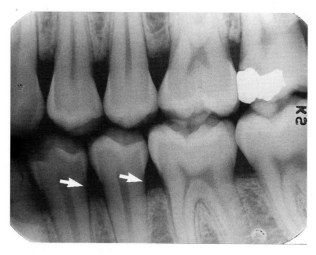

FIG. **9-2** Cervical burnout caused by overexposure of the lateral portion of teeth between the enamel and alveolar crest (*arrows*).

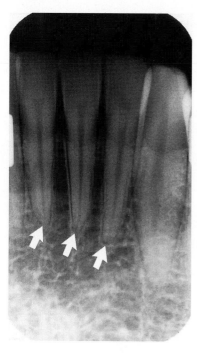

FIG. **9-3** Root canals open at the apices of adult incisors (*arrows*).

Diffuse radiolucent areas with ill-defined borders may be apparent radiographically on the mesial or distal aspects of teeth in the cervical regions between the edge of the enamel cap and the crest of the alveolar ridge (Fig. 9-2). This phenomenon, called *cervical burnout*, is caused by the normal configuration of the affected teeth, which results in decreased x-ray absorption in the areas in question. Furthermore, the perception of these radiolucent areas results from the contrast with the adjacent, relatively opaque enamel and alveolar bone. Such radiolucencies should be anticipated in almost all teeth and not confused with root surface caries, which frequently have a similar appearance.

The pulp of normal teeth is composed of soft tissue and consequently appears radiolucent. The chambers and root canals containing the pulp extend from the interior of the crown to the apices of the roots. Although the shape of most pulp chambers is fairly uniform within tooth groups, great variations exist among individuals in the size of the pulp chambers and the extent of pulp horns. The practitioner must anticipate such variations in the proportions and distribution of the pulp and verify them radiographically when planning restorative procedures.

In normal, fully formed teeth the root canal may be apparent, extending to the apex of the root; an apical foramen is usually recognizable (Fig. 9-3). In other normal teeth the canal may appear constricted in the region of the apex and not discernible in the last millimeter or so of its length (Fig. 9-4). In this case the canal may occasionally exit on the side of the tooth, just short of the radiographic apex. Lateral canals may occur as branches of an otherwise normal root canal. They may extend to the apex and end in a normal, discernible foramen or may exit the side of the root. In either case, two or more terminal foramina might cause endodontic treatment to fail if they are not identified.

At the end of a developing tooth root the pulp canal diverges and the walls of the root rapidly taper to a knife edge (Fig. 9-5). In the recess formed by the root walls and extending a short distance beyond is a small, rounded, ra-

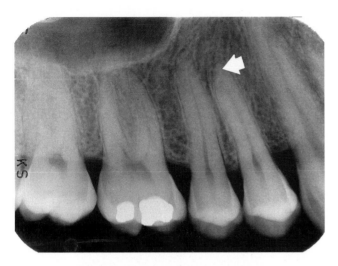

FIG. **9-4** Although the root canal is not radiographically visible in the apical 2 mm of a tooth, anatomically it is present *(arrow)*.

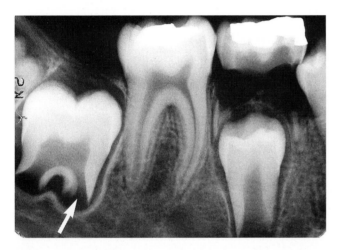

FIG. **9-5** A developing root shown by a divergent apex around the dental papilla *(arrow)*, which is enclosed by an opaque bony crypt.

diolucent area in the trabecular bone, surrounded by a thin layer of hyperostotic bone. This is the dental papilla bounded by its bony crypt. The papilla forms the dentin and the primordium of the pulp. When the tooth reaches maturity, the pulpal walls in the apical region begin to constrict and finally come into close apposition. Awareness of this sequence and its radiographic pattern is often useful in evaluating the stage of maturation of the developing tooth; it also helps avoid misidentifying the apical radiolucency as a periapical lesion.

In a mature tooth, the shape of the pulp chamber and canal may change. With aging occurs a gradual deposition of secondary dentin. This process begins apically, proceeds coronally, and may lead to pulp oblit-

eration. Trauma to the tooth (e.g., from caries, a blow, restorations, attrition, or erosion) also may stimulate dentin production, leading to a reduction in size of the pulp chamber and canals. Such cases usually include evidence of the source of the pathologic stimulus. In the case of a blow to the teeth, however, only the patient's recollection may suggest the true reason for the reduced pulp chamber size.

Supporting Structures

LAMINA DURA

A radiograph of sound teeth in a normal dental arch demonstrates that the tooth sockets are bounded by a thin radiopaque layer of dense bone (Fig. 9-6). Its name, *lamina dura* (hard layer), is derived from its radiographic appearance. This layer is continuous with the shadow of the cortical bone at the alveolar crest. It is only slightly thicker and no more highly mineralized than the trabeculae of cancellous bone in the area. Its radiographic appearance is caused by the fact that the x-ray beam passes tangentially through many times the thickness of the thin bony wall, which results in its observed attenuation. Developmentally the lamina dura is an extension of the lining of the bony crypt that surrounds each tooth during development.

The appearance of the lamina dura on radiographs may vary. When the x-ray beam is directed through a relatively long expanse of the structure, the lamina dura appears radiopaque and well defined. When the beam is directed more obliquely, however, the lamina dura appears more diffuse and may not be discernible. In fact, even if the supporting bone in a healthy arch is intact, identification of a lamina dura completely surrounding every root on each film is frequently difficult, although it usually is evident to some extent about the roots on each film (Fig. 9-7). In addition, small variations and disruptions in the continuity of the lamina dura may represent superimpositions of trabecular pattern and small nutrient canals passing from the mandibular bone to the periodontal ligament.

The thickness and density of the lamina dura on the radiograph vary with the amount of occlusal stress to which the tooth is subjected. The lamina dura is wider and more dense around the roots of teeth in heavy occlusion, and thinner and less dense around teeth not subjected to occlusal function.

The image of a double lamina dura is not uncommon if the mesial or distal surfaces of roots present two elevations in the path of the x-ray beam. A common example of this is seen on the buccal and lingual eminences on the mesial surface of mandibular first molar roots (Fig. 9-8).

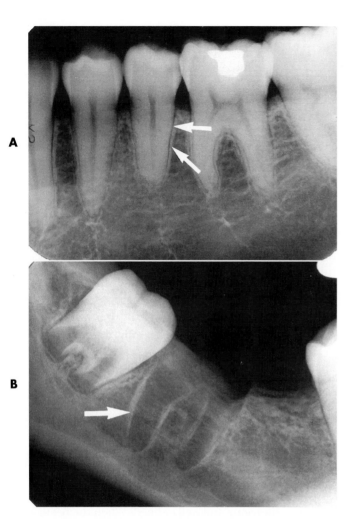

A

B

FIG. **9-6**   The lamina dura *(arrows)* appears as a thin opaque layer of bone around teeth, **A,** and around a recent extraction socket, **B.**

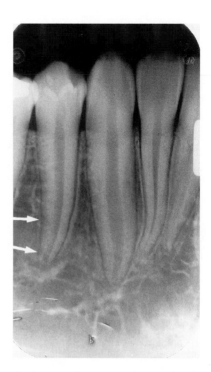

FIG. **9-7**   The lamina dura is poorly visualized on the distal surface of this premolar *(arrows)* but is clearly seen on the mesial surface.

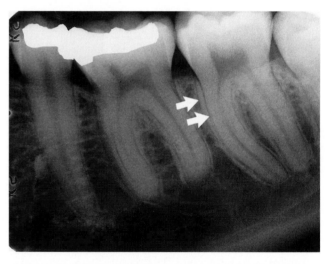

FIG. **9-8**   A double periodontal ligament space and lamina dura *(arrows)* may be seen when there is a convexity of the proximal surface of the root.

The appearance of the lamina dura is a valuable diagnostic feature. The presence of an intact lamina dura around the apex of a tooth strongly suggests a vital pulp. Because of the variable appearance of the lamina dura, however, the absence of its image around an apex on a radiograph may be normal. Rarely, in the absence of disease the lamina dura may be absent from a molar root extending into the maxillary sinus. The clinician is therefore advised to consider other signs and symptoms as well as the integrity of the lamina dura when establishing a diagnosis and treatment.

ALVEOLAR CREST

The gingival margin of the alveolar process that extends between the teeth is apparent on radiographs as a radiopaque line, the alveolar crest (Fig. 9-9). The level of this bony crest is considered normal when it is not more than 1.5 mm from the cementoenamel junction of the adjacent teeth. The alveolar crest may recede apically

with age and show marked resorption with periodontal disease. Radiographs can demonstrate only the position of the crest; determining the significance of its level is primarily a clinical problem. (See Chapter 16.)

The length of the normal alveolar crest in a particular region depends on the distance between the teeth in question. In the anterior region the crest is reduced to only a point of bone between the close-set incisors. Posteriorly it

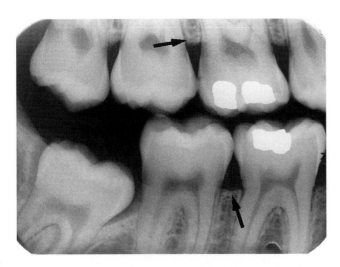

FIG. **9-9** The alveolar crests *(arrows)* are seen as cortical borders of the alveolar bone.

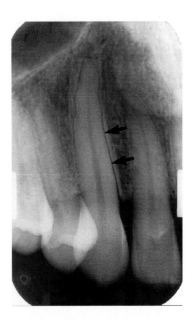

FIG. **9-11** The periodontal ligament space appears wide on the mesial surface of this canine *(arrows)* and thin on the distal surface.

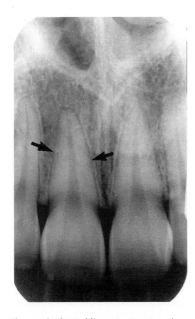

FIG. **9-10** The periodontal ligament space *(arrows)* is seen as narrow radiolucency between the tooth root and lamina dura.

is flat, aligned parallel with and slightly below a line connecting the cementoenamel junctions of the adjacent teeth. The crest of the bone is continuous with the lamina dura and forms a sharp angle with it. Rounding of these sharp junctions is indicative of periodontal disease.

The image of the crest varies from a dense layer of cortical bone to a smooth surface without cortical bone. In the latter case the trabeculae at the surface are of normal size and density. In the posterior regions this range of radiodensity of the crest is presumed to be normal if the bone is at a proper level in relation to the teeth. The absence of an image of cortex between the incisors, however, is considered by many to be an indication of incipient disease, even if the level of the bone is not abnormal.

PERIODONTAL LIGAMENT SPACE

Because the periodontal ligament (PDL) is composed primarily of collagen, it appears as a radiolucent space between the tooth root and the lamina dura. This space begins at the alveolar crest, extends around the portions of the tooth roots within the alveolus, and returns to the alveolar crest on the opposite side of the tooth (Fig. 9-10). The PDL varies in width from patient to patient, from tooth to tooth in the individual, and even from location to location around one tooth (Fig. 9-11). Usually it is thinner in the middle of the root and slightly wider near the alveolar crest and root apex, suggesting that the fulcrum of physiologic movement is in the region where the PDL is thinnest. The thickness of the ligament relates to the degree of function because the PDL is thinnest around the roots of embedded teeth and those that have lost their antagonists. The reverse is not necessarily true, however, because an appreciably wider space is not regularly observed in persons with especially heavy occlusion or bruxism.

The appearance of a double PDL space is created by the shape of the tooth. When the x-ray beam is directed so that two convexities of a root surface appear on a film, the double PDL space is seen (see Fig. 9-8).

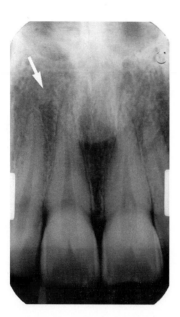

FIG. **9-12**   The trabecular pattern in the anterior maxilla is characterized by fine trabecular plates and multiple small trabecular spaces *(arrow)*.

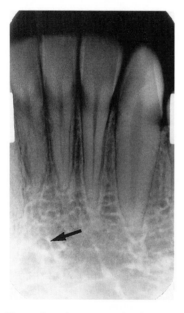

FIG. **9-13**   The trabecular pattern in the anterior mandible is characterized by coarser trabecular plates and larger marrow spaces *(arrow)* than in the anterior maxilla.

CANCELLOUS BONE

The cancellous bone (also called *trabecular bone* or *spongiosa*) lies between the cortical plates in both jaws. It is composed of thin radiopaque plates and rods (trabeculae) surrounding many small radiolucent pockets of marrow. The radiographic pattern of the trabeculae

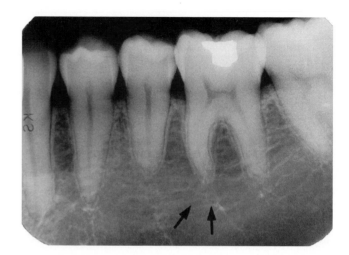

FIG. **9-14**   The trabecular pattern in the posterior mandible is quite variable, generally showing large marrow spaces and sparse trabeculation, especially inferiorly *(arrows)*.

shows considerable intrapatient and interpatient variability, which is normal and not a manifestation of disease. To evaluate the trabecular pattern in a specific area, the practitioner should examine the trabecular distribution, size, and density and compare them throughout both jaws. This frequently demonstrates that a particularly suspect region is characteristic for the individual.

The trabeculae in the anterior maxilla are typically thin and numerous, forming a fine, granular, dense pattern (Fig. 9-12), and the marrow spaces are consequently small and relatively numerous. In the posterior maxilla the trabecular pattern is usually quite similar to that in the anterior maxilla, although the marrow spaces may be slightly larger.

In the anterior mandible the trabeculae are somewhat thicker than in the maxilla, resulting in a coarser pattern (Fig. 9-13), with trabecular plates that are oriented more horizontally. The trabecular plates are also fewer than in the maxilla, and the marrow spaces are correspondingly larger. In the posterior mandible the periradicular trabeculae and marrow spaces may be comparable to those in the anterior mandible but are usually somewhat larger (Fig. 9-14). The trabecular plates are oriented mainly horizontally in this region also. Below the apices of the mandibular molars the number of trabeculae dwindles still more. In some cases the area from just below the molar roots to the inferior border of the mandible may appear to be almost devoid of trabeculae. The distribution and size of the trabeculae throughout both jaws show a relationship to the thickness (and strength) of the adjacent cortical plates. It may be speculated that where the cortical plates are thick (e.g., in the posterior region of the mandibular body), internal bracing by the trabeculae is not required, so there are relatively few except where required to support the alveoli. By contrast, in the maxilla and anterior region of the mandible, where the cortical plates are relatively thin and less rigid, trabeculae are more numerous and lend internal bolstering to the jaw. Occasionally the trabecular spaces in this region are very irregular, with some so large that they mimic pathologic lesions.

If trabeculae are apparently absent, suggesting the presence of disease, it is often revealing to examine previous radiographs of the region in question. This helps determine whether the current appearance represents a change from a prior condition. An abnormality is more likely when the comparison indicates a change in the trabecular pattern. If prior films are not available, it is frequently useful to repeat the radiographic examination at a reduced exposure because this often demonstrates the presence of an expected but sparse trabecular pattern that was overexposed and burned out in the initial projection. Finally, if prior films are not available and reduced exposure does not allay the examiner's apprehension, it may be appropriate to expose another radiograph at a later time to monitor for ominous changes. Again, considerable variation may exist in trabecular pattern among patients, so examining all regions of the jaws is important in evaluating a trabecular pattern for any individual. This enables the dentist to determine the general nature of the particular pattern and whether any areas deviate appreciably from that norm.

The buccal and lingual cortical plates of the mandible and maxilla do not cast a discernible image on periapical radiographs.

MAXILLA

Intermaxillary Suture

The intermaxillary suture (also called the *median suture*) appears on intraoral periapical radiographs as a thin radiolucent line in the midline between the two portions of the premaxilla (Fig. 9-15). It extends from the alveolar crest between the central incisors superiorly through the anterior nasal spine and continues posteriorly between the maxillary palatine processes to the posterior aspect of the hard palate. It is not unusual for this narrow radiolucent suture to terminate at the alveolar crest in a small rounded or V-shaped enlargement (Fig. 9-16). The suture is limited by two parallel radiopaque borders of thin cortical bone on each side of the maxilla. The radiolucent region is usually of uniform width. The ad-

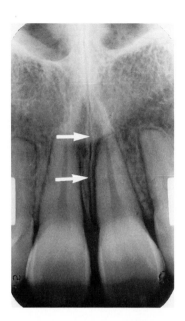

FIG. **9-15** The intermaxillary suture *(arrows)* appears as a curving radiolucency in the midline of the maxilla.

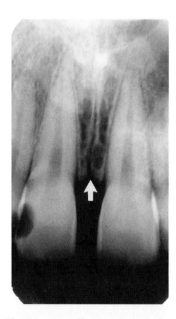

FIG. **9-16** The intermaxillary suture may terminate in a V-shaped widening *(arrow)* at the alveolar crest.

jacent cortical margins may be either smooth or slightly irregular. The appearance of the intermaxillary suture depends on both anatomic variability and the angulation of the x-ray beam through the suture.

Anterior Nasal Spine

The anterior nasal spine is most frequently demonstrated on periapical radiographs of the maxillary cen-

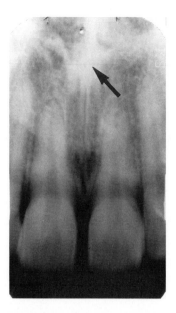

FIG. **9-17** The anterior nasal spine is seen as an opaque V-shaped projection from the floor of the nasal fossa in the midline *(arrow)*.

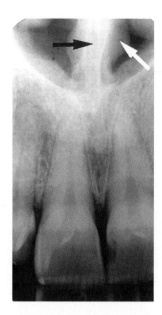

FIG. **9-19** The nasal septum *(black arrow)* arises directly above the anterior nasal spine and is covered on each side by nasal mucosa *(white arrow)*.

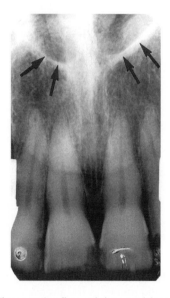

FIG. **9-18** The anterior floor of the nasal fossa *(arrows)* appears as opaque lines extending laterally from the anterior nasal spine.

Nasal Fossa

Because the air-filled nasal fossa (cavity) lies just above the oral cavity, its radiolucent image may be apparent on intraoral radiographs of the maxillary teeth, especially in central incisor projections. On periapical radiographs of the incisors the inferior border of the fossa appears as a radiopaque line extending bilaterally away from the base of the anterior nasal spine (Fig. 9-18). Above this line is the radiolucent space of the inferior portion of the fossa. If the radiograph was made with the x-ray beam directed in the sagittal plane, the relatively radiopaque nasal septum is seen arising in the midline from the anterior nasal spine (Fig. 9-19). The shadow of the septum may appear wider than anticipated, and not sharply defined because the image is a superimposition of septal cartilage and vomer bone. Also the septum frequently deviates slightly from the midline, and its plate of bone (the vomer) is somewhat curved.

The nasal cavity contains the hazy shadows of the inferior conchae extending from the right and left lateral walls for varying distances toward the septum. These conchae fill varying amounts of the lateral portions of the fossa (Fig. 9-20). The floor of the nasal fossa and a small segment of the nasal cavity not uncommonly are projected high onto a maxillary canine radiograph (Fig. 9-21). Also, in the posterior maxillary region, the floor of the nasal cavity and a portion of the fossa above it may be seen in the region of the maxillary sinus. (It is not possible from a single radiograph to determine which of two superimposed structures is in front of or behind

tral incisors (Fig. 9-17). Located in the midline, it lies some 1.5 to 2 cm above the alveolar crest, usually at or just below the junction of the inferior end of the nasal septum and the inferior outline of the nasal fossa. It is radiopaque because of its bony composition and is usually V-shaped.

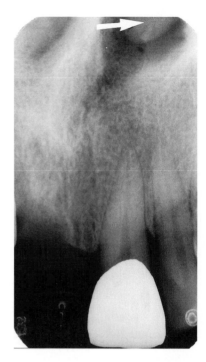

FIG. **9-20** The mucosal covering of the inferior concha *(arrow)* is occasionally visualized in the nasal fossa.

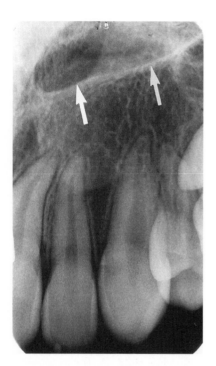

FIG. **9-21** The floor of the nasal fossa *(arrows)* may often be seen extending above the maxillary lateral incisor and canine.

the other unless the conclusion is based on an awareness of the anatomic features and relationships.) It may falsely convey the impression of a septum in the sinus or a limiting superior sinus wall (Fig. 9-22).

Incisive Foramen

The incisive foramen (also called the *nasopalatine* or *anterior palatine foramen*) in the maxilla is the oral terminus of the nasopalatine canal. It transmits the nasopalatine vessels and nerves (which may participate in the innervation of the maxillary central incisors) and lies in the midline of the palate behind the central incisors at approximately the junction of the median palatine and incisive sutures. Its radiographic image is usually projected between the roots and in the region of the middle and apical thirds of the central incisors (Fig. 9-23). The foramen varies markedly in its radiographic shape, size, and sharpness. It may appear smoothly symmetric, with numerous forms, or very irregular, with a well-demarcated or ill-defined border. The position of the foramen is also variable and may be recognized at the apices of the central incisor roots, near the alveolar crest, anywhere in between, or extending over the entire distance. The great variability of its radiographic image is primarily the result of (1) the differing angles at which the x-ray beam is directed for the maxillary central incisors, and (2) some variability in its anatomic size.

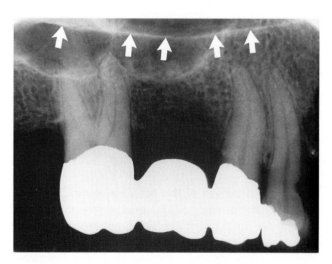

FIG. **9-22** The floor of the nasal fossa *(arrows)* extends posteriorly, superimposed with the maxillary sinus.

Familiarity with the incisive foramen is important because it is a potential site of cyst formation. An incisive canal cyst is radiographically discernible: it frequently causes a readily perceived enlargement of the foramen and canal. The presence of a cyst is presumed if the width of the foramen exceeds 1 cm or if enlargement can be demonstrated on successive radiographs. Also, if

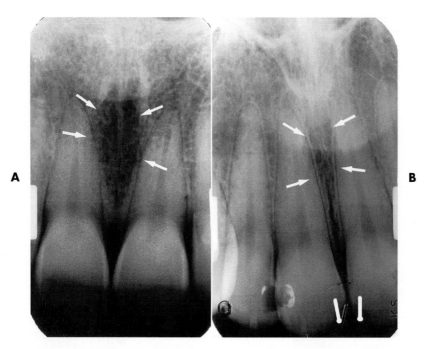

FIG. **9-23** **A,** The incisive foramen appears as an ovoid radiolucency *(arrows)* between the roots of the central incisors. **B,** Note its borders, which are diffuse but within normal limits.

the radiolucency of the normal foramen is projected over the apex of one central incisor, it may suggest a pathologic periapical condition. The absence of pathosis is indicated by a lack of clinical symptoms and an intact lamina dura around the central incisor in question.

The lateral walls of the nasopalatine canal are not usually seen but on occasion can be visualized on a projection of the central incisors as a pair of radiopaque lines running vertically from the superior foramina of the nasopalatine canal to the incisive foramen (Fig. 9-24).

Superior Foramina of the Nasopalatine Canal

The nasopalatine canal originates at two foramina in the floor of the nasal cavity. The openings are on each side of the nasal septum, close to the anteroinferior border of the nasal cavity, and each branch passes downward somewhat anteriorly and medially to unite with the canal from the other side in a common opening, the incisive (nasopalatine) foramen. The superior foramina of the canal occasionally appear in projections of the maxillary incisors, especially when an exaggerated vertical angle is used. When apparent radiographically, they can be recognized as two radiolucent areas above the apices of the central incisors in the floor of the nasal cavity near its anterior border and on both sides of the septum (Fig. 9-25). They are usually round or oval, al-

though they make take a variety of outlines depending on the angle of projection.

Lateral Fossa

The lateral fossa (also called *incisive fossa*) is a gentle depression in the maxilla near the apex of the lateral incisor (Fig. 9-26). On periapical projections of this region it may appear diffusely radiolucent. The image will not be misinterpreted as a pathologic condition, however, if the radiograph is examined for an intact lamina dura around the root of the lateral incisor. This finding, coupled with absence of clinical symptoms, suggests normalcy of the bone.

Nose

The soft tissue of the tip of the nose is frequently seen in projections of the maxillary central and lateral incisors, superimposed over the roots of these teeth. The image of the nose has a uniform, slightly opaque appearance with a sharp border (Fig. 9-27). Occasionally the radiolucent nares can be identified, especially when a steep vertical angle is used.

Nasolacrimal Canal

The nasolacrimal canal is formed by the nasal and maxillary bones. It runs from the medial aspect of the anteroinferior border of the orbit inferiorly, to drain under the inferior concha into the nasal cavity. Occasionally it

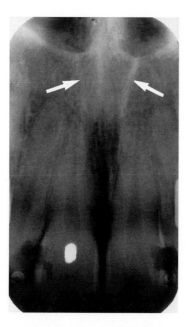

FIG. **9-24** The lateral walls of the nasopalatine canal *(arrows)* extend from the incisive foramen to the floor of the nasal fossa.

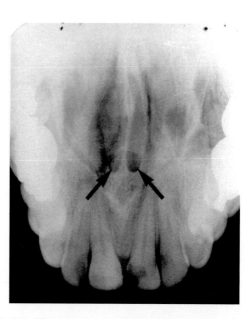

FIG. **9-25** The superior foramina of the nasopalatine canal *(arrows)* appear just lateral to the nasal septum and posterior to the anterior nasal spine.

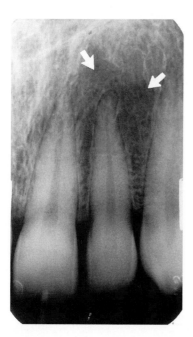

FIG. **9-26** The lateral fossa is a diffuse radiolucency *(arrows)* in the region of the apex of the lateral incisor. It is formed by a depression in the maxilla at this location.

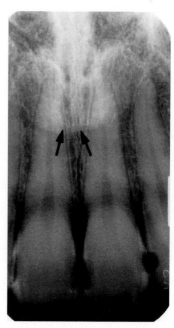

FIG. **9-27** The soft tissue outline of the nose *(arrows)* is superimposed on the anterior maxilla.

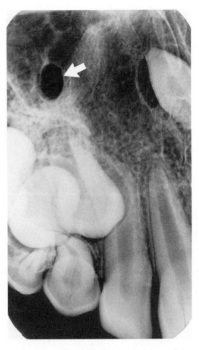

FIG. **9-28** The nasolacrimal canal *(arrow)* is occasionally seen near the apex of the canine when steep vertical angulation is used. Note the mesiodens (supernumerary tooth) superior to the central incisor.

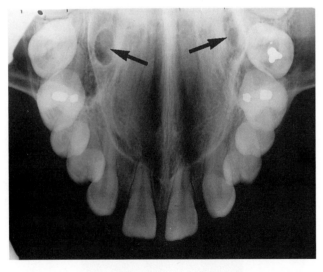

FIG. **9-29** The nasolacrimal canals are commonly seen as ovoid radiolucencies *(arrows)* on maxillary occlusal projections.

can be visualized on periapical radiographs in the region above the apex of the canine, especially when steep vertical angulation is used (Fig. 9-28). The nasolacrimal canals are routinely seen on maxillary occlusal projections (Chapter 8) in the region of the molars (Fig. 9-29).

Maxillary Sinus

The maxillary sinus, like the other paranasal sinuses, is an air-containing cavity lined with mucous membrane. It develops by the invagination of mucous membrane from the nasal cavity. Being the largest of the paranasal sinuses, it normally occupies virtually the entire body of the maxilla. Its function is unknown.

The sinus may be considered as a three-sided pyramid, with its base the medial wall adjacent to the nasal cavity and its apex extending laterally into the zygomatic process of the maxilla. Its three sides are (1) the superior wall forming the floor of the orbit, (2) the anterior wall extending above the premolars, and (3) the posterior wall bulging above the molar teeth and maxillary tuberosity. The sinus communicates with the nasal cavity via the ostium some 3 to 6 mm in diameter positioned under the posterior aspect of the middle turbinate.

The borders of the maxillary sinus appear on periapical radiographs as a thin, delicate, tenuous radiopaque line (actually a thin layer of cortical bone) (Fig. 9-30). In the absence of disease it appears continuous, but on close examination it can be seen to have small interruptions in its smoothness or density. These discontinuities are probably illusions caused by superimposition of small marrow spaces. In adults the sinuses are usually seen to extend from the distal aspect of the canine to the posterior wall of the maxilla above the tuberosity.

The maxillary sinuses show considerable variation in size. They enlarge during childhood, achieving mature size by the age of 15 to 18 years. They may change during adult life in response to environmental factors. The right and left sinuses usually appear similar in shape and size, although marked asymmetry is occasionally present. The floors of the maxillary sinus and nasal cavity are seen on dental radiographs at approximately the same level around the age of puberty. In older individuals the sinus may extend farther into the alveolar pro-cess, and in the posterior region of the maxilla its floor may appear considerably below the level of the floor of the nasal cavity. Anteriorly each sinus is restricted by the canine fossa and is usually seen to sweep superiorly, crossing the level of the floor of the nasal cavity in the premolar or canine region. Consequently, on periapical radiographs of the canine, the floors of the sinus and nasal cavity are often superimposed and may be seen crossing one another, forming an inverted Y in the area (Fig. 9-31).

The outline of the nasal fossa is usually heavier and more diffuse than that of the thin, delicate cortical bone denoting the sinus. The degree of extension of the maxillary sinus into the alveolar process is extremely variable. In some projections the floor of the sinus will be well above the apices of the posterior teeth; in others it may extend well beyond the apices toward the alveolar

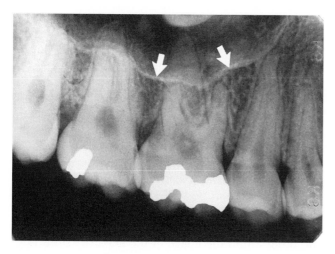

FIG. **9-30** The inferior border of the maxillary sinus *(arrows)* appears as a thin radiopaque line near the apices of the maxillary premolars and molars.

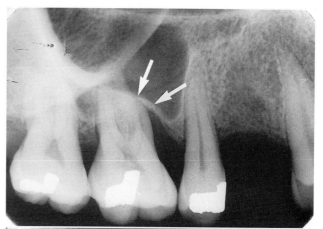

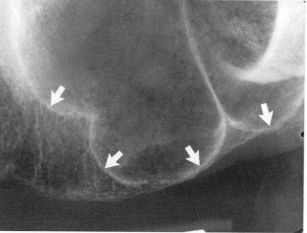

FIG. **9-32** The floor of the maxillary sinus *(arrows)* extends toward the crest of the alveolar ridge in response to missing teeth.

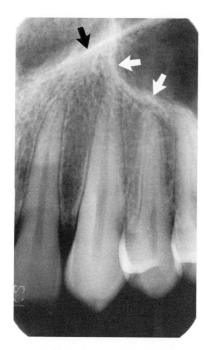

FIG. **9-31** The anterior border of the maxillary sinus *(white arrows)* crosses the floor of the nasal fossa *(black arrow).*

ridge. In response to a loss of function (associated with the loss of posterior teeth) the sinus may expand farther into the alveolar bone, occasionally extending to the alveolar ridge (Fig. 9-32).

The roots of the molars usually lie in close apposition to the maxillary sinus. Root apices may project anatomically into the floor of the sinus, causing small elevations

or prominences. The thin layer of bone covering the root is seen as a fusion of the lamina dura and the floor of the sinus. Rarely, defects may be present in the bony covering of the root apices in the sinus floor, and a periapical radiograph will fail to show lamina dura covering the apex.

When the rounded sinus floor dips between the buccal and palatal molar roots and is medial to the premolar roots, the projection of the apices is superior to the floor. This appearance conveys the impression that the roots project into the sinus cavity, which is an illusion. As the positive vertical angle of the projection is increased, the roots medial to the sinus appear to project farther into the sinus cavity. In contrast, the roots lateral to the sinus appear to move either out of the sinus or farther away from it as the angle is increased.

The intimate relationship between sinus and teeth leads to the possibility that clinical symptoms originat-

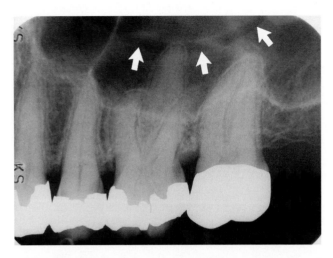

FIG. **9-33** Neurovascular canals *(arrows)* in the lateral wall of the maxillary sinus.

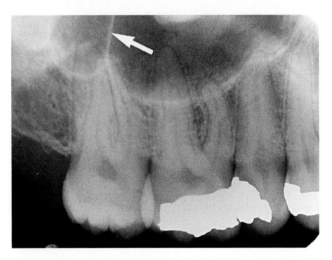

FIG. **9-34** A septum *(arrow)* in the maxillary sinus formed by a low ridge of bone on the sinus wall. (See also Figure 9-32, *lower illustration*).

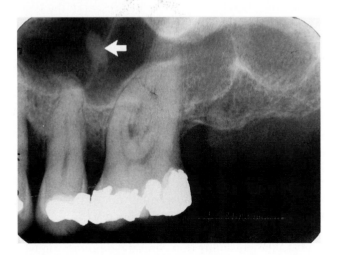

FIG. **9-35** This bony nodule *(arrow)* is a normal variant of the floor of the maxillary sinus.

ing in the sinus may be perceived in the teeth, and vice versa. This proximity of sinus and teeth is in part a consequence of the gradual developmental expansion of the maxillary sinus, which thins the sinus walls and opens the canals that traverse the anterolateral and posterolateral walls and carry the superior alveolar nerves. The nerves are then in intimate contact with the membrane lining the sinus. As a result, an acute inflammation of the sinus is frequently accompanied by pain in the maxillary teeth innervated by that portion of the nerve proximal to the insult. Subjective symptoms in the area of the maxillary posterior teeth may require careful analysis to differentiate tooth pain from sinus pain.

Frequently, thin radiolucent lines of uniform width are found within the image of the maxillary sinus (Fig. 9-33). These are the shadows of neurovascular canals or grooves in the lateral sinus walls that accommodate the posterior superior alveolar vessels, their branches, and the accompanying superior alveolar nerves. Although they may be found coursing in any direction (including vertically), they are usually seen running a curved posteroanterior course that is convex toward the alveolar process. On occasion they may be found to branch, and rarely also to extend outside the image of the sinus and continue as an interradicular channel. Because such vascular markings are not seen in the walls of cysts, they may serve to distinguish a normal sinus from a cyst.

Often the image of the maxillary sinus is found to be traversed by one or several radiopaque lines (Fig. 9-34). These septa represent folds of cortical bone projecting a few millimeters away from the floor and wall of the antrum. They are usually oriented vertically, although horizontal bony ridges also occur, and it is not uncommon for them to vary in number, thickness, and length. Septa are believed by some to have been formed through the uneven resorption of bone as the sinus was pneumatized, but others hold that they are remnants of incompletely fused cavities from which the sinus formed. They appear on many periapical intraoral radiographs, although seldom in extraoral projections because for this view the x-ray beam is rarely directed tangential to them. Although septa appear to separate the sinuses into distinct compartments, this is seldom the case because the septa are usually of limited extent. It has been reported, however, that in 1% to 10% of examined skulls, complete septa did in fact divide the sinus into individual compartments, each compartment with separate ostia for drainage. Septa deserve attention because they sometimes mimic periapical pathoses, and the chambers they create in the alveolar recess may complicate the search for a root fragment displaced into the sinus.

The floor of the maxillary sinus occasionally shows small radiopaque projections, which are nodules of bone (Fig. 9-35). These must be differentiated from root tips, which they resemble in shape. In contrast to a root frag-

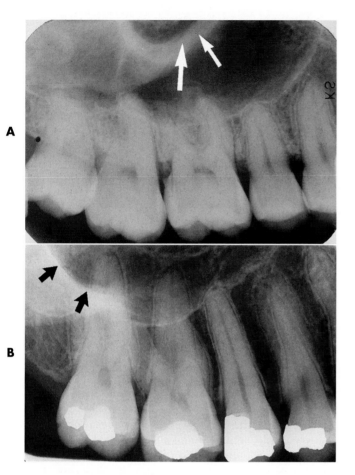

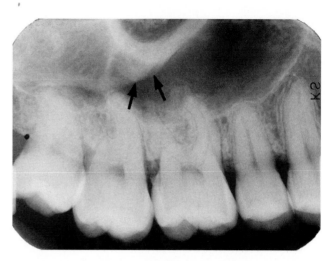

FIG. **9-37** The inferior border of the zygomatic arch *(arrows)* extends posteriorly from the inferior portion of the zygomatic process of the maxilla.

FIG. **9-36** The zygomatic process of the maxilla *(arrows)* protrudes laterally from the maxillary wall. Its size may be quite variable: small with thick borders, **A,** or large with thin borders, **B.**

ment, which is quite homogeneous in appearance, the bony nodules often show trabeculation; and although they may be quite well defined, at certain points on their surface they blend with the trabecular pattern of adjacent bone. A root fragment may also be recognized by the presence of a root canal. It is not uncommon to see the floor of the nasal fossa in periapical views of the posterior teeth superimposed on the maxillary sinus (see Fig. 9-22). The floor of the nasal fossa is usually oriented more or less horizontally, depending on film placement, and is superimposed high on maxillary views. The image, a solid opaque line, frequently appears somewhat thicker than the adjacent sinus walls and septa.

Zygomatic Process and Zygomatic Bone

The zygomatic process of the maxilla is an extension of the lateral maxillary surface that arises in the region of the apices of the first and second molars and serves as the articulation for the zygomatic bone. On periapical radiographs the zygomatic process appears as a U-shaped radiopaque line with its open end directed

superiorly. The enclosed rounded end is projected in the apical region of the first and second molars (Fig. 9-36). The size, width, and definition of the zygomatic process are quite variable, and its image may be large, depending on the angle at which the beam was projected. The maxillary antrum may expand laterally into the zygomatic process of the maxilla (and even into the zygomatic bone after the maxillozygomatic suture has fused), thereby resulting in a relatively increased radiolucent region within the U-shaped image of the process.

When the sinus is recessed deep within the process (and perhaps into the zygomatic bone), the image of the air space within the process is dark and typically the walls of the process are rather thin and well defined (in contrast to the very dark radiolucent air space). When the sinus exhibits relatively little penetration of the maxillary process (usually in younger individuals or those who have maintained their posterior teeth and vigorous masticatory function), the image of the walls of the zygomatic process tends to be somewhat thicker, and the appearance of the sinus in this region is somewhat smaller and more opaque.

The inferior portion of the zygomatic bone may be seen extending posteriorly from the inferior border of the zygomatic process of the maxilla (thereby completing the zygomatic arch between the zygomatic processes of the maxillary and temporal bones). It can be identified as a uniform gray or white radiopacity over the apices of the molars (Fig. 9-37). The prominence of the molar apices superimposed on the shadow of the zygomatic bone, and the amount of detail supplied by the radiograph, depends in part on the degree of aeration (pneumatization) of the zygomatic bone that has occurred, on the bony structure, and on the orientation of the x-ray beam.

Nasolabial Fold

Periapical radiographs of the premolar region are frequently traversed by an oblique line demarcating a region that appears to be covered by a veil of slight radiopacity (Fig. 9-38). The line of contrast is sharp, and the area of increased radiopacity is posterior to the line. The line is the nasolabial fold, and the opaque veil is the thick cheek tissue superimposed on the teeth and the alveolar process. The image of the fold becomes more evident with age, as the repeated creasing of the skin along the line (where the elevator of the lip, zygomatic head, and orbicularis all insert into the skin) and the degeneration of the elastic fibers finally lead to the formation and deepening of permanent folds. This radiographic feature frequently proves useful in identifying the side of the maxilla represented by a film of the area if it is edentulous and few other anatomic features are demonstrated.

Pterygoid Plates

The medial and lateral pterygoid plates lie immediately posterior to the tuberosity of the maxilla. The image of these two plates is extremely variable, and on many intraoral radiographs of the third molar area they do not appear at all. When they are apparent, they almost always cast a single radiopaque homogeneous shadow without any evidence of trabeculation (Fig. 9-39). Extending inferiorly from the medial pterygoid plate may be seen the hamular process (Fig. 9-40), which on close inspection can show trabeculae.

MANDIBLE

Symphysis

Radiographs of the region of the mandibular symphysis in infants demonstrate a radiolucent line through the midline of the jaw between the images of the forming deciduous central incisors (Fig. 9-41). This suture usually fuses by the end of the first year of life, after which it is no longer radiographically apparent. It is not frequently encountered on dental radiographs because few young patients have cause to be examined radiographically. If this radiolucency is found in older individuals, it is abnormal and may suggest a fracture or a cleft.

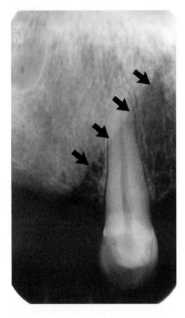

FIG. **9-38** The nasolabial fold *(arrows)* extends across the canine-premolar region.

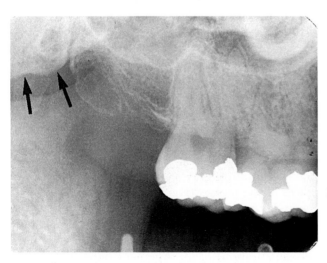

FIG. **9-39** Pterygoid plates *(arrows)* located posterior to the maxillary tuberosity.

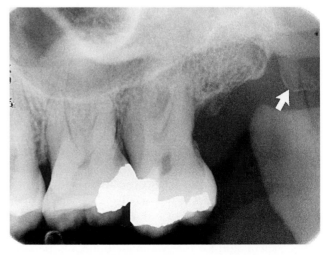

FIG. **9-40** The hamular process *(arrow)* extends downward from the medial pterygoid plate.

Genial Tubercles

The genial tubercles (also called the *mental spine*) are located on the lingual surface of the mandible slightly above the inferior border and in the midline. They are bony protuberances, more or less spine shaped, that often are divided into a right and left prominence and a superior and inferior prominence. They serve to attach the genioglossus muscles (at the superior tubercles) and the geniohyoid muscles (at the inferior tubercles) to the mandible. They are well visualized on mandibular occlusal radiographs as one or more small projections (Fig. 9-42). Their appearance on periapical radiographs of the mandibular incisor region may vary: a radiopaque mass (3 to 4 mm in diameter) in the midline below the incisor roots (Fig. 9-43), of nondescript shape or suggesting muscle attachments; they also may not be apparent at all. When not delineated on periapical films, a small radio-lucent dot (the lingual foramen) surrounded by the cortical wall of the termination of the incisive branch of the mandibular canal is usually quite apparent (Fig. 9-44).

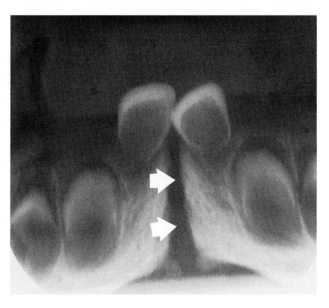

FIG. **9-41** Mandibular symphysis *(arrows)* in a newborn infant. Note the bilateral supernumerary primary incisors adjacent to it.

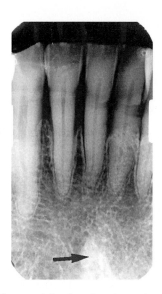

FIG. **9-43** The genial tubercles *(arrow)* appear as a radiopaque mass, in this case without evidence of the lingual foramen.

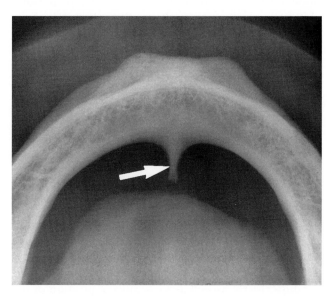

FIG. **9-42** Genial tubercles *(arrow)* on the lingual surface of the mandible in this cross-sectional mandibular occlusal view.

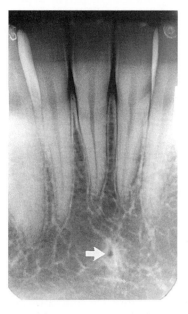

FIG. **9-44** Lingual foramen *(arrow)*, with a sclerotic border, in the symphyseal region of the mandible.

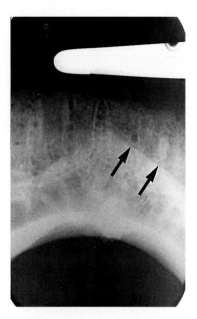

FIG. **9-45** Mental ridge *(arrows)* on the anterior surface of the mandible, seen as a radiopaque ridge.

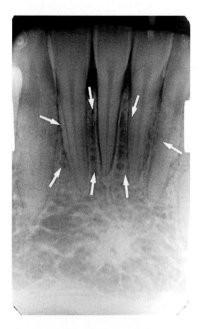

FIG. **9-46** The mental fossa is a radiolucent depression on the anterior surface of the mandible *(arrows)* between the alveolar ridge and mental ridge.

Mental Ridge

On periapical radiographs of the mandibular central incisors, the mental ridge (protuberance) may occasionally be seen as two radiopaque lines sweeping bilaterally forward and upward toward the midline (Fig. 9-45). They are of variable width and density and may be found to extend from low in the premolar area on each side up to the midline, where they lie just inferior to or are superimposed on the mandibular incisor tooth roots. The image of the mental ridge is most prominent when the beam is directed parallel with the surface of the mental tubercle (as when using the bisecting-angle technique).

Mental Fossa

The mental fossa is a depression on the labial aspect of the mandible extending laterally from the midline and above the mental ridge. Because of the resulting thinness of jawbone in this area, the image of this depression may be similar to that of the submandibular fossa (see below) and may, likewise, be mistaken for periapical disease involving the incisors (Fig. 9-46).

Mental Foramen

The mental foramen is usually the anterior limit of the inferior dental canal that is apparent on radiographs (Fig. 9-47). Its image is quite variable, and it may be identified only about half the time because the opening of the mental canal is directed superiorly and posteriorly. As a result, the usual view of the premolars is not pro-

jected through the long axis of the canal opening. This circumstance is responsible for the variable appearance of the mental foramen. Although the wall of the foramen is of cortical bone, the density of the foramen's image varies, as does the shape and definition of its border. It may be round, oblong, slitlike, or very irregular and partially or completely corticated. The foramen is seen about halfway between the lower border of the mandible and the crest of the alveolar process, usually in the region of the apex of the second premolar. Also, because it lies on the surface of the mandible, the position of its image in relation to the tooth roots is influenced by projection angulation. It may be projected anywhere from just mesial of the permanent first molar roots to as far anterior as mesial of the first premolar root. The image of two mental foramina, one above the other, has also been observed.

When the mental foramen is projected over one of the premolar apices, it may mimic periapical disease (Fig. 9-48). In such cases, evidence of the inferior dental canal extending to the suspect radiolucency or a detectable lamina dura in the area would suggest the true nature of the dark shadow. It is well to point out, however, that the relative thinness of the lamina dura superimposed with the radiolucent foramen may result in considerable "burnout" of the lamina dura image, which will complicate its recognition. Nevertheless, a second radiograph from another angle is likely to show the lamina dura clearly, as well as some shift in position of the radiolucent foramen relative to the apex.

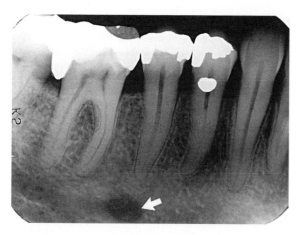

FIG. **9-47** The mental foramen *(arrow)* appears as an oval radiolucency near the apex of the second premolar.

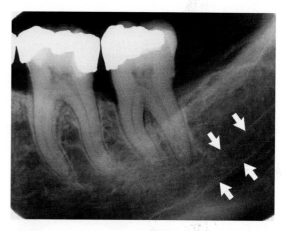

FIG. **9-49** Mandibular canal. Arrows denote its radiopaque superior and inferior cortical borders.

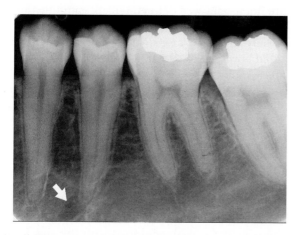

FIG. **9-48** The mental foramen *(arrow)* (over the apex of the second premolar) may simulate periapical disease. Continuity of the lamina dura around the apex, however, indicates the absence of periapical abnormality.

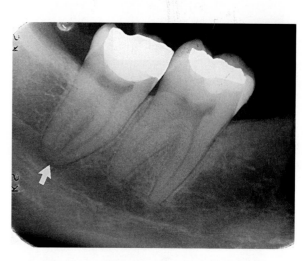

FIG. **9-50** The mandibular canal superimposed over the apex of a molar causes the image of the periodontal ligament space to appear wider *(arrow)*. The presence of an intact lamina dura, however, indicates that there is no periapical disease.

Mandibular Canal

The radiographic image of the mandibular canal is a dark linear shadow with thin radiopaque superior and inferior borders cast by the lamella of bone that bounds the canal (Fig. 9-49). Sometimes the borders are seen only partially or not at all. The width of the canal shows some interpatient variability but is usually rather constant anterior to the third molar region. The canal's course may be apparent between the mandibular foramen and the mental foramen. Only rarely is the image of its anterior continuation toward the midline discernible on the radiograph.

The relationship of the mandibular dental canal to the roots of the lower teeth may vary, from one in which there is close contact with all molars and the second premolar to one in which the canal has no intimate re-

lation to any of the posterior teeth. In the usual picture, however, the canal is in contact with the apex of the third molar, and the distance between it and the other roots increases as it progresses anteriorly. When the apices of the molars are projected over the canal, the lamina dura may be overexposed, conveying the impression of a missing lamina or a thickened PDL space that is more radiolucent than apparently normal for the patient (Fig. 9-50). To assure the soundness of such a tooth, other clinical testing procedures must be employed (e.g., vitality testing). Because the canal is usually located just inferior to the apices of the posterior teeth, altering the vertical angle for a second film of the area is not likely to separate the images of the apices and canal.

Nutrient Canals

Nutrient canals carry a neurovascular bundle and appear as radiolucent lines of fairly uniform width. They are most often seen on mandibular periapical radiographs running vertically from the inferior dental canal directly to the apex of a tooth (Fig. 9-51) or into the interdental space between the mandibular incisors (Fig. 9-52). They are visible in about 5% of all patients and are more frequent in blacks, males, older persons, and individuals with high blood pressure or advanced periodontal dis-

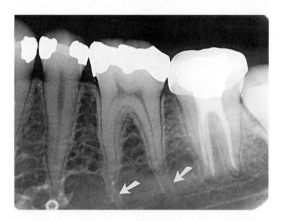

FIG. **9-51** Nutrient canals *(arrows),* demonstrated by radiopaque cortical borders, descend from the mandibular first molar.

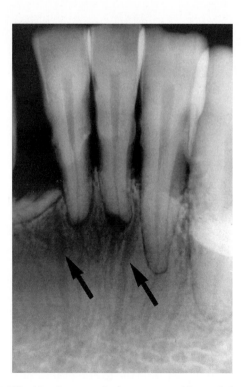

FIG. **9-52** Nutrient canals demonstrated by radiolucencies *(arrows)* in the anterior mandible of a patient with severe periodontal disease.

ease. They also indicate a thin ridge, useful in implant assessment. Because they are anatomic spaces with walls of cortical bone, their images occasionally have hyperostotic borders. At times a nutrient canal will be oriented perpendicular to the cortex and appear as a small round radiolucency simulating a pathologic radiolucency.

Mylohyoid Ridge

The mylohyoid ridge is a slightly irregular crest of bone on the lingual surface of the mandibular body. Extending from the area of the third molars to the lower border of the mandible in the region of the chin, it serves as an attachment for the mylohyoid muscle. Its radiographic image runs diagonally downward and forward from the area of the third molars to the premolar region, at approximately the level of the apices of the posterior teeth (Fig. 9-53). Sometimes this image is superimposed on the images of the molar roots. The margins of the image are not usually well defined but appear quite diffuse and of variable width. The contrary is also observed, however, where the ridge is relatively dense with sharply demarcated borders (Fig. 9-54). It will be more evident on periapical radiographs when the beam is positioned with excessive negative angulation. In general, as the ridge becomes less defined, its anterior and posterior limits blend gradually with the surrounding bone.

Submandibular Gland Fossa

On the lingual surface of the mandibular body, immediately below the mylohyoid ridge in the molar area, there is frequently a depression in the bone. This concavity accommodates the submandibular gland and often appears as a radiolucent area with the sparse trabecular pattern characteristic of the region (Fig. 9-55).

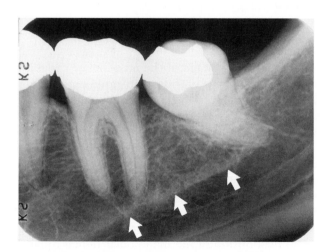

FIG. **9-53** Mylohyoid ridge *(arrows)* running at the level of the molar apices and above the mandibular canal.

This trabecular pattern is even less defined on radiographs of the area because it is superimposed on the relatively reduced mass of the concavity. The radiographic image of the fossa is sharply limited superiorly by the mylohyoid ridge and inferiorly by the lower border of the mandible, but is poorly defined anteriorly (in the premolar region) and posteriorly (at about the ascending ramus). Although the image may appear strikingly radiolucent, accentuated as it is by the dense mylohyoid ridge and inferior border of the mandible, awareness of its possible presence should preclude its being confused with a bony lesion by the inexperienced clinician.

External Oblique Ridge

The external oblique ridge is a continuation of the anterior border of the mandibular ramus. It follows an anteroinferior course lateral to the alveolar process, being relatively prominent in its upper part and jutting considerably on the outer surface of the mandible in the region of the third molar (Fig. 9-56). This bony elevation gradually flattens, and usually disappears, at about where the alveolar process and mandible join below the first molar. The ridge is a line of attachment of the buccinator muscle. Characteristically, it is projected onto posterior periapical radiographs superior to the mylohyoid ridge, with which it runs an almost parallel course. It appears as a radiopaque line of varying width, density, and length, blending at its anterior end with the shadow of the alveolar bone.

Inferior Border of the Mandible

Occasionally the inferior mandibular border will be seen on periapical projections (Fig. 9-57) as a characteristically dense, broad radiopaque band of bone.

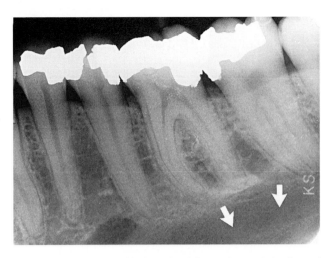

FIG. **9-55** Submandibular gland fossa *(arrows)*, indicated by a poorly defined radiolucency and sparse trabecular bone below the mandibular molars.

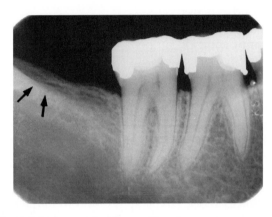

FIG. **9-56** External oblique ridge *(arrows)*, seen as a radiopaque line near the alveolar crest in the mandibular third molar region.

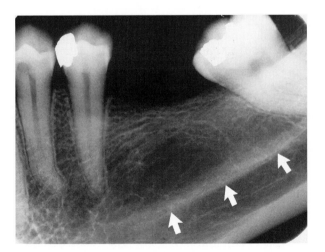

FIG. **9-54** The mylohyoid ridge *(arrows)* may be dense, especially when a radiograph is exposed with excessive negative angulation.

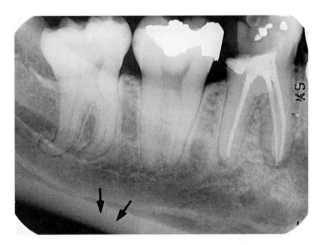

FIG. **9-57** The inferior border of the mandible *(arrows)* is seen as a dense, broad radiopaque band.

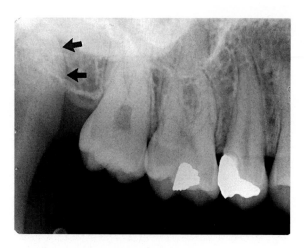

FIG. **9-58** Coronoid process of the mandible *(arrows)* superimposed on the maxillary tuberosity.

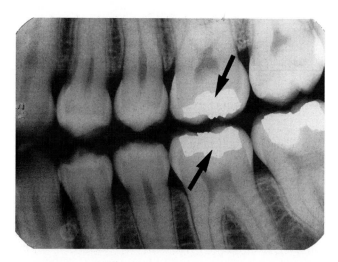

FIG. **9-59** Amalgam restorations appear completely radiopaque *(arrows)*.

Coronoid Process

The image of the coronoid process of the mandible is frequently apparent on periapical radiographs of the maxillary molar region as a triangular radiopacity, with its apex directed superiorly and somewhat anteriorly, superimposed on the region of the third molar (Fig. 9-58). In some cases it may appear as far forward as the second molar and be projected above, over, or below these molars, depending on the position of the jaw and the projection of the x-ray beam. Usually the shadow of the coronoid process is homogeneous, although internal trabeculation can be seen in some cases. Its appearance on maxillary molar radiographs results from the downward and forward movement of the mandible when the mouth is open. Consequently, if the opacity reduces the diagnostic value of a film and the film must be remade, the second view should be acquired with the mouth minimally open. (This contingency must be considered whenever this area is radiographically examined.) On occasion, and especially when its shadow is dense and homogeneous, the coronoid process is mistaken for a root fragment by the neophyte clinician. The true nature of the shadow can be easily demonstrated by obtaining two radiographs with the mouth in different positions and noting the change in position of the suspect shadow.

Restorative Materials

Restorative materials vary in their radiographic appearance, depending primarily on their thickness, density, and atomic number. Of these, the atomic number is most influential.

A variety of restorative materials may be recognized on intraoral radiographs. The most common, silver amalgam, is completely radiopaque (Fig. 9-59). Gold is

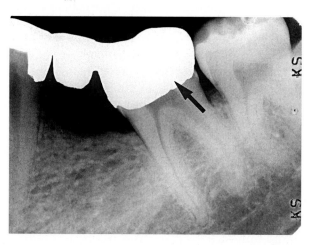

FIG. **9-60** A cast gold crown, appearing completely radiopaque *(arrow)*, serves as the terminal abutment of a bridge.

equally opaque to x-rays, whether cast as a crown or inlay (Fig. 9-60) or condensed as gold foil. Stainless steel pins also appear radiopaque (Fig. 9-61). Often a calcium hydroxide base is placed in a deep cavity to protect the pulp. Although such base material may be radiolucent, most is radiopaque (Fig. 9-62). Another material of comparable radiopacity is gutta-percha, a rubberlike substance used to fill tooth canals during endodontic therapy (Fig. 9-63). Silver points were also used during endodontic therapy (Fig. 9-64). Other restorative materials that appear rather radiolucent on intraoral films include silicates, usually in combination with a base but now little used (Fig. 9-65), composite, usually in anterior teeth (Fig. 9-66), and porcelain, now usually fused to a metallic coping (Fig. 9-67). Composite restorative materials may also be opaque (Fig. 9-68). In addition, stainless steel crowns (Fig. 9-69) and orthodontic appliances around teeth (Fig. 9-70) are relatively radiopaque.

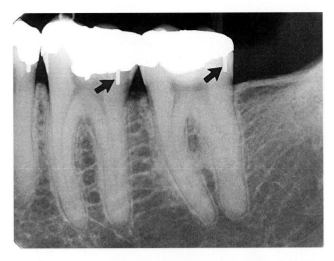

FIG. **9-61** Stainless steel pins *(arrows)* provide retention for amalgam restorations.

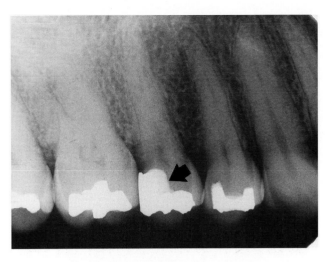

FIG. **9-62** Base material *(arrow)* is usually radiopaque.

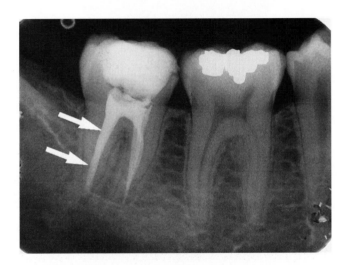

FIG. **9-63** Gutta-percha *(arrows)* is a radiopaque rubberlike material used in endodontic therapy.

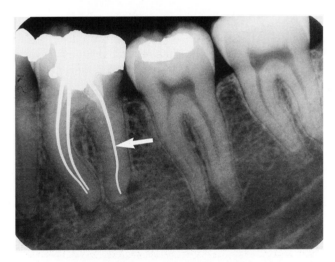

FIG. **9-64** Silver points *(arrow)* were used to fill the root canals in this patient.

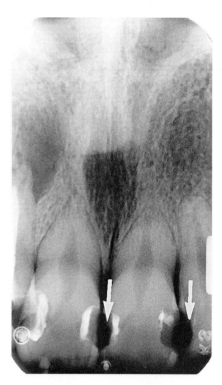

FIG. **9-65** Radiolucent silicate restorations *(arrows)* were placed over a base to protect the pulp in this patient.

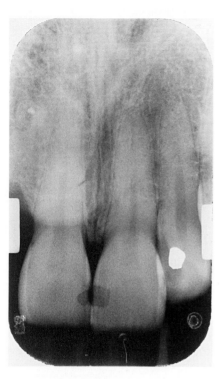

FIG. **9-66** Composite restorations may be radiolucent and may suggest caries but can be recognized by their well-demarcated border with dentin.

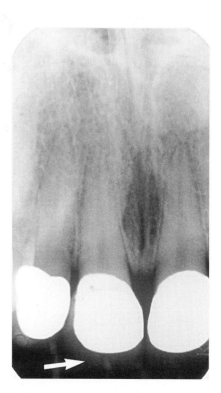

FIG. **9-67** Porcelain appears radiolucent *(arrow)* over a metal coping.

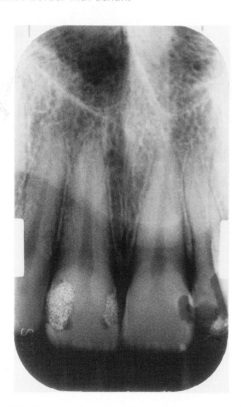

FIG. **9-68** Composite restorations containing particles of barium glass are radiopaque and not likely to be confused with caries.

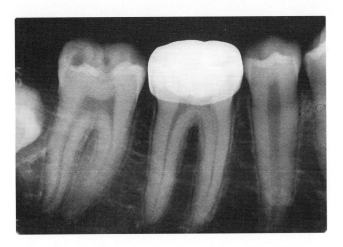

FIG. **9-69**   Stainless steel crowns appear mostly radiopaque.

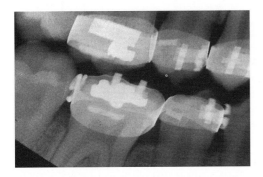

FIG. **9-70**   Orthodontic appliances have a characteristic radiopaque appearance.

BIBLIOGRAPHY

Britt G: A study of human mandibular nutrient canals, *Oral Surg* 44:635, 1977.

DuBrul EL: *Sicher's oral anatomy*, ed 7, St Louis, 1980, Mosby.

Elfenbaum A: Alveolar lamina dura, *Dent Radiogr Photogr* 31:21, 1958.

Fairbanks DNE: Embryology and anatomy. In Bluestone CD, Stool SE, editors: *Pediatric otolaryngology*, Philadelphia, 1983, WB Saunders.

Goldman HM, Millsap JS, Brenman HS: Origin of registration of the architectural pattern, the lamina dura and the alveolar crest in dental radiography, *Oral Surg* 10:749, 1957.

Greer D, Wege W, Wuehrmann A: The significance of nutrient canals appearing on intraoral radiographs, *IADR Abstr*, March 1968.

Ingram FL: *Radiology of the teeth and jaws*, London, 1950, Edward Arnold.

Killey HC, Kay LW: *The maxillary sinus and its dental implications*, Bristol, U.K., 1975, John Wright & Sons.

Manson JD: The lamina dura, *Oral Surg* 16:432, 1963.

Miller SC: *Oral diagnosis and treatment*, New York, 1957, McGraw-Hill.

Morse DR: Age-related changes of the dental pulp complex and their relationship to systemic aging, *Oral Surg* 72:721, 1991.

Patel J, Wuehrmann A: A radiographic study of nutrient canals, *Oral Surg* 42:693, 1976.

Wasson WW, Saunders SH, Cowen DE: *The lung and paranasal sinuses*, Springfield, Ill., 1969, Charles C Thomas.

SUGGESTED READINGS

Blackman S: *An atlas of dental and oral radiology*, Bristol, U.K., 1959, John Wright & Sons.

Kasle MJ: *An atlas of dental radiographic anatomy*, Philadelphia, 1993, WB Saunders.

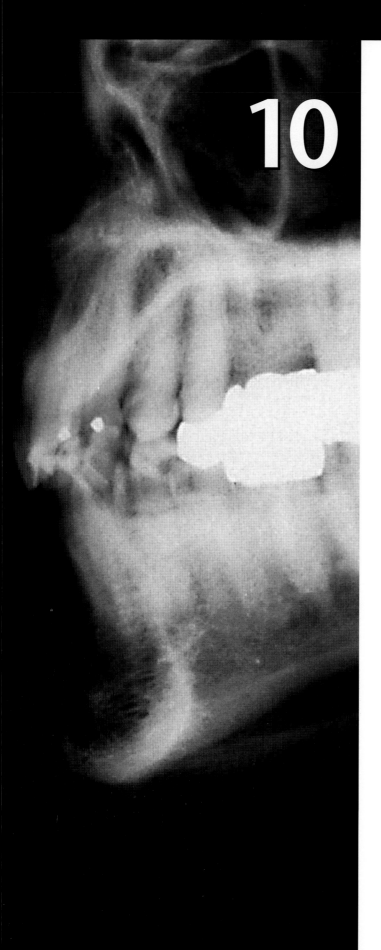

10 Extraoral Radiographic Examinations

Extraoral radiographic examinations include *all views* made of the orofacial region with films positioned extraorally. The dentist often uses these views to examine areas not fully covered by intraoral films or to visualize the skull and facial structures. When appropriate clinical signs or symptoms are present, it may be beneficial to examine the mandible, maxilla, and other facial bones for evidence of disease or injury. Orthodontists often use extraoral projections to evaluate skeletal growth. This chapter describes the standard views used for these purposes. Panoramic radiography is discussed in Chapter 11, and specific radiographic techniques for examining the temporomandibular joint are described in Chapter 24.

Film and Intensifying Screens

To achieve the best images with the lowest exposures, it is important to make all extraoral radiographic projections with the appropriate combination of film and intensifying screens (see Table 4-3). Medium- or high-speed rare earth screen-film combinations provide the optimal balance between loss of image detail and reduction of patient exposure. For lateral oblique views of the mandible, a 13 × 18 cm (5 × 7 inch) film and cassette are sufficient. A skull film requires at least a 20 × 25 cm (8 × 10 inch) film and cassette. Extraoral films usually can be processed either in conventional wet tanks or in an automatic processor. It is essential to place an *R* or *L* on the appropriate corner of the cassette to indicate the patient's right and left side on the resultant radiograph. Using grids reduces fog from scattered radiation, thereby increasing contrast. However, the use of grids approximately doubles the patient's exposure; therefore they should be used only when the highest contrast is necessary. The most common extraoral projection (the lateral cephalometric projection) can be made quite satisfactorily without a grid.

X-Ray Machines

Extraoral skull projections can be made with conventional dental x-ray machines, advanced types of panoramic x-ray machines, or larger x-ray units designed specifically for extraoral radiography. When a conventional dental x-ray machine is used for skull radiography (e.g., in an orthodontic practice), it is important to have some means of fixing the tube head in a standardized position. Wall-mounted brackets often are used for this purpose. Similarly, a device for positioning the head (a cephalostat) must be available for reproducible positioning of the patient. These devices can help achieve consistent, accurate positioning of the patient in relation to the tube head and film cassette. The more specialized types of equipment available for extraoral radiography provide the means for consistent positioning of the patient.

Skull Projections

Radiographic examination of the skull requires patience, attention to detail, and practice to achieve satisfactory results. Proper patient positioning requires the use of skeletal landmarks. The *Frankfort plane,* which connects the superior border of the external auditory meatus with the infraorbital rim, is the classic reference line. The canthomeatal line, which joins the central point of the external auditory meatus to the outer canthus of the eye, forms an angle of about 10 degrees with the Frankfort plane. Radiologists prefer using the canthomeatal line for patient positioning because it is more easily visualized. A cephalostat must be used to obtain consistent results.

POSTEROANTERIOR PROJECTION

The straight posteroanterior (PA) projection is so named because the x-ray beam passes in a posterior-to-anterior direction through the skull (Fig. 10-1). This projection is used to examine the skull for disease, trauma, or developmental abnormalities. It also provides a good record for detecting progressive changes in the mediolateral dimensions of the skull, including asymmetric growth. In addition, the PA projection offers good visualization of facial structures, including the frontal and ethmoid sinuses, nasal fossae, and orbits. Cephalometric examinations use a slight variation of this technique.

Film Placement
The cassette is positioned vertically in a holding device.

Head Position
For the straight PA projection the head is centered in front of the cassette with the canthomeatal line parallel to the floor. For cephalometric applications the nose should be a little higher so that the anterior projection of the canthomeatal line is 10 degrees above the horizontal plane and the Frankfort plane is perpendicular to the film (Fig. 10-2). On the resultant radiograph the superior border of the petrous ridge should lie in the lower third of the orbit. This orientation places the occlusal plane in a horizontal position.

Projection of the Central Ray
The central ray is directed perpendicular to the plane of the film in the horizontal and vertical dimensions from a source 91 to 102 cm (36 to 40 inches) away. The source should be coincident with the midsagittal plane of the head at the level of the bridge of the nose. For cephalometric applications the distance should be 152.4 cm (60 inches) between the x-ray source and the midcoronal plane of the patient.

Exposure Parameters
Exposure parameters vary considerably; they depend on the type of x-ray machine, the distance from the source to the patient, and the screen-film combination. When a film and screen combination with a speed class of 250 is used with a kVp of 70, the mAs should be about 30 to 50.

LATERAL SKULL PROJECTION (LATERAL CEPHALOMETRIC PROJECTION)

The lateral skull projection is used to survey the skull and facial bones for evidence of trauma, disease, or developmental abnormality. This view reveals the nasopharyngeal soft tissues, paranasal sinuses, and hard palate. Orthodontists use it to assess facial growth (Fig. 10-3), and it is used in oral surgery and prosthetics to es-

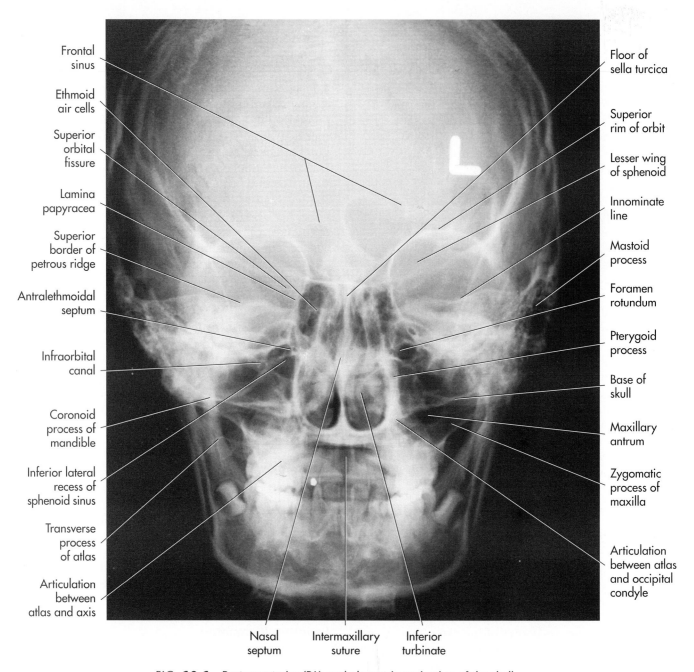

Frontal sinus

Ethmoid air cells

Superior orbital fissure

Lamina papyracea

Superior border of petrous ridge

Antralethmoidal septum

Infraorbital canal

Coronoid process of mandible

Inferior lateral recess of sphenoid sinus

Transverse process of atlas

Articulation between atlas and axis

Floor of sella turcica

Superior rim of orbit

Lesser wing of sphenoid

Innominate line

Mastoid process

Foramen rotundum

Pterygoid process

Base of skull

Maxillary antrum

Zygomatic process of maxilla

Articulation between atlas and occipital condyle

Nasal septum

Intermaxillary suture

Inferior turbinate

FIG. **10-1** Posteroanterior (PA) cephalometric projection of the skull.

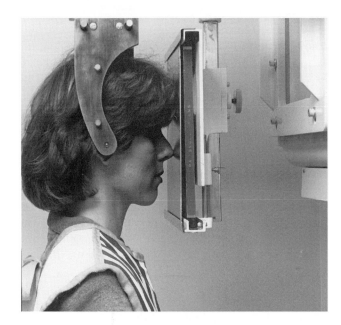

FIG. **10-2** Patient positioning for a PA cephalometric projection of the skull.

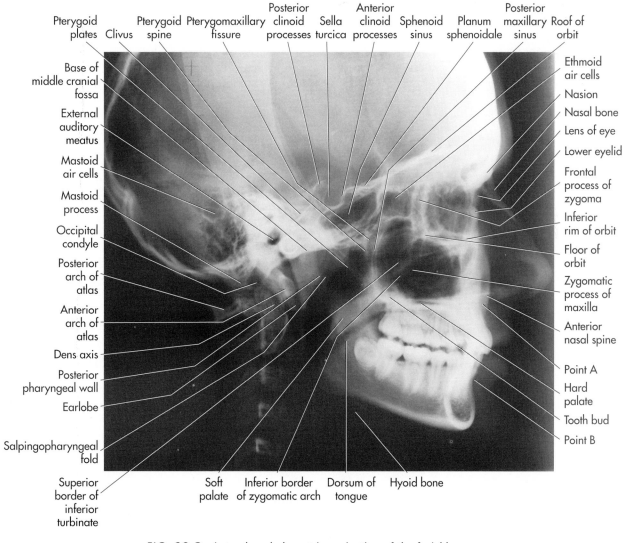

FIG. **10-3** Lateral cephalometric projection of the facial bones.

tablish pretreatment and posttreatment records. The lateral cephalometric projection reveals the facial soft tissue profile but otherwise is identical to the lateral skull view.

Film Placement
The film is positioned vertically in a cassette-holding device.

Head Position
The head should be positioned with the left side of the face near the cassette and the midsagittal plane parallel with the plane of the film (Fig. 10-4). A wedge filter is placed over the anterior side of the beam at the tube head. The filter absorbs some of the radiation striking the nose, lips, and chin, thereby reducing the intensity of radiation in the anterior region and helping to reveal the soft tissue outline of the patient's face on the radiograph.

Projection of the Central Ray
For cephalometric applications the distance between the x-ray source and the midsagittal plane is 152.4 cm (60 inches). The central ray is directed toward the external auditory meatus and perpendicular to the plane of the film and the midsagittal plane.

Exposure Parameters
Exposure parameters vary considerably according to the type of x-ray machine, the distance from the

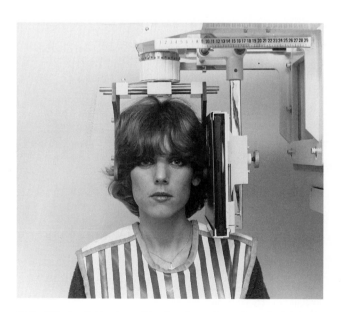

FIG. **10-4** Patient positioning for a lateral cephalometric projection of the facial bones.

source to the patient, and the screen-film combination. When a film and screen combination with a speed class of 250 is used with a kVp of 70, the mAs should be about 15 to 25.

WATERS' PROJECTION

The Waters' projection (also called the occipitomental projection) is a variation of the PA view. It is particularly useful for evaluating the maxillary sinuses. In addition, it demonstrates the frontal and ethmoid sinuses, the orbit, the zygomaticofrontal suture, and the nasal cavity (Fig. 10-5). It also demonstrates the position of the coronoid process of the mandible between the maxilla and the zygomatic arch.

Film Placement
The cassette is positioned vertically.

Head Position
The head should be oriented with the sagittal plane perpendicular to the plane of the film. The chin is raised high to elevate the canthomeatal line 37 degrees above horizontal (Fig. 10-6). If the petrous portion of the temporal bone lies over the apex of the maxillary sinus, the patient's chin must be elevated further. If the patient's mouth is open, the image of the sphenoid sinus will project onto the palate.

Projection of the Central Ray
The central ray should be perpendicular to the film, through the midsagittal plane, and at the level of the maxillary sinus.

Exposure Parameters
Exposure parameters vary considerably according to the type of x-ray machine, the distance from the source to the patient, and the screen-film combination and grid. When a film and screen combination with a speed class of 250 is used with a kVp of 70, the mAs should be about 100.

REVERSE-TOWNE'S PROJECTION

The reverse-Towne's projection is used to examine radiographically a patient suspected of having a condylar fracture of the neck (Fig. 10-7). This projection is particularly suitable for revealing a medially displaced condyle. The reverse-Towne's projection also reveals the posterolateral wall of the maxillary antrum.

Film Placement
The cassette is positioned in a holding device.

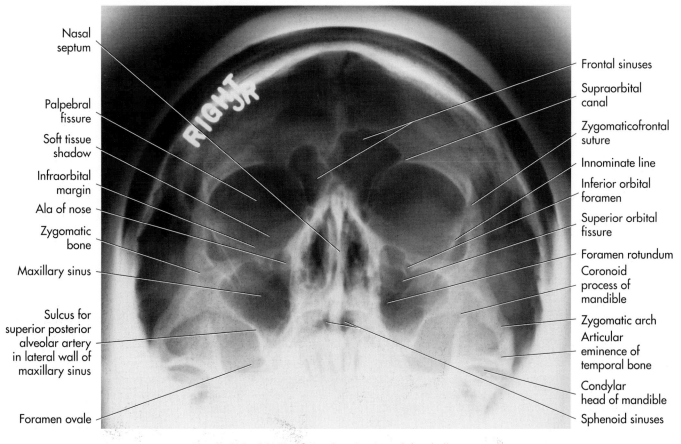

Nasal septum
Palpebral fissure
Soft tissue shadow
Infraorbital margin
Ala of nose
Zygomatic bone
Maxillary sinus
Sulcus for superior posterior alveolar artery in lateral wall of maxillary sinus
Foramen ovale

Frontal sinuses
Supraorbital canal
Zygomaticofrontal suture
Innominate line
Inferior orbital foramen
Superior orbital fissure
Foramen rotundum
Coronoid process of mandible
Zygomatic arch
Articular eminence of temporal bone
Condylar head of mandible
Sphenoid sinuses

FIG. **10-5** Waters' projection of the skull.

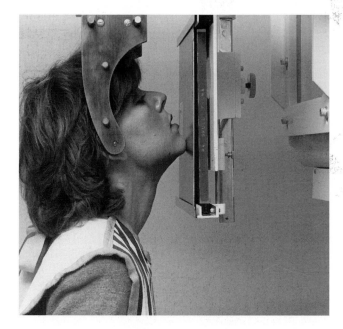

FIG. **10-6** Patient positioning for a Waters' projection of the skull.

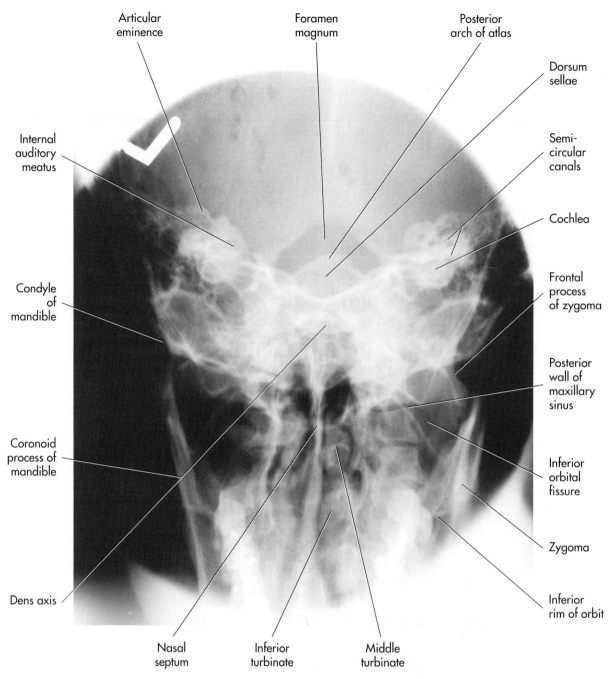

Articular eminence

Foramen magnum

Posterior arch of atlas

Dorsum sellae

Internal auditory meatus

Semi-circular canals

Cochlea

Condyle of mandible

Frontal process of zygoma

Posterior wall of maxillary sinus

Coronoid process of mandible

Inferior orbital fissure

Zygoma

Dens axis

Inferior rim of orbit

Nasal septum

Inferior turbinate

Middle turbinate

FIG. **10**-7   Reverse-Towne's projection of the skull.

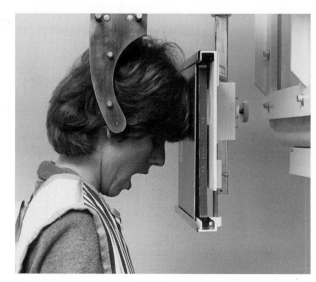

FIG. **10**-8   Patient positioning for a reverse-Towne's projection of the skull.

Head Position

The head should be centered in front of the cassette with the canthomeatal line oriented downward 25 to 30 degrees (Fig. 10-8). The condyles are better visualized if the patient opens the mouth as wide as possible.

Projection of the Central Ray

The central ray is directed toward the film in the sagittal plane through the occipital bone. The beam is collimated to the areas of interest to reduce patient exposure and film fog.

Exposure Parameters

Exposure parameters vary considerably according to the type of x-ray machine, the distance from the source to the patient, and the screen-film combination and grid. When a film and screen combination is used having a speed class of 250 with a kVp of 70, the mAs should be about 100.

SUBMENTOVERTEX PROJECTION

The submentovertex projection (also called the *base* or *full axial projection*) is used to demonstrate the base of the skull, the position and orientation of the condyles, the sphenoid sinus, the curvature of the mandible, the lateral wall of the maxillary sinuses, and any displacement of a fractured zygomatic arch (Fig. 10-9). Often this view also displays the medial and lateral pterygoid plates and foramina in the base of the skull.

Film Placement

The film cassette is placed vertically in a holding device.

Head Position

The patient's head and neck should be extended backward as far as possible, with the vertex of the skull on the center of the cassette. It usually is helpful to lean the patient's chair back as far as it will go to help patient orient the head. However, the midsagittal plane of the head must remain perpendicular to the floor. The can-

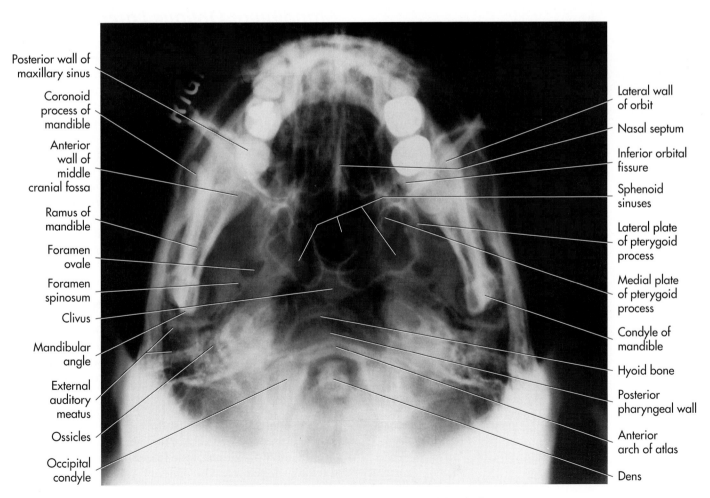

FIG. **10-9** Submentovertex projection of the skull.

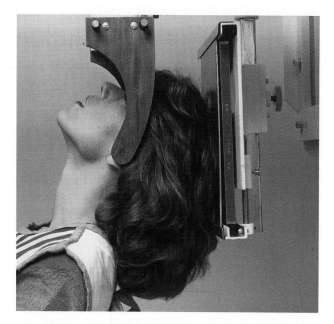

FIG. **10-10**   Patient positioning for a submentovertex projection of the skull.

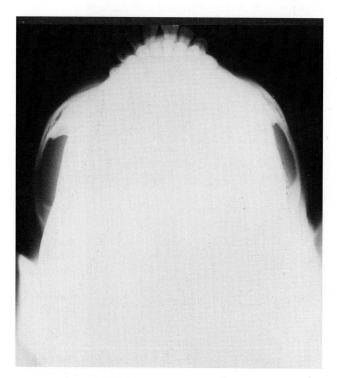

FIG. **10-11**   Submentovertex projection of the zygomatic arches.

thomeatal line should extend 10 degrees past vertical so that the Frankfort line is vertical and parallel to the film (Fig. 10-10).

Projection of the Central Ray

The central ray is directed from below the mandible upward, toward the vertex of the skull, and is positioned far enough anterior to pass about 2 cm in front of a line connecting the right and left condylar processes.

Exposure Parameters

Exposure parameters vary considerably according to the type of x-ray machine, the distance from the source to the patient, and the screen-film combination and grid. When a film and screen combination with a speed class of 250 is used with a kVp of 70, the mAs should be about 100. For viewing the zygomatic arches specifically, the exposure time is reduced to one third that used to visualize the skull (Fig. 10-11).

Mandibular Oblique Lateral Projections

Two oblique lateral projections commonly are used to examine the mandible, one for the body and one for the ramus. A dental x-ray machine with an open-ended aiming cylinder is best for these projections. The film usually is a screen film that is 13 × 18 cm (5 × 7 inches) or larger. Either fast or moderate-speed film and screens should be used. The patient should hold the cassette. Although these views largely have been replaced by panoramic radiographs, dentists still use the oblique lateral projections when an image with greater resolution than a panoramic view can provide is needed or when a panoramic machine is not available.

MANDIBULAR BODY PROJECTION

The mandibular body projection demonstrates the premolar-molar region and the inferior border of the mandible (Fig. 10-12). It provides much broader coverage than is possible with periapical projections.

Film Placement

The cassette is placed against the patient's cheek and centered over the first molar, its lower border parallel with the inferior border of the mandible and extending at least 2 cm below it. The patient can hold the cassette in place (Fig. 10-13).

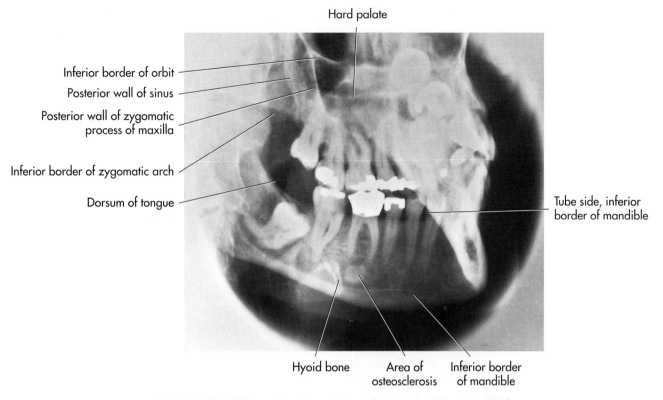

Hard palate

Inferior border of orbit

Posterior wall of sinus

Posterior wall of zygomatic process of maxilla

Inferior border of zygomatic arch

Dorsum of tongue

Tube side, inferior border of mandible

Hyoid bone

Area of osteosclerosis

Inferior border of mandible

FIG. **10-12** Oblique lateral projection of the body of the mandible.

Head Position

The head is tilted toward the side being examined, and the mandible is protruded.

Projection of the Central Ray

The central ray is directed toward the first molar region of the mandible from a point 2 cm below the angle on the tube side. The central ray should be as close to perpendicular to the plane of the film as possible.

Exposure Parameters

Although exposure parameters vary, it is customary to use 65 kVp, 10 mA, and about ¼ seconds for medium-speed screens and film.

MANDIBULAR RAMUS PROJECTION

The mandibular ramus projection gives a view of the ramus from the angle of the mandible to the condyle (Fig. 10-14). It often is very useful for examining the third molar regions of the maxilla and mandible.

Film Placement

The cassette is placed over the ramus and far enough posteriorly to include the condyle. The lower border of

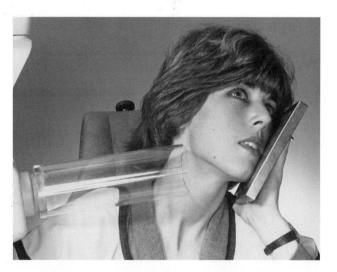

FIG. **10-13** Patient positioning for an oblique lateral projection of the mandibular body.

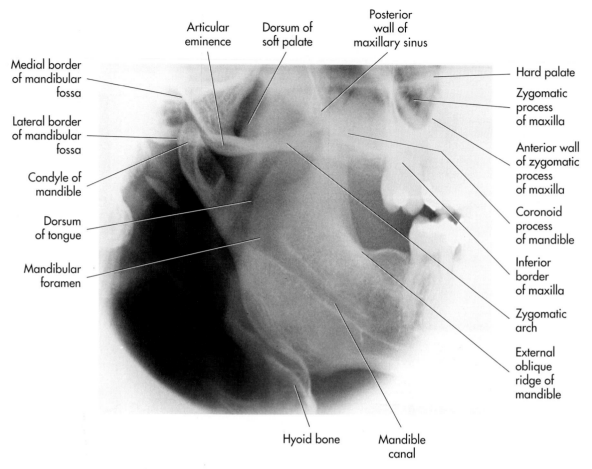

Articular eminence

Dorsum of soft palate

Posterior wall of maxillary sinus

Medial border of mandibular fossa

Lateral border of mandibular fossa

Condyle of mandible

Dorsum of tongue

Mandibular foramen

Hard palate

Zygomatic process of maxilla

Anterior wall of zygomatic process of maxilla

Coronoid process of mandible

Inferior border of maxilla

Zygomatic arch

External oblique ridge of mandible

Hyoid bone

Mandible canal

FIG. **10-14** Oblique lateral projection of the ramus of the mandible.

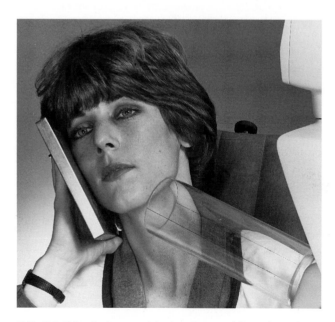

FIG. **10-15** Patient positioning for an oblique lateral projection of the mandibular ramus.

the cassette should be approximately parallel with the inferior border of the mandible and should extend at least 2 cm below the border (Fig. 10-15).

Head Position

The head is tilted toward the side of the mandible being examined until a line between the mandibular angle next to the tube and the condyle away from the tube is parallel with the floor. To prevent the cervical spine from being superimposed on the ramus, the patient should protrude the mandible.

Projection of the Central Ray

The central ray is directed posteriorly toward the center of the ramus on the side of interest from a point 2 cm below the inferior border of the first molar region of the mandible on the tube side.

Exposure Parameters

The usual exposure factors for this projection are 65 kVp, 10 mA, and about ¼ seconds for medium-speed screens and film.

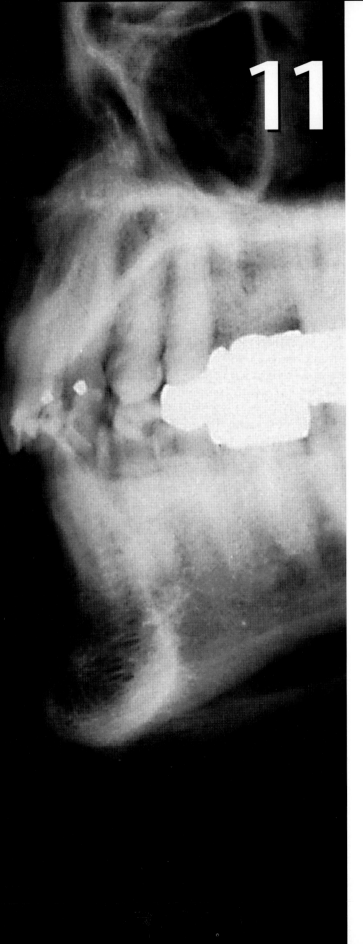

11 | *Panoramic Radiography*

Panoramic radiography (*also called* **pantomography**) is a radiologic technique for producing a single image of the facial structures that includes both the maxillary and mandibular dental arches and their supporting structures (Fig. 11-1). The principal advantages of panoramic images are (1) their broad coverage of the facial bones and teeth, (2) low patient radiation dose, (3) the convenience of the examination for the patient, (4) the fact that it can be used in patients unable to open their mouths, and (5) the short time required to make a panoramic image, usually in the range of 3 to 4 minutes. This includes the time necessary for positioning the patient and the actual exposure cycle. Panoramic films are readily understood by patients; thus they are also a useful visual aid in case presentation and patient education.

Panoramic radiographs are most useful clinically for diagnostic problems requiring broad coverage of the jaws. Common examples include evaluation of trauma, third molars, extensive disease, known or suspected large lesions, tooth development (especially in the mixed dentition), retained teeth or root tips (in edentulous patients), and developmental anomalies. These tasks do not require the high resolution and sharp detail available on intraoral radiographs. Panoramic radiography is often used as the initial survey film that can provide the required insight or assist in determining the need for other projections. Panoramic radiographs are also useful for patients who do not tolerate intraoral procedures well. However, when a full-mouth series of radiographs is available for a patient receiving general dental care, typically little or no additional useful information is gained from a simultaneous panoramic examination.

The main disadvantage of panoramic radiography is that the image does not display the fine anatomic detail available on intraoral periapical radiographs. Thus it is not as useful as periapical radiography for detecting small carious lesions or periapical disease. The proximal

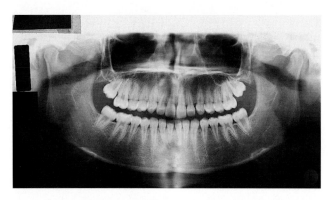

FIG. **11-1** Maxilla, mandible, and dentition in a 12-year-old child (panoramic view).

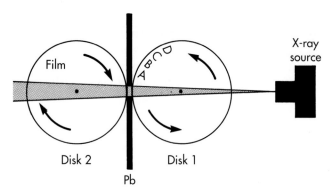

FIG. **11-2** Movement of the film and objects (*A, B, C,* and *D*) about two fixed centers of rotation. *Pb,* lead collimator.

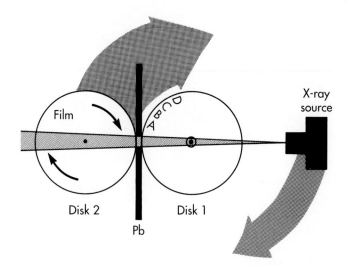

FIG. **11-3** Movement of the film and x-ray source about one fixed center of rotation. *Pb,* lead collimator.

surfaces of premolars also typically overlap. Accordingly, the availability of a panoramic radiograph for an adult patient often does not preclude the need for intraoral films for patient diagnosis. Other problems associated with panoramic radiography include uneven magnification and geometric distortion. Occasionally the presence of overlapping structures, such as the cervical spine, can hide odontogenic lesions, particularly in the incisor region. Further, clinically important objects may be situated outside the plane of focus (focal trough) and may appear distorted or not imaged at all.

Principles of Panoramic Image Formation

Paatero and, working independently, Hisatugu Numata, were the first to describe the principles of panoramic radiography. The following illustrations explain the operation of a panoramic machine. Two adjacent disks are rotating at the same speed in opposite directions as an

x-ray beam passes through their centers of rotation (Fig. 11-2). Lead collimators in the shape of a slit, located at the x-ray source and at the film, limit the central ray to a narrow vertical beam. Radiopaque objects *A, B, C,* and *D* stand upright on disk 1 and rotate past the slit. Their images are recorded on the film, which also moves past the slit at the same time. The objects are displayed sharply on the film because they are moving past the slit at the same rate and in the same direction as the film. This causes their moving shadows to appear stationary in relation to the moving film. Other objects between the letters and the center of rotation of disk 1 rotate with a slower velocity and are blurred on the film. Any objects between the x-ray source and the center of rotation of disk 1 move in the opposite direction of the film, and their shadows are also blurred on the film.

Fig. 11-3 shows that the same relationship of moving film to image is achieved if disk 1 is held stationary and the x-ray source is rotated so that the central ray constantly passes through the center of rotation of disk 1 and, simultaneously, both disk 2 and the lead film collimator (Pb) rotate around the center of disk 1. Note that although disk 2 moves, the film on this disk also rotates past the slit. In this situation, as before, the objects *A* through *D* move through the x-ray beam in the same direction and at the same rate as the film. To obtain optimal image definition, it is crucial that the speed of the film passing the collimator slit (Pb) be maintained equal to the speed at which the x-ray beam sweeps through the objects of interest.

Fig. 11-4 shows that a patient may replace disk 1 and that objects *A* through *D* represent teeth and surrounding bone. In practice, the center of rotation is located off to the side, away from the objects being imaged. Dur-

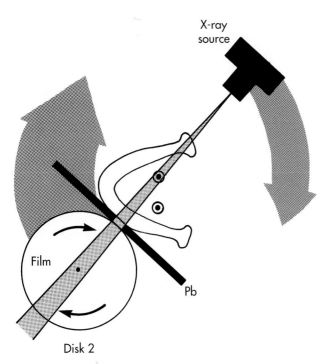

FIG. **11-4** Movement of the film and x-ray source about a shifting center of rotation. *Pb,* lead collimator.

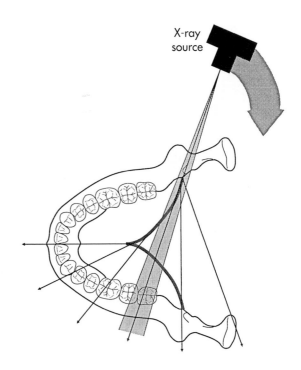

FIG. **11-5** *Movement of the x-ray source and beam.* The dark line shows a continuously moving center of rotation. As the source moves behind the patient's neck and the anterior teeth are imaged, the center of rotation moves forward along the arc *(dark line)* toward the sagittal plane. The x-ray source continues to move around the patient to image the opposite side.

ing the exposure cycle, the machine automatically shifts to other rotation centers. The rate of movement of the film behind the slit is regulated to be the same as that of the central ray sweeping through the dental structures on the side of the patient near the film. Structures on the opposite side of the patient (near the x-ray tube) are distorted and appear out of focus because the x-ray beam sweeps through them in the direction opposite that in which the film cassette is moving. In addition, structures near the x-ray source are so magnified (and their borders so blurred) that they are not seen as discrete images on the resultant radiograph. These structures appear only as diffuse phantom or ghost images. Because of both these circumstances, only structures near the film are usefully imaged on the resultant radiograph. Structures inside the jaws, such as the hyoid bone and epiglottis, appear as double images.

Most panoramic machines now use a continuously moving center of rotation rather than fixed locations. Fig. 11-5 shows a continually moving center of rotation. This feature optimizes the shape of the focal trough to reveal the teeth and supporting bone. This center of rotation is initially near the lingual surface of the right body of the mandible when the left temporomandibular joint (TMJ) is imaged. The rotation center moves forward along an arc that ends just lingual to the symphysis of the mandible when the midline is imaged. The arc is reversed as the opposite side of the face is imaged.

FOCAL TROUGH

The focal trough is a three-dimensional curved zone or image layer in which structures are reasonably well defined on panoramic radiographs. The image seen on a panoramic radiograph consists largely of the anatomic structures located within the focal trough. Objects outside the focal trough are blurred, magnified, or reduced in size and are sometimes distorted to the extent of not being recognizable. The shape of the focal trough varies with the brand of equipment used. Fig. 11-6 shows the general shape of the focal trough used in panoramic machines. The factors that affect its size are variables that influence image definition: arc path, velocity of the film and x-ray tube head, alignment of the x-ray beam, and collimator width. The location of the focal trough can change with extensive machine use, so recalibration may be necessary if consistently suboptimal images are produced.

As the position of an object is moved within the focal trough, the size and shape of the resultant image change. Fig. 11-7, *A* through *F,* illustrates the influence of patient positioning on image magnification. Fig. 11-7, *A* and *B,* shows a mandible supporting a brass ring

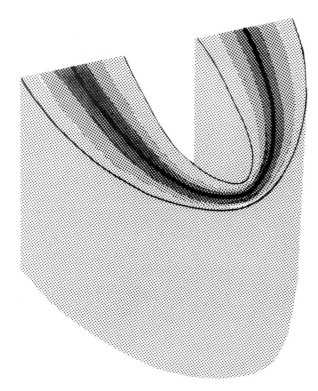

FIG. **11-6** *Focal trough.* The closer to the center of the trough *(dark zone)* an anatomic structure is positioned, the more clearly it is imaged on the resulting radiograph.

properly aligned in the middle of the focal trough. Note the even magnification of the ring and the images of the anterior teeth in proper proportion. Fig. 11-7, *C* and *D*, shows the same mandible positioned 5 mm anterior to the middle of the focal trough. This position causes distortion of the ring in the horizontal dimension with decreased width of the images of the teeth. Fig. 11-7, *E* and *F*, shows the same mandible positioned 5 mm posterior to the middle of the focal trough. Note the horizontal magnification of the ring and the increased width of the projected teeth. On these radiographs the vertical dimension, in contrast to the horizontal dimension, is little altered. These distortions result from the horizontal movement of the film and x-ray source. Thus as a general rule, when the object is displaced to the lingual side of its optimal position in the focal trough, toward the x-ray source, the beam passes more slowly through the mandible than the speed at which the film moves. Consequently, the image of the structures in this region is elongated horizontally on the film. Alternatively, when the mandible is displaced toward the buccal aspect of the focal trough, the beam passes at a rate faster than normal through the structures. In the example shown, because the film is moving at the proper rate, the image of the anterior teeth is compressed horizontally on the

film. Special attention must be paid to these considerations in following the progress of a bony lesion, especially in the anterior region. As a result of improper patient positioning the lesion may appear greater (enlarging) (see Fig. 11-7, *F*) or reduced (healing) (see Fig. 11-7, *D*) on successive radiographs. Thus the importance of careful alignment and positioning of the patient's dental arches within the area of the focal trough is apparent.

PANORAMIC MACHINES

A number of companies manufacture high-quality panoramic machines. The Orthopantomograph 100 (Sirona USA LLC, Charlotte, N.C.) (Fig. 11-8), the Orthophos Plus (Sirona), the Orthoralix S (Gendex Division, Dentsply International), and the PM 2002 CC Proline (Planmeca) (Fig. 11-9) are all highly versatile. In addition to producing standard panoramic images of the jaws, they have the capability of adjusting to patients of various sizes as well as making frontal and lateral images of the TMJs. These machines also make tomographic views through the sinuses and cross-sectional views of the maxilla and mandible. These views are accomplished by having special tube head and film movements programmed into the machine. Each machine also has the capability for adding on a cephalometric attachment to allow exposure of standardized skull views. Some machines further have the capability of automated exposure control. This is accomplished by measuring the amount of radiation passing through the patient's mandible during the initial part of the exposure and adjusting the imaging factors (kVp, mA, and speed of imaging movements) to obtain a correctly exposed image.

Recently a new line of computer-controlled multimodality machines has become available. In these machines, the direction and speed of movement of the tube head and film are highly variable, in some cases including multidirectional tomography. This allows the machines to be programmed to make tomographic views through many areas of the head. For instance, they can be programmed to image frontal or lateral views of the TMJs, coronal or sagittal sections through the maxillary sinuses, and cross-sectional cuts through a predetermined portion of the maxilla or mandible. These machines have much greater versatility than the conventional panoramic machines, and they are more expensive. The Scanora (Soredex) (Fig. 11-10) and Comm-CAT (Imaging Sciences International) (Fig. 11-11), for example, have the capability of making conventional panoramic images as well as many special-purpose examinations of the facial skeleton. Most of the special examinations made on these machines use circular or hypocycloidal tomography. (See Chapter 12.)

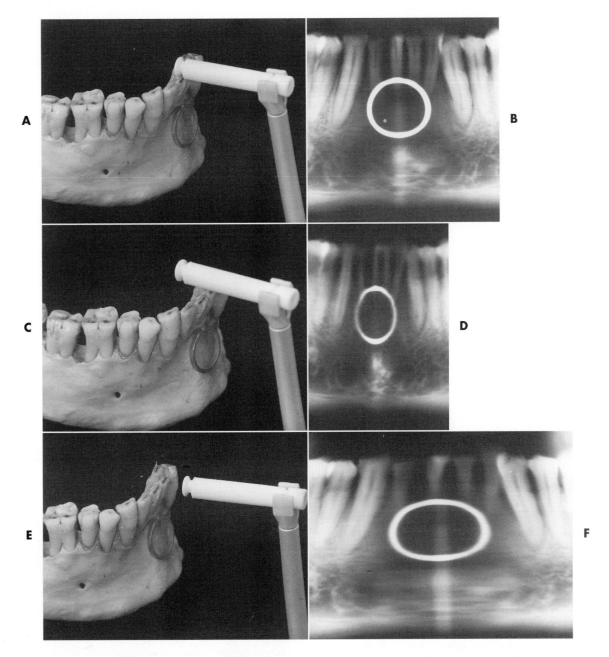

FIG. **11-7   A,** Mandible supporting a metal ring positioned at the center of the focal trough. The incisal edges of the mandibular teeth are indexed by a bite rod–positioning device. The mandible is positioned at the center of the trough. **B,** Resultant panoramic radiograph. **C,** Mandible and ring positioned 5 mm anterior to the focal trough. The incisal edges of the teeth are anterior to the trough. **D,** Resultant panoramic radiograph demonstrating the horizontal minification of both ring and mandibular teeth. **E,** Mandible and ring positioned 5 mm posterior to the focal trough. The incisal edges of the teeth are also posterior to the trough. **F,** Resultant panoramic radiograph demonstrating the horizontal magnification of both ring and mandibular teeth.

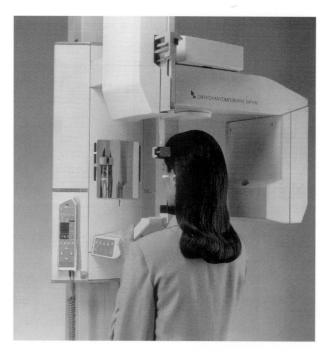

FIG. **11-8** Orthopantomograph 100 panoramic machine. (Courtesy Sirona USA LLC, Charlotte, N.C.)

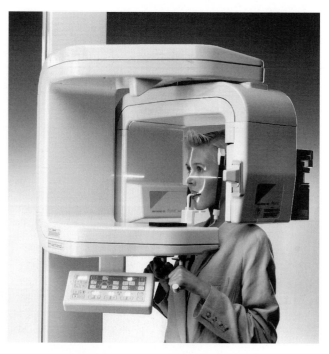

FIG. **11-9** PM 2002 CC Proline (Planmeca) panoramic machine. (Courtesy Planmeca Inc., Wood Dale, Ill.)

FIG. **11-10** Scanora multimodality machine. (Courtesy Soredex Inc., Marietta, Ga.)

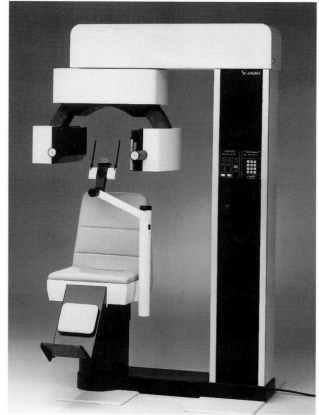

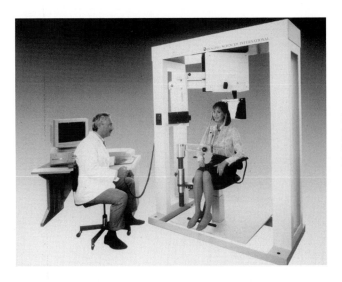

FIG. **11-11** The CommCAT Imaging System is capable of panoramic radiography as well as complex motion tomography of the TMJ and jaws. (Courtesy Imaging Sciences International, Roebling, N.J.)

Patient Positioning and Head Alignment

To obtain diagnostically useful panoramic radiographs, it is necessary to properly prepare patients and position their heads carefully in the focal trough. Remove dental appliances, earrings, necklaces, hairpins, and any other metallic objects in the head and neck region. It may also be wise to demonstrate the machine by cycling it while explaining the need to remain still during the procedure. This is particularly true for children, who may be anxious. Instruct children to look forward and not follow the tube head with their eyes.

The anteroposterior position radiograph of the patient is achieved typically by having patients place the incisal edges of their maxillary and mandibular incisors into a notched positioning device (the bite block). Be sure patients do not shift their mandible to either side when making this protrusive movement. The midsagittal plane must be centered within the focal trough of the particular x-ray unit. Failure to position the midsagittal plane in the rotational midline of the machine results in a radiograph showing right and left sides that are unequally magnified in the horizontal dimension. Poor midline positioning is a common error, causing horizontal distortion in the posterior regions and, on occasion, clinically unacceptable radiographs. A simple method for evaluating the degree of horizontal distortion of the image is to compare the apparent width of the mandibular first molars bilaterally. The smaller side is too close to the film.

The patient's chin and occlusal plane must be properly positioned to avoid distortion. The occlusal plane is aligned so that it is lower anteriorly, angled 20 to 30 degrees below the horizontal. A general guide for chin positioning is to place the patient so that a line from the tragus of the ear to the outer canthus of the eye is parallel with the floor. If the chin is tipped too high, the occlusal plane on the radiograph appears flat or inverted, and the image of the mandible is distorted (Fig. 11-12, *A*). In addition, a radiopaque shadow of the hard palate is superimposed on the roots of the maxillary teeth. If the chin is tipped too low, the teeth become severely overlapped, the symphyseal region of the mandible may be cut off the film, and both mandibular condyles may be projected off the superior edge of the film (Fig. 11-12, *B*).

Patients are positioned with their backs and spines erect and necks extended. Allowing patients to slump their heads and necks forward causes a large opaque artifact in the midline created by the superimposition of an increased mass of cervical spine. This shadow obscures the entire symphyseal region of the mandible and may require that the radiograph be retaken (Fig. 11-13). Proper positioning in seated units may be facilitated by having patients place their feet on a foot support and by using a cushion for back support. These devices help straighten the spine, minimizing the artifact produced by a shadow of the spine.

Finally, after patients are positioned in the machine, instruct them to swallow and hold the tongue on the roof of the mouth. This raises the dorsum of the tongue to the hard palate, eliminating the air space and providing optimal visualization of the apices of the maxillary teeth.

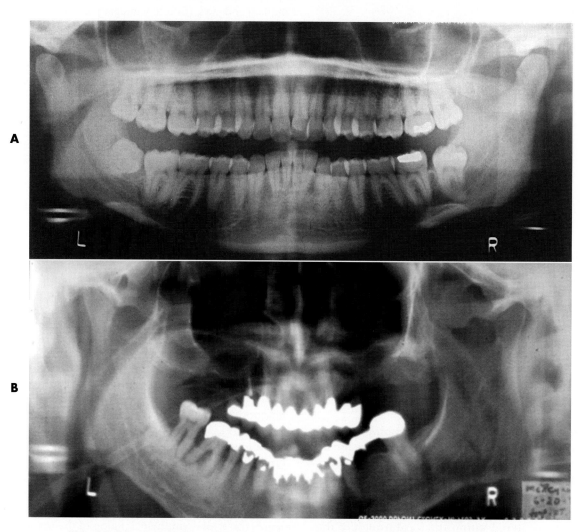

FIG. **11-12** *Panoramic radiographs demonstrating poor patient head alignment.* **A,** The chin and occlusal plane are rotated upward, resulting in overlapping images of the teeth and an opaque shadow (the hard palate) obscuring the roots of the maxillary teeth. **B,** The chin and occlusal plane are rotated downward, cutting off the symphyseal region on the radiograph and distorting the anterior teeth.

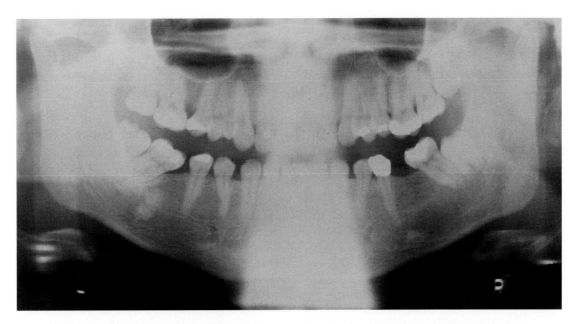

FIG. **11-13** *Panoramic radiograph of an improperly positioned patient.* Note the large radiopaque region in the middle. This artifact ("spine-shadow ghost") could have been eliminated by having the patient sit straight and align or stretch the neck.

Image Receptors

Intensifying screens (see Chapter 4) are routinely used in panoramic radiography because they significantly reduce the amount of radiation required for properly exposing a radiograph. Fast films combined with high-speed (rare earth) screens are indicated for most examinations. In most cases, the manufacturer provides panoramic machines with intensifying screens. The type of screen (manufacturer and model) is printed in black letters on each screen and clearly projected onto the radiograph. With rare earth screens and fast films, the patient's exposure from panoramic radiography is equivalent to four bitewing views.

Some new panoramic machines replace the film-screen combination with a linear charge-coupled device (CCD) sensor or a photostimulable phosphor (storage phosphor) screen. These systems produce direct digital panoramic images. These units will likely become more widely used as dentistry moves toward the use of intra-oral digital imaging and electronic patient records.

All panoramic radiographs should have some mechanism for automatically marking the patient's left and right sides on the image. Also, the patient's name, age, and the date the film was exposed should be indicated, with markers, photographic imprinting, or glued labels. The dentist's name must be on the film. No significant anatomic structures should be obscured by any of these labels or markings. Also, no parts of the image are trimmed to make the film fit the patient's chart.

Panoramic Film Darkroom Techniques

Special darkroom procedures are needed when panoramic film is being processed. These films are far more light sensitive than intraoral films, especially after they have been exposed. A reduction in darkroom lighting from that used for conventional intraoral film is necessary. A Kodak GBX-2 filter can be installed with a 15-watt bulb at least 4 feet from the working surface. An ML-2 filter should not be used because it fogs panoramic film. Panoramic film should be developed either manually or in automatic film processors using the manufacturer's recommendations. Obtaining optimal results relies on the same care to develop, rinse, fix, and wash panoramic films as is taken with intraoral films.

Radiographic Appearance of Normal Anatomy

Recognizing normal anatomic structures on panoramic radiographs is frequently challenging because of the complex anatomy of the midface, the superimposition of various anatomic structures, and the changing projection orientation. A systematic approach is useful in interpreting panoramic radiographs so as not to overlook structures. Place the radiograph on a viewbox as if you were looking at the patient, with the structures on the patient's right side positioned on your left (Fig. 11-14). Mask out extraneous light from around the film and dim the room lights. When possible, work seated in a quiet room. Consider the following method for examining panoramic radiographs.

APPEARANCE OF VARIOUS STRUCTURES

Mandibular Ramus

Begin viewing the radiograph at the superior aspect of the head of the right mandibular condyle (see Fig. 11-14, *1*). Follow the posterior border of the condyle past the condylar neck along the posterior border of the mandible to the mandibular angle. The condyle is usually positioned downward and forward in the mandibular fossa because the patient is protruded. Usually only fairly gross structural changes of the condyles can be seen. Corrected frontal and lateral tomographic views are recommended for detailed examination of the osseous structures of the TMJ. Note also the posterior wall of the nasopharynx (Fig. 11-15, *3*), ear lobe (see Fig. 11-15, *1*), soft palate (see Fig. 11-14, *24*), dorsum of the

tongue (see Fig. 11-14, *9*), and ghost shadow opposite the mandible in this region (see Fig. 11-14, *23*).

Mandibular Body

From the angle of the mandible, continue viewing anteriorly toward the symphyseal region. A fracture often manifests as a discontinuity in the inferior border and a sharp change in the level of the occlusal plane. The width of the cortical bone at the inferior border of the mandible should be at least 3 mm in adults and of uniform density. The bone may be thinned locally by an expansile lesion such as a cyst or generally by systemic disease such as hyperparathyroidism and osteoporosis. Compare the outlines of both sides of the mandible for symmetry, noting any changes. Asymmetry of size may result from improper patient positioning or conditions such as hemifacial hyperplasia or hypoplasia. The hyoid bone may be projected below or onto the inferior border of the mandible.

Assess the medullary bone of the mandible. Examine each mandibular canal (see Figs. 11-14, *20*, and 11-15, *7*) and mental foramen (see Fig. 11-14, *21*). The mandibular canal is usually easily visualized in the ramus and molar

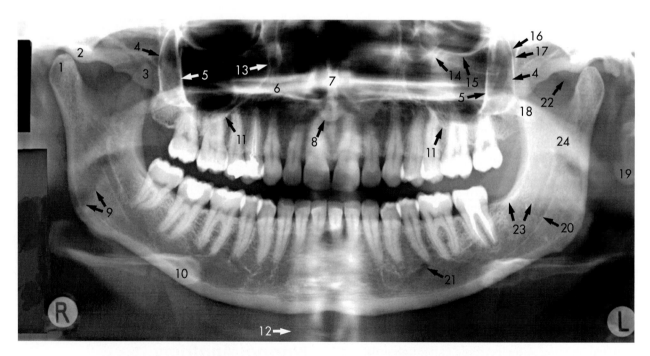

FIG. **11-14** *1*, Mandibular condyle. *2*, Articular eminence. *3*, Coronoid process of mandible superimposed on zygomatic arch. *4*, Posterior wall of maxillary sinus. *5*, Posterior wall of zygomatic process of maxilla. *6*, Hard palate. *7*, Nasal septum. *8*, Tip of nose. *9*, Dorsum of tongue. *10*, Hyoid superimposed over inferior border of mandible. *11*, Inferior border of maxillary sinus. *12*, Image of cervical spine. *13*, Medial border of maxillary sinus. *14*, Infraorbital canal. *15*, Infraorbital rim. *16*, Pterygomaxillary fissure. *17*, Anterior border of the pterygoid plates. *18*, Lateral pterygoid plate superimposed over soft palate and coronoid process of mandible. *19*, Ear lobe. *20*, Inferior border of mandibular canal. *21*, Mental foramen. *22*, Posterior wall of nasopharynx. *23*, Inferior border of mandible superimposed from opposite side. *24*, Soft palate over mandibular foramen of mandible.

region of the body of the mandible. Typically it exhibits a uniform width or gentle tapering from the mandibular foramen to the mental foramen. It may be less well seen in the first molar and premolar region. It usually rises to meet the mental foramen, sometimes looping a few millimeters anterior of the mental foramen. A bulging of the canal suggests a neural tumor; however, it should be noted that slight widening at the point that the canal bends to enter the body of the mandible from the ramus is a variation of normal. Examine the mandible for radiolucencies or opacities. The midline is more opaque because of the mental protuberance and superimposition of the cervical spine (see Fig. 11-14, *12*). The regions of the submandibular gland and sublingual gland fossae are more radiolucent. Trabeculation is most evident within the alveolar process, less so inferiorly.

Maxilla

Examine the cortical outline of the maxilla. Trace the posterior border of the maxilla (see Figs. 11-14, *4,* and 11-15, *11*), beginning from the superior portion of the pterygomaxillary fissure (see Fig. 11-15, *10*) down to the tuberosity region and around to the other side. The posterior border of the pterygomaxillary fissure is the pterygoid spine of the sphenoid bone (the anterior border of the pterygoid plates) (see Fig. 11-15, *9*). Occasionally the sphenoid sinus may extend into this structure. Examine the trabecular bone for evidence of abnormali-

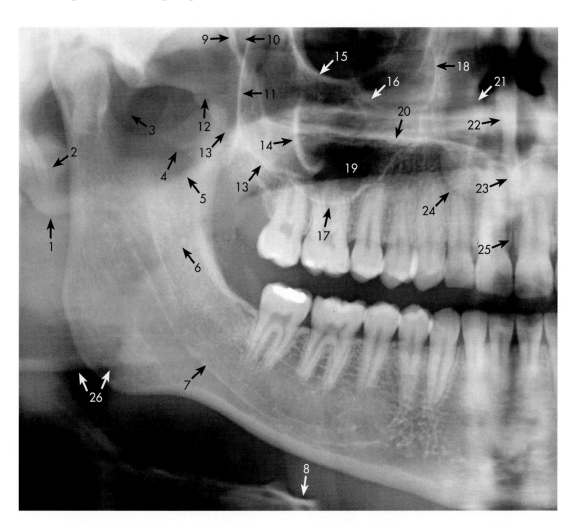

FIG. **11-15** *1,* Ear lobe. *2,* Styloid process. *3,* Posterior wall of nasopharynx. *4,* Inferior border of lateral pterygoid plate. *5,* Dorsum of soft palate. *6,* Dorsum of tongue. *7,* Inferior border of mandibular canal. *8,* Hyoid. *9,* Posterior border of the pterygomaxillary fissure. *10,* Pterygomaxillary fissure. *11,* Posterior wall of maxillary sinus. *12,* Zygomaticotemporal suture. *13,* Inferior border of zygoma. *14,* Posterior wall of zygomatic process of maxilla. *15,* Infraorbital rim. *16,* Infraorbital canal. *17,* Inferior border of maxillary sinus. *18,* Medial border of maxillary sinus. *19,* Maxillary sinus. *20,* Hard palate. *21,* Inferior concha. *22,* Nasal septum. *23,* Anterior nasal spine. *24,* Ala of nose. *25,* Intermaxillary suture. *26,* Inferior border of mandible superimposed from opposite side.

ties. The nasal fossa may show the nasal septum (see Fig. 11-14, *7*) and inferior concha (see Fig. 11-15, *21*), including both the bone and its mucosal covering.

Examine both maxillary sinuses (see Fig. 11-15, *19*), first by identifying each of the borders and then by noting whether they are entirely outlined with cortical bone, roughly symmetric, and comparable in radiographic density. The borders should be present and intact. It is often useful to compare both right and left maxillary sinuses when looking for abnormalities. The posterior aspect of the sinuses is more opaque because of superimposition of the zygoma. Examine each sinus for evidence of a mucous retention cyst, mucoperiosteal thickening, and other sinus conditions.

Zygoma

The zygomatic process of the maxilla (see Figs. 11-14, *5*, and 11-15, *14*) arises over the maxillary first and second molar. The inferior border of the zygomatic arch (see Fig. 11-15, *13*) extends posteriorly from the inferior portion of the zygomatic process of the maxilla and extends posteriorly to the articular tubercle (see Fig. 11-14, *2*) and mandibular (glenoid) fossa. Note also the superior border of the zygomatic arch. The zygomaticotemporal suture (see Fig. 11-15, *12*) often lies in the middle of the zygomatic arch and may simulate a fracture.

Soft Tissues

A number of opaque soft tissue structures may be identified on panoramic radiographs, including the tongue (see Figs. 11-14, *9*, and 11-15, *6*, arching across the film under the hard palate, roughly from the region of the right angle of the mandible to the left angle), lip markings (in the middle of the film), the soft palate (see Figs. 11-14, *24*, and 11-15, *5*) extending posteriorly from the hard palate (see Fig. 11-14, *6*) over each ramus, the posterior wall of the oral and nasal pharynx (see Fig. 11-15, *3*), the nasal septum (see Fig. 11-15, *22*), ear lobes (see Fig. 11-15, *1*), nose (see Figs. 11-14, *8*, and 11-15, *24*), and nasolabial folds. Radiolucent airway shadows superimpose on normal anatomic structures and may be demonstrated by the borders of adjacent soft tissues. They include the nasal fossa, nasal pharynx, oral cavity, and oral pharynx. Occasionally the air space between the dorsum of the tongue and the soft palate simulates a fracture through the angle of the mandible.

Superimpositions

Many radiopaque objects out of the focal trough superimpose on the image of normal anatomic structures.

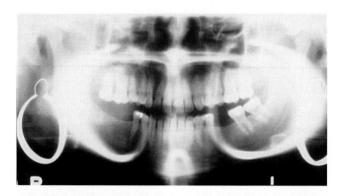

FIG. **11-16** Radiograph taken with large earrings in place. Note the opaque shadows present in the right and left mandibular ramus and body regions. These obscuring artifacts could have been eliminated by having the patient remove her earrings before the radiographic examination.

They result when the x-ray beam projects through a dense object (e.g., an earring, the spinal column, the mandibular ramus, or the hard palate) that is in the path of the x-ray beam but out of the portion of the focal trough being imaged. The object typically appears blurred and projects onto the opposite side of the radiograph (Fig. 11-16). These ghostlike opaque images may obscure normal anatomy.

Dentition

Finally, evaluate the teeth and immediate periapical bone. If the anterior teeth are excessively wide or narrow, this suggests malposition of the patient. Similarly, if the teeth are wider on one side than the other, this suggests that the patient's head was not aligned straight. Although gross caries and periapical and periodontal disease may be evident, subtle disease requires intraoral images for diagnosis. The proximal surfaces of the premolar teeth often overlap, which further interferes with caries interpretation.

BIBLIOGRAPHY

Chomenko AG: *Atlas for maxillofacial pantomographic interpretation,* Chicago, 1985, Quintessence Publishing.

Langland OE et al: *Panoramic radiology,* ed 2, Philadelphia, 1989, Lea & Febiger.

Numata H: Consideration of the parabolic radiography of the dental arch, *J Shimazu Stud* 10:13, 1933.

Paatero YV: A new tomographic method for radiographing curved outer surfaces, *Acta Radiol* 32:177, 1949.

Paatero YV: The use of a mobile source of light in radiography, *Acta Radiol* 29:221, 1948.

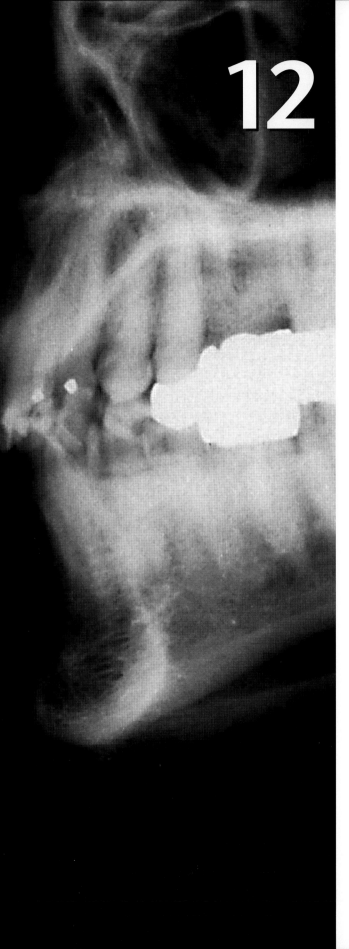

12

Specialized Radiographic Techniques

NEIL L. FREDERIKSEN

The techniques described in this chapter are used to address specific diagnostic tasks. Some have been available to the clinician for years; others are more recent innovations made possible through computer technology. Although most of these techniques are not used routinely by general dental practitioners, all are used occasionally to aid in diagnosis of conditions in the oral cavity. For this reason, all involved in providing oral health care must have a basic understanding of these operating principles and their clinical applications.

Film Radiography

TOMOGRAPHY

Conventional film-based tomography, also called *body section radiography*, is a radiographic technique designed to image more clearly objects lying within a plane of interest. This is accomplished by blurring the images of structures lying superficial and deep to the plane of interest through the process of motion "unsharpness." Since the introduction of computed tomography and magnetic resonance imaging, which have superior low-contrast resolution, film-based tomography has been used less frequently. Conventional tomography now is applied primarily to high-contrast anatomy, such as that encountered in temporomandibular joint (TMJ) and dental implant diagnostics.

217

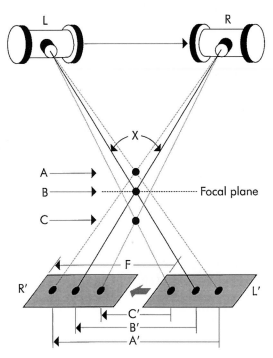

FIG. 12-1 *Tomographic techniques.* As the x-ray tube moves from left to right, the film moves in the opposite direction. In the figure, points *A* and *C* lie outside the focal plane (the plane that contains the fulcrum), whereas object *B* lies at the center of tube/film movement. Only objects that lie in the focal plane (i.e., *B*) remain in sharp focus because the image of *B* moves exactly the same distance *(B')* as the film travels *(F)*, and thus its image remains stationary on the film. The image of point *A* moves more than the film (distance *A'*) and the image of point *C* less than the film (distance *C'*); therefore the images of both are blurred. The figure illustrates a parallel movement of tube and film. *X* is the tomographic angle. The greater the tomographic angle, the thinner the plane of focus.

Essential equipment for tomography includes an x-ray tube and radiographic film rigidly connected and capable of moving about a fixed axis or fulcrum (Fig. 12-1). The examination begins with the x-ray tube and film positioned on opposite sides of the fulcrum, which is located within the plane of interest (focal plane). As the exposure begins, the tube and film move in opposite directions simultaneously through a mechanical linkage. With this coordinated movement of tube and film, the images of objects located within the focal plane (at the fulcrum) remain in fixed positions on the radiographic film throughout the length of tube and film travel, and are clearly imaged. On the other hand, the images of objects located either superficial or deep to the focal plane have continuously changing positions on the film; as a result, the images of these objects are blurred beyond recognition by motion unsharpness.

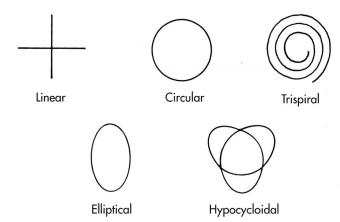

FIG. 12-2 *Tomographic movements.* The more complex the motion, the smaller the likelihood the x-ray beam will strike an object of importance at the same tangent through the entire exposure. (Therefore blurring depends less on the orientation of the object under study.)

The objective of tomography, then, is to blur the images of structures not located in the focal plane both as much and as uniformly as possible. Blurring is greater under the following conditions:

- The farther the structure lies from the focal plane and the greater the distance between the structure and the film (this is determined by the physical location of the fulcrum within the object to be imaged and hence the diagnostic task to be accomplished)
- The more closely the long axis of the structure to be blurred is oriented perpendicular to the direction of tube travel (this is accomplished by the tomographic movement)
- The greater the amplitude of tube travel (this is determined by the tomographic angle or arc)

There are at least five types of tomographic movement: linear, circular, elliptical, hypocycloidal, and spiral (Fig. 12-2). Mechanically, the simplest tomographic motion is linear. Linear tomography can be accomplished in two ways: (1) the x-ray tube and film move in opposite directions about a fixed fulcrum in paths of travel parallel with one another, or (2) both the x-ray tube and the film move along concentric arcs rather than in straight lines. Both methods, which give similar results, are used by currently available x-ray units (Fig. 12-3).

The image quality of linear tomograms has several deficiencies compared with tomograms produced by other types of movement. With linear motion, tomograms often appear streaked (Fig. 12-4). These streaks, called *parasite lines*, appear when the long axis of a structure lying outside the focal plane is oriented parallel with the movement of the tube. As a result, linear motion, whether it be the parallel or arc type, fails to satisfy a requirement

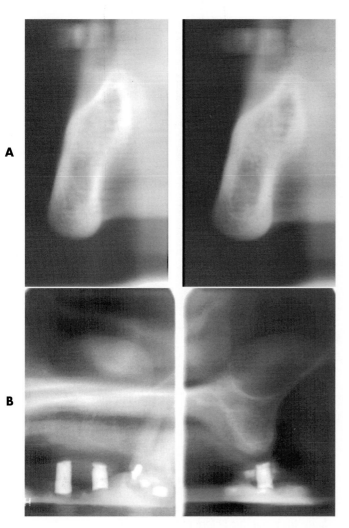

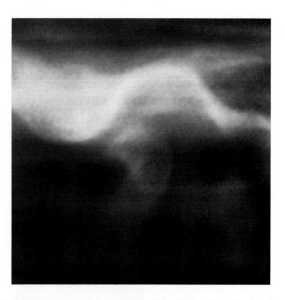

FIG. **12-4** *Linear tomogram of the TMJ.* Note the horizontal radiopaque streaks in this image. These streaks, called *parasite lines*, represent the blurred image of objects lying outside the focal plane. They are evident in the image when the long axes of objects located superficial or deep to the focal plane lie parallel with the path of the x-ray tube and film movement. Compare with Fig. 12-5.

FIG. **12-3** *Linear tomographic images made by panoramic units.* **A,** Mandibular tomograms acquired using a Planmeca PM 2002 CC Proline panoramic unit. **B,** Maxillary tomograms in the premolar region acquired using an Instrumentarium Orthopantomograph 100 panoramic unit. Note the dome-shaped opacity in the floor of the maxillary sinus consistent with a mucous retention cyst. (**A,** Courtesy Planmeca, Inc.; **B,** Courtesy Brad Potter, DDS, Augusta, Ga.)

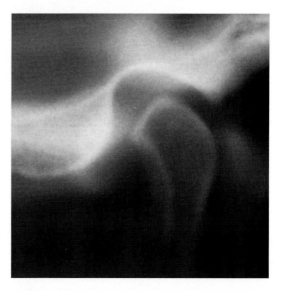

FIG. **12-5** *Spiral tomogram of the TMJ.* Complex tomographic movements result in maximal blurring of the images of objects lying superficial and deep to the plane of focus; the streaking parasite lines, therefore, are absent.

for optimal blurring. In addition, because the distance from the tube to the patient, the patient to the film, and the tube to the film changes constantly and because the angulation of the x-ray beam through the focal plane changes during exposure with the parallel type of motion, inconsistent magnification, dimensional instability, and a nonuniform density may be seen across the linear tomographic image. For some applications these deficiencies may be acceptable; if sharper tomographic images of more uniform density, consistent magnification, and dimensional stability are required, a multidirectional tomographic motion is necessary (Fig. 12-5).

The thickness of tissue in the focal plane is called the *tomographic layer.* The location of the tomographic layer within the object is determined by the position of the fulcrum and its width (described numerically as the thickness of cut) by the tomographic angle or arc (see

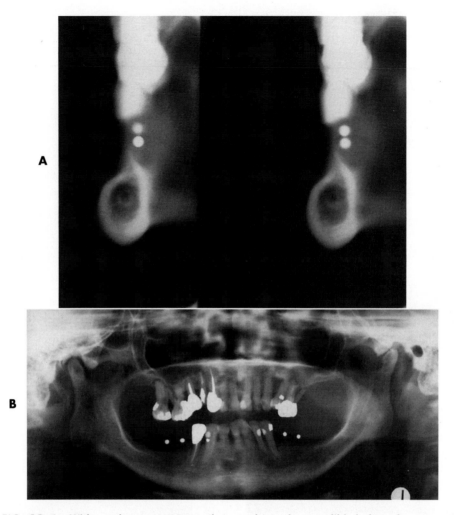

FIG. **12-6** *Wide-angle tomograms made to evaluate the mandible before placement of a dental implant.* The mandibular right premolar-molar area in cross-section at the radiopaque markers is demonstrated on both the panoramic radiograph and the tomograms. Note the clarity with which the inferior alveolar canal is imaged in the tomograms acquired with a spiral movement. **A,** Each slice is 4 mm thick. **B,** The metallic markers are for orientation of the cross-sectional images.

Fig. 12-1). The relationship between the tomographic angle and the thickness of cut is inverse: the greater the tomographic angle, the thinner the thickness of cut. Selection of the tomographic angle, and hence the thickness of cut, depends on the objective of the diagnostic task and the type of tissue being examined.

Wide-angle tomography, which by definition uses tomographic angles greater than 10 degrees, allows visualization of fine structures that normally would be obscured by superimposition in conventional radiography. Using this technique, layers as thin as 1 mm can be imaged. A disadvantage of this technique, however, is that it produces images of decreased contrast. Subject contrast results partly from the different thickness of adjacent structures. Because wide-angle tomography reduces these differences by the thinness of its cut, subject contrast is decreased. Wide-angle tomography is most useful when tissues of greater physical density (another contributor to subject contrast), such as bone, are studied. Thus wide-angle tomography is an excellent technique for evaluating the maxilla and mandible before placing dental implants (Fig. 12-6).

Narrow-angle tomography uses an angle of less than 10 degrees. Called *zonography* because a relatively thick zone of tissue (up to 25 mm) is sharply imaged, it is particularly useful when subject contrast is low because of little difference in physical density between adjacent structures (Fig. 12-7). Because subject contrast is low in soft tissue, zonography is the preferred tomographic technique when this tissue is imaged.

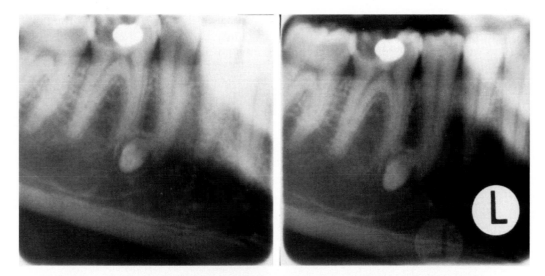

FIG. **12-7** *Narrow-angle tomograms (zonograms).* This pair of images, with a plane of focus tangent to the mandible, was made with narrow-angle tomographic techniques. The thick plane of focus (25 mm) allowed the supernumerary tooth and adjacent permanent teeth to be imaged clearly in one depth of the field. The diagnostic value of these images is increased by their having been made stereoscopically, allowing for localization of the supernumerary tooth relative to clinically erupted teeth. Also see Fig. 12-8.

STEREOSCOPY

Stereoscopy is not a new technique. It was introduced in 1898 by J. MacKenzie Davidson, only 3 years after Röntgen's discovery of x-rays. Over the next 30 to 40 years it grew in popularity among radiologists because of its educational value; understanding normal anatomy is simplified with stereoscopic images. Stereoscopy also was widely used to determine the location of small intracranial calcifications and multiple foreign bodies in dense or thick body sections, cases in which the interpretation of images produced at right angles might be difficult, and to evaluate the relationships of margins of bony fractures. Despite these advantages, stereoscopy fell from favor for several reasons, among which were the introduction of more sophisticated and less time-consuming imaging techniques and, by the 1930s, a greater awareness of the possible adverse biologic effects of x-rays. Stereoscopic imaging requires the exposure of two films, one for each eye, and thus delivers twice the amount of radiation to the patient. Between exposures the patient is maintained in position, the film is changed, and the tube is shifted from the right eye to the left eye position. Although the magnitude of the tube shift is empiric, it must be sufficient to form slightly different or discrepant images. A tube shift equal to 10% of the focal-film distance has been found to produce satisfactory results. After processing, the films commonly are viewed with a stereoscope that uses either mirrors or prisms to coordinate the accommodation and convergence of the viewer's eyes so that the brain can fuse the two images (see Figs. 12-7 and 12-8).

Stereoscopy currently enjoys a renewed interest for evaluation of bony pockets in patients with periodontal disease, determination of root configuration of teeth that require endodontic therapy, assessment of the relationship of the mandibular canal to the roots of unerupted mandibular third molars, and assessment of bone shape when placement of dental implants is considered.

SCANOGRAPHY

Scanography is a technique that uses a narrowly collimated, fan-shaped beam of radiation to scan an area of interest, sequentially projecting image data relative to this area onto a moving film, much the same as in panoramic radiography. Compared with images produced by standard radiography using round or rectangular collimation, scanograms demonstrate higher contrast with the perception of greater detail. Image contrast is greater in scanography because collimation of the x-ray beam reduces the amount of radiation scattered to the film during exposure. Therefore the major advantage of scanography over standard transmission radiography is image quality.

The Soredex Scanora (Soredex Inc., Marietta, Ga.) (see Fig 11-10) is a commercially available x-ray unit capable of performing both rotational and linear scan–

ography. In rotational scanography the beam of radiation rotates about a fixed axis that is predetermined based on the area to be imaged. The imaging sequence used by this unit results in the production of two or four scanograms, each made with the x-ray tube in a different position; thus multiple images are made, any two of which can be viewed as stereoscopic pairs (see Fig. 12-8). Rotational scanography has been found to be as effective as intraoral periapical films in the assessment of peri-odontal disease and the detection of periapical lesions. In linear scanography the x-ray beam and film move in a linear fashion, scanning the area of interest. Linear scanography can be thought of as panoramic radiography that has been "straightened out." The Scanora system is capable of both posteroanterior and lateral linear scanning of the maxillofacial complex. Although these views are not produced stereoscopically, they have the advantage of optimal image contrast (Fig. 12-9).

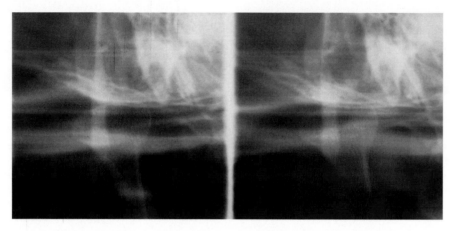

FIG. **12-8** *Posteroanterior rotational stereoscopic scanogram of the right TMJ.* Compared with a standard posteroanterior view of the condyle, this view demonstrates higher contrast and greater detail. The diagnostic value of such images is increased by their having been made stereoscopically, which allows for the perception of depth.

FIG. **12-9** *Lateral linear scanogram of the maxillofacial area.* Maximal image contrast is obtained by using linear scanning techniques rather than standard radiography.

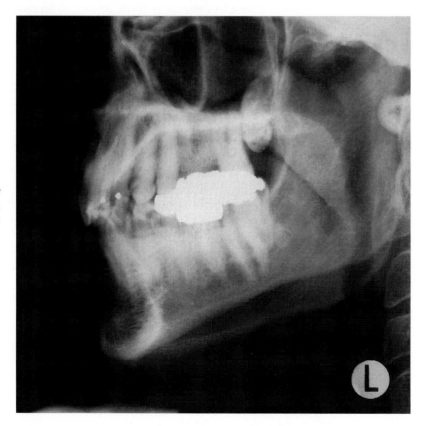

Digital Imaging

From the time of Röntgen's discovery of x-rays, some type of photographic film has been the most commonly used image receptor. As an image receptor, radiographic film is versatile; it serves as the recording, display, and storage medium for diagnostic images. Yet, however advantageous this versatility, film has a number of disadvantages. It is relatively inefficient as a detector of radiation, requiring relatively high doses for exposure, and it requires chemical processing by solutions that are potentially allergenic and polluting. Perhaps even more significantly, film provides the clinician with a static image that allows for little manipulation because of the inherent union of its image recording and display functions. Because these two functions are linked, neither can be optimized independently. As a result, if the exposure latitude over which a film responds with densities in the diagnostically useful range were increased, film contrast may be reduced to a point where information is lost. Conversely, inherent film contrast may be increased only by reducing the exposure latitude.

The application of computer technology to radiography has allowed image acquisition, manipulation, storage, retrieval, and transmission (teleradiography) to remote sites in a digital format. Potentially, one of the greatest advantages of digital imaging over film radiography is the separation of the image recording and display functions. Digital techniques produce a dynamic, rather than static, image in which the visual characteristics of density and contrast can be manipulated after acquisition to meet specific diagnostic tasks or to correct errors in exposure techniques. The capability for postacquisition manipulation provides the clinician with the potential to obtain more information from the image and should reduce the number of images that need to be remade because of overexposure or underexposure. The use of digital technology also results in a 50% to 95% reduction in patient exposure because of the greater sensitivity of the digital receptor, elimination of wet processing and the need for a darkroom, and considerable reduction in the time lapse between image acquisition and display.

Several techniques use images recorded in digitized form, such as intraoral and extraoral radiography, computed tomography, and magnetic resonance imaging. Digital imaging requires a number of components, including some form of electronic sensor or detector, a computer with an analog-to-digital converter, and a monitor or printer (or both) for image display (Fig. 12-10). In each of these techniques, data acquired by an electronic sensor is presented to the computer as analog information, or data that is represented in a continuous fashion. For this information to be useful, it must be converted into discrete units, since computers function only with digital information, represented by

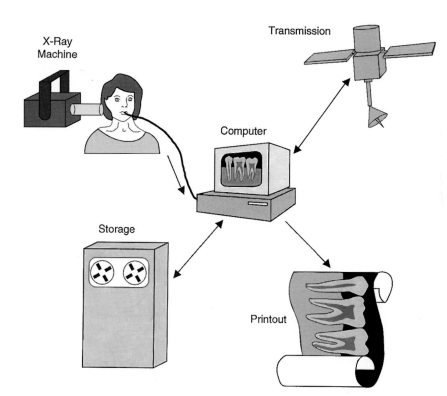

FIG. **12-10** *Digital image acquisition and display.* In this instance the image is captured directly on a charge-coupled device (CCD) in the patient's mouth. The signal from the CCD is sent to the computer, where it is digitized into 256 gray levels. The image can then be displayed on a monitor, where it can be enhanced by varying the density and contrast. The image may also be stored for future use, printed if a hard copy is required, or transmitted electronically to a remote site.

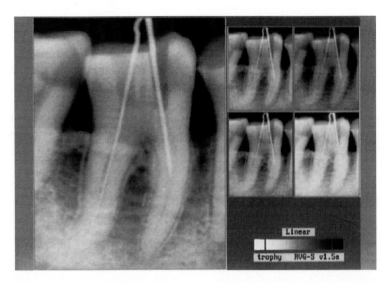

FIG. **12-11** *Direct digital intraoral radiographs.* Advantages of digital radiography include rapid image acquisition, the ability to manipulate image contrast and density, and significant radiation dose reduction compared with direct exposure film. (Courtesy Trex Trophy Radiology, Marietta, Ga.)

either a 0 or a 1. Computer "language" is based on the binary number system, in which two digits (0 and 1) are used to represent information. These two characters are called *bits,* for *bi*nary digi*t.* In typical computer language, these characters form words eight or more bits in length, called *bytes.* With every bit of an 8-bit word being either 0 or 1, the number of possible words, or bytes, in this language is 2^8 (256). Using a 12-bit language increases the number of possible bytes dramatically, to 2^{12} (4096).

The analog-to-digital converter (A/D converter or digitizer) is used to change the analog output signal from these detector systems to a numeric representation based on the binary number system recognizable by the computer. This task is accomplished by measuring the voltage of the output signal at discrete intervals and then assigning a number (0 to 255 with an 8-bit language) to the intensity of the voltage. Thus 256 voltage levels may be discriminated that ultimately are displayed in image form, after computer manipulation, as 256 shades of gray. The sensitivity that can be achieved with even this relatively short 8-bit system can be appreciated when one considers that the human eye can distinguish only about 32 shades of gray!

The methods by which digital images are produced, manipulated, stored, retrieved, and transmitted are similar for all techniques, from computed tomography to intraoral radiography, differing only in the means by which they are acquired. In the context of this section, digital radiography is considered as either direct or indirect radiography. In direct digital radiography the image is acquired by some detector that is sensitive to elec-

tromagnetic energy either in the range of visible light or x-rays (Fig. 12-11). Indirect digital radiography uses radiographic film as the image receptor; the image is digitized from the output signal of either a video camera, a charge-coupled device (CCD) scanner, or a laser scanner that views the processed radiograph.

DIRECT DIGITAL RADIOGRAPHY

The most widely used detector in digital medical radiography is the photostimulable phosphor (PSP), also known as the *storage phosphor.* PSPs, which have x-ray absorption mechanisms similar to those of phosphors used in intensifying screens, usually are of the barium fluorohalide family. They differ from intensifying-screen phosphors in that the useful optical signal is not derived from the light emitted in response to the incident x-radiation, but rather from the subsequent emission, when electrons are released from traps in the phosphor. The initial interaction between x-ray photons and crystals of PSP excites the electrons in the phosphor. Although some of these electrons produce light in the usual manner, a significant proportion are trapped within the phosphor. When the phosphor subsequently is stimulated by irradiation with a ruby laser in the read-out unit, the trapped electrons are released, causing emission of shorter-wavelength light in the blue region of the spectrum. This process is called *photostimulated luminescence.* The emitted blue light, which has an intensity proportional to the amount of x-rays absorbed by the phosphor, is detected by a photomultiplier tube, and the output of the tube is digitized to form the image (Fig. 12-12).

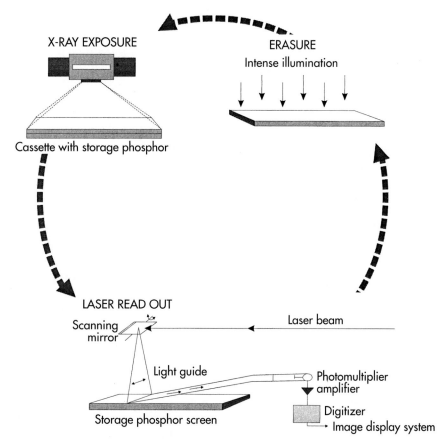

FIG. **12-12** *Digital imaging with PSP.* After the PSP has been exposed to x-ray beams, it is placed in the read-out unit and scanned by a laser beam. Laser scanning causes the release of energy from the PSP. This energy, the intensity of which is directly proportional to the quantity of x-rays absorbed by the PSP, is in the form of visible light, which is detected by a photomultiplier and digitized to form an image. After the PSP has been read, it is erased by illumination with visible light and exposed again.

Another type of detector is the CCD. A CCD consists of a chip of pure silicon with an active area that has been divided into a two-dimensional array of elements called *pixels* (*pic*ture *el*ements). When either electromagnetic energy in the range of visible light that has been emitted from an intensifying screen or x-rays interact with pixels of a CCD, an electric charge is created that the pixels are able to store in much the same fashion as an electrical capacitor. The total charge developed and stored by a pixel is proportional to the light or x-ray energy incident on the pixel. After exposure of the CCD to radiation, charges stored by the individual pixels are sequentially removed electronically, creating an analog output signal with a voltage proportional to the charge on each of the pixels in succession.

Both the PSP and CCD detectors described previously have been incorporated into systems that are available today to the dental practitioner for intraoral, panoramic, and cephalometric radiography. Because all systems are computer based, they have certain similarities.

They all ultimately can be linked with electronic record systems so that all patient data can be stored in the same computer memory, easily accessed, and displayed or transmitted. They all have capabilities for a range of image manipulations, including density and contrast enhancement, magnification, and distance and angle measurements. Typically, intraoral digital images occupy data files of 100 to 400 Kb in uncompressed format. All systems achieve image resolution in the range of 6 to 12 line pairs per millimeter. This range of resolution is similar to that in extraoral images acquired with screen-film combinations and considerably less than the 20 line pairs per millimeter capability of direct exposure intraoral radiographic film. Print images may be acquired with all systems, but prints generally are of lesser quality than monitor-displayed images.

Any perceived advantage or disadvantage of one system over the other (PSP versus CCD) is directly related to the detector. CCD detectors generally have a smaller active surface area than PSP detectors, which approxi-

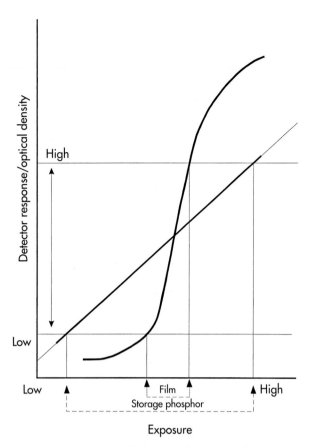

FIG. **12-13** *Exposure latitude.* The range of x-ray exposures over which PSPs respond with densities in the diagnostically useful range is wider than that of radiographic film. This gives PSPs a much wider exposure latitude than film.

mate intraoral film in size. CCDs require a direct wire connection to the computer, whereas PSPs are independent of the read-out unit. This means that the computer of the CCD-based system must be relatively close to the patient when the exposure is made, and it cannot be used to service more than one operatory without physically moving the equipment. A single, centrally located PSP read-out unit can provide service to the entire dental suite. However, the CCD system's direct connection to the computer allows almost instantaneous image display, whereas PSP systems require about 25 seconds for the readout to be completed and the image to be displayed.

The dynamic range of PSP systems is much wider than that of radiographic film, giving this system a much broader exposure latitude (Fig. 12-13). The range of latitude achieved by PSP systems is partly the result of a prescan operation that serves as an automatic gain control. The practical significance of this procedure is that images that were underexposed or overexposed ultimately are displayed with equal density as correctly exposed images. Because of this capability, only rarely does

an image need to be remade because of incorrect exposure techniques. In contrast to PSP systems, the dynamic range of CCDs is less than that of radiographic film. Practically this means that the range of exposures over which CCD systems respond with images in the diagnostically useful density range is less than that of both PSP systems and radiographic film. The increased latitude achieved by PSP systems also allows for image acquisition with less radiation exposure than with CCD systems.

Current evidence suggests that digital systems perform comparably with film radiography for detection of periodontal bone lesions and dental caries. Also, rapid image acquisition and reduced radiation exposure per image may prove to be advantageous for imaging during the course of endodontic therapy.

New technologies constantly are being developed to improve direct digital image quality and convenience. One such technology uses amorphous selenium as the detector. The first medical application of this detector was in xeroradiography, a technique in which a latent image charge on the surface of an amorphous selenium plate was read out to create an image with toner, much like the making of a photocopy. This imaging technology was used in mammography and briefly in intraoral radiography, but it is no longer viable, not because of the amorphous selenium but because of the toner read-out. The technology today uses a thin layer of amorphous selenium on an aluminum support. The selenium is rendered sensitive to x-rays by charging its surface to a high potential. When x-rays strike the charged surface, electron-hole pairs are created in the selenium, and the freed electrons migrate to the surface, resulting in a latent image charge. The detector is then passed under an array of electrometers, which scan the image and read it into a computer. To date, this detector system has been used only in chest radiography, but the technology may be adapted for use in oral radiography.

INDIRECT DIGITAL RADIOGRAPHY

Digital processing of images recorded by radiographic film may serve several useful purposes. First, because digital images can be manipulated, digitization allows optimization of image quality in terms of contrast and density, with the potential for enhanced perception of detail and improved diagnosis. Second, as does direct digital radiography, digitization of radiographic images provides for storage of information. Third, this information can be transmitted to remote sites for consultation. Unfortunately, digital image processing of direct exposure nonscreen films may result in loss of information because the digitized image represents a second generation.

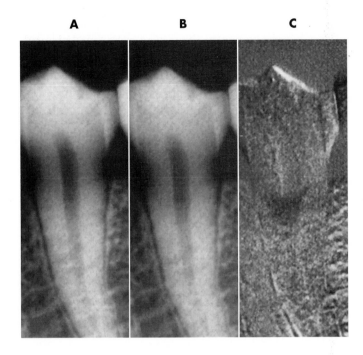

A   B   C

FIG. **12-14** *Digital subtraction radiographs.* Subtraction radiography requires two images (**A** and **B**), which are exposed with the same geometry. In this instance the loss of alveolar bone in **B** is too subtle to be seen. However, the subtracted image (**C**) displays the differences between **A** and **B**; the bone loss is seen as a dark structure superimposed over the pulp. (Courtesy Dr. H.G. Gröndahl, Göteborg, Sweden.)

The ability to digitize information contained in the remnant x-ray beam relative to the subject has made possible digital subtraction radiography and digitized image interpretation.

Digital Subtraction Radiography

Subtraction radiography requires two identical images. The subtracted image is a composite of these two, representing their differing densities (Fig. 12-14). Although visual examination of standard radiographs cannot detect a 0.85-mm change in the thickness of cortical bone, digital subtraction radiography is so sensitive it can detect a 0.12-mm change. The ability of digital subtraction to record minute differences depends on the degree of matching of the two images. However, techniques have been developed to correct differences in image contrast, projection geometry, and hardening of the x-ray beam caused by tissues through which the x-rays travel.

Digital subtraction radiography has been reported to be useful in the diagnosis of periodontal and carious lesions, both of which may be characterized by their sometimes insidious and relatively slow rate of progression. Some have suggested that contrast enhancement of the subtracted image with color aids the observation of small periodontal defects. Subtraction radiography also has been reported to have potential for evaluation of small changes in the mandibular condyle position and the integrity of the articular surface, as well as for assessment of osseous remodeling around granular hydroxyapatite implants. Digital subtraction radiography is difficult to use in clinical practice because each occa-

sion requires reproducible alignment of the central ray of the x-ray beam, the teeth, and the film.

Digitized Image Interpretation

With the advent of digital imaging has come the possibility of computer interpretation of the image. Systems and programs have been developed for recognizing anatomy as imaged radiographically, detecting carious and periodontal lesions, and assessing periapical regions of teeth and bone quality. Computer interpretation may prove to play a significant role in diagnoses of the future.

Computed Tomography

In 1972 Godfrey Hounsfield announced the invention of a revolutionary imaging technique, which he referred to as *computerized axial transverse scanning*. With this technique he was able to produce an axial cross-sectional image of the head using a narrowly collimated, moving beam of x-rays. The remnant radiation of this beam was detected by a scintillation crystal; the resulting analog signal was fed into a computer, digitized, and analyzed by a mathematical algorithm, and the data were reconstructed as an axial tomographic image. The image produced by this technique was like no other x-ray image. Claimed to be 100 times more sensitive than conventional x-ray systems, it demonstrated differences between various soft tissues never before seen with x-ray imaging techniques. Since 1972 computed tomography has had many names, each of which referred to at least one as-

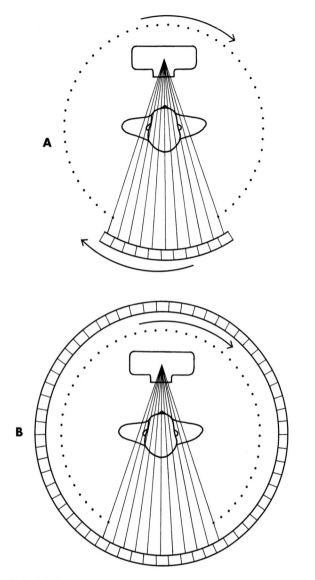

FIG. 12-15 *Mechanical geometry of CT scanners.* **A,** Both the x-ray tube and the detector array revolve around the patient. **B,** Only the x-ray tube rotates; radiation detection is accomplished by the use of a fixed circular array of as many as 1000 detectors.

pect of the technique: computerized axial tomography, computerized reconstruction tomography, computed tomographic scanning, axial tomography, and computerized transaxial tomography. Currently the preferred name is *computed tomography,* abbreviated as *CT.*

In its simplest form a CT scanner consists of a radiographic tube that emits a finely collimated, fan-shaped x-ray beam that is directed to a series of scintillation detectors or ionization chambers. Depending on the scanner's mechanical geometry, both the radiographic tube and detectors may rotate synchronously about the patient, or the detectors may form a continuous ring about the patient and the x-ray tube may move in a circle

within the detector ring (Fig. 12-15). Regardless of the mechanical geometry, the transmission signal recorded by the detectors represents a composite of the absorption characteristics of all elements of the patient in the path of the x-ray beam.

The CT image is reconstructed by the computer, which mathematically manipulates the transmission data obtained from multiple projections (Fig. 12-16). For example, if one projection is made every one third of a degree, 1080 projections result during the course of a single 360-degree rotation of the scanner about the patient. Data derived from these 1080 projections (1080 projections constitute one scan) contain all the information necessary to construct one image. The CT image is recorded and displayed as a matrix of individual blocks called *voxels* (*vo*lume *el*ements). Each square of the image matrix is a pixel. Whereas the size of the pixel (about 0.1 mm) is determined partly by the computer program used to construct the image, the length of the voxel (about 1 to 20 mm) is determined by the width of the x-ray beam, which in turn is controlled by the prepatient and postpatient collimators. Voxel length is analogous to the tomographic layer in film tomography. For image display, each pixel is assigned a CT number representing density. This number is proportional to the degree to which the material within the voxel has attenuated the x-ray beam. It represents the absorption characteristics, or linear attenuation coefficient, of that particular volume of tissue in the patient. CT numbers, also known as *Hounsfield units* (named in honor of the inventor Godfrey Hounsfield), may range from −1000 to +1000, each constituting a different level of optical density. This scale of relative densities is based on air (−1000), water (0), and dense bone (+1000).

CT has several advantages over conventional film radiography and film tomography. First, CT completely eliminates the superimposition of images of structures superficial or deep to the area of interest. Second, because of the inherent high-contrast resolution of CT, differences between tissues that differ in physical density by less than 1% can be distinguished; conventional radiography requires a 10% difference in physical density to distinguish between tissues. Third, data from a single CT imaging procedure consisting of multiple contiguous scans can be viewed as images in the axial, coronal, or sagittal planes, depending on the diagnostic task. This is referred to as *multiplanar reformatted imaging.*

Primarily because of its high-contrast resolution and ability to demonstrate small differences in soft tissue density, CT has become useful for the diagnosis of disease in the maxillofacial complex (Fig. 12-17), including the salivary glands and TMJ. However, with the advent of magnetic resonance imaging, which has proved superior to CT for depicting soft tissue, the use of CT scanning for assessment of internal derangements of the TMJ has de-

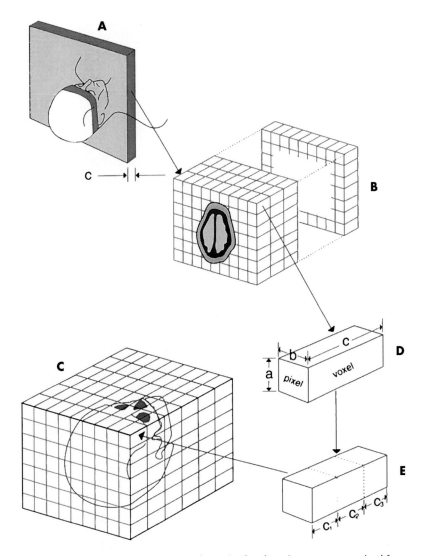

FIG. **12-16** *CT image formation.* **A,** Data for a single-plane image are acquired from multiple projections made during the course of a 360-degree rotation around the patient. Dimension *c* is controlled by prepatient and postpatient collimators. **B,** A single-plane image is constructed from absorption characteristics of the subject and displayed as differences in optical density, ranging from −1000 to +1000 Hounsfield units. Several planes may be imaged from multiple contiguous scans. **C,** The image consists of a matrix of individual pixels representing the face of a volume called a *voxel.* Although dimensions *a* and *b* are determined partly by the computer program used to construct the image, dimension *c* is controlled by the collimators as in **A**. **D,** Cuboid voxels can be created from the original rectangular voxel by computer interpolation. This allows the formation of multiplanar and three-dimensional images **(E).**

creased significantly. Additionally, CT has been shown useful for evaluation of patients before placement of endosseous oral implants. Despite the fact that similar information about maxillary and mandibular anatomy can be obtained with film tomography, CT allows reconstruction of cross-sectional images of the entire maxilla or mandible or both from a single imaging procedure.

Multiplanar CT imaging has made a significant contribution to diagnosis. However, these images are two-dimensional and require a certain degree of mental in-

tegration by the viewer for interpretation; this limitation has led to the development of computer programs that reformat data acquired from axial CT scans into three-dimensional images (3D CT).

Three-dimensional CT requires that each voxel, shaped as a rectangular parallelepiped or rectangular solid, be dimensionally altered into multiple cuboidal voxels. This process, called *interpolation*, creates sets of evenly spaced cuboidal voxels (cuberilles) that occupy the same volume as the original voxel (see Fig. 12-16).

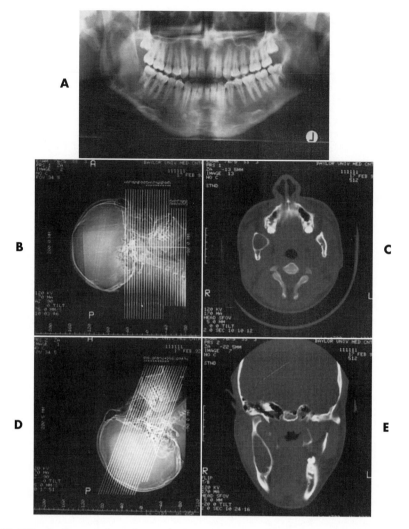

FIG. **12-17** **A,** Panoramic radiograph showing a unilocular radiolucent lesion involving the right mandibular ramus. **B,** Lateral scout radiograph for planning the location of contiguous CT scans. **C,** Reconstructed axial image at the level of scan 13 in **B.** Note the faciolingual extent of the radiolucent lesion on the right side. **D,** The patient is repositioned for oblique scans through the area of the lesion. **E,** Reconstructed oblique image at the level of scan 7 in **D.** Note the superior extent of the lesion into the condylar neck. (**B** through **E,** Courtesy Radiology Department, Baylor University Medical Center, Dallas, Tex.)

The CT numbers of the cuberilles represent the average of the original voxel CT numbers surrounding each of the new voxels. Creation of these new cuboidal voxels allows the image to be reconstructed in any plane without loss of resolution by locating their position in space relative to one another. In construction of the 3D CT image, only cuberilles representing the surface of the object scanned are projected onto the viewing monitor. The surface formed by these cuberilles then appears as if illuminated by a light source located behind the viewer. In this manner the visible surface of each pixel is assigned a gray-level value, depending on its distance from and orientation to the light source. Thus pixels that face the light source and/or are closer to it appear brighter than those that are turned away from the source and/or are farther away. The effects of this shading and the resulting image perceived by the viewer have been described as similar to an artist's three-dimensional rendering of an object within a two-dimensional medium. Once constructed, 3D CT images may be further manipulated by rotation about any axis to display the structure imaged from many angles (Fig. 12-18). Also, external portions of the image can be removed electronically to reveal concealed deeper anatomy.

One of the first applications of 3D CT was the study of patients with suspected intervertebral disk hernia-

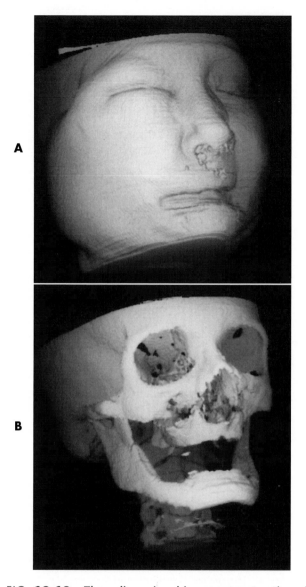

FIG. **12-18** *Three-dimensional image reconstruction of a patient following facial trauma.* By computer manipulation of the data acquired from a CT scanner, both soft tissue and hard tissue three-dimensional images can be constructed. Note the facial swelling in **A** and the Le Fort I fracture in **B** (with the maxillary alveolar ridge separated from the midface). (Courtesy Columbia Scientific Inc., Columbia, Md.)

tion and spinal stenosis. Since that time 3D CT has been applied to craniofacial reconstructive surgery and has been used both for treatment of congenital and acquired deformities and for evaluation of intracranial tumors, benign and malignant lesions of the maxillofacial complex, cervical spine injuries, pelvic fractures, and deformities of the hands and feet. The availability of data in a three-dimensional format also has allowed the construction of life-sized models that can be used for trial surgeries and the construction of

surgical stents and creation of accurate implanted prostheses.

CT technology is being advanced continuously. Imatron (San Francisco) has developed a CT scanner capable of acquiring data up to 10 times faster than conventional CT. Its Ultrafast CT, which has scan times on the order of 50 msec, is able to freeze cardiac and pulmonary motion, enhancing the quality without motion artifacts. Other manufacturers have developed spiral CT scanners. With these, while the gantry containing the x-ray tube and detectors revolves around the patient, the table on which the patient is lying continuously advances through the gantry. This results in the acquisition of a continuous spiral of data as the x-ray beam moves down the patient. It is reported that, compared with conventional CT scanners, spiral scanners provide improved multiplanar image reconstructions, reduced examination time (12 seconds versus 5 minutes), and a reduced radiation dose (up to 75%).

Magnetic Resonance Imaging

In contrast to the techniques described above, which use x-rays for acquisition of information pertaining to an object studied, magnetic resonance imaging (MRI) uses nonionizing radiation from the radiofrequency (RF) band of the electromagnetic spectrum. To produce an MR image, the patient is placed inside a large magnet, which induces a relatively strong external magnetic field. This causes the nuclei of many atoms in the body, including hydrogen, to align themselves with the magnetic field. After application of an RF signal, energy is released from the body, detected, and used to construct the MR image by computer. The high contrast sensitivity of MRI to tissue differences and the absence of radiation exposure are the reasons MRI for the most part has replaced CT for imaging soft tissue. CT remains an important technique for imaging bony tissues.

The theory of MRI is based on the magnetic properties of an atom. Atomic nuclei spin about their axes much as earth spins about its axis. In addition, individual protons and neutrons (nucleons), which make up the nuclei of atoms, each possess a spin, or angular momentum. In nuclei in which the protons and neutrons are evenly paired, the spin of each nucleon cancels that of another, producing a net spin of zero. In nuclei that contain an unpaired proton or neutron, a net spin is created. Because spin is associated with an electrical charge, a magnetic field is generated in nuclei with unpaired nucleons, causing these nuclei to act as magnets with north and south poles (magnetic dipoles).

The nucleus of the element hydrogen contains a single, unpaired proton and therefore acts as a magnetic

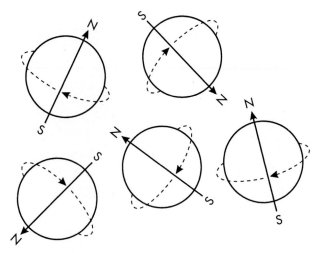

FIG. **12-19**   A sample of hydrogen nuclei with net spins showing these dipoles to be randomly oriented.

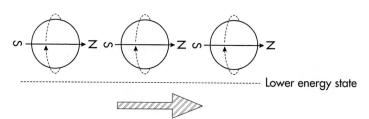

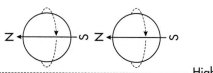

FIG. **12-20**   *Hydrogen nuclei in an external magnetic
field.* Most nuclei are in the lower energy state and are
aligned parallel with the magnetic field.

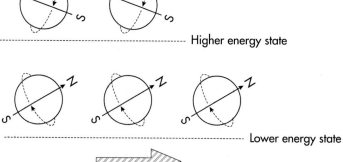

FIG. **12-21**   *Hydrogen nuclei in an external magnetic
field.* The magnetic dipoles are not aligned exactly with
the external magnetic field. Instead, the axes of spinning
protons actually oscillate or wobble with a slight tilt from
being absolutely parallel with the flux of the external
magnet.

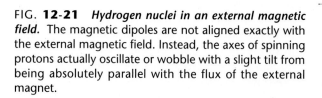

dipole. A sample containing many hydrogen atoms would find these magnetic dipoles to be randomly oriented. This results in a total magnetization for the sample of zero (Fig. 12-19). In this natural state, if an external magnetic field is applied to the sample, all the hydrogen nuclear axes line up in the direction of the magnetic field, producing a quantity of net magnetization. However, not all north poles point in the same direction. Rather, two states are possible: spin-up, which parallels the external magnetic field, and spin-down, which is antiparallel with the field. Because more energy is required to align antiparallel with the magnetic

field, those hydrogen nuclei are considered to be at a higher energy state than those aligned parallel with the field. Nuclei prefer to be in a lower energy state, and usually more are aligned parallel with the magnetic field (Fig. 12-20). Nuclei can be made to undergo transition from one energy state to another by absorbing or releasing a certain quantity of energy. Energy required for transition from the lower to the higher or from the higher to the lower energy level can be supplied or recovered in the form of electromagnetic energy in the RF portion of the electromagnetic spectrum. The transition from one energy level to another is called *resonance*.

When an external magnetic field is applied to a sample of nuclei, their north and south poles do not align exactly with the direction of the magnetic field (Fig. 12-21). The axes of spinning protons actually oscillate or wobble with a slight tilt from being absolutely parallel with the flux of the external magnet (Fig. 12-22). This tilting or wobbling, called *precession*, is similar to that of a spinning toy top, which does not spin in a perfectly upright position as it slows down because of the effect of the earth's gravitational field. The axis of the spinning top wobbles about the direction of the local gravitational field, and the axis of the spinning proton wobbles (or precesses) about the applied magnetic field. Because of the spin-up and spin-down states, the spinning protons precess together in the direction of their spin states, which can be visualized as two cones placed end to end (Fig. 12-23). The rate or frequency of precession is called the *resonant* or *Larmor frequency;* it depends on the species of nucleus and is proportional to the strength of

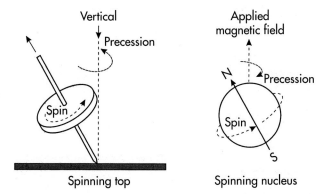

FIG. **12-22** *Precession.* The tilting or wobbling of the spinning hydrogen nuclei around the direction of the external magnetic field is called *precession.* The rate or frequency of precession is called the *resonant* or *Larmor frequency.* The Larmor frequency is specific for the nuclear species and depends on the strength of the external magnetic field.

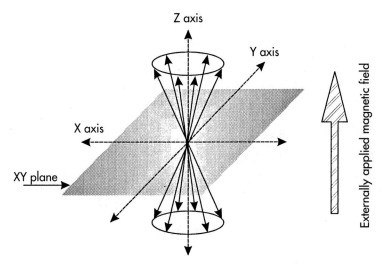

FIG. **12-23** *Spin-up and spin-down.* Because of the spin-up and spin-down states, the spinning hydrogen nuclei precess together in the direction of their spin states, which can be visualized as two cones placed end to end.

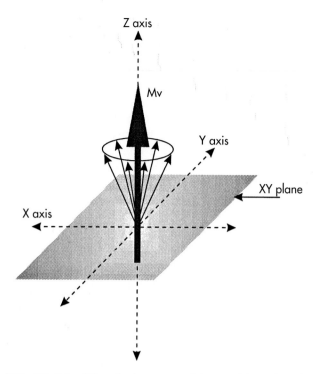

FIG. 12-24 When hydrogen nuclei are subjected to the flux of an external magnetic field, two energy states result: spin-up, which is in the direction of the field, and spin-down, which is in the opposite direction of the field. The combined effect of these two energy states is a weak net magnetic moment, or magnetization vector (Mv), parallel with the applied magnetic field.

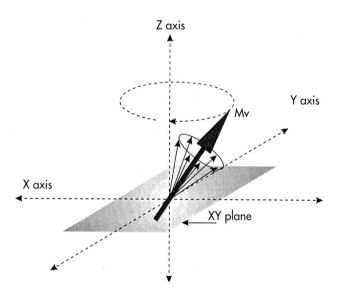

FIG. 12-25 When energy in the form of an electromagnetic wave in the radiofrequency (RF) range from an RF antenna coil is directed to tissue with hydrogen nuclei that are aligned in the Z axis by an external static magnetic field, the protons in the tissue that have a Larmor frequency matching that of the electromagnetic wave absorb energy and shift or rotate away from the direction induced by the imaging magnet.

the external magnetic field. The Larmor frequency of hydrogen is 42.58 MHz in a magnetic field of 1 Tesla (T). One Tesla is 10,000 times the earth's magnetic field. The magnetic field strengths used for MR imaging range from 0.15 to 1.5 T.

In summary, when nuclei are subjected to the flux of an external magnetic field, two energy states result: spin-up, which is in the direction of the field, and spin-down, which is in the opposite direction of the field. The combined effect of these two energy states is a weak net magnetic moment, or magnetization vector (Mv), parallel with the applied magnetic field (Fig. 12-24).

When energy in the form of an electromagnetic wave in the radiofrequency range from an RF antenna coil is directed to tissue with protons (hydrogen nuclei) that are aligned in the Z axis by an external static magnetic field (by the imaging magnet), the protons in the tissue that have a Larmor frequency matching that of the electromagnetic wave absorb energy and shift or rotate away from the direction induced by the imaging magnet (Fig. 12-25). The longer the RF pulse is applied, the greater the angle of rotation. If the pulse is of sufficient intensity (duration), it will rotate the net tissue magnetization vector into the transverse plane (XY plane), which is perpendicular to longitudinal alignment (Z axis), and cause all the protons to precess in phase. This is referred to as a *90-degree RF pulse* or a *flip angle of 90 degrees*. During an MR imaging sequence, many RF pulses with different intensities can be used, along with different times between repetition of the pulse.

The net magnetization of the tissue in the transverse plane and the amount of transverse magnetization that exists at the termination of the RF pulse are equal to the amount of longitudinal magnetization that existed just before the pulse. Both are directly proportional to the strength of the static magnetic field and the number of hydrogen nuclei (protons) present in the tissue. At this precise moment, a maximal RF signal is induced in a receiver coil. The magnitude of this signal represents information about the overall concentration of hydrogen nuclei (proton density) in a sample of tissue, or about the number of hydrogen nuclei in a sample of different types of tissue. This signal depends not only on the presence or absence of hydrogen but also on the degree to which hydrogen is bound within a molecule. Tightly bound hydrogen atoms, such as those present in bone, do not align themselves with the external magnetic field and do not produce a usable signal. Loosely bound or mobile hydrogen atoms such as those present in soft tissues and liquids tilt and align to produce a detectable signal. The measure of the concentration of loosely bound hydrogen nuclei available to create the signal is referred to as the *proton density* or *spin density* of the tissue in question. The higher the concentration of these nuclei of loosely bound hydrogen atoms, the stronger the net magnetization at equilibrium and at all degrees of excitement, the more intense the recovered signal, and the lighter the MR image.

As soon as the radio waves (the resonant RF pulse) are turned off, two events occur simultaneously—the radiation of energy and the return of the nuclei to their original spin state at a lower energy. This process is called *relaxation*, and the energy loss is detected as a signal, which is called *free induction decay (FID)*:

- First, the nuclei in transverse alignment begin to re-align themselves with the main magnetic field (i.e., to relax), and net magnetization regrows to the original longitudinal orientation. This relaxation is accomplished by a transfer of energy from individual hydrogen nuclei (spin) to the surrounding molecules (lattice). The time constant that describes the rate at which net magnetization returns to equilibrium by this transfer of energy is called the *T1 relaxation time* or *spin-lattice relaxation time*. T1 varies with different tissues and the ability of nuclei to transfer their excess energy to their environment. A T1-weighted image is produced by a short repetition time between RF pulses and a short signal recovery time. Because T1 is an exponential growth time constant, a tissue with a short T1 produces an intense MR signal, displayed as bright white in a T1-weighted image. A tissue with a long T1 produces a low-intensity signal and appears dark in the MR image.
- Second, the magnetic moments of adjacent hydrogen nuclei begin to interfere with one another; this causes the nuclei to dephase, with a resultant loss of transverse magnetization. The time constant that describes the rate of loss of transverse magnetization is called the *T2 relaxation time* or *transverse (spin-spin) relaxation time*. The transverse magnetization rapidly decays (exponentially) to zero, as do the amplitude and duration of the detected radio signal. A T2-weighted image is acquired using a long repetition time between RF pulses and a long signal recovery time. A tissue with a long T2 produces a high-intensity signal and is bright in the image. One with a short T2 produces a low-intensity signal and is dark in the image.

The FID relates signal intensity to time. A mathematical technique called the *Fourier transform* converts the relationship of signal intensity versus time to signal intensity versus resonant frequency, transforming the oscillating FID signal to a pulse of energy (current), the MR signal. When FIDs are received from a mixture of tissues, as is the case when a section of the body is examined, each volume of tissue generates a different radio signal at different frequencies. The individual signals are not separated by the antenna; rather, they are summed to form a complex FID signal. The Fourier transform also separates the complex FID signal from the different tissues into its various frequency components. This procedure is coupled with reconstruction techniques used in CT to produce diagnostic images.

Image contrast among the various tissues in the body is manipulated in MRI by varying the rate at which the RF pulses are transmitted. A short repetition time (TR) of 500 msec between pulses and a short echo or signal recovery time (TE) of 20 msec produce a T1-weighted image; a long TR (2000 msec) and a long TE (80 msec) produce a T2-weighted image. For every diagnostic task, the operator must decide which imaging sequence will bring out optimal image contrast. T1-weighted images are called *fat images* because fat has the shortest T1 relaxation time and the highest signal relative to other tissues and thus appears bright in the image. High anatomic detail is possible in this type of image because of good image contrast. T1-weighted images thus are useful for depicting small anatomic regions (e.g., the TMJ) where high spatial resolution is required. T2-weighted images are called *water images* because water has the longest T2 relaxation time and thus appears bright in the image. In general, the T2 time of abnormal tissues is longer than that of normal tissues. Images with T2 weighting are most commonly used when the practitioner is looking for inflammatory changes and tumors. T1-weighted images are more commonly used to demonstrate anatomy. In practice, images often must be acquired with both T1 and T2 weighting to separate the several tissues by contrast resolution.

Localization of the MR image to a specific part of the body (selecting a slice) and the ability to create a three-dimensional image depend on the fact that the Larmor frequency of a nucleus is governed in part by the strength of the external magnetic field. When this strength is changed in a gradient across a body of tissue (selectively exciting the image slice), the Larmor frequency of individual nuclei or groups of nuclei (voxels) in the gradient also changes.

This magnetic gradient is produced by three electromagnetic coils within the bore of the imaging magnet. The coils surround the patient and produce magnetic fields that oppose and redirect the magnetic flux in three orthogonal or right-angle directions to delineate individual volumes of tissue (voxels), which are subjected to magnetic fields of unique strength. Partitioning the local magnetic fields tunes all the hydrogen protons in a particular voxel to the same resonant frequency. This is called *selective excitation*. When an RF pulse with a range of frequencies is applied, a voxel of tissue tuned to one of the frequencies is excited; when the RF radiation is terminated, the excited voxel radiates that distinctive frequency, identifying and localizing it. The bandwidth or spectrum of frequencies of the RF pulse and the magnitude of the slice-selecting gradient determine the slice thickness. Slice

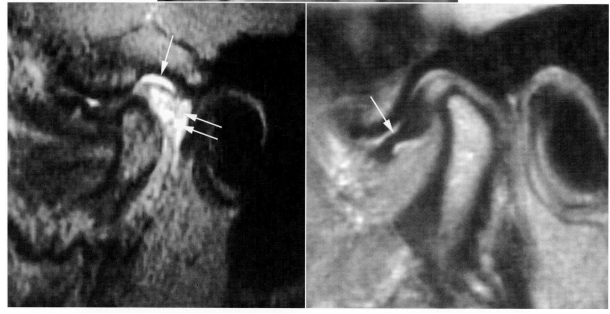

FIG. **12-26** **A,** T1-weighted MR image of the TMJ. The MR signal depends not only on the presence or absence of hydrogen nuclei (protons) but also on the degree to which hydrogen is bound within a molecule. Tightly bound hydrogen atoms such as those in bone do not align themselves with the external magnetic field and do not produce a usable signal (the cortical outlines of the condyles appear black). In this image the jaw is partly open, as indicated by the location of the condyle relative to the articular eminence. The articular disk, which has a "bow tie" appearance *(arrows),* is in a normal position relative to the translating condyle. **B,** T2-weighted MR image of the TMJ. Loosely bound or mobile hydrogen atoms such as those in soft tissues and liquids tilt and align, producing a detectable signal *(varying shades of gray).* This image illustrates both inflammatory effluent in the superior joint space *(arrow)* and hyperemia caused by increased vasculature in the retrodiskal tissues *(double arrows).* **C,** Proton or spin density MR image of the TMJ. The normal position of the posterior band of the articular disk is at the 11 to 12 o'clock position relative to the superior aspect of the condyle. In this image the disk is anteriorly displaced *(arrow),* with the posterior band in the 9 o'clock position relative to the condylar head. (**B** and **C,** Courtesy Richard Harper, DDS, Dallas, Tex.)

thickness can be reduced by increasing gradient strength or decreasing the RF bandwidth (frequency range).

MRI has several advantages over other diagnostic imaging procedures. First, it offers the best resolution of tissues of low inherent contrast. Although the x-ray attenuation coefficient may vary by no more than 1% between soft tissues, the spin density and T1 and T2 relaxation times may vary by up to 40%. Second, no ionizing radiation is involved with MRI. Third, because the region of the body imaged in MRI is controlled electronically, direct multiplanar imaging is possible without reorienting the patient. Disadvantages of MRI include relatively long imaging times and the potential hazard imposed by the presence of ferromagnetic metals in the vicinity of the imaging magnet. This latter disadvantage excludes from MRI any patient with implanted metallic foreign objects or medical devices that consist of or contain ferromagnetic metals (e.g., cardiac pacemakers, some cerebral aneurysm clips). Finally, some patients suffer from claustrophobia when positioned in a MRI machine.

Because of its excellent soft tissue contrast resolution, MRI has proved useful in a variety of circumstances (Fig. 12-26): diagnosing a suspected internal derangement of the TMJ and evaluating the treatment of that derangement after surgery; identifying and localizing orofacial soft tissue lesions; and providing images of salivary gland parenchyma.

Nuclear Medicine

Film radiography, CT, MRI, and diagnostic ultrasonography are considered morphologic imaging techniques; that is, each requires some specific structural difference or anatomic change for information to be recorded by an image receptor. In film radiography, for example, perception of an image depends on contrast, which in turn partly depends on the differential absorption of x-rays. The dependence of x-ray imaging on differential absorption essentially limits this technique to a single variable (tissue electron density), which in turn is presented as a structural or anatomic difference. However, human disease can exist with no specific anatomic changes. Changes that are seen may simply be later effects of some biochemical process that remains undetected until physical symptoms develop. Radionuclide imaging (or functional imaging techniques) provides the only means of assessing physiologic change that is a direct result of biochemical alteration (Fig. 12-27).

Radionuclide imaging is based on the radiotracer method, which assumes that radioactive atoms or molecules in an organism behave in a manner identical to that of their stable counterparts because they are chemically indistinguishable. Radiotracers allow measurement of tissue function in vivo and provide an early marker of disease through measurement of biochemical change.

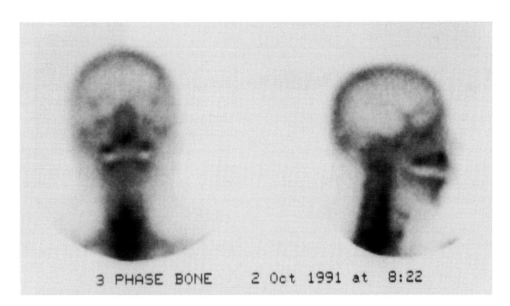

3 PHASE BONE   2 Oct 1991 at   8:22

FIG. **12-27** *Radionuclide image.* The increased uptake of isotope in the region of the maxilla and mandible was attributed to an inflammatory response caused by poorly fitting complete dentures. (Courtesy Radiology Department, Baylor University Medical Center, Dallas, Tex.)

Radionuclide-labeled tracers are used in quantities well below amounts that are lethal to cells. Although radionuclide imaging is considered noninvasive, the radiation dose the patient receives as a result of intravenous injection of radionuclide-labeled tracers should be considered. It has been reported that injection of 3.7×10^8 Bq of ^{99m}Tc-pertechnetate delivers a whole-body radiation dose of 1 mGy. This quantity is about one third the average annual effective dose resulting from natural radiation (see Chapter 3). Although many gamma-emitting isotopes have been used in radionuclide imaging, including iodine (^{131}I), gallium (^{67}Ga), and selenium (^{74}Se), the one most commonly used is technetium 99m (^{99m}Tc). As technetium pertechnetate, ^{99m}Tc mimics iodine distribution when injected intravenously. Additionally, when it is manipulated chemically and attached to other compounds, it can be used to perform scans of virtually every organ of the body.

The use of tracers for diagnostic imaging became possible with the development of, first, the rectilinear scanner and, later, the Anger or gamma scintillation camera. Both these instruments record the gamma emissions from patients injected with appropriate tracers. The cameras use a scintillation crystal that has the ability to fluoresce on interaction with gamma rays. This flash of light (or fluorescence) is detected by a photomultiplier tube that magnifies and amplifies the signal many times to produce an image. Use of a scintillation crystal for acquisition of data for image formation has led to the labeling of this technique as *scintigraphy.*

A stationary Anger camera or a rectilinear scanner is capable of producing a flat-plane image of an area or organ in question. Use of an Anger camera with the capacity to rotate 360 degrees about the patient or specialized ring detectors makes single photon emission computed tomography (SPECT) possible. In this technique, either multiple detectors or a single moving detector allows acquisition of data from a number of contiguous transaxial slices, similar to CT by x-ray. These data can then be used to construct multiplanar images of the area of study.

An even more recent development than SPECT in the field of nuclear medicine is positron emission computed tomography (PET). PET, which is reported to have a sensitivity nearly 100 times that of a gamma camera, relies on positron-emitting radionuclides generated in a cyclotron. As a positron is emitted within tissue, it meets a free electron and mutual annihilation occurs, resulting in the production of two 551 keV photons emitted at 180 degrees to each other. When electronically coupled opposing detectors simultaneously identify this pair of gamma photons, the annihilation event is known to have occurred along the line joining the two detectors. Raw PET scan data consist of a number of these coincidence lines, which are reorganized into projections that identify where activity is concentrated within the patient. The utility of PET is based not only on its sensitivity but also on the fact that the most commonly used radionuclides (^{11}C, ^{13}N, ^{15}O, ^{18}F) are isotopes of elements that occur naturally in organic molecules. Although fluorine does not technically fit into this category, it is a chemical substitute for hydrogen.

Ultrasonography

The phenomenon perceived as sound is the result of periodic changes in the pressure of air against the eardrum. The periodicity of these changes lies anywhere between 1500 and 20,000 cycles per second (hertz [Hz]). By definition, ultrasound has a periodicity greater than 20 kHz. Thus it is distinguished from other mechanical waveforms simply by having a vibratory frequency greater than the audible range. Diagnostic ultrasonography (sonography), the clinical application of ultrasound, uses vibratory frequencies in the range of 1 to 20 MHz.

Scanners used for sonography generate electrical impulses that are converted into ultra–high-frequency sound waves by a transducer, which is a device that can convert one form of energy into another; in this case, electrical energy into sonic energy. The most important component of the transducer is a thin piezoelectric crystal or material made up of a great number of dipoles arranged in a geometric pattern. A dipole may be thought of as a distorted molecule that appears to have a positive charge on one end and a negative charge on the other. Currently, the most widely used piezoelectric material is lead zirconate titanate (PZT). The electrical impulse generated by the scanner causes the dipoles in the crystal to realign themselves with the electrical field and thus suddenly change the crystal's thickness. This abrupt change begins a series of vibrations that produce the sound waves that are transmitted into the tissues being examined.

As the ultrasonic beam passes through or interacts with tissues of different acoustic impedance, it is attenuated by a combination of absorption, reflection, refraction, and diffusion. Sonic waves that are reflected back (echoed) toward the transducer cause a change in the thickness of the piezoelectric crystal, which in turn produces an electrical signal that is amplified, processed, and ultimately displayed on a monitor. In this system the transducer serves as both a transmitter and a receiver. Current techniques permit echoes to be processed at a sufficiently rapid rate to allow perception of motion; this is referred to as *real-time imaging.*

In contrast to x-ray imaging, in which the image is produced by transmitted radiation, the image in sonography is produced by the reflected portion of the beam. The fraction of the beam that is reflected back to the transducer

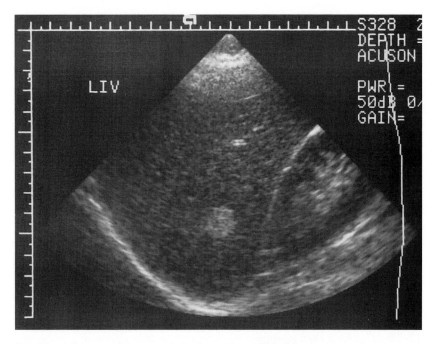

FIG. **12-28** *Ultrasound image of the liver.* The gallbladder is the oval structure on the right side of the image. Note the round radiopacity within the lower center of the image; this is a cavernous hemangioma. (Courtesy Radiology Department, Baylor University Medical Center, Dallas, Tex.)

depends on the acoustic impedance of the tissue, which is a product of its density (and thus the velocity of sound through it) and the beam's angle of incidence. Because of its acoustic impedance, a tissue has a characteristic internal echo pattern. Consequently, not only can changes in echo patterns delineate different tissues, they also can be correlated with pathologic changes in a tissue. Interpretation of sonograms, therefore, relies on knowledge of both the physical properties of ultrasound and the anatomy of the tissues being scanned (Figs. 12-28 and 12-29).

Electronic Thermography

Thermography is a term given to methods of temperature pattern resolution and analysis. The utility of thermography in diagnosis is based on the fact that disease processes and abnormal conditions may result in different temperature patterns because of alterations in blood supply or the presence of inflammation. Sensors used to record temperatures may be small electronic probes called *thermistors* (which are used for point determinations), liquid crystals, or infrared scanners, which are used to record temperatures over wide areas. Infrared scanners look like small television cameras. When an individual is viewed by such a scanner in a draft-free, temperature-controlled environment, the temperature differences recorded are displayed

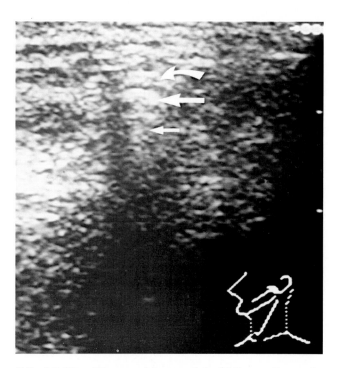

FIG. **12-29** *Ultrasound image of the TMJ area.* Parasagittal image of the TMJ area showing the articular disk in its normal location superior to the condyle in the closed-mouth position. Glenoid fossa *(curved arrow)*, articular disk *(long arrow)*, and condyle *(short arrow)*. (Courtesy Rüdiger Emshoff, MD, DMD, Innsbruck, Austria.)

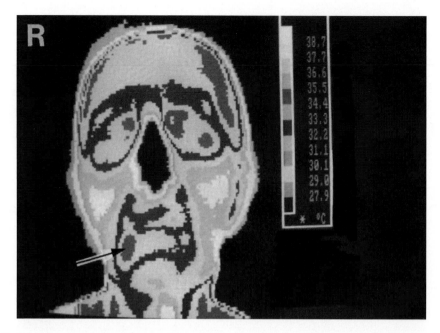

FIG. **12-30** *Electronic thermography.* Black and white photograph of a multicolored facial thermogram. The arrow indicates heat emission over the right mentum. This patient has a deficit of the right inferior alveolar nerve, the result of surgical implant trauma. (Courtesy Barton M. Gratt, DDS, PhD, Seattle, Wash.)

as a color image on a video monitor (Fig. 12-30). Color differences may represent temperature changes as little as 0.1° C. Although the technique is still in the prototype stage for diagnosing disease of the maxillofacial complex, it has been suggested as a method useful in determining a tooth's vitality, evaluating a case of atypical odontalgia, or assessing an internal derangement of the TMJ.

BIBLIOGRAPHY

Bushberg JT et al: *The essential physics of medical imaging,* Baltimore, 1994, Williams & Wilkins.

Curry TS et al: *Christensen's physics of diagnostic radiology,* ed 4, Philadelphia, 1990, Lea & Febiger.

Fahey FH: State of the art in emission tomography equipment, *Radiographics* 16:409, 1996.

Patton JA: MR imaging instrumentation and image artifacts, *Radiographics* 14:1083, 1994.

Reiderer SJ, Wood ML, editors: *Categorical course in physics: the basic physics of MR imaging,* Oak Brook, Ill., 1997, RSNA Publications.

Rowlands JA et al: Flat-panel digital radiology with amorphous selenium and active-matrix readout, *Radiographics* 17:753, 1997.

Wenzel A: Digital radiography and caries diagnosis, *Dentomaxillofac Radiol* 27:3, 1998.

Wenzel A, Gröndahl HG: Direct digital radiography in the dental office, *Int Dent J* 45:27, 1995.

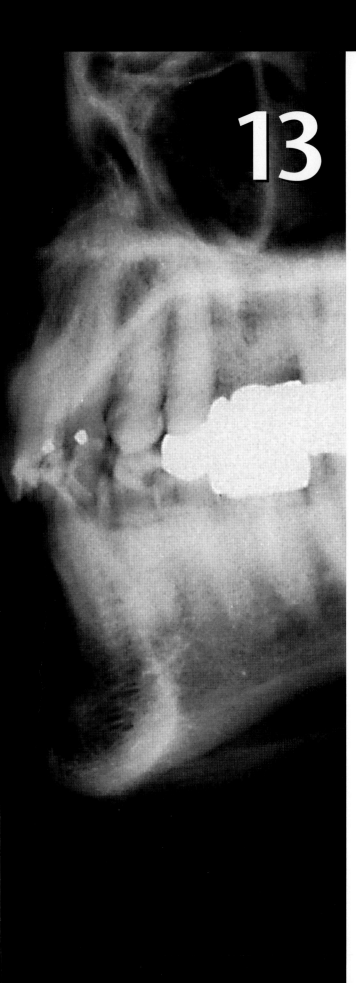

13 Guidelines for Prescribing Dental Radiographs

KATHRYN A. ATCHISON
SHARON L. BROOKS

The decision to conduct a radiographic examination is based on the individual characteristics of the patient. These include age, general health, clinical findings, and dental history. At the first patient visit it is necessary to obtain the patient's medical and dental history. After the recording of this information the patient is clinically examined. This examination may disclose dental problems that will prove crucial to decisions relevant to the radiographic examination. A radiographic examination is necessary when the history and clinical examination have not provided enough information to evaluate completely a patient's condition and formulate an appropriate treatment plan. Radiographic exposures are necessary only when the patient will potentially benefit by the discovery of clinically useful information on the radiograph.

Role of Radiographs in Disease Detection and Monitoring

The goal of dental care is to preserve and improve patients' oral health while minimizing other health-related risks. Although the diagnostic information provided by radiographs may be of definite benefit to the patient, the radiographic examination does carry the potential for harm from exposure to ionizing radiation. One of the most effective means of reducing possible harm is to avoid making radiographs that will not contribute information pertinent to patient care. The judgment that underlies the decision to make a radiographic examination centers on several factors, including the following:

- Prevalence of the diseases that may be detected radiographically in the oral cavity
- Ability of the clinician to detect these diseases clinically and radiographically
- Consequences of undetected and untreated disease

As a general principle, radiographs are indicated when a high probability exists that they will provide valuable information about a disease that is not evident clinically. Conversely, radiographs are not indicated when they are unlikely to yield information contributing to patient care. Information sought from radiographs includes both detecting disease and monitoring the progression of detected diseases.

For many clinical situations it is not readily apparent to the practitioner whether radiographs have a high probability of providing valuable information. In these situations it is up to the practitioner's clinical judgment after weighing the patient factors to decide whether radiographs are indicated.

In the next section guidelines are presented for obtaining radiographs for various clinical situations. Decisions regarding the appropriateness of type and frequency of radiographic examinations for individual patients must be made by the dentist on a case-by-case basis.

CARIES

Dental caries is the most common dental disease, affecting people of all ages. The caries prevalence rates of developed countries have been decreasing since the 1970s, probably partially as a result of the widespread use of fluoride. However, increasing numbers of older adults are maintaining their teeth throughout their lifetime, leaving them at risk of developing both coronal and root caries. These factors reinforce the need to select individually the radiographs most appropriate for an individual's age and oral health condition. Occlusal, buccal, and lingual carious lesions are reasonably easy to detect clinically. Interproximal caries and caries associated with existing restorations are much more difficult to detect with only a clinical examination (see Chapter 15). Studies have repeatedly demonstrated that clinicians using radiographs detect caries not evident clinically, including both enamel and dentinal caries.

Although a radiographic examination is very important for diagnosis of dental caries, consider mitigating features when determining the optimal frequency for such an examination. These features include the patient's medical condition, diet, oral hygiene practices, oral health status, and the nature of the carious process.

Carious lesions demonstrate one of three behaviors: progression, arrest, or regression. Only about 50% of lesions progress beyond the initial, just detectable defect, and in most instances the lesions demonstrate a slow rate of progression through enamel (months to years). The rate of caries progression is significantly faster in deciduous than in permanent enamel. Patients vary widely in their rates of formation of caries and in their rates of caries progression.

Because the presence of caries cannot be determined with confidence by clinical examination, it is necessary to expose patients periodically through radiography to monitor dental caries. The length of the exposure intervals varies considerably because of different patient circumstances. For most patients in good physical health with adequate oral hygiene, an infrequent radiographic examination is needed to monitor dental caries. However, if the patient history and clinical examination suggest that the individual has a relatively high caries experience, shorter intervals allow careful monitoring of disease.

PERIODONTAL DISEASES

Over the course of a person's lifetime one can expect to encounter some form of periodontal disease. Generally, gingival manifestations are present in younger ages, and periodontal manifestations, including gingival recession and alveolar bone loss, are more common in older adults. Periodontal diseases are responsible for a substantial portion of all teeth lost. A consensus exists among practitioners that radiographic examinations play an important role in the evaluation of patients with periodontal disease (see Chapter 16). In addition to providing a picture of the extent of alveolar bone support for the dentition, radiographic examinations help demonstrate local factors that complicate the disease, including the presence of gingival irritants such as calculus and faulty restorations. Occasionally the length and morphology of roots are crucial factors that are apparent on periapical films. These observations suggest that when clinical evidence of periodontal disease exists, other than nonspecific gingivitis, it is appropriate to make radiographs to help establish the severity of the disease. Using follow-up radiographs after completed therapy is a recommended procedure to monitor the progression of disease and determine whether the destruction of alveolar bone has been halted.

DENTAL ANOMALIES

Abnormal formation of teeth may be apparent as deviations in number, size, and composition. These abnormalities in dental development occur less frequently in the primary than in the permanent dentition. Also, the impact of a dental anomaly in the permanent dentition is more serious, leading to a requirement to consider replacement or removal of teeth. The most frequently encountered anomalies are the presence of supernumerary teeth, usually mesiodens, or developmentally absent teeth, usually second premolars (see Chapter 17).

Few anomalies exist for which orthodontic treatment or surgical correction or modification must start at an early age. When the dentist suspects an abnormality requiring treatment, radiographs to confirm and localize it are not required until the time when the treatment is most appropriate. For example, a panoramic examination of a 5-year-old individual to determine the presence or absence of permanent teeth may be ill timed. Even though the examination provides evidence that one or more second premolars or lateral incisors are developmentally missing, this information usually does not influence the current treatment plan. When examination for dental anomalies is appropriate, consider both the radiation dose and anticipated diagnostic benefit. Select the projections that best demonstrate the required diagnostic information. A panoramic radiograph of the lower face is usually best for observing the presence or absence of teeth in all quadrants, although a periapical film or an occlusal film is sufficient for an examination limited to one area.

GROWTH AND DEVELOPMENT AND DENTAL MALOCCLUSION

Children and adolescents are often examined to assess the growth and development of the teeth and jaws. This assessment considers the relationship of one jaw to the other and to the soft tissues. An examination of occlusion, growth, and development requires an individualized radiographic examination that may include periapicals or a panoramic examination to supplement any radiographs ordered to assess dental disease. In addition, a patient of any age group who is being considered for orthodontic treatment may need other radiographs such as a lateral or frontal cephalograph, occlusal view, carpal index, or temporomandibular joint (TMJ) radiograph (Fig. 13-1).

The dentist who is the primary provider of orthodontic treatment should select the number and type of radiographs needed. The needs of each patient are considered individually. Selected radiographs must allow a maximal diagnostic yield with a minimal radiographic exposure after considering the clinical examination, the

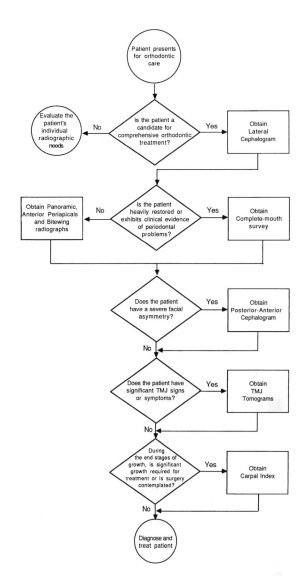

FIG. **13-1** *An example of a clinical algorithm to order radiographs for orthodontic patients.* Selected radiographs are ordered after the dentist's consideration of the patient's history and clinical characteristics.

study of plaster models and photographs, and the optimal time to initiate treatment.

OCCULT DISEASE

Occult disease refers to disease presenting no clinical signs or symptoms. Occult diseases include a combination of dental and intraosseous findings. Dental findings may include incipient carious lesions, resorbed or dilacerated roots, and hypercementosis. Intraosseous findings include osteosclerosis, unerupted teeth, periradicular disease, and a wide variety of cysts and benign and malignant tumors. Small carious lesions, resorption of root structure, cysts, and tumors may go unnoticed until signs and symptoms develop.

Although the consequences of some occult diseases may be quite serious, most serious diseases other than caries and periodontal disease are rare. Often a historical or clinical sign or symptom of intraosseous disease suggests its presence. For instance, an unusual contour of bone or an absent third molar, not explained by a history of extraction, suggests the possibility of an impaction with the potential for an associated dentigerous cyst. However, patient history and clinical signs and symptoms do not always accurately predict the finding of dental and intraosseous findings. The majority of these true occult diseases are not clinically relevant or are so rare that, except for caries as described previously, one need not obtain a radiographic examination of the jaws solely to look for occult disease in dentate individuals in the absence of a patient history or unusual clinical signs or symptoms. Caries is an exception because of its much higher prevalence than other occult diseases.

The situation is also different for edentulous patients. In this group of patients the high number of dental problems justifies an initial radiographic examination to look for occult disease. Edentulous patients tend to be older individuals who may be medically compromised and have a higher risk of accompanying oral disease. In addition, the risk of radiation-induced disease is lower for older adults.

JAW PATHOLOGY

Imaging of known jaw lesions, such as fibroosseous diseases or neoplastic diseases, before biopsy and definitive treatment is also important for appropriate management of the patient. For small lesions of the jaws, periapical and/or panoramic radiographs may be enough as long as the lesion can be seen in its entirety. If clinical evidence exists of swelling, some type of radiograph at 90 degrees to the original plane should be made to detect evidence of expansion of the jaw and perforation of the buccal or lingual cortical bone. If lesions are too large to fit on standard dental films, extend into the maxillary sinus or other portions of the head outside the jaws, or are suspected of malignancy, additional imaging such as computed tomography (CT) is appropriate before biopsy (see Chapter 12). This type of imaging can define the extent of the lesion, suggest an operative approach, and provide information about the nature of the lesion. The person performing the biopsy or managing the patient should order the advanced images to decrease confusion and increase coordination of care.

TEMPOROMANDIBULAR JOINT

A wide variety of diseases affect the TMJ, including congenital and developmental malformations of the man-

dible and cranial bones; acquired disorders such as disk displacement, neoplasms, fractures, and dislocations; inflammatory diseases that produce capsulitis or synovitis; and arthritides of various types, including rheumatoid and osteoarthritis. The goal of TMJ imaging, similar to that for imaging other body parts, should be to obtain new information that will influence patient care. Radiologic examination may not be needed for all patients with signs and symptoms referable to the TMJ region, particularly if no treatment is contemplated (see Chapter 24). The decision of whether and how to image the joints should depend on the results of the history and clinical findings, the clinical diagnosis, and results of prior examinations, as well as the tentative treatment plan and expected outcome.

The cost of the examination and the radiation dose should also influence the decision if more than one type of examination can provide the desired information. For example, information about the status of the osseous tissues can be obtained from panoramic radiographs, plain films, conventional tomography, CT, and magnetic resonance imaging (MRI). The subtlety of the expected findings and the amount of detail required should be considered when selecting the examination to perform. If soft tissue information such as disk position is necessary for patient care, MRI or arthrography is appropriate.

IMPLANTS

An increasingly common method of replacing missing teeth is with osseointegrated implants, metal screws that are inserted into the mandible or maxilla. Prosthetic appliances are then affixed to the screws after a period of healing. Preoperative planning is crucial to ensure success of the implants. The dentist must evaluate the adequacy of the height and thickness of bone for the desired implant; the quality of the bone, including the relative proportion of medullary and cortical bone; the location of anatomic structures such as the mandibular canal or maxillary sinus; and the presence of structural abnormalities such as undercuts that may affect placement or angulation of the implant (see Chapter 30).

Standard periapical and panoramic radiographs can supply information regarding the vertical dimensions of the bone in the proposed implant site. However, some type of cross-sectional imaging, either conventional tomography or CT, is recommended before implant placement for visualization of important anatomic landmarks, determination of size and path of insertion of implant, and evaluation of the adequacy of the bone for anchorage of the implant. Postoperative evaluation of implants may be needed at later times to judge healing, complete seating of fixtures, and continued health of the surrounding bone.

PARANASAL SINUSES

Because dentists are not usually the primary provider of treatment for acute or chronic sinus disease, the necessity to perform sinus imaging may be limited in general dental practice. However, because sinus disease can present as pain in the maxillary teeth and because periapical inflammation of maxillary molars and premolars can also lead to changes in the mucosa of the maxillary sinus, circumstances occur in which the dentist needs to obtain an image of the maxillary sinus. Periapical and panoramic radiographs demonstrate the floor of the maxillary sinus well, but visualization of other walls requires additional imaging techniques such as occipitomental (Waters') view or CT. These radiographs are best ordered by the person treating the patient so that diagnostic and therapeutic measures may be coordinated (see Chapter 25).

TRAUMA

Patients who experience trauma to the oral region may report to a dentist for evaluation and management of the injuries. For proper management it is important to determine the full extent of the injuries. Periapical and/or panoramic radiographs are helpful for evaluation of fractures of the teeth. If a suspected root fracture is not visible on a periapical radiograph, a second radiograph made with a different angulation may be helpful. A fracture that is not perpendicular to the beam may not be detectable unless root resorption is associated. Thus a tooth with a history of trauma but no associated clinical finding should be monitored and evaluated radiographically on a periodic basis.

Fractures of the mandible can frequently be detected with panoramic radiographs, supplemented by images at 90 degrees such as a posteroanterior or modified Towne's view (see Chapter 27). Trauma to the maxilla and midface may require CT for a thorough evaluation. Affected patients are more likely to report to a hospital emergency department than to a general dental office. The hospital may have a standard protocol for trauma cases. Ideally the clinician responsible for managing care determines the appropriate radiographs for the specific case.

Radiographic Examinations

After concluding that a patient requires a radiograph, the dentist should consider which radiographic examination is most appropriate to meet all the patient's diagnostic and treatment planning needs. A variety of radiographic projections are available. In choosing one, the dentist considers the anatomic relationships, the size of the field, and the radiation dose from each view. Table 13-1 summarizes the more common types of radiographic examinations for general dental patients and factors to consider in choosing the most appropriate one. For example, a panoramic radiograph provides broad area coverage with moderate resolution. Intraoral films give more detailed information but a significantly higher radiation dose per unit area exposed. The clinician must use clinical judgment to weigh these factors. Fig. 13-2 shows examples of each of the radiographic examinations.

INTRAORAL RADIOGRAPHS

Intraoral radiographs are examinations made by placing the x-ray film within the patient's mouth during the exposure. They offer the dentist a high-detail view of the teeth and bone in the area exposed. Such views are most appropriate for revealing caries and periodontal and periapical disease in a localized region. A complete-mouth or full-mouth examination (FMX) consists of periapical views of all the tooth-bearing regions as well as interproximal views (see Chapter 8).

Periapical Radiographs
Periapical views show all of a tooth and the surrounding bone. They are very useful for revealing caries and periodontal and periapical disease.

Interproximal Radiographs
Interproximal views (bitewings) show the coronal aspects of both the maxillary and mandibular dentition in a region as well as the surrounding crestal bone. They are most useful for revealing proximal caries and evaluating the height of the alveolar bony crest. They can be made in either the anterior or posterior region of the mouth.

Occlusal Radiographs
Occlusal views are intraoral radiographs in which the film is positioned in the occlusal plane. They are often used in children in place of periapical views because of the small size of the patient's mouth. In adults, occlusal radiographs may supplement periapical views, providing visualization of a greater area of teeth and bone. They are useful for demonstrating impacted or abnormally placed maxillary anterior teeth or visualizing the region of a palatal cleft. They may also demonstrate buccal or lingual expansion of bone.

EXTRAORAL RADIOGRAPHS

Extraoral radiographs are examinations made of the orofacial region (e.g., the jaws, skull, TMJ) using films located extraorally. The relationships among patient position, film location, and beam direction vary depending on the specific radiographic information desired. The standard

TABLE 13-1
Common Dental Radiographic Examinations and Their Properties

TYPE OF EXAMINATION	COVERAGE	RESOLUTION	RELATIVE PATIENT EXPOSURE*	DETECTABLE DISEASES
Intraoral Radiographs				
Individual periapical	Limited	High	1	Caries, periodontal disease, periapical disease, dental anomalies, occult disease
Interproximal bitewings	Limited	High	10	Caries, periodontal bone level
Full-mouth	Limited	High	14 to 17	Caries, periodontal disease, periapical disease, dental anomalies, occult disease
Occlusal	Moderate	High	2.5	Dental anomalies, occult disease, salivary stones, expansion of jaw
Extraoral Radiographs				
Panoramic	Broad	Moderate	1 to 2	Dental anomalies, occult disease, extensive caries, periodontal disease, periapical disease, TMJ
Conventional tomography/slice	Moderate	Moderate	0.2 to 0.6	TMJ, implant site assessment
CT/head	Broad	High	25 to 800	Extent of craniofacial pathology, fracture, implants
MRI	Broad	Moderate	—	Soft tissue disease
Skull	Broad	Moderate	31	Fracture, anatomic relation, jaw pathology

*The parameters assume use of E-speed film and rectangular collimation for periapical films, round collimation for bitewings and occlusal views, and rare-earth screens for the panoramic examination. With D-speed film the intraoral values are doubled compared with E-speed film, and with round collimation the periapical values increase by 2.5 times compared with using rectangular collimation. Frederiksen N, Benson B, Sokolowski T: Effective dose and risk assessment from computed tomography of the maxillofacial complex, *Dentomaxillofac Radiol* 24:55, 1995; Scaf G et al: Dosimetry and cost of imaging osseointegrated implants with film-based and computed tomography, *Oral Surg Oral Med Oral Pathol Oral Radiol and Endod* 83:41, 1997; White SC: 1992 assessment of radiation risks from dental radiology, *Dentomaxillofac Radiol* 21:118, 1992.

technique for making several extraoral radiographs is discussed in Chapter 10. Only the panoramic radiograph is described here because it has common use as a radiographic examination for general dental patients.

Panoramic Radiographs

Panoramic radiographs provide a broad view of the jaws, teeth, maxillary sinuses, nasal fossa, and TMJs (see Chapter 11). They show which teeth are present, their relative state of development, presence or absence of dental abnormalities, and many traumatic and pathologic lesions in bone. They are the examination of choice for initial examinations of edentulous patients. Because this system is an extraoral technique and uses intensifying screens, the resolution of the images is less than with the intraoral nonscreen films (see Chapter 4). Consequently it is generally inadequate for independent diagnosis of caries, root abnormalities, and periapical changes.

In the great majority of dental patients, oral disease involving the teeth or jaw bones lies within the area imaged by periapical radiographs. Therefore when a full-mouth set of radiographs is available, a panoramic examination is usually redundant because it does not add information that alters the treatment plan. However, situations may exist in which a panoramic radiograph may be preferred over a periapical examination such as for a patient with unerupted third molars that will be surgically removed. Panoramic views are most useful when the required field of view is large. Although the selection of a radiographic examination should be based on the extent of the expected information it is likely to provide, the relatively low dose of radiation from the panoramic examination should be a qualifying factor.

Advanced Imaging Procedures

A variety of advanced imaging procedures such as CT, MRI, ultrasonography, and nuclear medicine scans may be required in specific diagnostic situations. These techniques are discussed in Chapter 12, although in general the dentist refers the patient to a hospital or other imaging center for these procedures, rather than performing them in the dental office.

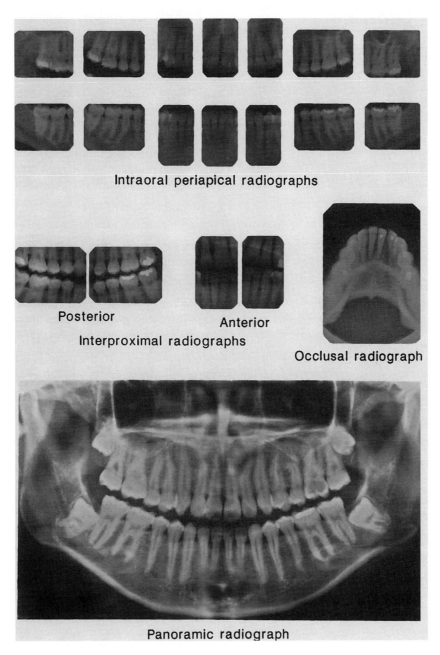

FIG. **13-2** Comparative size and coverage of common intraoral and extraoral radiographs.

Guidelines for Ordering Radiographs

The profession has issued guidelines recommending which radiographs to make and how often to repeat them:

- Make radiographs only after a clinical examination.
- Order only those radiographs that directly benefit the patient's diagnosis or treatment plan.
- Use the least amount of radiation exposure necessary to generate an acceptable view of the imaged area.

PREVIOUS RADIOGRAPHS

Most patients have been seen previously by a dentist and have had radiographs made. These radiographs are helpful regardless of when they were exposed. If they are relatively recent, they may be adequate to the diagnostic problem at hand. Even if they were made so long ago that they are not likely to reflect the current status of the patient, they may still prove useful. They may demonstrate whether a condition has worsened, has remained unchanged, or has shown healing, such as the progression of caries or periodontal disease.

TABLE **13-2**
Guidelines for Prescribing Dental Radiographs

The recommendations in this table are subject to clinical judgment and may not apply to every patient. They are to be used by dentists only after reviewing the patient's health history and completing a clinical examination. They do not need to be altered because of pregnancy.

	CHILD	
	PRIMARY DENTITION (BEFORE ERUPTION OF FIRST PERMANENT TOOTH)	TRANSITIONAL DENTITION (AFTER ERUPTION OF FIRST PERMANENT TOOTH)
New Patient		
All new patients to assess dental diseases and growth and development	Posterior bitewing examination if proximal surfaces of primary teeth cannot be visualized or probed	Individualized radiographic examination consisting of periapical and/or occlusal views, posterior bitewing or panoramic examination, and posterior bitewings
Recall Patient		
Clinical caries or high-risk factors for caries†	Posterior bitewing examination at 6-month intervals or until no carious lesions are evident	
No clinical caries and no high-risk factors for caries	Posterior bitewing examination at 12- to 24-month intervals if proximal surfaces of primary teeth cannot be visualized or probed	Posterior bitewing examination at 12- to 24-month intervals
Periodontal disease or history of periodontal treatment	Individualized radiographic examination consisting of selected periapical and/or bitewing radiographs for areas where periodontal disease (other than nonspecific gingivitis) can be demonstrated clinically	
Growth and development assessment	Usually not indicated	Individualized radiographic examination consisting of a periapical and/or occlusal or panoramic examination

*Clinical situations for which radiographs may be indicated include the following:

Positive historical findings:
1. Previous periodontal or endodontic therapy
2. History of pain or trauma
3. Familial history of dental anomalies
4. Postoperative evaluation of healing
5. Presence of implants

Positive clinical signs or symptoms:
1. Clinical evidence of periodontal disease
2. Large or deep restorations
3. Deep carious lesions
4. Malposed or clinically impacted teeth
5. Swelling
6. Evidence of facial trauma
7. Mobility of teeth
8. Fistula or sinus tract infection

9. Clinically suspected sinus pathology
10. Growth abnormalities
11. Oral involvement in known or suspected systemic disease
12. Positive neurologic findings in the head and neck
13. Evidence of foreign objects
14. Pain and/or dysfunction of the TMJ
15. Facial asymmetry

ADMINISTRATIVE RADIOGRAPHS

Administrative radiographs are those made for reasons other than diagnosis. Examples may include making radiographs for an insurance company or for an examining board. The authors believe that it is appropriate to expose patients only when it benefits their health care. Most administrative radiographs do not serve such an objective. Unfortunately, this recommendation is often not adhered to in practice, and dentists are left to sort out the most appropriate criteria to use in their practices.

Use of Guidelines to Order Dental Radiographs

At any time patients generally have a combination of diseases that the clinician must consider. Therefore guidelines specify not only which examinations to order but also which specific patient factors influence the number and type of x-ray films to order.

A panel of individuals was convened in the mid-1980s at the request of a branch of the Food and Drug Administration to develop a set of guidelines (Table 13-2)

ADOLESCENT	ADULT	
PERMANENT DENTITION (BEFORE ERUPTION OF THIRD MOLARS)	DENTULOUS	EDENTULOUS
Individualized radiographic examination consisting of posterior bitewings and selected periapicals; a full-mouth intra-oral radiographic examination is appropriate whenpatient presents with clinical evidence of generalized dental disease or a history of extensive dental treatment*		Full-mouth intraoral radiographic examination or panoramic examination
Posterior bitewing examination at 6- to 12-month intervals or until no carious lesions are evident	Posterior bitewing examination at 12- to 18-month intervals	Not applicable
Posterior bitewing examination at 18- to 36-month intervals	Posterior bitewing examination at 24- to 36-month intervals	Not applicable
Individualized radiographic examination consisting of selected periapical and/or bitewing radiographs for areas where periodontal disease (other than non-specific gingivitis) can be demonstrated clinically		Not applicable
Periapical or panoramic examination to assess developing third molars	Usually not indicated	Usually not indicated

16. Abutment for fixed or removable partial prosthesis
17. Unexplained bleeding
18. Unexplained sensitivity of teeth
19. Unusual eruption, spacing or migration of teeth
20. Unusual tooth morphology, calcification, or color
21. Missing teeth with unknown reason

†Patients at high risk for caries may demonstrate any of the following:
1. High level of caries experience
2. History of recurrent caries
3. Existing restoration of poor quality
4. Poor oral hygiene
5. Inadequate fluoride exposure
6. Prolonged nursing (bottle or breast)
7. Diet with high sucrose frequency

8. Poor family dental health
9. Developmental enamel defects
10. Developmental disability
11. Xerostomia
12. Genetic abnormality of teeth
13. Many multisurface restorations
14. Chemotherapy or radiation therapy

for the making of dental radiographs. The panel addressed the topic of appropriate radiographs for an adequate evaluation of a new or recall asymptomatic patient seeking general dental care. The guidelines describe circumstances (patient age, medical and dental history, and physical signs) that suggest the need for radiographs. These circumstances are called *selection criteria*. The guidelines also suggest the types of radiographic examinations most likely to benefit the patient in terms of yielding diagnostic information. They recommend that radiographs not be made unless some expectation exists that they will provide evidence of diseases that will affect the treatment plan. The American Dental Association (ADA) recommends use of the guidelines.

Central to the guidelines is the idea that dentists should expose patients to radiation only when they reasonably expect that the resulting radiograph will benefit patient care. Accordingly, two situations mandate a radiograph: some clinical evidence of an abnormality or a high probability of disease.

Selection criteria for radiographs are those signs or symptoms found in the patient history or clinical examination that suggest that a radiographic examination will yield clinically useful information. For example, a clinical examination may disclose a disease that is clinically apparent, but the nature and extent of which is not possible to evaluate clinically. Such situations frequently require a radiographic examination for adequate assessment. (This chapter considers the choice of appropriate radiographic examinations. Other chapters of this book address the means for conducting the examination and interpreting the resulting radiographs.)

A key concept in the use of selection criteria is recognition of the need to consider each patient individually. Prescription of radiographs is on an individual basis according to the patient's demonstrated need. The ADA's recommendations on the use of radiography include the following:

- The nature and extent of diagnosis required for patient care constitute the only rational basis for determining the need, type, and frequency of radiographic examination.
- Because each patient is different from the next, radiographic examinations should be individualized for each patient.
- The ADA specifically cautions against the routine use of radiography as a part of periodic examination of all patients.

The guidelines include a description of clinical situations in which radiographs are likely to contribute to the diagnosis, treatment, or prognosis. Two examples highlight the differences between ordering radiographs for dental diseases with clinical signs and symptoms and dental diseases with no clinical indicators but high prevalences. In the first case, consider a patient with a hard swelling in the premolar region of the mandible with expansion of the buccal and lingual cortical plates. The clinical sign of swelling alerts the dentist to the need for a radiograph. A radiograph of this region is indicated to determine whether the abnormality in the region causing the swelling involves the bone.

A more common example is the patient who has not seen a dentist for many years who comes seeking general dental care. Even without clinical evidence of caries, bitewings are indicated. Because this patient has not had interproximal radiographs for many years, it is reasonable that the patient may benefit from the radiograph by the detection of interproximal caries. Although no clinical signs exist that predict the presence of caries, the dentist relies on clinical knowledge of the prevalence of caries to decide that this radiograph has a reasonable probability of finding disease.

Without some specific indication it is inappropriate to expose the patient "just to see if there is something there." The major exception to this rule is the use of interproximal films for caries, in which no clinical signs exist of early lesions. The probability of finding occult disease in a patient with all permanent teeth erupted and no clinical or historical evidence of abnormality or risk factors is so low that making a periapical radiographic survey just to look for such disease is not indicated.

PATIENT EXAMINATION

Ordering radiographs requires a reasonable expectation that they will provide information that will contribute to exposing the diagnostic problem at hand. Accordingly, the first step is a careful examination of the patient. The clinical examination provides indications as to the nature and extent of the radiographic examination appropriate to the situation. Transillumination of anterior teeth should be conducted to evaluate for interproximal decay. Posterior interproximal radiographs form the foundation of the ADA guidelines. They are useful to detect interproximal caries and periodontal disease. Other intraoral or extraoral radiographs should be added as indicated by the clinical examination.

A team of dentists tested the ability of the ADA guidelines to reduce the number of intraoral radiographs while still offering adequate diagnostic information. This testing of the use of selection criteria demonstrated that a small but significant amount of radiographic findings were not 100% covered in the anterior region if only posterior interproximal and selected periapical radiographs were used. The testing suggested that anterior interproximal radiographs or anterior periapicals are also indicated to detect interproximal caries and periodontal disease in the anterior region, specifically for patients with high levels of dental disease. A panoramic radiograph could be made in place of the periapical radiographs to supplement the posterior bitewings if the totality of the disease expected indicates a broad area of coverage.

A footnote to Table 13-2 outlines some clinical findings that indicate when radiographs are likely to contribute to a complete description of the asymptomatic patient. In the guidelines patients are classified by stage of dental development, whether they are being evaluated for the first time (without previous documentation) or being reevaluated during the clinical examination, and by an estimate of their risk of having dental caries or periodontal disease.

Applying these guidelines to the specific circumstances with each patient requires clinical judgment and an amalgamation of knowledge, experience, and concern. Recognizing situations not described by the guidelines in which patients will need radiographs also requires clinical judgment.

Initial Visit

The guidelines recommend that a child with primary dentition who is cooperative and has closed posterior contacts have only interproximal radiographs to examine for caries. Additional periapical views are recommended only in the case of clinically evident diseases and/or specific historical or clinical indications such as those listed at the footnote of Table 13-2. If the molar contacts are not closed, interproximal radiographs are not necessary because the proximal surfaces may be examined directly.

The guidelines recommend radiographic coverage of all tooth-bearing areas for a child with transitional dentition (after eruption of the first permanent tooth, 6 to 8 years of age). This usually consists of bitewings supplemented with either periapical or occlusal views (8 to 12 exposures) or a panoramic view. At this stage of development a panoramic projection is usually the view of choice because it offers the most general information with the lowest dose of ionizing radiation. Some express concern that complete coverage of all tooth-bearing areas is not warranted without a specific indication.

The guidelines group adolescents and dentate adults together to identify the kind and extent of appropriate radiographic examination. The guidelines recommend that these patients receive an individualized examination consisting of interproximal views and periapical views selected on the basis of specific historical or clinical indications. The presence of generalized dental disease often indicates the need for a full-mouth examination. Alternatively, the presence of only a few localized abnormalities or diseases suggests that a more limited examination consisting of interproximal and selected periapical views may suffice. In circumstances with no evidence of current or past dental disease, only interproximal views may be necessary for caries examination.

For the edentulous patient it is appropriate to obtain a radiographic examination of all the tooth-bearing areas, either by periapical or panoramic radiographs. If available, the panoramic projection usually provides the required information at a reduced radiation dose.

Recall Visit

Patients who are returning after initial care require careful examination. As at the initial examination, obtain selected periapical views if any of the historical or clinical signs or symptoms that are listed in the footnote to Table 13-2 are present.

The guidelines recommend interproximal radiographs for recall patients to detect interproximal caries and monitor the status of alveolar bone loss. The optimal frequency for these views depends on the age of the patient and the probability of finding these two diseases. If the patient has clinically demonstrable caries or the presence of high-risk factors for caries (poor diet, poor oral hygiene and those listed in the footnote to Table 13-2), then bitewings are exposed at fairly frequent intervals. Obtain bitewings for children at 6-month intervals until no carious lesions are clinically evident. For the adolescent at high risk of caries, the guidelines recommend bitewings at 6- to 12-month intervals; for the high risk adult, at 12- to 18-month intervals. The recommended intervals are longer for individuals not at high risk for caries; 12 to 24 months for the child, 18 to 36 months for the adolescent, and 24 to 36 months for the adult. Note that individuals can change their risk category, going from high to low risk or the reverse. Similarly, recall that patients with a history or clinical evidence of periodontal disease more serious than nonspecific gingivitis should have a combination of periapical and interproximal radiographs to allow appropriate monitoring.

A radiographic examination may be required in a number of other situations such as for patients contemplating orthodontic treatment or patients with intraosseous lesions. The goal should be to obtain the necessary diagnostic information with the minimal radiation dose and financial cost, which can be substantial for advanced imaging procedures such as MRI. The dentist should determine specifically what type of information is needed and the most appropriate technique for obtaining it. An example of a clinical algorithm for ordering radiographs before orthodontic treatment is shown in Fig. 13-1, using guidelines endorsed by the American Academy of Orthodontics. Because guidelines for ordering radiographs for other situations are not as well developed, the dentist must rely on clinical judgment.

SPECIAL CONSIDERATIONS

Pregnancy

Occasionally it is desirable to obtain radiographs of a woman who is pregnant. The x-ray beam is largely confined to the head and neck region in dental x-ray examinations; thus the fetal exposure is only about 1 mGy for a full-mouth examination. This exposure is quite small compared with that received normally from natural background sources. Accordingly, apply the guidelines to pregnant patients just as with other patients, using an appropriate leaded apron to shield the abdominal area.

Radiation Therapy

Patients with a malignancy in the oral cavity or perioral region often receive radiation therapy for their disease. Some oral tissues receive 50 Gy or more. Although such patients are often apprehensive about receiving additional exposure, dental exposure is insignificant compared with what they have already received. The average skin dose from a dental radiograph is approximately 3 mGy. Further, patients who have received radiation therapy may suffer from radiation-induced xerostomia and thus are at a high risk of developing radiation caries. Accordingly, carefully follow patients who have had radiation therapy to the oral cavity because they are at special risk for dental disease.

EXAMPLES OF USE OF THE GUIDELINES

Consider the ways the guidelines can be applied to different clinical situations:

- *The first visit of a 5-year-old boy to a dental office*—A careful clinical examination reveals that the patient is cooperative and that the posterior teeth are in contact. Posterior bitewings are recommended to detect caries. If all of this patient's teeth are present, no evidence exists of decay, a reasonably good diet is being observed, and the parent(s) seems well motivated to promote good oral hygiene, no further radiographic examination is required at this time. Radiographs for the detection of development abnormalities are not in order at this age because a complete appraisal cannot be made at 5 years. Even if it could be made, it is too early to initiate treatment for such abnormalities.

- *A 25-year-old woman receiving a 6-month checkup after her last treatment for a fractured incisor*—No caries is evident on interproximal radiographs made 6 months ago; currently no clinical signs suggest caries, nor does the patient have high-risk factors for caries. No evidence exists of periodontal disease or other remarkable signs or symptoms in general or associated with the recently fractured tooth. As long as the fractured incisor shows normal vitality testing, no radiographs are recommended for this patient. If it is nonvital, expose a periapical view of this tooth.

- *A 45-year-old man returning to the dentist's office after 1 year*—At his last visit you placed two mesial, occlusal, distal (MOD) amalgam restorations on premolars and performed root canal therapy on number 30. The patient has a 5-mm pocket in the buccal furcation of number 3 but no other evidence of periodontal disease. The guidelines recommend that this patient receive interproximal radiographs to see whether he still has active caries and periapical views of numbers 3 and 30 to evaluate the extent of the periodontal disease and periapical disease, respectively.

- *A 65-year-old woman coming to your office for the first time*—No previous radiographs are available. A history exists of root canal therapy in two teeth, although the patient is not aware which teeth were treated. Clinical examination reveals multiple carious teeth, multiple missing teeth, and pockets of more than 3 mm involving most of the remaining teeth. The guidelines recommend a full-mouth examination, including interproximal radiographs, for this patient because of the high probability of finding caries, periodontal disease, and periapical disease.

SUGGESTED READINGS

GUIDELINES FOR ORDERING RADIOGRAPHS

Åerblom A, Rohlin M, Hasselgren G: Individualised restricted intraoral radiography versus full-mouth radiography in the detection of periradicular lesions, *Swed Dent J* 12:151, 1988.

Atchison KA, Luke LS, White SC: An algorithm for ordering pretreatment orthodontic radiographs, *Am J Orthod Dentofac Orthop* 102:29, 1992.

Atchison KA et al: Assessing the FDA guidelines for ordering dental radiographs, *JADA* 126:1372, 1995.

Brooks SL: A study of selection criteria for intraoral dental radiography, *Oral Surg Oral Med Oral Pathol* 62:234, 1986.

Brooks SL et al: Imaging of the temporomandibular joint: a position paper of the American Academy of Oral and Maxillofacial Radiology, *Oral Surg Oral Med Oral Pathol Oral Radiol and Endod* 83:609, 1997.

Brooks SL, Joseph L: Basic concepts in the selection of patients for dental x-ray examinations, U.S. Department of Health and Human Services, PHS, FDA, DHHS Publication 85-8249, Rockville, Md., 1985.

Council on Dental Materials, Instruments, and Equipment: Recommendations in radiographic practices: an update, 1988, *JADA* 118:115, 1989.

Hollender L: Decision making in radiographic imaging, *J Dent Educ* 56: 834, 1992.

Keur JJ: Radiographic screening of edentulous patients: sense or nonsense? A risk-benefit analysis, *Oral Surg Oral Med Oral Pathol* 62:463, 1986.

Molander B: Panoramic radiography in dental diagnostics, *Swed Dent J Suppl* 119:1, 1996.

Pitts NB, Kidd EA: Some of the factors to be considered in the prescription and timing of bitewing radiography in the diagnosis and management of dental caries, *J Dent* 20:74, 1992.

Rushton VE, Horner K: The use of panoramic radiology in dental practice, *J Dent* 24:185, 1996.

Stephens RG, Kogon SL: New U.S. guidelines for prescribing dental radiographs: a critical review, *J Can Dent Assoc* 56:1019, 1990.

U.S. Department of Health and Human Services: The selection of patients for x-ray examinations: dental radiographic examinations, DHHS Publication FDA 88-8273, Rockville, Md., 1987.

DISEASE DETECTION

Atchison K et al: Efficacy of the FDA selection criteria for radiographic assessment of the periodontium, *J Dent Res* 74:1424, 1995.

Backer Dirks O: Posteruptive changes in dental enamel, *J Dent Res* 45(suppl):503, 1966.

Featherstone JDB, Mellberg JR: Relative rates of progress of artificial carious lesions in bovine and human enamel, *Caries Res* 15:109, 1981.

Hall WB: *Decision making in periodontology*, ed 3, St Louis, 1998, Mosby.

Leverett DH: Fluorides and the changing prevalence of dental caries, *Science* 217:26, 1982.

Shwartz M et al: A longitudinal analysis from bite-wing radiographs of the rate of progression of approximal carious lesions through human dental enamel, *Archs Oral Biol* 29:529, 1984.

White SC et al: Clinical and historical predictors of dental caries on radiographs, *Dentomaxillofac Radiol* 24:121, 1995.

White SC et al: Efficacy of FDA guidelines for ordering radiographs for caries detection, *Oral Surg Oral Med Oral Pathol* 77:531, 1994.

RADIATION DOSAGE AND EFFECTS

Frederiksen N, Benson B, Sokolowski T: Effective dose and risk assessment from computed tomography of the maxillofacial complex, *Dentomaxillofac Radiol* 24:55, 1995.

Gonad doses and genetically significant dose from diagnostic radiology: U.S., 1964 and 1970, DHEW Publication (FDA) 76-8034, Washington, D.C., 1976.

Scaf G et al: Dosimetry and cost of imaging osseointegrated implants with film-based and computed tomography, *Oral Surg Oral Med Oral Pathol Oral Radiol Endod* 83:41, 1997.

White SC: 1992 assessment of radiation risks from dental radiology, *Dentomaxillofac Radiol* 21:118, 1992.

Radiographic Interpretation of Pathology

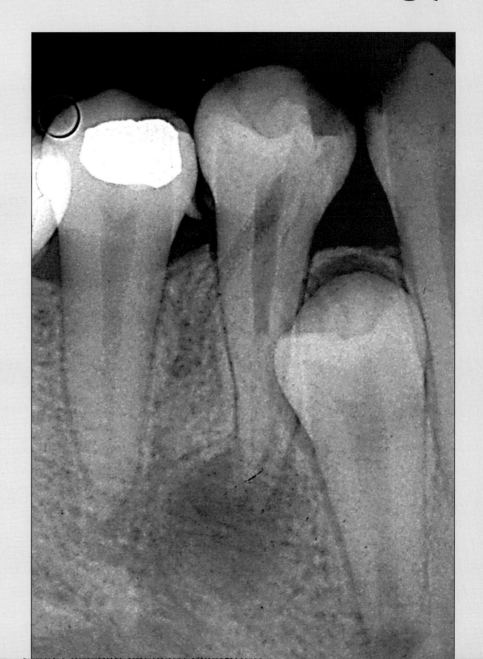

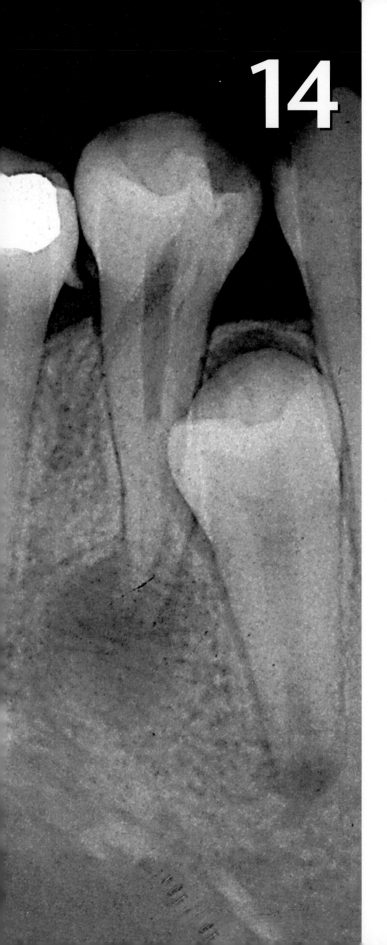

14 Principles of Radiographic Interpretation

The objective of this chapter is to provide a step-by-step, analytic process that can be applied to the interpretation of diagnostic images. However, reading this chapter, by itself, will not instantly bestow the ability to interpret radiographic films correctly; rather, it will equip the reader with a systematic method of image analysis. Proficiency comes only with practice.

Clinical Examination

Radiographs are prescribed when the dentist thinks that they are likely to offer useful diagnostic information that will influence the treatment plan. Often some clinical sign or symptom or finding from the patient's history indicates the need for a radiologic examination. This clinical information should be used first to select the type of radiographs and later to aid in their interpretation.

ACQUIRING APPROPRIATE DIAGNOSTIC IMAGES

An insufficient number or inadequate quality of radiographs limits the information available from diagnostic imaging. Because the general practitioner often is responsible both for prescribing and interpreting radiographs, inadequate films should be identified and supplemental images obtained before proceeding with the analysis.

Quality of the Diagnostic Image
Before the analysis is started, the quality of the images is examined. Is the image distorted? For instance, if the im-

age is elongated, greater error occurs in measuring the length of a root canal. Because of the inherent frequency of image distortion in panoramic films, this factor must always be taken into consideration. For example, a region of image magnification involving the mandibular condyle may be diagnosed erroneously as condylar hyperplasia. For this reason, a thorough knowledge of all possible image distortions is a prerequisite for analysis of panoramic images.

The practitioner also should check to see if the density or contrast of the image has been degraded by exposure or developing errors. It may be impossible, for example, to diagnose osteoporosis in an overexposed image, or detail may be obscured in an underexposed film. If the images are of poor quality, it might be prudent to obtain better quality images before proceeding to the analysis.

Number and Type of Available Images

Initially the clinical examination indicates the number and types of films required (see Chapter 13). The interpretation of these films in turn may suggest the need for additional imaging. Caution should be exercised in attempting to make an interpretation based on a single film, especially if the only film is a panoramic view. Also, a bitewing or periapical projection often can be supplemented by another view produced by altering the horizontal or vertical angulation of the x-ray beam. For example, detection of recurrent caries around a heavily restored dentition may benefit from an additional view taken by altering the angle of the x-ray beam. One of the benefits of a full-mouth series of intraoral films is that it provides a second view of most areas at a slightly different angle.

Conventional dental radiography produces images in only two dimensions, usually in the mesiodistal direction. In some cases a view at right angles to the plane of the original film is beneficial. For instance, if a condylar neck fracture is suspected, a lateral view of the condylar region (e.g., a panoramic view) should be supplemented with an anteroposterior (AP) view. In a similar fashion, occlusal projections of the jaws can provide a supplementary right-angle view for the periapical film. Use of a vertex occlusal view follows this principle in establishing the location of impacted maxillary cuspids. In some cases an investigation requires other images in addition to intraoral radiography or panoramic images. Techniques such as tomography, sialography, arthrography, nuclear imaging, computed tomography, and magnetic resonance imaging may be required (see Chapter 12). These techniques are available through consultation with an oral and maxillofacial radiologist.

Diagnostic imaging should be completed before a biopsy procedure or treatment is done. Diagnostic imaging can aid in the selection of the most appropriate anatomic site for a biopsy procedure. Also, the biopsy procedure may alter the tissue by inducing inflammatory changes, which in turn alter the imaging characteristics of the tissue. This compromises the diagnostic information that can be obtained, such as determining the extent of a disease.

Viewing Conditions

Ideally, viewing conditions should include the following characteristics:

- Ambient light in the viewing room should be reduced.
- Intraoral radiographs should be mounted in a film holder.
- Light from the viewbox should be of equal intensity across the viewing surface.
- The size of the viewbox should accommodate the size of the film. If the viewing area is larger than the film, an opaque mask should be used to eliminate all light from around the periphery of the film. This mask can be fabricated from a sheet of opaque material cut to fit the entire view-box, leaving an opening for one film.
- An intense light source is essential for evaluating dark regions of the film.
- A magnifying glass allows detailed examination of small regions of the film.

Image Analysis

When the quality and number of films are satisfactory, analysis of the image begins.

SYSTEMATIC RADIOGRAPHIC EXAMINATION

The first step in image analysis is to use a systematic approach to identify all the normal anatomy present in an image or set of images. A profound knowledge of the variation of normal appearance is required to be able to recognize an abnormal appearance. Because no textbook can display all possible variations, the best learning method is to identify normal anatomy in every film analyzed. In this way the observer can build up a large mental database of the spectrum of normal anatomic appearances. An additional benefit of this procedure is that it forces the observer to examine the entire film. Practitioners should avoid limiting their attention to one particular region of the film; rather, all aspects of each image should be examined systematically. More than one abnormality may be present. For instance, a bitewing radiograph made to detect caries and alveolar bone loss also may reveal just the edge of an unsuspected intraosseous lesion that will be seen only if the dentist examines the radiograph thoroughly.

INTRAORAL IMAGES

For almost all dental patients, treatment planning includes some combination of periapical and bitewing images. We present here a systematic method for analyzing these images. This method may be used to analyze a single image or a full-mouth set. It is most important for the practitioner to develop a particular method and to use it regularly. A thorough examination is best accomplished when a specific sequence of analysis is used to enhance the scrutiny of all parts of images.

To follow the method presented here, examine the periapical images before the bitewing images, starting in the right maxilla and working across to the left, then dropping down and continuing in the left mandible to the right. Concentrate on one anatomic structure at a time. First, examine the bone. Identify all anatomic landmarks appropriate for the region. In the posterior maxilla, for example, examine the maxillary sinus, tuberosity, and zygomatic process of the maxilla. In what way does their appearance change as the angle of each projection is altered? Also examine the character of the trabecular bone. Are the density and size of the trabeculae normal for the region? Compare the same areas on adjacent images and with the corresponding area on images of the other side.

Next, make a second visual circuit through all the images, examining the bone of the alveolar process. Examine in particular the height of the alveolar crest and its cortication. Loss of height of the alveolar bone (more than 1.5 mm from the adjacent cementoenamel junctions) may indicate active or past periodontal disease. Examine all regions of the alveolar process to gain an overall appreciation for the extent and severity of alveolar bone loss. Note any areas of erosion of the alveolar crest and the thickness of the overlying mucosa. Carcinomas arising from the epithelial covering may cause erosive lesions with ill-defined borders in the alveolar bone. Examine the trabecular pattern of the alveolar process. The lamina dura may be examined later with the periodontal membrane space and tooth roots.

Finally, make a third visual circuit, examining the dentition and associated structures. Study each tooth in sequence, using all images available. Note the way the tooth's appearance and root structure change with dif-

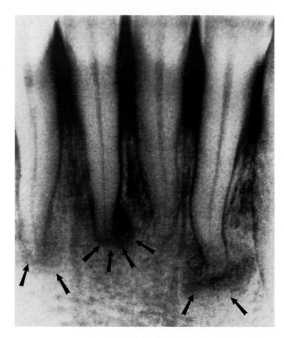

FIG. **14-1** The typical location of lesions of periapical cemental dysplasia. Early lesions are radiolucent *(arrows)*.

ferent orientations of the x-ray beam. Count the teeth, looking for missing or supernumerary teeth. Examine the crowns for normal development of the enamel and for caries. Pay particular attention to the interproximal regions at or below the contact points. Check restorations carefully for signs of recurrent caries. Often lesions found on one view cannot be detected on another because of superimposition of the restoration. Examine the pulp chamber for size and contents. Examine the roots for shape and form to detect developmental or acquired abnormalities such as external resorption. Inspect the width of the periodontal ligament space around the root of the tooth. The width should be fairly uniform, with very subtle widening toward the cervical region of the tooth. Examine particularly the lamina dura around each tooth. Is it intact? The most common abnormalities found in the bone are radiolucent or radiopaque lesions at the apices of teeth.

EXTRAORAL RADIOGRAPHY

The extraoral radiographs most commonly used in dentistry are panoramic images, cephalometric views, and examinations of the temporomandibular joint (TMJ). Specific methods for examining these images are covered in the chapters pertaining to these types of images. The same general principles of thorough, systematic coverage described earlier should be used. For viewing each of these types of images, it is important to develop a definite sequence that considers all the hard and soft

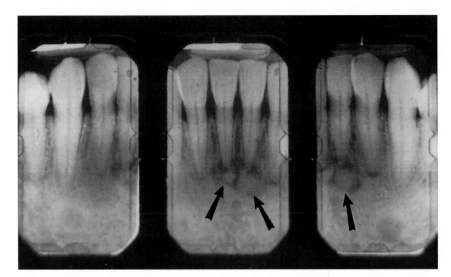

FIG. **14**-2 Late lesions of periapical cemental dysplasia have a more radiopaque interior.

tissues in the field. Always focus on one component at a time and examine it thoroughly. Only with such a pattern can the practitioner maximize the likelihood of detecting all abnormalities.

When an intraosseous lesion is identified, the following five steps should be used to analyze the lesion as fully as possible.

Analysis of Intraosseous Lesions

Two basic approaches can be used to analyze images of a lesion. One is the picture matching, or "Aunt Minnie," method. This involves trying to match the radiographic image with a mental picture or with an image in a favorite textbook. Although all radiologists probably use this technique to a certain extent, it has significant limitations. For instance, the observer's experience and memory limit the mental image of a particular disorder. Similarly, the appearance of different abnormalities in a textbook is limited by the author's knowledge and experience and, of course, by the number of images printed. Also, figures in a textbook usually represent the most ideal examples of the abnormality. For example, the term *periapical cemental dysplasia* often evokes a mental image of a radiolucent or mixed radiolucent-radiopaque lesion at the apex of a mandibular incisor because this appearance is the one used most often in textbooks (Figs. 14-1 and 14-2). Although this is a common location, this concept limits recognition and acceptance of this lesion in other areas of the jaws or where teeth have been extracted (Fig. 14-3). Therefore using this technique limits the scope of possible entities to be considered in the interpretation.

The preferred method of radiographic interpretation is presented here. It is a step-by-step analysis of all the

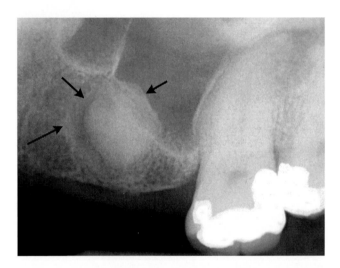

FIG. **14**-3 A periapical film revealing a lesion of cemental dysplasia left behind after extraction of the associated tooth.

radiographic characteristics of the abnormality and production of a radiographic interpretation based on these findings. This procedure helps ensure recognition and collection of all the information contained in the image and in turn improves the accuracy of interpretation.

STEP 1: LOCALIZE THE ABNORMALITY

Localized or generalized—Attempt to describe the anatomic location and limits of the abnormality. This information aids in starting to select various disease categories. Many abnormalities are localized to a specific region. If an abnormal appearance affects all the osseous structures of the maxillofacial region, generalized conditions such as metabolic or endocrine abnormalities of bone are considered. If the abnormality is localized, it may be unilat-

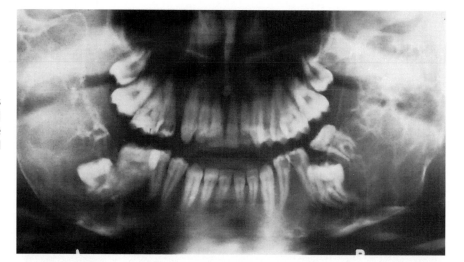

FIG. **14-4** This lesion, cherubism, is bilateral, manifesting in both the left and right mandibular rami. Note that the mandibular molars have been displaced anteriorly on both sides.

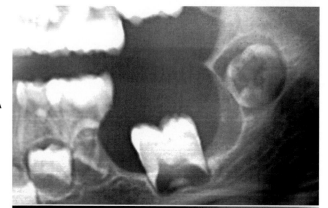

A

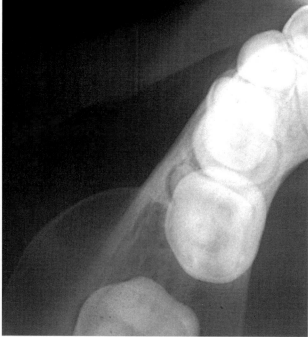

B

FIG. **14-5** **A,** A cropped panoramic image of a lesion related to the unerupted mandibular first molar. **B,** An occlusal projection providing a right-angled view of the same lesion.

eral or bilateral (Fig. 14-4). Often variations of normal anatomy are bilateral, whereas abnormal conditions are unilateral. For instance, a bilateral mandibular radiolucency may indicate normal anatomy, such as extensive submandibular gland fossa, whereas fibrous dysplasia commonly is unilateral. However, a few abnormalities such as Paget's disease are always seen bilaterally in the mandible.

Position in the jaws—Is the abnormality in soft tissue or is it contained within the jaws? When the lesion is in bone, the point of origin, or epicenter, can be estimated based on the assumption that the abnormality grew equally in every direction (this becomes less accurate with very large lesions). The point of origin may indicate the tissue types that compose the abnormality. However, determining the exact location may be difficult in some circumstances if the nature of the abnormality is not well defined. The following are a few examples:

- If the epicenter is coronal to a tooth, the lesion probably is composed of odontogenic epithelium (Fig. 14-5, *A*).
- If it is above the inferior alveolar nerve canal (IAC), the likelihood is greater that it is composed of odontogenic tissue (Fig. 14-6).
- If the epicenter is below the IAC, it is unlikely to be odontogenic in origin (Fig. 14-7).
- If it originates within the IAC, the tissue of origin probably is neural or vascular in nature (Fig. 14-8).
- The probability of cartilaginous lesions and osteochondromas occurring is greater in the condylar region.
- If the epicenter is within the maxillary antrum, the lesion is not of odontogenic tissue, as opposed to a lesion that has grown into the antrum from the alveolar process of the maxilla (Fig. 14-9).

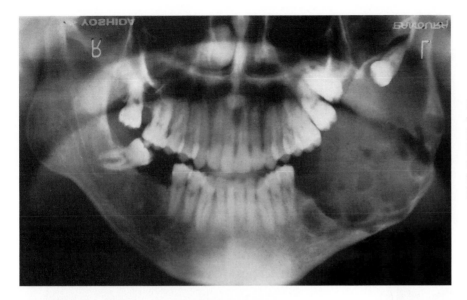

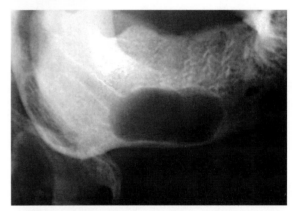

FIG. **14-6** A panoramic image revealing an ameloblastoma within the body and ramus of the left mandible. Note that the inferior alveolar nerve canal has been displaced inferiorly into the inferior cortex, indicating that the lesion started superior to the canal.

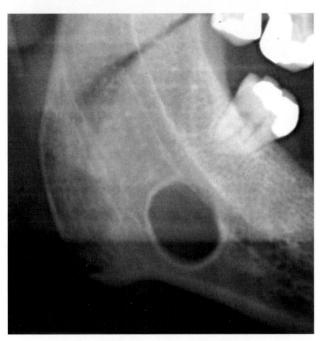

FIG. **14-7** A cropped panoramic image displaying a lesion (developmental salivary gland defect) below the inferior alveolar canal and thus unlikely to be of odontogenic origin.

FIG. **14-8** A lateral oblique view of the mandible revealing a lesion within the inferior alveolar canal. The smooth fusiform expansion of the canal indicates a neural lesion.

Particular lesions tend to be found in specific locations:

- Central giant cell granulomas tend to be located anterior to the first molars in the mandible and anterior to the cuspid in the maxilla.
- Osteomyelitis occurs in the mandible and rarely in the maxilla.
- Periapical cemental dysplasia occurs in the periapical region of teeth (see Figs. 14-1 and 14-2).

Single or multifocal—Establishing whether an abnormality is multifocal aids in interpretation because the list of possible multifocal abnormalities is short. Some examples are periapical cemental dysplasia, odontogenic keratocysts, metastatic lesions, multiple myeloma (Fig. 14-10), and leukemic infiltrates.

Occasionally exceptions to all these points occur. However, the following observational criteria can serve as a guide to a final interpretation.

Size—Finally, consider the size of the lesion. There are very few size restrictions for a particular lesion, but the size may aid in the differential diagnosis. For instance, a dentigerous cyst is often larger than a hyperplastic follicle.

STEP 2: ASSESS THE PERIPHERY AND SHAPE

Study the periphery of the lesion. Is the periphery well defined or ill defined? If an imaginary pencil can be used to draw confidently the limits of the lesion, the

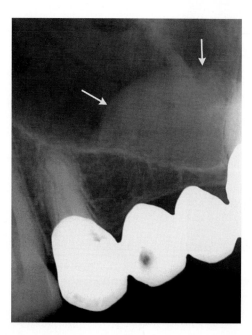

FIG. **14-9**   The lack of a peripheral cortex on this benign cyst indicates that it originated in the sinus and not in the alveolar process. It therefore is unlikely to be of odontogenic origin.

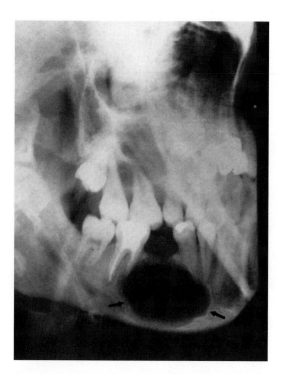

FIG. **14-11**   A lateral oblique projection of the mandible showing the well-defined border of a residual cyst.

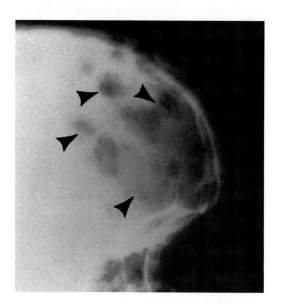

FIG. **14-10**   A cropped lateral projection of the skull revealing several punched-out lesions of multiple myeloma.

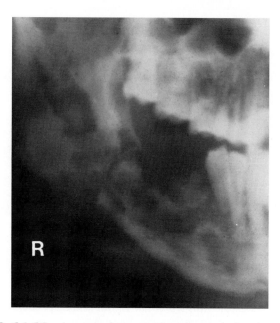

FIG. **14-12**   A cropped panoramic radiograph showing the poorly defined border of a malignant neoplasm (leiomyosarcoma).

margin is well defined (Fig. 14-11). Do not become concerned if some small regions are ill defined; these may be due to the shape or direction of the x-ray beam at that particular location. A well-defined lesion is one in which most of the periphery is well defined. In contrast, it is difficult to draw an exact delineation around most of an ill-defined periphery (Fig. 14-12). These two types of peripheries or borders can be further broken down into two subcategories: well-defined borders and ill-defined borders.

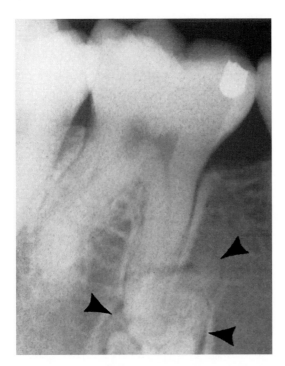

FIG. **14-13** Note the thin, radiolucent periphery positioned between the internal radiopaque structure of this odontoma and the radiopaque outer cortical boundary.

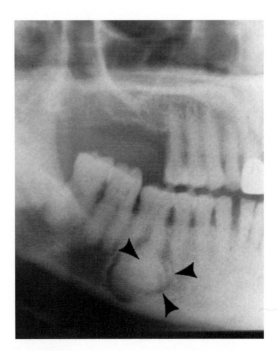

FIG. **14-14** A cropped panoramic film revealing a radiopaque mass associated with the roots of the first molar. Note the prominent radiolucent periphery of this benign cementoblastoma.

Well-Defined Borders

A punched-out border is one that has a sharp boundary in which no bone reaction is apparent immediately adjacent to the abnormality. This is analogous to punching a hole in a radiograph with a paper punch. The border of the resulting hole is well defined, and the surrounding bone has a normal appearance up to the edge of the hole. This type of border sometimes is seen in multiple myeloma (see Fig. 14-10).

A corticated margin is a thin, fairly uniform radiopaque line of reactive bone at the periphery of a lesion. This is commonly seen with cysts (see Fig. 14-5).

A sclerotic margin is a wide, radiopaque border of reactive bone that usually is not uniform in width. This may be seen with periapical cemental dysplasia and may indicate a very slow rate of growth or the potential for the lesion to stimulate the production of surrounding bone (see Fig. 14-3).

A radiopaque lesion may have a soft tissue capsule, which is indicated by the presence of a radiolucent line at the periphery. This may be seen in conjunction with a corticated periphery, as is observed with odontomas (Figs. 14-13 and 14-14).

Ill-Defined Borders

A blending margin is ill defined because of the gradual transition between normal-appearing bone trabeculae and the abnormal-appearing trabeculae of the lesion.

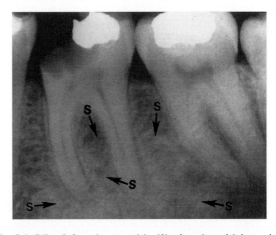

FIG. **14-15** Sclerosing osteitis (S), showing thickened trabeculae. Note that the periphery is ill defined as the normal surrounding trabeculae gradually blend with the abnormal sclerotic bone pattern.

Some conditions with this type of margin are sclerosing osteitis (Fig. 14-15) and fibrous dysplasia.

An invasive border usually is associated with rapid growth and can be seen with malignant lesions. Usually an area of radiolucency representing bone destruction can be seen just behind the margin (Fig. 14-16). These borders have also been described as permeative because the lesion grows around existing trabeculae, producing radiolucent, fingerlike or bay-type extensions at the pe-

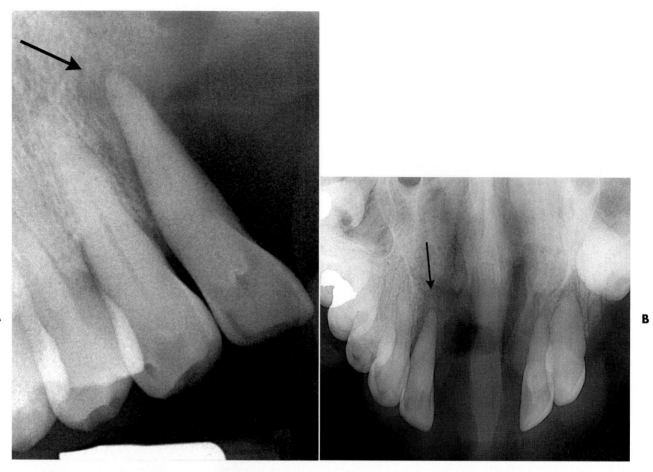

A

B

FIG. **14-16**   Periapical **(A)** and occlusal **(B)** films revealing a squamous cell carcinoma in the anterior maxilla. Note the invasive margin that extends beyond the lateral incisor *(arrow)* and the bone destruction immediately behind this margin.

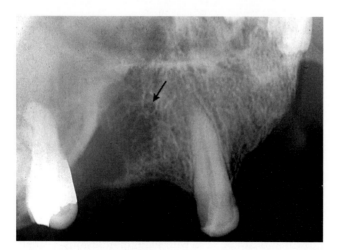

FIG. **14-17**   Occlusal view of a lesion revealing an ill-defined periphery with enlargement of the small marrow spaces at the margin *(arrow)*. This is characteristic of a malignant neoplasm, in this case a lymphoma.

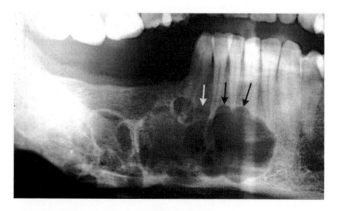

FIG. **14-18**   A cropped panoramic film of an odontogenic keratocyst displaying a scalloped border, especially around the apex of the associated teeth *(arrows)*.

riphery. This may result in enlargement of the marrow spaces at the periphery (Fig. 14-17).

Shape

The lesion may have a particular shape, or it may be irregular. The following are some examples:

- A circular or fluid-filled shape, much like an inflated balloon, which sometimes is referred to as *hydraulic*, is characteristic of a cyst (see Fig. 14-5).
- A scalloped shape is a series of contiguous arcs or semicircles that may reflect the mechanism of growth (Fig. 14-18). This shape may be seen in cysts (e.g., odontogenic keratocysts), cystlike lesions (e.g., simple bone cysts), and some tumors. Occasionally a lesion with a scalloped periphery is referred to as *multilocular*; however, in this text the term *multilocular* is reserved for the description of the internal structure.

STEP 3: ANALYZE THE INTERNAL STRUCTURE

The internal appearance of a lesion can be classified into one of three basic categories: totally radiolucent, totally radiopaque, or mixed radiolucent and radiopaque (mixed density).

A radiolucent interior is common in cysts (see Fig. 14-5, *A*), and a totally radiopaque interior is observed in osteomas. The mixed density internal structure is seen as the presence of calcified structures against a radiolucent (black) backdrop. A challenging aspect of this analysis may be the decision concerning whether a calcified structure is in the internal aspect of the lesion or resides on either side. This is difficult to determine using images that are two-dimensional representations of three-dimensional structures. Examine the calcified structures and attempt to identify the structure by its shape, size, and pattern. For example, bone can be identified by the presence of trabeculae.

The following list presents a few possible internal structures that may be seen in mixed density lesions:

- Abnormal bone may have a variety of trabecular patterns different from normal bone. These variations result from a difference in the number, length, and orientation of the trabeculae. For instance, in fibrous dysplasia the trabeculae usually are greater in number, shorter, and not aligned in response to applied stress to the bone but are randomly oriented, resulting in patterns described as have an orange-peel or a ground-glass appearance (Fig. 14-19). Another example is the stimulation of new bone formation on existing trabeculae in response to inflammation. This

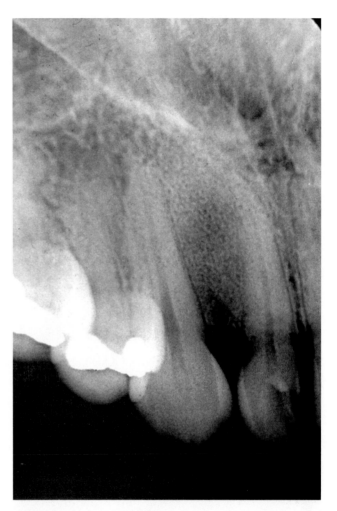

FIG. **14-19** A periapical film of a small lesion of fibrous dysplasia between the lateral incisor and cuspid demonstrating a change in bone pattern. Note the presence of a greater number of trabeculae per unit area and that the trabeculae are small and thin and randomly oriented in an orange-peel pattern.

results in thick trabeculae, giving the area a more radiopaque appearance (see Fig. 14-15).
- Septa represent bone that has been organized into long strands. If these septa divide the internal structure into at least two compartments, the term *multilocular* is used. The length, width, and orientation of the septa can be assessed. For instance, curved, coarse septa may be seen in ameloblastoma and sometimes in odontogenic keratocysts (Fig. 14-20), giving the internal pattern a multilocular, "soap bubble" appearance. The septa seen in giant cell granulomas are described as wispy or granular; odontogenic myxomas may display a small number of straight, thin septa.
- Dystrophic calcification is a calcification that occurs in damaged soft tissue. This is most commonly seen in calcified lymph nodes that appear as dense, cauliflower-

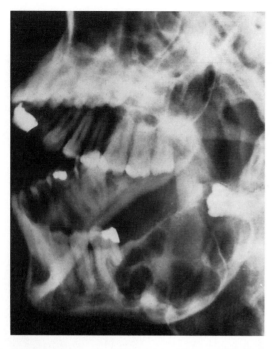

FIG. **14-20**   A lateral oblique view of a mandibular lesion showing an internal septa that divides the lesion into several compartments.

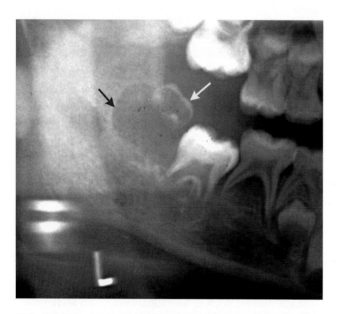

FIG. **14-21**   Leukemic infiltration of the mandible showing coronal displacement of the developing second molar *(white arrow)* from the remnants of its crypt *(black arrow)*. Note the lack of a lamina dura around the apex of the first molar and widening of the periodontal ligament space around the second deciduous molar.

like masses in the soft tissue. In chronically inflamed cysts the calcification may have a very delicate, particulate appearance without a recognizable pattern.

- Cementum usually has a homogeneous, dense, amorphous structure and sometimes is organized into round or oval shapes (see Figs. 14-2 and 14-3).
- Tooth structure usually can be identified by the organization into enamel, dentin, and pulp chambers. Also, the internal density is equivalent to tooth structure and greater than the surrounding bone (see Fig. 14-13).

STEP 4: ANALYZE THE EFFECTS OF THE LESION ON SURROUNDING STRUCTURES

Evaluating the effects of the lesion on surrounding structures allows the observer to infer its behavior. The behavior may aid in identification of the disease, but this requires knowledge of the mechanisms of various diseases. For instance, inflammatory disease, as is seen in periapical osteitis, can stimulate bone resorption or formation. Bone formation may occur on the surface of existing trabeculae, resulting in thick trabeculae, which is reflected in the trabecular pattern and in an overall increase in the radiopacity of the bone (see Fig. 14-15). The term *space-occupying* is used to describe a lesion that slowly creates its own space by displacing teeth and other surrounding structures. The following sections give examples of effects on surrounding structures and the conclusions that may be inferred from the behavior of the lesions.

Teeth, Lamina Dura, and Periodontal Membrane Space

Displacement of teeth is seen more commonly with slower-growing, space-occupying lesions. The direction of tooth displacement is significant. Lesions with an epicenter above the crown of a tooth (i.e., follicular cysts and occasionally odontomas) displace the tooth apically (see Fig. 14-5, *A*). Lesions that start in the ramus such as cherubism (see Fig. 14-4) may push teeth in an anterior direction. Some lesions grow in the papilla of developing teeth (i.e., lymphoma, leukemia, Langerhans' cell histiocytosis) and may push the developing tooth in a coronal direction (Fig. 14-21).

Widening of the periodontal membrane space may be seen with many different kinds of abnormalities. It is important to observe whether the widening is uniform or irregular and whether the lamina dura is still present. For instance, orthodontic movement of teeth results in widening of the periodontal membrane space, but the lamina dura remains intact. Malignant lesions can quickly grow down the ligament space, resulting in an irregular widening and destruction of the lamina dura (Fig. 14-22).

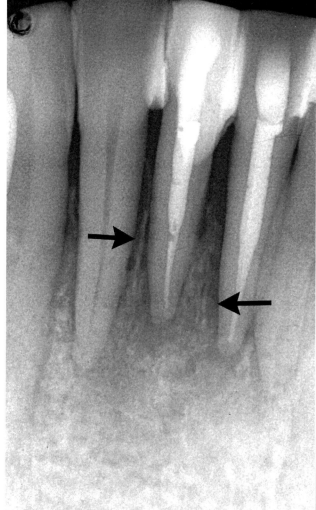

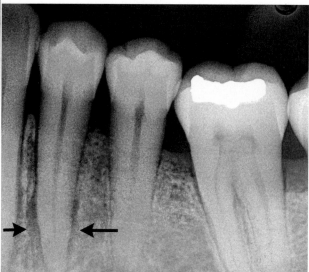

A

B

FIG. **14-22** **A** and **B,** Periapical films revealing a malignant lymphoma that has invaded the mandible. Note the irregular widening of the periodontal ligament spaces *(arrows).*

Resorption of teeth usually occurs with a more chronic or slowly growing process (see Fig. 14-5) and may result from chronic inflammation. Although tooth resorption is more commonly related to benign processes, malignant tumors occasionally resorb teeth.

Surrounding Bone Density and Trabecular Pattern

The presence of reactive bone at the periphery of a lesion, whether corticated or sclerotic, usually signifies slow, benign growth and possibly the ability to stimulate osteoblastic activity in the surrounding bone (see Fig. 14-3).

Inferior Alveolar Nerve Canal and Mental Foramen

Some changes tend to be characteristic. For example, superior displacement of the inferior alveolar canal is strongly associated with fibrous dysplasia. Widening of

the inferior alveolar canal with the maintenance of a cortical boundary may indicate the presence of a benign lesion of vascular or neural origin (see Fig. 14-8). Irregular widening with cortical destruction may indicate the presence of a malignant neoplasm growing down the length of the canal.

Outer Cortical Bone and Periosteal Reactions

The cortex of bone may remodel in response to a lesion. A slowly growing lesion may allow time for the outer periosteum to manufacture new bone so that the resulting expanded bone appears to have maintained an outer cortical plate (see Fig. 14-5). On the other hand, a rapidly growing lesion outstrips the ability of the periosteum to respond, and the cortical plate may be missing (see Fig. 14-12). Exudate from an inflammatory lesion can lift the periosteum off the surface of the cortical bone and then stimulate the periosteum to lay down

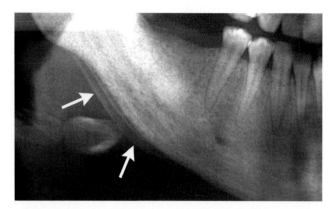

FIG. **14-23** A panoramic image of osteomyelitis revealing at least two layers of new bone *(arrows)* produced by the periosteum at the inferior aspect of the mandible.

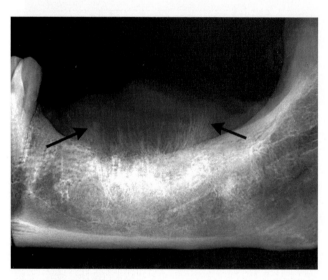

FIG. **14-24** Specimen radiograph of a resected mandible with an osteosarcoma. Note the fine linear spicules of bone at the superior margin of the alveolar process.

BOX 14-1
Analysis of Intraosseous Lesions

Step 1: Localize the Abnormality
Anatomic position (epicenter)
Localized or generalized
Unilateral or bilateral
Single or multifocal

Step 2: Assess the Periphery and Shape
PERIPHERY
Well defined
   Punched out
   Corticated
   Sclerotic
   Soft tissue capsule
Ill defined
   Blending
   Invasive

SHAPE
Circular
Scalloped
Irregular

Step 3: Analyze the Internal Structure
Totally radiolucent
Totally radiopaque
Mixed (describe pattern)

Step 4: Analyze the Effects of the Lesion on Surrounding Structures
Teeth, lamina dura, periodontal membrane space
Inferior alveolar nerve canal and mental foramen
Maxillary antrum
Surrounding bone density and trabecular pattern
Outer cortical bone and periosteal reactions

Step 5: Formulate a Radiographic Interpretation

---

new bone (Fig. 14-23). When this process occurs more than once, an onion-skin type of pattern can be seen. This is most commonly seen in inflammatory lesions and more rarely in some malignant lesions (e.g., leukemia) and in Langerhans' cell histiocytosis. Some periosteal reactions are very specific, such as spiculated new bone formed at right angles to the outer cortical plate, which is seen with metastatic lesions of the prostate gland and in osteogenic sarcoma (Fig. 14-24).

STEP 5: FORMULATE A RADIOGRAPHIC INTERPRETATION

The preceding steps enable the observer to collect all the radiographic findings in an organized fashion (Box 14-1 presents the process in abbreviated form). Now the significance of each observation must be determined.

The algorithm shown in Fig. 14-25 should be used as a dynamic guide to accommodate new observations and change incorrect concepts. The ability to stress some observations over others comes with experience. For instance, in the analysis of a hypothetical lesion, the observations of tooth movement, tooth resorption, and an invasive destructive border are made. The effects on the teeth in this example may indicate a benign process; however, the invasive border and bone destruction are more important characteristics and indicate a malignant process. Avoid making an interpretation from a single observation. In the analysis, all the accumulated characteristics point the way to the diagnosis. Also, occasionally any algorithm may fail because lesions sometimes do not behave as expected.

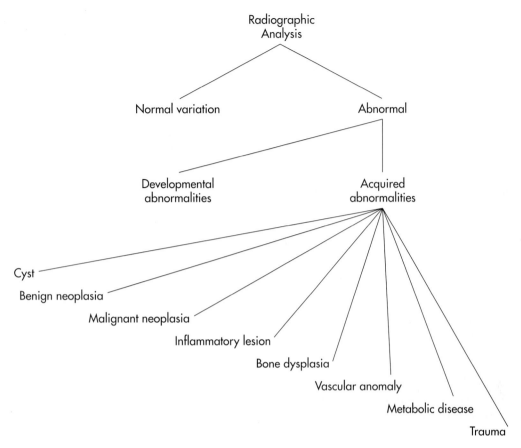

FIG. **14-25** An algorithm representing the diagnostic process that follows evaluation of the radiographic features of an abnormality.

Decision 1: Normal Versus Abnormal

Determine whether the structure of interest is a variation of normal or represents an abnormality. This is a crucial decision because variations of normal do not require treatment or further investigation. However, as previously stated, to be proficient in the interpretation of diagnostic images, the practitioner needs an in-depth knowledge of the various appearances of normal anatomy.

Decision 2: Developmental Versus Acquired

If the area of interest is abnormal, the next step is to decide whether the radiographic characteristics (location, periphery, shape, internal structure, and effects on surrounding structures) indicate that the region of interest represents a developmental abnormality or an acquired change. For instance, the observation that a tooth has an abnormally short root leads to the pertinent question, "Did the tooth develop a short root, or was the root at one time of normal length?" If the answer is the latter, then the process must be external root resorption and hence an acquired abnormality. If the tooth merely developed a short root, the pulp canal should not be visible to the very end of the root because of normal apexification. In contrast, external root resorption may

shorten the root, but the canal remains visible to the end of the root.

Decision 3: Classification

If the abnormality is acquired, the next step is to select the most likely category of acquired abnormality: cysts, benign tumors, malignant tumors, inflammatory lesions, bone dysplasias (fibroosseous lesions), vascular abnormalities, metabolic diseases, or physical changes such as fractures. Other chapters describe the characteristic radiographic findings of these abnormalities. The analysis should strive at least to narrow the interpretation to one of these groups because this directs the next course of action for continued investigation and treatment. This is a good time to bring the clinical information such as patient history and clinical signs and symptoms into the decision-making process. Introducing this information at the end helps avoid the problem of trying to make the radiographic characteristics fit a preconceived diagnosis.

Decision 4: Ways to Proceed

After analyzing the images, the clinician must decide in what way to proceed. This may require further imaging, treatment, biopsy, or observation of the abnormality (watchful waiting). For example, if the lesion fits in the malignant category, the patient first should be referred to an oral and maxillofacial radiologist to complete the diagnostic imaging in order to stage the lesion and select the biopsy site and then should be referred to a surgeon for biopsy and treatment. Cemental dysplasia may not require any further investigation or treatment. In other cases a period of watchful waiting, followed by reexamination in a few months, may be indicated if the abnormality appears benign and no clear need for treatment exists.

With advanced training or experience in diagnostic imaging, the practitioner may be able to name one specific abnormality or at least make a short list of entities from one of the divisions of acquired abnormalities.

SELF-TEST

Using the following illustrated case, practice the analytic technique. Look at Fig. 14-5, *A* and *B*, and write down all your observations and the results of your diagnostic algorithm before reading the following section.

Description
Location. The abnormality is singular and unilateral, and the epicenter lies coronal to the mandibular first molar.

Periphery and shape. The lesion has a well-defined cortical boundary and a spherical or round shape. The periphery also attaches to the cementoenamel junction.

Internal structure. The internal structure is totally radiolucent.

Effects. This lesion has displaced the first molar in an apical direction, which reinforces the decision that the origin was coronal to this tooth. Also, the lesion has displaced the second molar distally and the second premolar in an anterior direction. Apical resorption of the distal root of the second deciduous molar has occurred. The occlusal radiograph reveals that the buccal cortical plate has expanded in a smooth, curved shape, and a thin cortical boundary still exists.

Analysis. Making all the observations is an important first step; the following is an analysis built on these observations. To accomplish this next step, further knowledge of pathologic conditions and a certain amount of practice are required. The first objective is to select the correct category of diseases (e.g., inflammatory, benign tumor, cyst); at this point, try not to let all the names of specific diseases overwhelm you.

These images reveal an abnormal appearance. The coronal location of the lesion suggests that the tissue making up this abnormality probably is derived from a component of the dental follicle. The effects on the surrounding structures indicate that this abnormality is acquired. The displacement and resorption of teeth, intact peripheral cortex, curved shape, and radiolucent internal structure all indicate a slow-growing, benign, space-occupying lesion, most likely in the cyst category. Odontogenic tumors such as an ameloblastic fibroma may be considered but are less likely because of the shape. The most common type of cyst in a follicular location is a follicular or dentigerous cyst. Odontogenic keratocysts occasionally are seen in this location, but the tooth resorption and degree of expansion are not characteristic of that pathologic condition. Therefore the final interpretation is a follicular cyst; with odontogenic keratocyst and ameloblastic fibroma as possibilities in the differential diagnosis but less likely. Treatment usually is indicated for follicular cysts; therefore the patient is referred for surgical consultation.

BIBLIOGRAPHY

Worth HM: *Principles and practice of oral radiologic interpretation,* Chicago, 1972, Mosby.

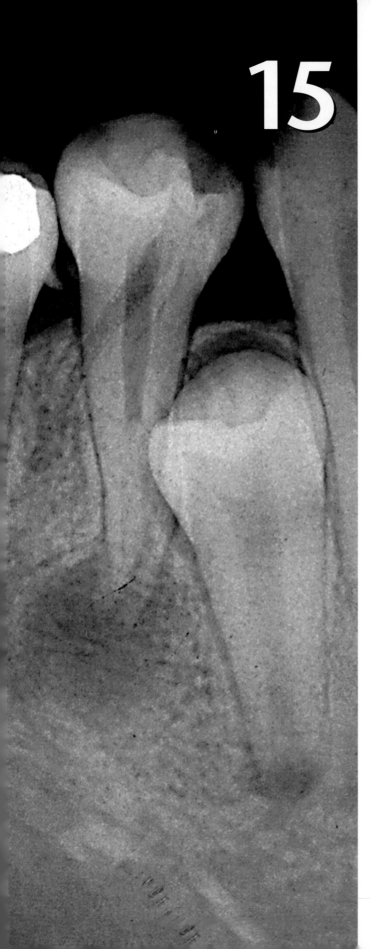

15

Dental Caries

In collaboration with
BARTON M. GRATT

Dental caries is a common infectious disease, strongly influenced by diet, affecting 95% of the population. It is caused primarily by the mutans streptococci, including *Streptococcus mutans, S. sobrinus, S. rattus, S. cricetus, and S. downei. Actinomyces viscosus* is also involved in root surface caries. These bacteria grow on specific tooth sites as an adherent gelatinous mat known as *bacterial plaque.* Cariogenic plaque may contain more than 2×10^8 bacteria per milligram wet weight. The formation of caries requires both the presence of bacteria and a diet containing fermentable carbohydrates. In susceptible individuals the bacterial plaque ferments sucrose, glucose, and fructose, with a resultant production of lactic acid and a drop in plaque pH. A pH of 5.5 is usually considered to be the crucial threshold for acid demineralization of enamel.

Repeated cycles of acid generation can, in time (usually 18 ± 6 months), cause an incipient carious lesion. The initial lesion appears as an opaque white or brown spot beneath the plaque layer. The chalky white spots are areas of subsurface demineralization. In most individuals early lesions progress slowly, often requiring 6 to 8 years to progress through the enamel. As more intercrystalline voids form, mineral loss occurs faster. In time the surface enamel loses hardness, bacteria penetrate into the enamel, and a microscopic cavity develops. Without treatment, carious lesions may progress through the enamel, the dentin, and eventually into the pulp and may destroy the entire tooth (Fig. 15-1).

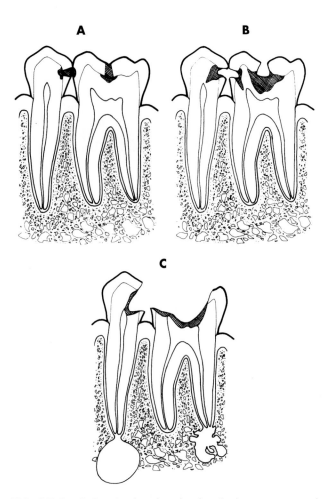

FIG. 15-1   A, Proximal and occlusal caries have penetrated through tooth enamel and into the dentin. **B,** Severe proximal and occlusal caries nearing the pulp chamber of two vital teeth. **C,** Severe proximal and occlusal caries that invaded the pulp chambers result in two nonvital pulps and periapical disease.

Rationale for the Use of Intraoral Radiographs

Radiography is useful for detecting dental caries because the carious process causes tooth demineralization. The carious lesion (the demineralized area of the tooth that allows greater infiltration of x-rays) is darker (i.e., more radiolucent) than the unaffected portion and may be detected on radiographs. An early carious lesion may not have yet caused sufficient demineralization to be detected radiographically. The practitioner should recognize that because caries is an active process, it can be accurately diagnosed only when evidence exists of progression of the lesion—that is, evidence that the defect is enlarging. An enamel defect that was created by caries several decades ago but is now arrested is not caries. It is

often useful to mount successive sets of bitewing radiographs in one film holder to facilitate comparison and evaluation of evidence of progression.

Intraoral radiography can reveal carious lesions that otherwise might go undetected during a thorough clinical examination. A number of studies have shown the value of dental radiographs by repeatedly demonstrating that approximately half of all proximal surface lesions cannot be seen clinically and may be detected only with radiographs. This is especially true for individuals older than the age of 12 years. On the other hand, early carious lesions are difficult to detect with radiographs, particularly when they are small and limited to the enamel. Therefore both clinical examination and x-ray examination are necessary in the detection of dental caries.

In recent years the use of digital imaging technology for dental radiographic examinations has increased. Most studies comparing digital systems have been conducted in the laboratory environment. These studies show that the digital systems are essentially comparable to film for caries diagnosis. Algorithms that perform computer-aided diagnosis of caries using digital images are available. They generally perform comparably to dentists. Other detection methods, such as bacteriologic testing, fiberoptic transillumination and electrical resistance methods, are likely to provide a significant contribution to the diagnosis of caries in the future.

Detecting caries on radiographs is a difficult task. If the amount of demineralization is fairly slight, radiographs are not sensitive enough to detect the lesion. However, even when different experienced dentists examine a set of radiographs, they often do not agree on the presence or absence of caries, especially when the lesions are limited to the enamel. Some dentists may identify lesions on surfaces that are actually intact (false-positive errors), whereas other dentists may fail to detect lesions that are present (false-negative errors). The difficulties in detecting small lesions, combined with the knowledge that caries progresses slowly in most individuals, argue for a conservative approach to caries diagnosis and treatment.

Examinations

Posterior bitewing radiographs are the most useful x-ray projections for detecting caries in the distal third of a canine and the interproximal and occlusal surfaces of premolars and molars. Periapical radiographs are useful primarily for detecting changes in the periapical and interradicular bone. Use of a paralleling technique for obtaining periapical radiographs increases the value of this projection in detecting caries of both anterior and posterior teeth.

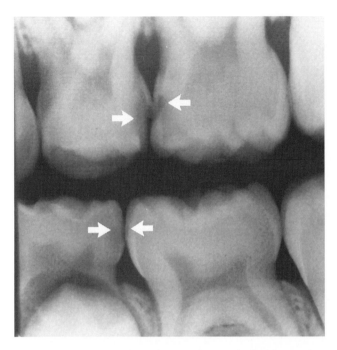

FIG. **15-2** Posterior bitewing radiograph demonstrating both permanent and deciduous teeth. Note the proximal caries *(arrows)*.

Radiographic examination for caries in children should include bitewing films (Fig. 15-2). Dentists may not be able to use the larger no. 2 size film or even the smaller no. 1 size in examining children younger than 3 years of age because of their small mouths. However, the cooperation of children may be gained by using a small no. 0 film. As children grow, they should be able to tolerate a no. 1 size; by age 6, 7, and 8, they should willingly accept the no. 2 size film. The larger the film used, the greater the chance of projecting the appropriate anatomic structures onto it. The smaller the film, the less discomfort is felt and the better the child's acceptance of the procedure.

The most useful adult bitewing examination consists of four no. 2 size films for separate premolar and molar projections.

Frequency

Radiographs are useful for detecting proximal caries when the teeth are in contact and cannot be directly inspected. The frequency of any radiographic procedure must be decided on the basis of a patient's needs, considering factors such as oral hygiene, fluoride exposure, diet, caries history, extent of restorative care, and age (see Chapter 13).

Radiographic Appearance of Caries

OCCLUSAL CARIES

New carious lesions in children and adolescents most often occur on the occlusal surfaces of posterior teeth. Bitewing radiographs are useful in detecting them on the occlusal surfaces of premolars and molars. The demineralization process originates in enamel pits and fissures and penetrates to the dentinoenamel junction (DEJ). The carious lesion spreads along the DEJ and is seen as a thin radiolucent line between enamel and dentin. In most cases no early radiographic evidence of enamel involvement exists (Fig. 15-3) because the lesion is in a pit or fissure surrounded by dense sound enamel. The enamel obscures the small lesion, which penetrates only a thin layer. Although radiographs may provide the first indication of occlusal caries, a careful clinical examination reveals most destruction. As the carious process spreads, the thin radiolucent line extends below the enamel and extends pulpally in a spherical pattern (Fig. 15-4). The margin of the expanding radiolucent area between the carious and noncarious dentin is very diffuse. As the lesion spreads through the dentin, it undermines the enamel, and masticatory forces frequently cause cavitation (Fig. 15-5).

Interpretation of Incipient Occlusal Lesions
Radiographs are usually not effective for the detection of an occlusal carious lesion until it reaches the dentin. Fig. 15-3 shows examples of teeth requiring restorations that exhibit little or no radiographic changes. The only detectable evidence of an early lesion at the occlusal surface may be a fine gray shadow just under the DEJ. A similar but usually less broad shadow, however, is frequently apparent on the images of unaffected teeth below (or above) the occlusal enamel. This line of increased density at the junction represents an optical illusion referred to as a *mach band*. The occlusal carious lesion generally starts in the sides of a fissured wall rather than at the base, and it tends to penetrate nearly perpendicularly toward the DEJ. The clinician usually makes the radiographic decision of normal or equivocal for caries and performs a careful clinical evaluation before deciding to restore the tooth. Visual changes such as chalkiness or yellow, brown, or black discoloration may develop on the occlusal surface of the tooth, although a stained fissure is not a reliable criterion for caries.

Interpretation of Moderate Occlusal Lesions
The moderate occlusal lesion is usually the first to induce specific radiographic changes, prompting a definitive decision regarding the presence of caries. The

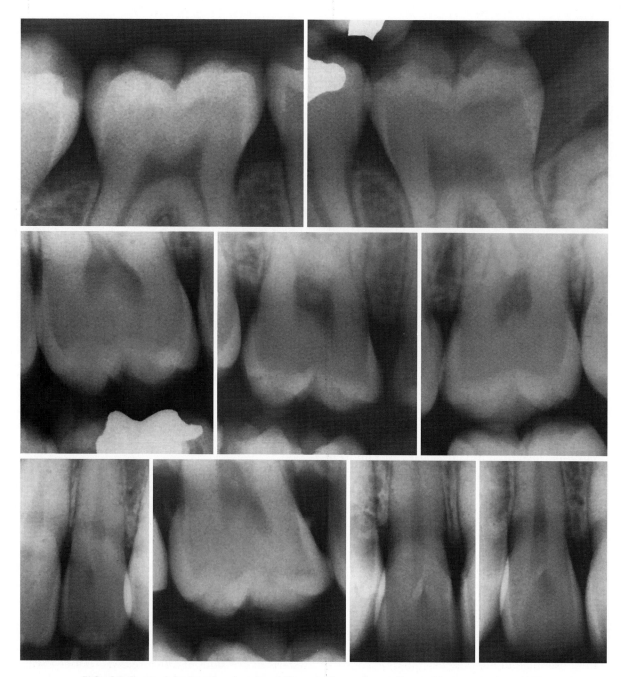

FIG. **15-3** *Incipient occlusal caries.* Although these nine radiographic images show little or no change, occlusal caries requiring treatment is present in each case.

classic radiographic change is a broad-based, thin radiolucent zone in the dentin with little or no changes apparent in the enamel. Fig. 15-4 shows examples of moderate occlusal caries with minor radiolucent changes. If a radiolucent region is present in the region next to the DEJ, a decision of either equivocal or positive for caries is necessary. Another significant manifestation of occlusal caries in the dentin is a band of increased opacity between the lesion and pulp chamber. This light band, which represents calcification within the primary dentin, is not usually seen with buccal caries. Careful clinical evaluation of the area must precede a treatment decision.

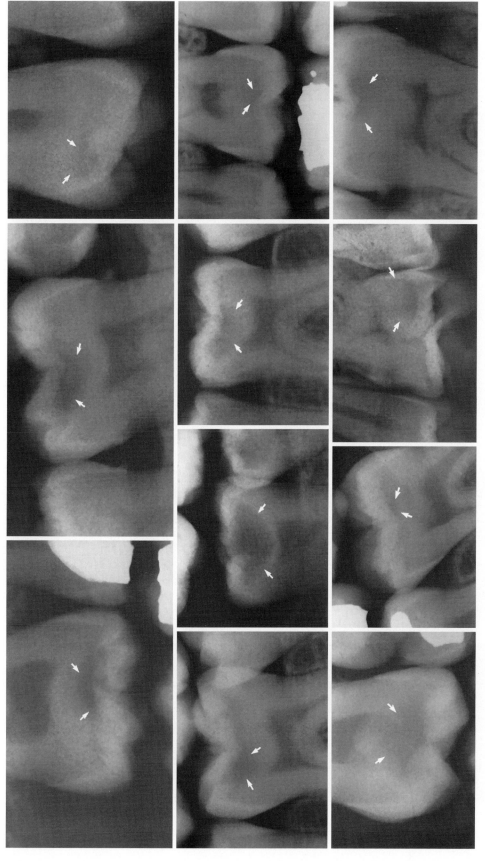

FIG. **15-4** *Moderate occlusal caries.* Eleven radiographs show a radiolucent zone within dentin but little or no changes apparent in the overlying enamel.

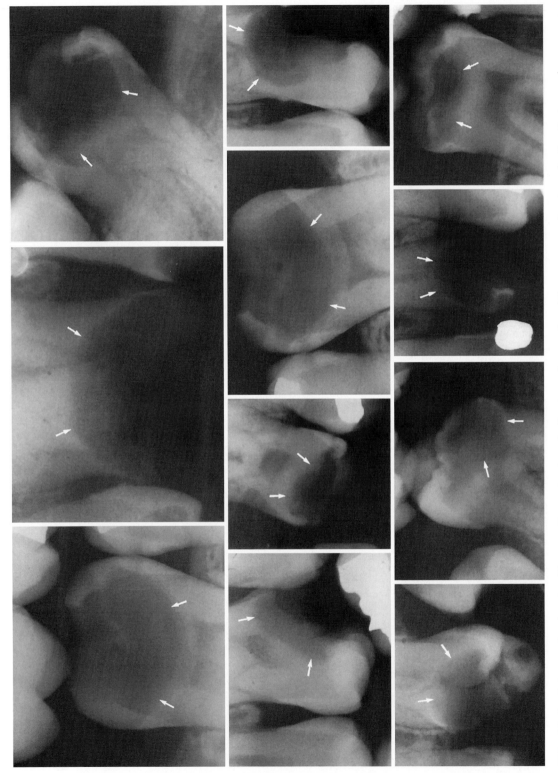

FIG. **15-5** *Severe occlusal caries.* Eleven radiographs show both a loss of enamel and the presence of carious dentin. Carious pulp exposures, however, cannot be determined by these radiographs. Only with clinical evaluation is it possible to substantiate the extent of a carious process and the accuracy of its x-ray appearance.

Interpretation of Severe Occlusal Lesions

Severe occlusal lesions are readily observed both clinically and radiographically. They appear as large holes, or cavities, in the crowns of teeth. Because the underlying dentin is carious and cannot support the enamel, masticatory forces cause a collapse of the occlusal surface. Fig. 15-5 shows examples of the radiographic appearance of such severely carious teeth. Pulp exposures cannot be determined by radiographs, however; only clinical evidence can substantiate the radiographic impression.

Radiographic Pitfalls in the Interpretation of Occlusal Lesions

Three common errors are made in interpreting occlusal caries. First is the failure to recognize that occlusal caries of enamel is not ordinarily detectable on radiographs because of the superimposition of heavy cuspal enamel over the fissured (carious) areas. Second is the carelessness of not observing the rather long, thin radiolucency that first appears at the DEJ as a sign of occlusal caries. Third is the confusion shown by many clinicians in distinguishing between occlusal and buccal caries. This occurs when lesions in the buccal grooves of molars are superimposed on the occlusal area and simulate occlusal lesions. A direct clinical inspection of the tooth eliminates any such confusion.

PROXIMAL CARIES

Radiographic detection of carious lesions on the proximal surfaces of teeth depends on loss of enough mineral to result in a detectable change in radiographic density. Because the proximal surfaces of posterior teeth are often broad, the loss of small amounts of mineral from incipient lesions or the advancing front of more advanced lesions is often difficult to detect on a radiograph. For this reason, the actual depth of penetration of a carious lesion is deeper than may be detected radiographically. Approximately 40% demineralization is required for radiographic detection of a lesion.

Interpretation of Incipient Proximal Lesions

Interproximal carious lesions develop slowly, taking 3 to 4 years to become clinically apparent. Clinically the lesions are first seen as having a loss of enamel transparency, resulting in an opaque chalky region ("white spot"). These generally occur on the outer surface of the enamel between the contact point and the height of the free gingival margin. Proximally this caries-susceptible zone has a vertical dimension on the radiograph of 1 to 1.5 mm that continues to enlarge with receding of the gingiva (Fig. 15-6). Because caries does not begin below the free margin of the gingiva, recognition of this zone

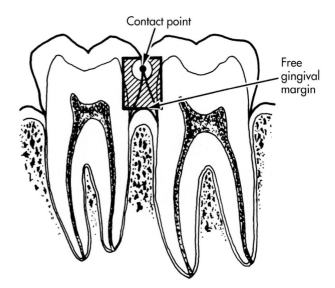

FIG. **15-6** *Proximal caries–susceptible zone.* This region extends from the contact point down to the height of the free gingival margin. It increases with recession of the alveolar bone and gingival tissues.

minimizes difficulties in differentiating caries from cervical burnout. (See Chapter 9.) The early lesions are radiolucent and do not appear radiographically to penetrate more than half the thickness of the enamel. The general radiographic appearance of an incipient lesion is of a radiolucent "notch" on the outer surface of the tooth (Fig. 15-7). Often, incipient lesions may not be visualized radiographically because of the small volume of tooth mineral lost.

A magnifying glass is useful for examining the film when evaluating the extent of incipient carious lesions and any of the other fine details that appear on a radiograph. Fig. 15-8 is a series of radiographs showing early lesions with and without magnification.

Interpretation of Moderate Proximal Lesions

Moderate proximal lesions are those that involve more than the outer half of the enamel but are not seen radiographically to extend into the DEJ. These lesions generally have one of three radiographic appearances: first, and most common (67%), is a triangle with its broad base at the surface of the tooth; second, and less common (16%), is a diffuse radiolucent image; and third (17%) is a combination of these two types. The larger the radiolucent area is, the larger is the lesion found on clinical examination. Fig. 15-9 is a series of radiographs showing moderate proximal carious lesions.

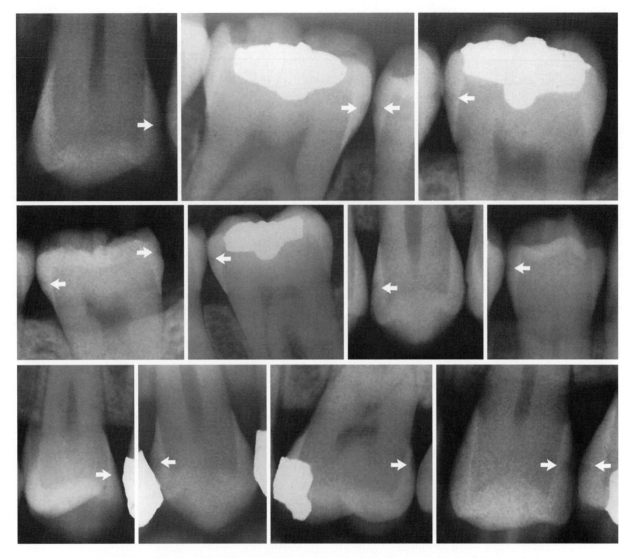

FIG. **15-7** "Notched" incipient proximal enamel caries. (*Arrows* indicate the areas showing demineralization.) Note the shape, size, and location of these 14 early lesions.

Interpretation of Advanced Proximal Lesions

Advanced proximal lesions are those that have invaded the DEJ. The description of an advanced lesion classically includes a radiolucent penetration through the enamel. The configuration is usually triangular, but it may be diffuse or a combination of triangular and diffuse. In addition, the demineralization process spreads at the DEJ, undermining the enamel and subsequently extending into the dentin. This forms a second triangular radiolucent image in the dentin with its base at the DEJ and its apex directed toward the pulp cavity. Fig. 15-10 presents examples of advanced lesions that can be seen radiographically not to have spread through more than half the thickness of the dentin. Oc-

casionally, lesions that have penetrated into the dentin appear not to have penetrated from the enamel.

Interpretation of Severe Proximal Lesions

A severe carious proximal lesion is one that can be seen radiographically to penetrate more than half the dentin and is approaching the pulp chamber. Examination of the image usually reveals a narrow path of destruction through the enamel, an expanded radiolucency at the DEJ (forming the base of its triangular shape), and lesional development toward the pulp chamber. The lesion may or may not appear to involve the pulp. An important point to stress is that it is not possible to identify pulp exposures by radiographs

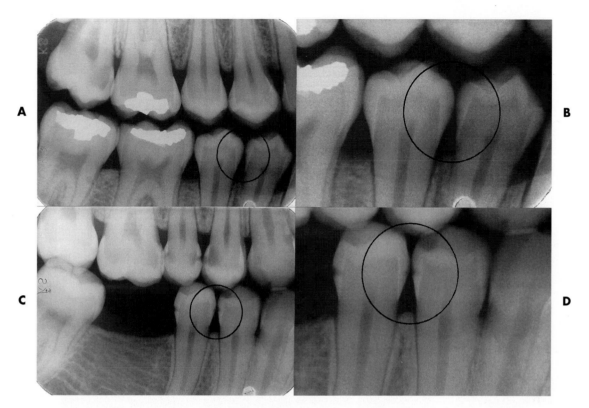

FIG. **15-8** **A,** A magnifying glass is important for examining the extent of dental caries. **A** and **C** are not magnified. **B** and **D** are magnified.

alone. The relationship of caries to the pulp is important, and certain information may be gained from a radiograph, but care must be taken not to place too great a reliance on the film. Because a radiograph is a two-dimensional image on which all parts of the tooth are projected, the full extent of the carious process may not be revealed. A lesion far removed from the pulp chamber may be superimposed on it. Only by clinical appraisal can the impression conveyed by the x-ray interpretation be substantiated.

Severe interproximal lesions with much dentinal destruction also undermine the enamel. Subsequently forces of mastication cause the enamel to collapse, leaving a large cavity in the tooth. Fig. 15-11 shows examples of severe proximal dental caries.

Radiographic Pitfalls in the Interpretation of Proximal Caries

Accurate radiographic detection of proximal surface caries is challenging. One must differentiate cervical burnout from proximal caries. Also, various dental anomalies such as hypoplastic pits or concavities produced by wear on the proximal surfaces can mimic caries on sound surfaces. Accordingly, the clinician must diagnose proximal caries cautiously and with the benefit of a careful clinical and radiographic examination.

FACIAL, BUCCAL, AND LINGUAL CARIES

Facial, buccal, and lingual carious lesions occur in enamel pits and fissures of teeth. When small, these lesions are usually round; as they enlarge, they become elliptic or semilunar. They demonstrate sharp, well-defined borders.

It is difficult to differentiate between buccal and lingual caries on a radiograph. When viewing buccal, lingual, or palatal caries, the clinician should look for a uniform noncarious region of enamel surrounding the apparent radiolucency. This well-defined circular area represents parallel noncarious enamel rods surrounding the buccal or palatal decay. It is necessary to examine more than one view of the area because a margin of a buccal or lingual lesion may be superimposed on the DEJ and suggest occlusal caries. Also, a buccal or lingual lesion at or near the mesial or distal line angle of the tooth may project onto a proximal surface and appear as a proximal lesion. Occlusal caries, however, ordinarily is more extensive than lingual or buccal caries, and its outline is not as well defined (Fig. 15-12). Clinical evalua-

Text continued on p. 283.

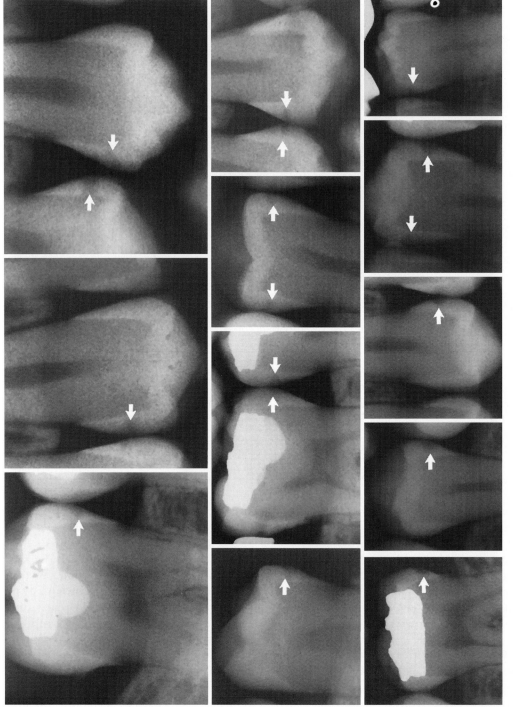

FIG. **15-9** *Moderate enamel proximal caries.* Note that these 17 lesions involve more than the outer half of the enamel but do not involve the DEJ to a radiographically detectable extent.

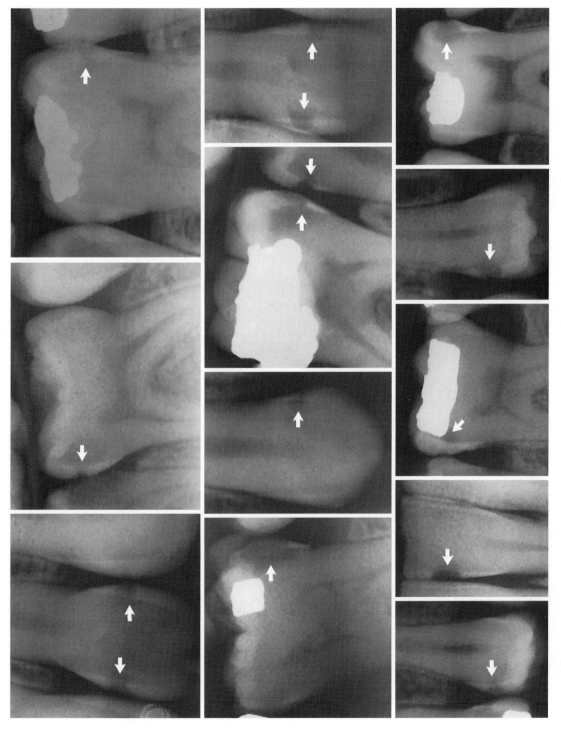

FIG. **15-10** *Advanced proximal caries.* Note the size, shape, and location of these 15 lesions and the radiographic changes (increased radiolucency) of both enamel and dentin.

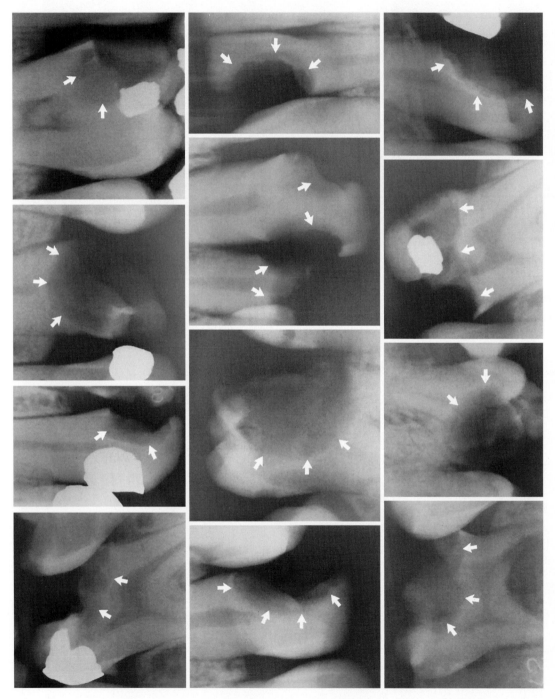

FIG. **15-11** *Severe proximal caries.* Note the loss of enamel structure in these 12 examples. Only an approximation of the degree of dentinal involvement toward the pulp can be made.

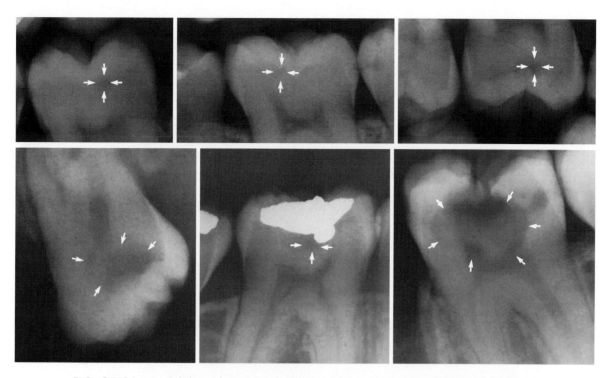

FIG. **15-12** *Facial, buccal, and lingual caries.* Note in these six examples the uniform enamel surrounding each radiolucent lesion. Clinical observation is the definitive method for making treatment decisions.

tion and probing of buccal or lingual caries are usually straightforward and the definitive method of diagnosis.

ROOT SURFACE CARIES

Root surface caries (also called *cemental caries*) involves both cementum and dentin. Its prevalence is approximately 40% to 70% in an aged population. The tooth surfaces most frequently affected are, in order, buccal, lingual, and proximal. The exposed cementum is relatively soft and usually only 20 to 50 mm thick near the cementoenamel junction, so it rapidly degrades by attrition, abrasion, and erosion. Consequently, root caries is a lesion of dentin associated with gingival recession. The carious process is a scooping out that results in a radiographic appearance usually described as *ill-defined, saucerlike,* and *radiolucent.* If the peripheral surface area is small, the appearance of the carious lesion is more notched than saucerlike. Root surface caries does not involve enamel except by extension into the dentin immediately under the enamel along the DEJ. In such cases fracturing of the unsupported enamel frequently occurs. Fig. 15-13 shows examples of typical root surface dental caries.

Pitfalls in the Interpretation of Root Surface Caries

Intact root surfaces may appear to be carious as a result of the phenomenon called *cervical burnout* (see Fig. 9-2). The true carious lesion may be distinguished from the intact surface primarily by the absence of an image of the root edge and by the appearance of a diffuse rounded inner border where the tooth substance has been lost. Clinical evaluation and probing of root surface caries are the definitive method of diagnosis.

RECURRENT CARIES

Recurrent caries is that occurring immediately next to a restoration. It may result from poor adaptation of a restoration, which allows for marginal leakage, or from inadequate extension of a restoration. In addition, caries may remain if the original lesion is not completely evacuated, which later may appear as residual or recurrent caries. Approximately 16% of restored tooth surfaces have recurrent caries. These lesions should be treated without delay because they are a frequent cause of pulp necrosis.

The radiographic appearance of recurrent caries depends on the amount of decalcification present and

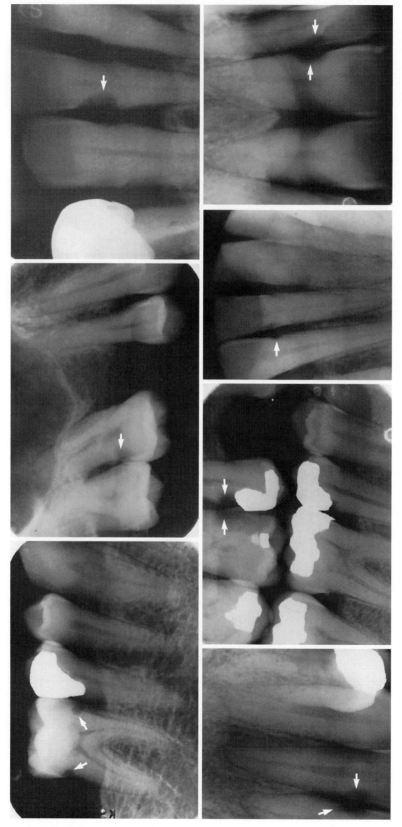

FIG. **15-13** *Root surface (cementum) caries.* Note the radiographic appearance of these 11 ill-defined, saucer-shaped defects on the mesial and distal portions of the root exposed as a result of gingival recession.

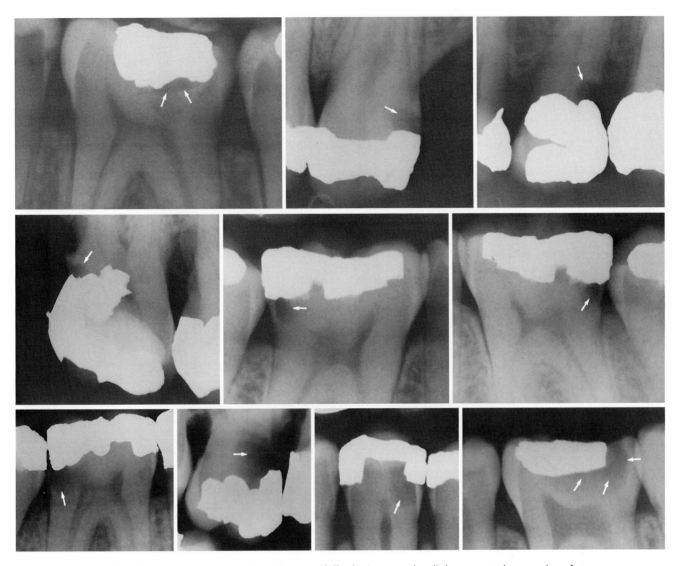

FIG. **15-14** *Recurrent caries.* Note carefully the increased radiolucency at the margins of existing restorations in these 10 examples.

whether a restoration is obscuring the lesion. Radiopaque restorations often hide small and large regions of demineralized (radiolucent) dentin. Thus the discovery and conformation of recurrent caries depend on careful clinical examination. Recurrent lesions at the mesiogingival, distogingival, and occlusal margins are most frequently discovered radiographically. In contrast, considerable destruction may occur around the margins of buccal, facial, and lingual restorations before it becomes apparent radiographically. Fig. 15-14 demonstrates several examples of recurrent dental caries as seen on the mesial, distal, and occlusal borders of amalgam, gold, and composite dental restorations.

RESTORATIVE AND BASE MATERIALS

Restorative materials vary in their radiographic appearance depending on thickness, density, atomic number, and the photon energy used to make the radiographic projection. Some can be confused with caries. Older calcium hydroxide preparations without barium, lead, or zinc (added to lend radiopacity) appear radiolucent and may resemble recurrent caries. Despite the calcium present, the relatively large proportion of low atomic number material in calcium hydroxide causes its radiodensity to approximate that of a carious lesion. Composite, plastic, or silicate restorations also may simulate caries (Fig. 15-15). It is often possible, however, to identify and

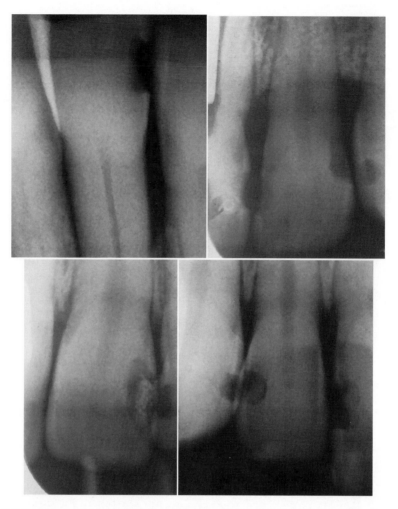

FIG. **15-15** *Restorative materials resembling radiolucent dental caries.* Note the smooth classic outlines of these radiolucent areas, which are actually prepared cavity preparations.

differentiate these radiolucent materials from caries by their well-defined and smooth classic outline. Again, although the radiographic interpretation may be equivocal for recurrent caries, it is possible to make treatment decisions on the basis of dental history and a careful clinical examination.

RAMPANT CARIES

Rampant caries usually occurs in children with poor dietary habits who generally demonstrate extensive interproximal and smooth surface caries. This condition, however, is becoming increasingly rare because of the extensive availability of water fluoridation and the more widespread and enlightened practices of good nutrition and oral hygiene. Radiographs (Fig. 15-16) demonstrate severe (advanced) carious lesions, especially of the

mandibular anterior teeth. Treatment requires extensive dental care and education of the child's parents.

RADIATION CARIES

Patients who have received therapeutic radiation to the head and neck may suffer a loss of salivary gland function, leading to xerostomia (or dry mouth). Untreated, this induces rampant destruction of the teeth, termed *radiation caries.* (See Chapter 2.) Typically the destruction begins at the cervical region and may aggressively encircle the tooth, causing the entire crown to be lost, with only root fragments remaining in the jaws. The radiographic appearance of radiation caries is characteristic: dark radiolucent shadows appearing at the necks of teeth, most obvious on the mesial and distal aspects. Variations in the depth of destruction

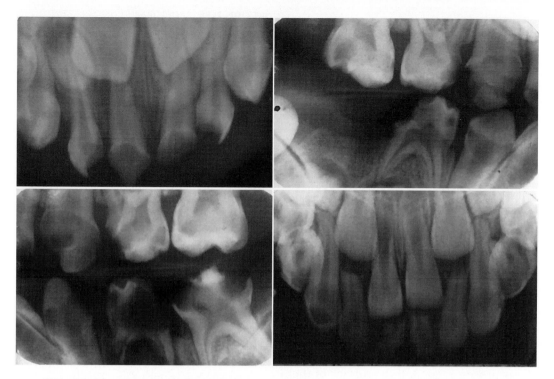

FIG. **15-16** *Rampant (advanced) caries.* These four examples were found in young children. (Courtesy Raphael Yeung, DDS, Alhambra, Calif.)

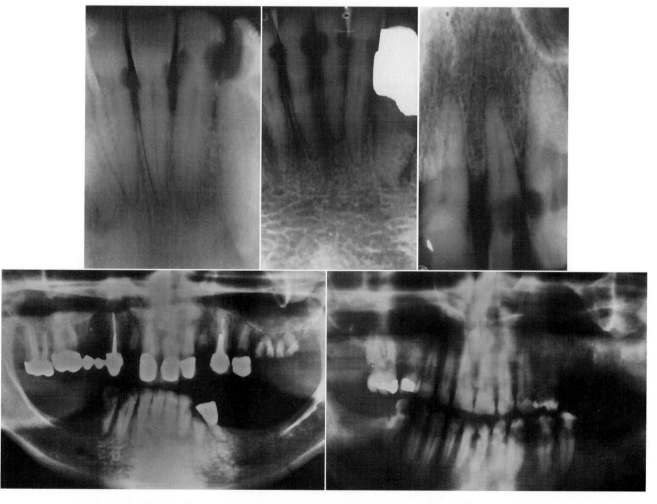

FIG. **15-17** *Radiation caries.* The five postirradiation patients presented here experienced a loss or decrease of salivary gland function (xerostomia).

may be present, but generally there is uniformity within a given region of the mouth. Fig. 15-17 shows examples of radiation caries in patients with xerostomia following therapeutic radiation for cancer of the head and neck. Use of topical fluorides, remineralizing solutions, and meticulous oral hygiene can markedly reduce the radiation damage to teeth resulting from xerostomia.

Treatment Considerations

Incipient (or early) dental caries may require only preventive and/or remineralizing treatment. Many of the small demineralization defects identified radiographically impose the obligation of deciding whether this represents active caries or static defects. When the radiograph shows a lesion limited to enamel, the probability of cavitation is low and the prospect of arresting or reversing the decay process is good. If the surface of the tooth is intact, treatment should include means to stop the microbiologic activity and possibly reverse the demineralization. Treatment of such lesions may include dietary modification to remove sugar, proper oral hygiene to reduce bacteria, and use of topical fluoride to inhibit microbiologic activity, retard demineralization, and promote remineralization of enamel and dentin. If subsequent radiographic examinations show no change in these incipient lesions, preventive or remineralizing methods can be considered to have been proper and effective. However, the consensus dictates that when the surface of a lesion is no longer intact, meaning that cavitation has occurred, a restoration is required. Remineralization techniques are ineffective when a radiograph of the carious lesion indicates it has progressed into dentin and cavitation is certain. The treatment of severe and even moderate dental caries requires removal of the lesion and restoration of the tooth to form and function.

BIBLIOGRAPHY

Mandel ID: Caries prevention: current strategies, new directions, *J Am Dent Assoc* 127:1477, 1996.
Newbrun E: *Cariology,* ed 3, Baltimore, 1989, Williams & Wilkins.
Nikiforuk G: *Understanding dental caries: 1 etiology and mechanisms,* Basel, 1985, Karger.
Nikiforuk G: *Understanding dental caries: 2 prevention,* Basel, 1985, Karger.
Schachtele CF: Dental caries. In Schuster GS, editor: *Oral microbiology and infectious disease,* ed 2, Baltimore, 1983, Williams & Wilkins.
Tanzer JM: Understanding dental caries: an infectious disease, not a lesion, *Int J Oral Biol* 22:205, 1997.

SUGGESTED READINGS

CARIES RADIOGRAPHY

Berry H: Cervical burnout and mach band: two shadows of doubt in radiologic interpretation of carious lesions, *J Am Dent Assoc* 106:622, 1983.
de Vries HCB et al: Radiographic versus clinical diagnosis of proximal carious lesions, *Caries Res* 24:364, 1990.
Gibilisco JA: *Stafne's oral radiographic diagnosis,* ed 5, Philadelphia, 1985, WB Saunders.
Gröndahl HJ, Hollender L: The value of the radiographic examination in caries diagnosis. In Thylstrup A, Fejerskov O, editors: *Textbook of cariology,* Copenhagen, 1986, Munksgaard.
Kidd EAM, Pitts NB: A reappraisal of the value of the bitewing radiograph in the diagnosis of posterior proximal caries, *Br Dent J* 1689:195, 1990.
Mileman PA, van der Weele LT: Accuracy in radiographic diagnosis: Dutch practitioners and dental caries, *J Dent* 18:130, 1990.
Murray J, Shaw L: Errors in diagnosis of approximal caries on bitewing radiographs, *Comm Dent Oral Epidemiol* 3:276, 1975.
Pitts NB: Current methods and criteria for caries diagnosis in Europe, *J Dent Edu* 57:409, 1993.
Wenzel A: Current trends in radiographic caries imaging, *Oral Surg Oral Med Oral Pathol Oral Radiol Endod* 80:527, 1995.

CARIES DECISION MAKING

Anusavice KJ: Decision analysis in restorative dentistry, *J Dent Educ* 56:812, 1992.
Bader JD, Shugars DA: Variation in dentists' clinical decisions, *J Public Health Dent* 55:181, 1995.
Bader JD, Shugars DA: What do we know about how dentists make caries-related treatment decisions? *Comm Dent Oral Epidemiol* 25:97, 1997.
Beck JD, Kohout F, Hunt RJ: Identification of high caries risk adults: attitudes, social factors and diseases, *Int Dent J* 38:231, 1988.
Caries diagnosis and risk assessment. A review of preventive strategies and management, *J Am Dent Assoc* 126 Suppl:1S, 1995.
de Vries H et al: Radiographic versus clinical diagnosis of approximal carious lesions, *Caries Res* 24:364, 1990.
Douglass C et al: Clinical indicators of radiographically detectable dental diseases in the adult patient, *Oral Surg Oral Med Oral Pathol* 65:474, 1988.
Espelid I, Tveit A: Clinical and radiographic assessment of approximal carious lesions, *Acta Odontol Scand* 44:31, 1986.
Hollender L: Decision making in radiographic imaging, *J Dent Educ* 56:834, 1992.
Kidd EA, Pitts NB: A reappraisal of the value of the bitewing radiograph in the diagnosis of posterior approximal caries, *Br Dent J* 169:195, 1990.
Petersson GH, Bratthall D: The caries decline: a review of reviews, *Eur J Oral Sci* 104:436, 1996.
Pitts NB: The use of bitewing radiographs in the management of dental caries: scientific and practical considerations, *Dentomaxillofac Radiol* 25:5, 1996.

Steiner M, Helfenstein U, Marthaler TM: Dental predictors of high caries increment in children, *J Dent Res* 71:1926, 1992.

Woodward GL, Leake JL: The use of dental radiographs to estimate the probability of cavitation of carious interproximal lesions. Part I: evidence from the literature, *J Can Dent Assoc* 62:731, 1996.

ALTERNATIVE DIAGNOSTIC TOOLS

De Araujo F et al: Diagnosis of approximal caries: radiographic versus clinical examination using tooth separation, *Am J Dent* 5:245, 1992.

Duncan RC et al: Using computers to diagnose and plan treatment of approximal caries detected in radiographs, *J Am Dent Assoc* 126:873, 1995.

Molander B et al: Comparison of panoramic and intraoral radiography for the diagnosis of caries and periapical pathology, *Dentomaxillofac Radiol* 22:28, 1993.

Møystad A et al: Detection of approximal caries with a storage phosphor system. A comparison of enhanced digital images with dental X-ray film, *Dentomaxillofac Radiol* 25:202, 1996.

Naitoh M et al: Observer agreement in the detection of proximal caries with direct digital intraoral radiography, *Oral Surg Oral Med Oral Pathol Oral Radiol Endod* 85:107, 1998.

Nielsen LL, Hoernoe M, Wenzel A: Radiographic detection of cavitation in approximal surfaces of primary teeth using a digital storage phosphor system and conventional film, and the relationship between cavitation and radiographic lesion depth: an in vitro study, *Int J Paediatr Dent* 6:167, 1996.

Nyvad B, Fejerskov O: Assessing the stage of caries lesion activity on the basis of clinical and microbiological examination, *Comm Dent Oral Epidemiol* 25:69, 1997.

Pine CM, ten Bosch JJ: Dynamics of and diagnostic methods for detecting small carious lesions, *Caries Res* 30:381, 1996.

Pitts NB: Diagnostic tools and measurements—impact on appropriate care, *Comm Dent Oral Epidemiol* 25:24, 1997.

van Papenrecht F et al: Computer-aided detection of approximal caries in dental radiographs, *Dentomaxillofac Radiol* 24:89, 1995.

Verdonschot EH et al: Performance of electrical resistance measurements adjunct to visual inspection in the early diagnosis of occlusal caries, *J Dent* 21:332, 1993.

Webber RL et al: Tuned-aperture computed tomography (TACT). Theory and application for three-dimensional dento-alveolar imaging, *Dentomaxillofac Radiol* 26:53, 1997.

Wenzel A: Digital radiography and caries diagnosis, *Dentomaxillofac Radiol* 27:3, 1998.

White SC, Yoon DC: Comparative performance of digital and conventional images for detecting proximal surface caries, *Dentomaxillofac Radiol* 26:32, 1997.

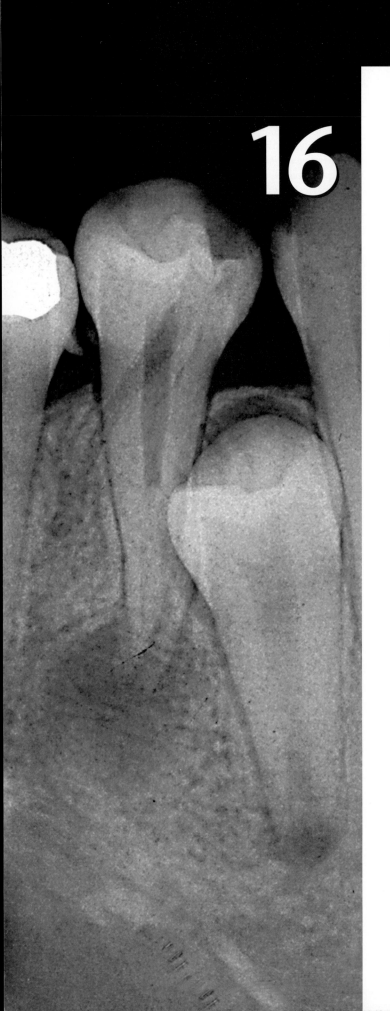

16 Periodontal Diseases

Several distinct yet related disorders of the *periodontium* are collectively known as *periodontal disease.* The most common of these are gingivitis and periodontitis. Gingivitis is a sequela of infection. It is limited to the marginal gingiva and usually is seen as a common, nonspecific form of the disease. Periodontitis is also the result of infection, but it differs from gingivitis in that loss of alveolar bone also occurs. The various types of periodontal disease are caused by different specific infections, which are classified according to their distinctive clinical manifestations. Some examples are localized and generalized forms of prepubertal periodontitis (patients 1 to 12 years), localized and generalized forms of juvenile periodontitis (patients 13 to 20), a rapidly progressing periodontitis, and localized and generalized forms of adult periodontitis (usually occurring after 30 years). These various periodontal diseases all are caused by an infection and all result in deleterious changes in the supporting tissues of the dentition. They differ with respect to cause, pathogenesis, progression, natural history, and response to treatment.

Approximately half the population is free of any sign of periodontal disease, and probably fewer than 20% of American adults have active periodontitis. The prevalence of adult periodontitis increases with age. The prevalence of juvenile periodontitis is less than 1%. It also seems that the prevalence of gingivitis in the United States is declining, apparently because of the extensive use of fluoride and antibiotics. As the elderly population increases, and with increased retention of their teeth as a result of improved preventive and restorative measures, the prevalence of periodontal disease will likely increase. However, the development of improved treatment methods may well modify this picture.

The causes of periodontal disease arise from an interplay of various host and environmental factors. Plaque-forming bacteria play an intimate role in the initiation and progression of periodontal destruction. They colonize the root surface, spread into the region between the root and the gingival margin, and stimulate a chronic inflammatory response. This results in pocket formation, subsequent apical migration of the epithelial attachment, and loss of bone. Those more prone to periodontal disease include smokers; older individuals; and people with poor education, neglected dental care, previous periodontal destruction, and diabetes. The immune system plays a primarily protective role. Bacterial antigens stimulate antibody responses that promote destruction and elimination of the bacteria. Neutrophilic granulocytes and monocytes are important to the destruction of bacteria; many patients with periodontitis are found to have functional defects in these cells. However, the immune system may contribute to the destruction of the periodontium through the release of tissue-destructive lymphokines.

The clinical manifestation of the presence of bacteria and the host response is an inflammatory reaction in the periodontium. Gingivitis is the most common first clinical sign, although some forms of periodontitis may be seen without gingivitis. Progression of these diseases leads to pocket formation, the universal manifestation of periodontal disease. Other clinical signs include bleeding, purulent exudate, edema, resorption of the alveolar crest, and tooth mobility. Rather than progressing smoothly from mild to moderate to severe, adult periodontitis often progresses in bursts. There are active periods of inflammation and loss of attachment followed by periods (often years) of no appreciable change. The extent of disease activity is best measured by longitudinal probing of periodontal attachment level. This cycle of disease activity may repeat. The relative duration of the destructive and quiescent phases depends on the form of periodontitis, the nature of the bacterial pathogens, and the host response. Host factors such as systemic disease, age, immune system status, occlusal trauma, and stress influence the course of the disease. Spontaneous remission of the destructive process may even occur. The disease usually is painless, and most patients are unaware of its presence. Various forms of therapy are effective, including oral hygiene, scaling, and surgical treatment.

Assessment of Periodontal Disease

CONTRIBUTIONS OF RADIOGRAPHS

Radiographs play an integral role in the assessment of periodontal disease. They provide unique information about the status of the periodontium and a permanent record of the condition of the bone throughout the course of the disease. Radiographs aid the clinician in identifying the extent of destruction of alveolar bone, local contributing factors, and features of the periodontium that influence the prognosis. Radiographs often are valuable in assessing specific points, which are presented in Box 16-1.

It is important to emphasize that the clinical and radiographic examinations are complementary. The clinical examination should include periodontal probing, a gingival index, mobility charting, and an evaluation of the amount of attached gingiva. Features that are not well delineated by the radiograph are most apparent clinically, and those that the radiograph best demonstrates are difficult to identify and evaluate clinically. Radiographs are an adjunct to the diagnostic process. Although a radiograph demonstrates advanced periodontal lesions well, other equally important changes in the periodontium may not be seen radiographically. Therefore a complete diagnosis of periodontal disease requires insight from a clinical examination of the patient combined with radiographic evidence.

BOX **16-1**
*Radiographic Assessment
of Periodontal Conditions*

Radiographs are especially helpful in the evaluation of the following points:

- Amount of bone present
- Condition of the alveolar crests
- Bone loss in the furcation areas
- Width of the periodontal ligament space
- Local initiating factors that cause or intensify periodontal disease
    Calculus
    Poorly contoured or overextended restorations
- Root length and morphology and the crown-to-root ratio
- Anatomic considerations
    Position of the maxillary sinus in relation to a periodontal deformity
    Missing, supernumerary, or impacted teeth
- Pathologic considerations
    Caries
    Periapical lesions
    Root resorptions

LIMITATIONS OF RADIOGRAPHS

Radiographs may provide an incomplete presentation of the status of the periodontium. They have three broad limitations:

1. Radiographs provide a two-dimensional view of a three-dimensional situation. Because the radiographic image fails to reveal the three-dimensional structure, bony defects overlapped by higher bony walls may be hidden. Also, because of overlapping tooth structure, only the interproximal bone is seen clearly. However, subtle changes in the density of the root structure (which is more radiolucent) may indicate bone loss on the buccal or lingual aspect of the tooth. Furthermore, use of multiple images made at different angulations, as in a full-mouth set, allows the viewer to use the buccal object rule to obtain three-dimensional information such as whether cortical plate loss has occurred on the buccal or lingual aspects.
2. Radiographs typically show less severe bone destruction than is actually present. The earliest (incipient) mild destructive lesions in bone do not cause a sufficient change in density to be detectable.
3. Radiographs do not demonstrate the soft-tissue-to-hard-tissue relationships and thus provide no information about the depth of soft tissue pockets.

For these reasons, although radiographs play an invaluable role in treatment planning, their use must be supplemented by careful clinical examination.

Technical Procedures

The usefulness of radiographs in the evaluation of periodontal disease can be improved by making radiographs with high technical quality. Interproximal (bitewing) and periapical radiographs both are useful for evaluating the periodontium. This material is covered in greater detail in the chapters on projection geometry and intraoral radiographic technique (Chapters 5 and 8, respectively), but the features that are particularly important for imaging the alveolar bone are emphasized here.

FILM PLACEMENT AND BEAM ALIGNMENT

Place the film parallel with the long axis of the teeth or as near to this ideal position as the size and structure of the mouth permit. Direct the x-ray beam perpendicular to the long axis of the tooth and the plane of the film. These measures result in the best, undistorted images of the teeth and periodontal tissues. Interproximal (bitewing) images more accurately record the distance between the cementoenamel junction (CEJ) and the crest of the interradicular alveolar bone because with interproximal views the beam is oriented at right angles to the long axis of the teeth, thus providing an accurate view of the relation of the height of the alveolar bone to the roots. Periapical views, especially in the posterior maxilla, may present a distorted view of the relationship between the teeth and the height of the alveolar bone because the presence of the hard palate often requires the x-ray tube to be oriented slightly downward toward the posterior teeth to see the apices of these teeth. In this circumstance the level of the buccal alveolar bone may be projected near or even above the level of the lingual CEJ, thus making the bone height appear greater than it actually is.

The teeth will be depicted in their correct positions relative to the alveolar process when there is (1) no overlapping of the proximal contacts between crowns, (2) no overlapping of roots of adjacent teeth, and (3) overlapping of the buccal and lingual cusps of molars.

In recent years some periodontists have recommended the use of vertical interproximal radiographs for patients with periodontal disease. This method uses seven no. 2 films as vertical interproximal radiographs to cover the molar, premolar, canine, and midline regions. These views have the advantageous orientation of the interproximal views yet show the reduced alveolar bone level even when bone loss has been considerable. Panoramic radiographs are not recommended for evaluation of periodontal disease because panoramic views tend to lead the clinician to underestimate minor marginal bone destruction and overestimate major destruction.

FILM EXPOSURE AND PROCESSING

For radiography of the alveolar bone, a beam energy of 80 kVp or more should be used. This increased pentration provides a longer gray scale and better visualization of the extent of bony detail and tooth roots. Films that are slightly light are more useful for examining cortical margins of bone. A properly collimated beam reduces scattered radiation and improves image definition.

SPECIAL CONSIDERATIONS AND TECHNIQUES

The dentist must determine the optimal frequency of radiographic examination for patients with periodontal disease. Certainly, radiographs of all diseased areas must be available at the beginning of periodontal therapy to allow treatment planning and provide a baseline for later comparisons. The extent of continued disease activity should dictate the frequency of subsequent radiographic examinations.

Some clinicians have found it useful to superimpose fine wire grids when exposing radiographs to aid the measurement of relative bone height. Typically the grids form 1-mm squares (which show as fine, radiopaque lines on the resultant radiograph) that allow quantitative measurement of the position of the alveolar bone with respect to the dentition. This procedure is particularly useful in evaluating osseous changes on radiographs made at different times with a reproducible positioning technique.

In recent years computers and image-processing techniques have been used to enhance radiographs to achieve improved detection of alveolar bone loss associated with periodontal disease. The most widely used of these techniques is subtraction radiography (see Chapter 12). The advantage of this method is that it allows better detection of small amounts of bone loss between radiographs made at different times than may be achieved by visual inspection. However, radiographic subtraction is difficult to use because the images must be made with the same orientation of the x-ray machine, bone, and film at each examination, which is quite impractical and difficult to accomplish in general practice.

Normal Anatomy

The normal alveolar bone that supports the dentition has a characteristic radiographic appearance. A thin layer of opaque cortical bone often covers the alveolar crest. The height of the crest lies at a level approximately 1 to 1.5 mm below the level of the cementoenamel junctions (CEJs) of adjacent teeth. Between posterior teeth the alveolar crest also is parallel to a line connecting adjacent CEJs (Fig. 16-1). Between anterior teeth the alveolar crest usually is pointed and has a dense cortex. As between the posterior teeth, the alveolar crest between anterior teeth lies within 1 to 1.5 mm of a line connecting the adjacent CEJs (Fig. 16-2). A well-mineralized cortical outline of the alveolar crest indicates the absence of periodontitis activity. However, lack of a well-mineralized alveolar crest may be found in patients with or without periodontitis.

The alveolar crest is continuous with the lamina dura of adjacent teeth. In the absence of disease, this bony junction between the alveolar crest and lamina dura of posterior teeth forms a sharp angle next to the tooth root. The periodontal ligament space may be widened slightly around the cervical portion of the tooth root, especially

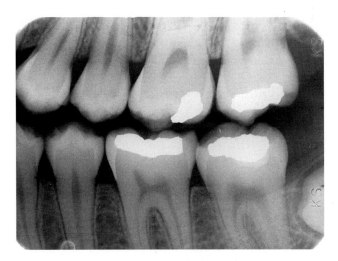

FIG. **16-1** The normal alveolar crest lies 1 to 1.5 mm below the adjacent CEJs and forms a sharp angle with the lamina dura of the adjacent tooth.

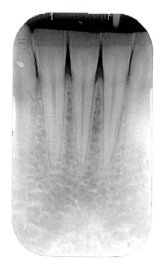

FIG. **16-2** Between the anterior teeth the alveolar crest normally is pointed and well corticated, coming to within 1 to 1.5 mm of the adjacent CEJs.

in adolescents with erupting teeth. In this situation, if the lamina dura still forms a sharp, well-defined angle with the alveolar crest, the condition is a variant of normal and is not an indication of disease. The density of alveolar crests varies widely, with no clear correlation between the density of the crestal lamina dura and periodontal status.

Gingivitis is an inflammatory condition of the gingiva caused by bacterial plaque. In this early condition the destruction has not spread to the underlying bone. When only gingivitis is present, the bone appears normal radiographically because by definition gingivitis shows no radiographic evidence of bone loss.

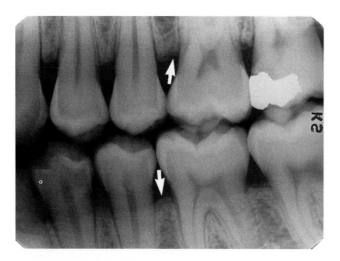

FIG. 16-3 Initial periodontal disease is seen as a loss of cortical density *(arrows)* and a rounding of the junction between the alveolar crest and the lamina dura.

Mild Adult Periodontitis

The early lesions of adult periodontitis appear as areas of localized erosion of the interproximal alveolar bone crest (Fig. 16-3). The anterior regions show blunting of the alveolar crests and slight loss of alveolar bone height. The posterior regions may also show a loss of the normally sharp angle between the lamina dura and alveolar crest. In early periodontal disease, this angle may lose its normal cortical surface (margin) and appear rounded off, having an irregular and diffuse border. If only slight radiographic changes are apparent, the disease process may not be of recent onset because significant loss of attachment must be present for 6 to 8 months before radiographic evidence of bone loss appears. Also, variations in the x-ray beam's angle of projection can cause a slight change in the apparent height of the alveolar bone. The presence of a slight lesion does not necessarily mean more severe involvement later. Small regions of bone loss on the buccal or lingual aspects of the teeth are much more difficult to detect.

Moderate Adult Periodontitis

If the lesions of adult periodontitis progress, the destruction of alveolar bone extends beyond early changes in the alveolar crest and may induce a variety of defects. The buccal or lingual cortical plate adjacent to the teeth may resorb. This type of loss is indicated by an increase in the radiolucency of the root of the tooth near the alveolar crest. The shape seen usually is a semicircular shadow with the apex of the radiolucency directed api-

cally in relation to the tooth. Defects of bone between the buccal and lingual plates also may be seen.

The overall pattern of bone loss may appear as generalized horizontal erosion of bone in a region or as localized vertical (angular) defects involving just one or two teeth. With moderate periodontitis, clinical evidence of tooth mobility may be seen. A radiograph is valuable in showing the extent of residual bone, but complete assessment of bone loss requires a clinical examination.

HORIZONTAL BONE LOSS

Horizontal bone loss is a term used to describe the radiographic appearance of loss in height of the alveolar bone around multiple teeth; the crest is still horizontal (i.e., parallel with the occlusal plane) but is positioned apically more than a few millimeters from the line of the CMJs. Horizontal bone loss may be mild, moderate, or severe, depending on its extent. *Mild bone loss* is defined as approximately 1 mm of attachment loss, and moderate loss is anything greater than 1 mm up to the midpoint of the length of the roots or to the furcation level of the molars. Severe loss is anything beyond this point. Evidence of furcation involvement is seen around molars.

In horizontal bone loss the occlusal surfaces of the buccal and lingual cortical plates and the intervening interdental bone have been resorbed (Fig. 16-4). The extent of bone loss evident at a single examination does not indicate the current activity of the disease. For example, a patient who previously had generalized periodontal disease that resulted in moderate horizontal bone loss may have undergone successful periodontal therapy with elimination of all pockets and inflammation. Such a patient will continue to show a moderate degree of horizontal bone loss, but the condition is stable. The return of a relatively dense alveolar cortex suggests the absence of active periodontitis. However, the lack of reformation of a distinct cortex does not indicate that healing has not occurred after treatment. Healing is best determined clinically.

VERTICAL OSSEOUS DEFECTS

The term *vertical* (or *angular*) *osseous defect* describes the types of bony lesions that are localized to one or two teeth. (An individual may have multiple osseous defects.) With these defects the occlusal border of the remaining alveolar bone typically displays an oblique angulation to the line of the CMJs in the area of involved teeth.

Vertical osseous defects can be divided into two primary types. The *interproximal crater* is a two-walled, troughlike depression that forms in the crest of the interdental bone between adjacent teeth (Fig. 16-5). The *infrabony defect* is a

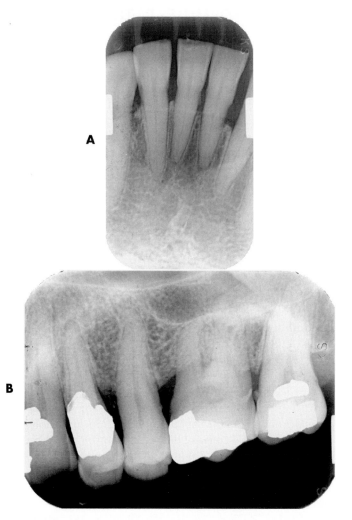

FIG. **16-4** Horizontal bone loss is seen in the anterior region **(A)** and the posterior region **(B)** as a loss of the buccal and lingual cortical plates and interdental alveolar bone.

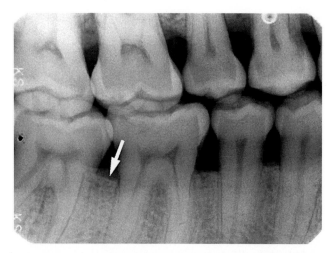

FIG. **16-5** An interproximal crater, seen through a defect between the buccal and lingual cortical plates, shows as a radiolucency below the level of the crestal edges *(arrow)*.

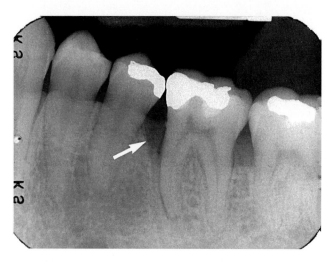

FIG. **16-6** A two-walled infrabony defect *(arrow)* has one side wall remaining and one wall lost.

vertical deformity within bone that extends apically along the root from the alveolar crest. The infrabony defect is described as *three-walled* (surrounded by three bony walls) when both buccal and lingual cortical plates remain; it is described as *two-walled* when one of these plates has been resorbed (Fig. 16-6) and as *one-walled* when both plates have been lost. The distinctions among these groups are important in designing the treatment plan.

Often infrabony defects are difficult or impossible to recognize on a radiograph because one or both of the cortical bony plates remain superimposed with the defect. Clinical and surgical inspections are the best means of determining the number of remaining bony walls. Visualization of the depth of pockets may be aided by inserting a gutta-percha point. The point follows the defect and appears on the radiograph because gutta-percha is relatively inflexible and radiopaque (Fig. 16-7).

SURROUNDING BONE

As with all other inflammatory lesions, the inflammation may stimulate a reaction in the bone surrounding the periodontal lesion. The peripheral bone may appear more sclerotic (radiopaque), or radiolucent, or a mixture of both reactions. In the sclerotic reaction, additional bone is added to existing trabeculae, increasing their size and reducing the volume of the radiolucent marrow. This reaction may extend a great distance from the focus of the periodontal disease (e.g., down into the middle portion of the body of the mandible). This type of reaction is seen more commonly in chronic cases. The other type of reaction is decalcification of adjacent bone, which results in an increased radiolucency (the

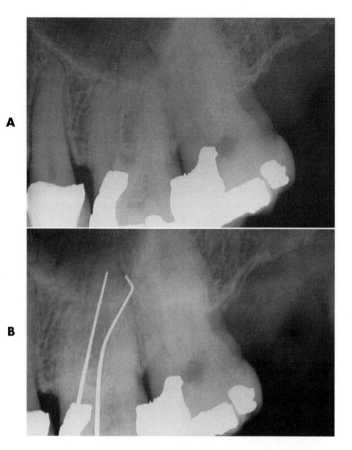

A

B

FIG. **16-7**   Gutta-percha may be used to visualize the depth of infrabony defects. **A,** Radiograph fails to show the osseous defect without the use of the gutta-percha points. **B,** Radiograph reveals an osseous defect extending to the region of the apex. (Courtesy H. Takei, DDS, Los Angeles, Calif.)

trabeculae are difficult to see or are very faint). This reaction is more common in acute cases. Most cases show a mixture of sclerosis and decalcification. Inflammatory products from a periodontal lesion can even pass through the cortex of the maxillary sinus and cause a secondary mucositis.

Severe Adult Periodontitis

In advanced adult periodontitis the bone loss is so extensive that the remaining teeth show excessive mobility and drifting and are in jeopardy of being lost because of inadequate support. Extensive horizontal bone loss or extensive vertical osseous defects may be present. As with moderate bone loss, the lesions seen during surgery usually are more extensive than is suggested by the radiographs alone.

OSSEOUS DEFORMITIES IN THE FURCATIONS OF MULTIROOTED TEETH

Progressive periodontal disease and its associated bone loss may invade the furcations of multirooted teeth. As bone resorption extends down the side of a multirooted tooth, eliminating the marginal cortical bone over the root, it can reach the level of the furcation and beyond. Widening of the periodontal ligament space at the apex of the interradicular bony crest is strong evidence that the periodontal disease process involves the furcation. If sufficient bone loss has occurred on the lingual and buccal aspects of a mandibular molar furcation, the radiolucent image of the lesion is sharply outlined between the roots (Fig. 16-8). The bony defect may involve either the buccal or lingual cortical plate and extend under the roof of the furcation. In such a case if the defect does not extend through to the other cortical plate, it appears more irregular and radiolucent than the adjacent normal bone (Fig. 16-9). By using the buccal object rule with films of different angulations, it may be possible to determine whether the septal bone has been lost from the buccal or lingual cortical plate.

If the crestal bone is below the furcation but the disease process has not extended into the interradicular bone, the width of the periodontal membrane space appears normal. Also, the septal bone may appear radiolucent or faint but otherwise be normal. In the mandible the external oblique ridge may mask furcation involvement of the third molars. Convergent roots may also obscure furcation defects in maxillary and mandibular second and third molars.

Furcation defects involve maxillary molars about three times as often as mandibular molars. The loss of interradicular bone in the furcation of a maxillary molar may originate from the buccal, mesial, or distal surface of the tooth. The most common route for furcation involvement of the maxillary permanent first molar is from the mesial side. However, the image of furcation involvement is not as sharply defined around maxillary first molars as around mandibular molars because the palatal root is superimposed on the defect. Mesial or distal furcation involvement of the maxillary molars also is not usually apparent on periapical radiographs because of the superimposition of one or both cortical plates. However, occasionally this pattern of bone destruction appears as an inverted "J" shadow with the hook of the J extending into the trifurcation.

PERIODONTAL ABSCESS

A periodontal abscess is a rapidly progressing, destructive lesion that usually originates in a deep soft tissue pocket. It occurs when the coronal portion of the pocket

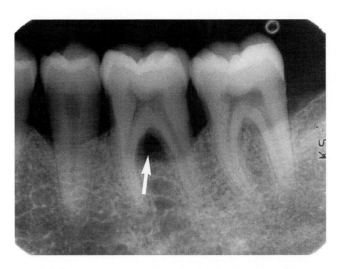

FIG. **16-8**   Advanced destruction of the periodontal bone has led to destruction of both cortical plates and interradicular bone in the furcation region of the first molar *(arrow).*

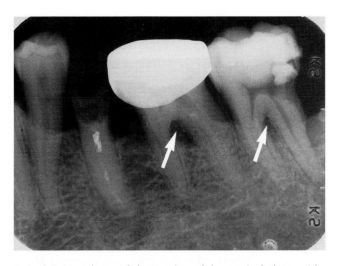

FIG. **16-9**   Advanced destruction of the cortical plates without complete destruction of interradicular bone in the furcation region is revealed as a reduction in normal bone density in this region *(arrows).*

becomes occluded or when foreign material becomes lodged between a tooth and the gingiva. Clinically, pain and swelling are present in the region. If the lesion persists, a radiolucent region appears, often superimposed over the root of a tooth. A bridge of bone may be present over the coronal aspect of the lesion, separating it from the crestal bone. After treatment, some of the lost bone may regenerate.

Early-Onset Periodontitis

Early-onset periodontitis is an aggressive but uncommon form of periodontal disease found in children, adolescents, and young adults. It may progress rapidly and result in the loss of several teeth. The condition is described in three forms. The *incidental form* is identified in children with attachment loss of 3 mm or more around one to three teeth. The incidental form is by far the most common. The *localized form* is identified with attachment loss of four or more teeth, primarily the incisors and first molars. In this form the amount of bone loss correlates with the time of tooth eruption—the teeth that erupt first (incisors and first molars) have the most bone loss. The *generalized form* involves most of the dentition, including the canines, premolars, and second molars. Whether the generalized form of juvenile periodontitis is an outgrowth of the localized form or a separate disease is not clear. In generalized forms the possible diagnosis of Papillon-Lefèvre syndrome should be considered.

CLINICAL PRESENTATION

Early-onset periodontitis begins as early as 12 to 13 years of age, and its prevalence increases in older age groups. It is found in 2.7 % of 13- to 15-year-olds and in 4% of 16- to 17-year-olds. The disease is slightly more common in males. In a recent survey, some form of early-onset periodontitis was found in 10% of African-American, 5% of Hispanic, and 1.3% of white U.S. adolescents.

Individuals with early-onset periodontitis have more gingival bleeding sites and more teeth with subgingival calculus than do individuals without periodontitis. Gingival bleeding and subgingival calculus are more prevalent in individuals with the generalized and localized forms of early-onset periodontitis than in individuals with the incidental form. Individuals with early-onset periodontitis also have a greater prevalence of tooth loss than do individuals without periodontitis. Molars are the teeth most commonly lost. Individuals with this condition are also more likely to have high levels of caries and many restorations.

RADIOGRAPHIC APPEARANCE

The radiographic appearance of the bone loss in the localized form of early-onset periodontitis typically is vertical (Fig. 16-10). This form results in severe and rapid loss of alveolar bone. Maxillary teeth are involved slightly more often than mandibular teeth, and strong left-right symmetry is common. The generalized form of juvenile periodontitis also displays the rapid and typically angular loss of alveolar bone that may progress to tooth loss.

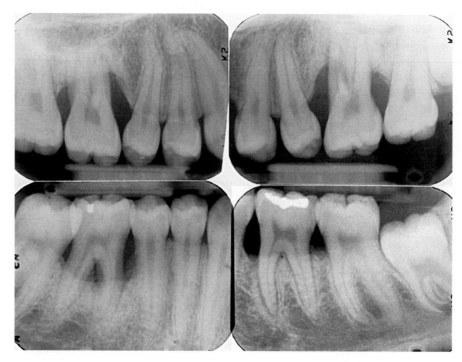

FIG. **16-10** Typical vertical bone loss in juvenile periodontitis. Note the localization to the region of the first molars. (Courtesy T.D. Charbeneau, DDS, Dallas, Tex.)

TREATMENT

Early identification and treatment of early-onset periodontitis is important because of the rapid progression of this condition and the associated tooth loss. It responds to total plaque control, just as adult periodontitis does. Treatment often consists of scaling, curettage, and administration of antibiotics.

Dental Conditions Associated with Periodontal Diseases

Various changes in the dentition and its supporting structures that frequently are associated with periodontal disease include overhanging and faulty restorations, occlusal trauma, tooth mobility, open contacts, and local irritation. These conditions usually are apparent on radiographs.

OCCLUSAL TRAUMA

Traumatic occlusion causes degenerative changes in response to occlusal pressures that are greater than the physiologic tolerances of the tooth's supporting tissues. These lesions occur as a result of malfunction caused by

excessive occlusal force on teeth or by normal forces on a periodontium compromised by bone loss. In addition to clinical symptoms such as increased mobility, wear facets, unusual response to percussion, and a history of contributing habits, radiographic evidence may suggest increased tooth mobility, including widening of the periodontal ligament (PDL) space, widening of the lamina dura, bone loss, and an increase in the number and size of trabeculae. Other sequelae of traumatic occlusion include hypercementosis and root fractures. However, traumatic occlusion can be diagnosed only by clinical evaluation. Traumatic occlusion does not cause gingivitis or periodontitis, affect the epithelial attachment, or lead to pocket formation.

TOOTH MOBILITY

Widening of the PDL space suggests tooth mobility, which may result from occlusal trauma or a lack of bone support arising from advanced bone loss. If the affected tooth has a single root, the socket may develop an hourglass shape. If the tooth is multirooted, it may show widening of the PDL space at the apices and in the region of the furcation. These changes result when the tooth moves about an axis of rotation at some midpoint on the roots. The widened PDL results from resorption of both the root and alveolar

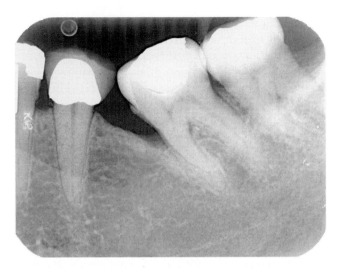

FIG. **16-11** Loss of the first molar has resulted in mesial tipping of the second and third molars. This condition resulted in an infrabony defect. Note also the calculus on the mesial surface of the second molar. The crown on the second premolar was constructed with an enlarged distal contour to stop further tipping of the molar.

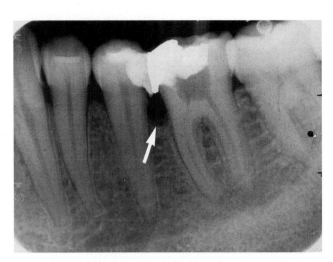

FIG. **16-12** Overhanging amalgam restoration has resulted in loss of alveolar bone (arrow).

bone (lamina dura). In addition, the radiographic image of the lamina dura may appear broad and hazy and show increased density (osteosclerosis). In some cases, if the trauma is extensive, no lamina dura may be evident. In the case of multirooted teeth, the interradicular bone may be reduced in height and density, especially if the trauma has moved the tooth buccally and lingually.

OPEN CONTACTS

When the mesial and distal surfaces of adjacent teeth do not touch, the patient has an open contact. This condition is potentially dangerous to the periodontium because of the potential for food debris to become trapped in the region. Trapped food particles may damage the soft tissue and induce an inflammatory response leading to periodontal disease. Areas with open contacts and early periodontal disease show more bone loss than areas of closed contacts. Similar problems may follow if a discrepancy exists in the height of two adjacent marginal ridges or tipped teeth (Fig. 16-11). These conditions are examples of the importance of proper tooth alignment in the prevention of periodontal disease.

LOCAL IRRITATING FACTORS

Local irritating factors may cause or aggravate periodontal defects. Calculus deposits prevent effective cleansing of a sulcus and lead to the progression of periodontal disease. Similarly, defective restorations

with overhanging or poorly contoured margins can lead to the accumulation of bacterial deposits and periodontal disease (Fig. 16-12). Radiographs often reveal these conditions. Occasionally crowns have insufficient contour and fail to protect the gingiva. Gingivitis and periodontitis may then result from trauma to the tissues. Previous surgical removal of an impacted third molar is associated with a higher incidence of plaque, gingivitis, and pockets on the distal surface of the second molar than on other surfaces of the first and second molars.

Evaluation of Periodontal Therapy

Radiographs may show signs of successful treatment of periodontal disease. The relatively radiolucent margins of bone that were undergoing active resorption before treatment may become more sclerotic (radiopaque) after successful therapy. In other cases, however, the radiographic appearance of the alveolar process may not change after successful periodontal treatment. The enlarged marrow spaces are reduced, and the bone becomes denser, creating the illusion of vertical bone growth (bone regeneration after therapy). Other changes may not be seen. For instance, radiographs do not disclose the therapeutic elimination of (radiolucent) soft tissue periodontal pockets; healing therefore is best assessed by clinical evaluation.

Radiographs made with poor technique may not accurately demonstrate the condition of bone after treatment. Even though periodontal therapy does not restore marginal bone or bone in the furcation region, changes in the beam orientation may give the false impression that such additive changes have taken place. The effect of exposure and processing also must be critically controlled and evaluated when assessing the result of treatment. Too high an x-ray exposure and too long a developing time create the impression of destroyed bone as a result of alveolar crest burnout. If followed (after treatment) by too low an exposure and too short a developing time, the denser-appearing image may suggest vertical bone growth.

The clinical crown-to-tooth ratio is a useful criterion not only for determining the nature of the restorative treatment to be performed on a tooth but also for deciding on the prognosis of an individual tooth. It is a measure of the tooth's bony support, relating the proportion of tooth length that is beyond the level of bone (clinical crown) to that supported by the lowest level of bone (bony investment). Teeth have an unfavorable crown-to-root ratio when the length of the tooth out of bone exceeds the length of root supported by bone.

Differential Diagnosis

Although the vast majority of bone loss around teeth is caused by one of the periodontal diseases, other diseases that manifest as bone destruction around the roots of the teeth should always be considered in the diagnosis. Occasionally, more serious diseases are missed or recognized late. The most likely clinical sign of disease other than periodontal disease is the presence of one or a few adjacent loose teeth when the rest of the mouth shows no signs of periodontal disease. Radiographically, suspicion should be heightened if the clinician sees localized saucerization of bone. Squamous cell carcinoma of the alveolar process occasionally is treated as periodontal disease, resulting in an unfortunate delay in diagnosis and treatment. This malignancy may display characteristics that suggest its true nature, such as extensive osteolytic destruction of a localized region (see Chapter 21), or it may mimic periodontal disease. In some cases only the clinical characteristics of the lesion and the failure to respond to treatment indicate the presence of malignancy.

Any lesion of bone destruction that has ill-defined borders and a lack of peripheral bone response (sclerosis) should be viewed with suspicion. Another disease to be considered is Langerhans' cell histiocytosis (eosinophilic granuloma). Often this disease may manifest as single or multiple regions of bone destruction around the roots of teeth, similar to periodontal disease. The condition may appear similar to juvenile periodontitis

except that the bone destruction does not correlate with the time of tooth eruption, as is seen in periodontitis. Also, in histiocytosis the midroot region is the epicenter of bone destruction, which gives early lesions an "ice cream scoop" appearance (see Chapter 22). The alveolar crest may remain intact.

Effect of Systemic Diseases on Periodontal Disease

Although systemic diseases do not cause periodontal disease, they do influence its course by interfering with the natural defenses against irritants or limiting the body's capacity to repair. Although any systemic disease may have some influence on other body systems, only a few appear to influence the periodontium and periodontal treatment. These include diabetes mellitus, hematologic disorders (e.g., monocytic conditions and, less often, myelogenous leukemia, neutropenia, hemophilia, abnormal bleeding, and nonhemophilic polycythemia vera), genetic and hereditary disturbances (e.g., hyperkeratosis palmoplantaris, Down syndrome, hypophosphatemia, Chédiak-Higashi syndrome), hormonal changes (e.g., puberty, pregnancy, menopause), and stress.

ACQUIRED IMMUNODEFICIENCY SYNDROME

The incidence and severity of periodontal disease have increased in patients with acquired immunodeficiency syndrome (AIDS). In these individuals the disease process is characterized by a rapid progression that leads to bone sequestration and loss of several teeth. The patient does not respond to standard periodontal therapy.

DIABETES MELLITUS

Diabetes mellitus is the most common and important systemic disease to influence the onset and course of periodontal disease. Uncontrolled, it may result in protein breakdown, degenerative vascular changes, lowered resistance to infection, and increased severity of infections. Consequently, patients with diabetes are more disposed to develop periodontal disease than are those with normal glucose metabolism. Patients with uncontrolled diabetes and periodontal disease also show more severe and rapid alveolar bone resorption and are more prone to develop periodontal abscesses. In patients whose diabetes is under control, periodontal disease responds normally to traditional treatment.

BIBLIOGRAPHY

CLINICAL CHARACTERISTICS OF PERIODONTAL DISEASES

Armitage GC: Clinical evaluation of periodontal diseases, *Periodontol 2000* 7:39, 1995.

Armitage GC: Periodontal diseases: diagnosis, *Ann Periodontol* 1:1, 1996.

Page RC: Periodontal research: implications for the future of academic dentistry, *J Dent Educ* 47:226, 1983.

Page RC, Schroeder HE: *Periodontitis in man and other animals*, Basel, 1982, S Karger.

Walsh TF et al: The relationship of bone loss observed on panoramic radiographs with clinical periodontal screening, *J Clin Periodontol* 24:153, 1997.

EPIDEMIOLOGY

American Academy of Periodontology, Research, Science, and Therapy Committee: Epidemiology of periodontal diseases, *J Periodontol* 67:935, 1996.

Beck JD et al: Prevalence and risk indicators for periodontal attachment loss in a population of older community-dwelling blacks and whites, *J Periodontol* 61:521, 1990.

Brown LJ et al: Evaluating the periodontal status of US employed adults, *J Am Dent Assoc* 121:226, 1990.

Melvin WL et al: The prevalence and sex ratio of juvenile periodontitis in a young racially mixed population, *J Periodontol* 62:330, 1991.

Page RC: Oral health status in the United States: prevalence of inflammatory periodontal disease, *J Dent Educ* 49:354, 1985.

ETIOLOGY

Bergström J et al: Cigarette smoking and periodontal bone loss, *J Periodontol* 62:242, 1991.

Bimstein E, Garcia-Godoy F: The significance of age, proximal caries, gingival inflammation, probing depths, and the loss of lamina dura in the diagnosis of alveolar bone loss in the primary molars, *ASDC J Dent Child* 61:125, 1994.

Fox CH: New considerations in the prevalence of periodontal disease, *Curr Opin Dent* 2:5, 1992.

Page RC et al: Advances in the pathogenesis of periodontitis: summary of developments, clinical implications and future directions, *Periodontol 2000* 14:216, 1997.

Salvi GE et al: Influence of risk factors on the pathogenesis of periodontitis, *Periodontol 2000* 14:173, 1997.

Schwartz Z et al: Mechanisms of alveolar bone destruction in periodontitis, *Periodontol 2000* 14:158, 1997.

RADIOGRAPHIC MANIFESTATIONS

Goodson JM et al: The relationship between attachment level loss and alveolar bone loss, *J Clin Periodontol* 11:348, 1984.

Gutteridge DL: The use of radiographic techniques in the diagnosis and management of periodontal diseases, *Dentomaxillofac Radiol* 24:107, 1995.

Jeffcoat MK et al: Radiographic diagnosis in periodontics, *Periodontol 2000* 7:54, 1995.

Khocht A et al: Screening for periodontal disease: radiographs vs PSR, *J Am Dent Assoc* 127:749, 1996.

Koral SM et al: Alveolar bone loss due to open interproximal contacts in periodontal disease, *J Periodontol* 52:477, 1981.

Kugelberg CF et al: Periodontal healing after impacted lower third molar surgery: a retrospective study, *Int J Oral Surg* 14:29, 1985.

Mann J et al: Investigation of the relationship between clinically detected loss of attachment and radiographic changes in early periodontal disease, *J Clin Periodontol* 12:247, 1985.

Nielsen IM et al: Interproximal periodontal intrabony defects: prevalence, localization, and etiological factors, *J Clin Periodontol* 7(3):187, 1980.

Rams TE et al: Utility of radiographic crestal lamina dura for predicting periodontitis disease activity, *J Clin Periodontol* 21:571, 1994.

Rushton VE, Horner K: The use of panoramic radiology in dental practice, *J Dent* 24:185, 1996.

Tammisalo T et al: Detailed tomography of periapical and periodontal lesions: diagnostic accuracy compared with periapical radiography, *Dentomaxillofac Radiol* 25:89, 1996.

Waite IM et al: Relationship between clinical periodontal condition and the radiological appearance at first molar sites in adolescents: a 3-year study, *J Clin Periodontol* 21:155, 1994.

EARLY-ONSET PERIODONTITIS

Albandar JM et al: Dental caries and tooth loss in adolescents with early onset periodontitis, *J Periodontol* 67:960, 1996.

Albandar JM et al: Clinical features of early onset periodontitis, *J Am Dent Assoc* 128:1393, 1997.

Brown LJ et al: Early onset periodontitis: progression of attachment loss during 6 years, *J Periodontol* 67:968, 1996.

Davies R et al: Destructive forms of periodontal disease in adolescents and young adults, *Br Dent J* 158:429, 1985.

Liljenberg B, Lindhe J: Juvenile periodontitis: some microbiological, histopathological, and clinical characteristics, *J Clin Periodontol* 7:48, 1980.

Liljenberg B, Lindhe J: Treatment of localized juvenile periodontitis: results after 5 years, *J Clin Periodontol* 11:399, 1984.

Page RC et al: Rapidly progressive periodontitis: a distinct clinical condition, *J Periodontol* 54:197, 1983.

Page RC et al: Clinical and laboratory studies of a family with a high prevalence of juvenile periodontitis, *J Periodontol* 56:602, 1985.

RADIOGRAPHIC TECHNIQUE

Bragger I: Radiographic diagnosis of periodontal disease progression, *Curr Opin Periodontol* 3:59, 1996.

Duckworth J et al: A method for the geometric and densitometric standardization of intraoral radiographs, *J Periodontol* 54:435, 1983.

Gröndahl K et al: Influence of variations in projection geometry on the detectability of periodontal bone lesions: a comparison between subtraction radiography and conventional radiographic technique, *J Clin Periodontol* 11:411, 1984.

Pepelassi EA, Diamanti-Kipioti A: Selection of the most accurate method of conventional radiography for the assessment of periodontal osseous destruction, *J Clin Periodontol* 24:557, 1997.

Reed B, Polson A: Relationships between bitewing and periapical radiographs in assessing crestal alveolar bone levels, *J Periodontol* 55:22, 1984.

SUBTRACTION RADIOGRAPHY

Griffiths GS et al: Use of an internal standard in subtraction radiography to assess initial periodontal bone changes, *Dentomaxillofac Radiol* 25:76, 1996.

Gröndahl HG, Gröndahl K: Subtraction radiography for the diagnosis of periodontal bone lesions, *Oral Surg* 55:208, 1983.

Jeffcoat MK: Diagnosing periodontal disease: new tools to solve an old problem, *J Am Dent Assoc* 122:55, 1991.

Stassinakis A et al: Accuracy in detecting bone lesions in vitro with conventional and subtracted direct digital imaging, *Dentomaxillofac Radiol* 24:232, 1995.

OCCLUSAL TRAUMA

Burgett FG: Trauma from occlusion: periodontal concerns, *Dent Clin North Am* 39:301, 1995.

Wank GS, Kroll YJ: Occlusal trauma: an evaluation of its relationship to periodontal prostheses, *Dent Clin North Am* 25:511, 1981.

SYSTEMIC DISEASE

Emrich LJ et al: Periodontal disease in non-insulin-dependent diabetes mellitus, *J Periodontol* 62:123, 1991.

Farzim I, Edalat M: Periodontosis with hyperkeratosis palmaris and plantaris (the Papillon-Lefèvre syndrome): a case report, *J Periodontol* 45:316, 1974.

Nelson RG et al: Periodontal diseases and NIDDM in Pima Indians, *Diabetes Care* 13:836, 1990.

Rateitschak-Pluss EM, Schroeder HE: History of periodontitis in a child with Papillon-Lefèvre syndrome, *J Periodontol* 55:35, 1984.

Winkler JR et al: Clinical description and etiology of HIV-associated periodontal disease. In Robinson PB, Greenspan JS, editors: *Prospectus on oral manifestations of AIDS*, Littleton, Mass, 1988, PSG Publishing.

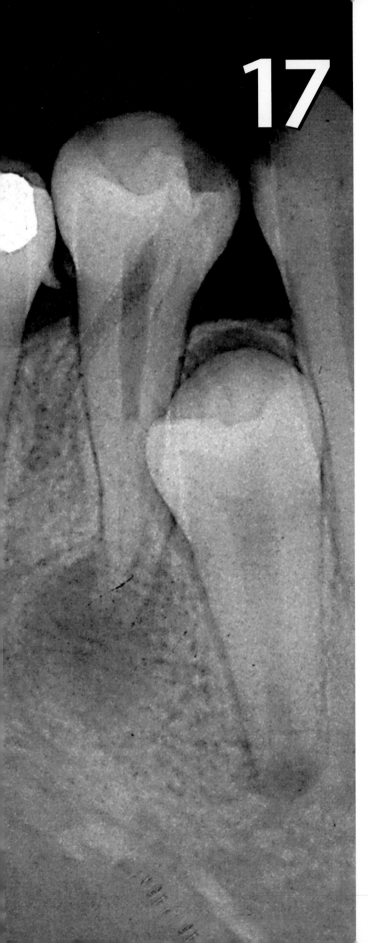

17 Dental Anomalies

Dental anomalies include variations in normal number, size, eruption, or morphology of the teeth. In this chapter these anomalies have been divided into either developmental abnormalities or acquired abnormalities. The term *developmental* indicates that the particular anomaly occurred during the formation of the tooth or teeth. Given the complexities and interactions involved in tooth development, from initiation at about the sixth week in utero to eruption, the small number of various anomalies is surprising. Most of the defects considered are inherited. In contrast, *acquired* abnormalities result from changes to teeth after normal formation. For instance, teeth that form abnormally short roots represent a developmental anomaly, whereas the shortening of normal tooth roots by external resorption represents an acquired change.

Developmental Abnormalities

NUMBER OF TEETH

Supernumerary Teeth
Synonyms. *Hyperdontia, distodens, mesiodens, parateeth, peridens,* and *supplemental teeth*

Definition. Supernumerary teeth are those that develop in addition to the normal complement. The tooth form may be normal or abnormal. When the extra teeth have normal morphology, the term *supplemental* is sometimes used. Although the cause is unknown, the tendency is familial. Most cases are polygenetic and represent initial spontaneous gene mutations. When the anomaly is restricted to supernumerary teeth, it is inherited as an autosomal recessive trait. The supernumerary teeth that occur between the maxillary central incisors are *mesio-*

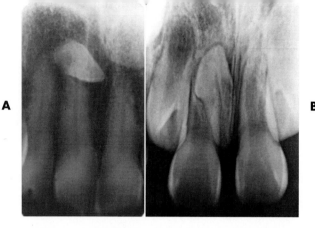

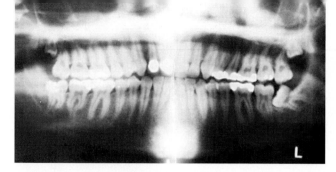

FIG. **17-3** Distomolars or fourth molars may be seen in both maxillary quadrants. Note the coincidental mucous retention cysts in both maxillary antra.

FIG. **17-1** *A mesiodens is a supernumerary tooth in the midline of the maxilla.* **A,** Mesiodens in the region of the maxillary central incisor apex. **B,** Mesiodens inverted and lying just lateral to the intermaxillary suture.

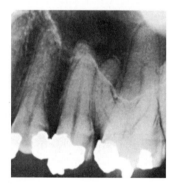

FIG. **17-2** A paramolar blocking the path of eruption of the third molar.

dens (Fig. 17-1); those occurring in the molar area are *parateeth* (Fig. 17-2). Those that erupt distal to the third molar are called *distodens* or *distomolar teeth* (Fig. 17-3). Also, supernumerary teeth that erupt ectopically either buccally or lingually to the normal arch are *peridens*.

Clinical features. Supernumerary teeth occur in 1% to 4% of the population. Although they may develop in both dentitions, they are more common in the permanent. Supernumerary teeth may occur anywhere in either jaw. Single teeth are most common in the anterior maxilla (mesiodens) and in the maxillary molar region. Multiple supernumerary teeth occur most frequently in the premolar regions, usually in the mandible (Fig. 17-4). The mandibular counterpart of the mesiodens is rare. Supernumerary teeth occur twice as often in males and

have a greater incidence in Asians and Native Americans. They usually do not erupt but are discovered radiographically. Occasionally a patient may appear clinically to be missing one or more teeth; however, an appropriate radiographic examination may reveal a supernumerary tooth interfering with normal tooth eruption (Fig. 17-5). When a supernumerary tooth is erupted and clinically evident, it is commonly positioned outside the normal arch because of space restriction.

Radiographic features. The radiographic features of the supernumerary tooth may vary from normal-appearing tooth structure to a conical tooth form and, in extreme cases, to grossly deformed tooth structure. The size varies but usually is smaller than the surrounding normal dentition. The supernumerary tooth is easily identified by counting and identifying all the teeth. The supernumerary tooth can interfere with normal eruption; therefore the radiograph often reveals an unerupted permanent tooth in close proximity to the supernumerary tooth. Radiographs may reveal supernumerary teeth in the deciduous dentition (Fig. 17-6) after 3 or 4 years of age, when the deciduous teeth have formed. They may be detected in the permanent dentition of children older than 9 to 12 years.

Care must be taken not to miss supernumerary teeth in the panoramic image, especially when the image of the tooth is distorted as a result of the position of the tooth outside the focal trough, for instance in the palate. Besides the periapical intraoral examination, occlusal radiographs aid in determining the location and number of unerupted supernumerary teeth.

Differential diagnosis. Multiple supernumerary teeth have been associated with a number of syndromes. For

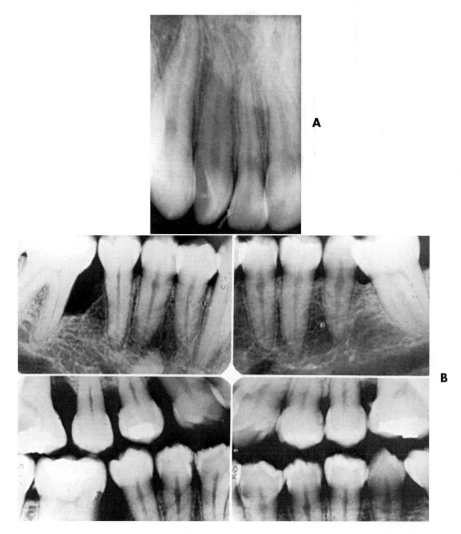

FIG. **17-4** Supernumerary or supplemental lateral incisors, **A,** and premolars, **B.** Note the presence of four mandibular left premolars.

instance, multiple teeth, especially bicuspids, have been associated with cleidocranial dysplasia (see Chapter 28). Supernumerary teeth have also been reported in Gardner's syndrome (see Chapter 20).

Management. The management of supernumerary teeth depends on many factors, including their potential effect on the developing normal dentition, their position and number, and the complications that may result from surgical intervention. If they erupt, they can cause malalignment of the normal dentition. Those that remain in the jaws may cause root resorption or interfere with the normal eruption sequence. Follicles of unerupted supernumerary teeth occasionally develop into dentigerous cysts. All of the preceding factors in-

fluence the decision to either remove a supernumerary tooth or keep it under observation.

Missing Teeth
Synonyms. *Hypodontia, oligodontia,* and *anodontia*

Definition. The expression of developmentally missing teeth may range from the absence of one or a few teeth *(hypodontia),* to the absence of numerous teeth *(oligodontia),* to the failure of all teeth to develop *(anodontia).* Developmentally missing teeth may also be the result of numerous independent pathologic mechanisms that can affect the orderly formation of the dental lamina (e.g., orofaciodigital syndrome), failure of a tooth germ to develop at the optimal time, lack of necessary space im-

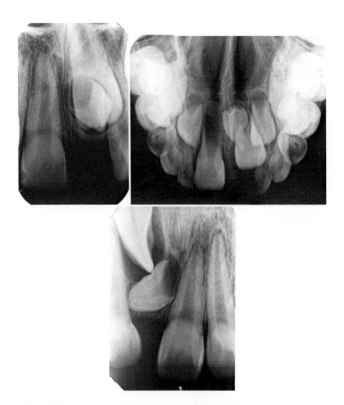

FIG. **17-5** Mesiodens may retard the eruption or cause impaction of permanent teeth.

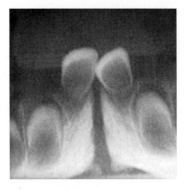

FIG. **17-6** Supernumerary primary central incisors that erupted soon after birth. Note the open mandibular suture, normal for an infant.

posed by a malformed jaw, and a genetically determined disproportion between tooth mass and jaw size.

Clinical features. Hypodontia in the permanent dentition, excluding third molars, is found in 3% to 10% of the population. Hypodontia is more frequently found in Asians and Native Americans. Although missing primary teeth are relatively uncommon, when one tooth

is missing, it is usually a maxillary incisor. The most commonly missing teeth are third molars, second premolars (Fig. 17-7), and maxillary lateral and mandibular central incisors. The absence may be either unilateral or bilateral. Children who have developmentally missing teeth tend to have more than one absent and more than one morphologic group (incisors, premolars, and molars) involved.

Radiographic features. Missing teeth are recognized by identifying and counting the existing teeth. However, it must be kept in mind that the development of teeth may vary markedly among patients. Eruption of some teeth may be developmentally delayed by a number of years after the established time (especially mandibular second bicuspids) and others may show evidence of development as late as a year after the contralateral tooth.

Differential diagnosis. A tooth may be considered to be developmentally missing when it cannot be discerned clinically or radiographically and no history exists of its extraction. Anodontia or oligodontia frequently occurs in patients with ectodermal dysplasia (Fig. 17-8). This inherited disorder results in the absence of at least two ectodermally derived structures, such as sweat glands, hair, skin, nails, and teeth. The severity of the condition is variable and may result in multiple missing teeth and malformed teeth, often having a conical shape or a notable decrease in size. Many other syndromes and conditions may interfere with the development of teeth.

Management. Missing teeth, abnormal occlusion, or altered facial appearance may cause some patients psychologic distress. If the extent of hypodontia is mild, the associated changes may likewise be slight and manageable by orthodontics. In more severe cases restorative, implant, and prosthetic procedures can be undertaken.

SIZE OF TEETH

A positive correlation exists between tooth size (mesiodistal diameter $\times$ buccolingual diameter) and body height. Males also have larger primary and permanent teeth than females. Beyond these normal variations, however, individuals may occasionally develop unusually large or small teeth.

Macrodontia
Definition. In macrodontia the teeth are larger than normal. When the teeth are of normal size but occur in smaller than normal jaws, the condition is relative macrodontia. Macrodontia may rarely affect the entire

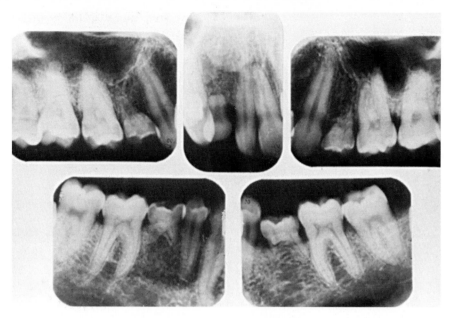

FIG. **17-7**   Developmental absence of all maxillary premolars and both mandibular second premolars. Note the retention of the maxillary primary canine as a result of the posterior position of the maxillary permanent canine.

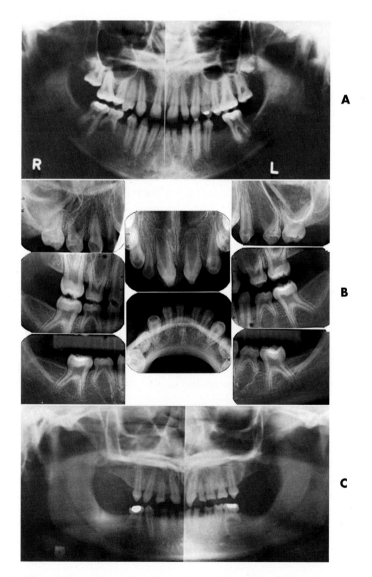

FIG. **17-8**   **A, B,** and **C** are examples of ectodermal dysplasia displaying various degrees of missing and malformed teeth.

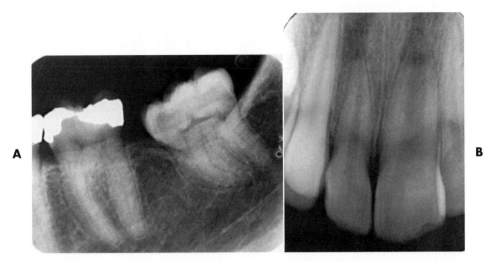

FIG. **17-9**   *Macrodontia is a condition that results in enlarged teeth.* **A,** The macrodont molar shows an increased mesiodistal dimension. **B,** The macrodont central incisor shows enlargement of both its mesiodistal and longitudinal dimension. (**A** courtesy B. Gratt, DDS, Los Angeles.)

dentition, but more commonly it involves a group of teeth, individual contralateral teeth, or a single tooth (Fig. 17-9). The presence of a hemangioma (either intraosseous or in the soft tissues) can result in an increase in the size and advanced development of adjacent teeth. Also localized true macrodontia can occur in hemihypertrophy of the face. True generalized macrodontia may also occur with pituitary giantism. The cause of macrodontia is unknown.

Clinical features.   The large size of the teeth is apparent on clinical examination. Associated crowding, malocclusion, or impaction may occur.

Radiographic features.   Radiographs reveal the increased size of both erupted and unerupted macrodont teeth. The crowding may cause impaction of other teeth. The shape of the tooth is usually normal, but some cases may exhibit a mildly distorted morphology.

Differential diagnosis.   The macrodont may resemble gemination or fusion. When fusion occurs there is a missing tooth. In gemination all the teeth may be present and often evidence exists of a division or cleft of the coronal or root segment of the tooth. However, the differentiation between these three conditions may not influence the treatment provided.

Management.   In most cases macrodontia does not require treatment. Orthodontic treatment may be necessary, however, in the case of malocclusion.

Microdontia

Definition.   In microdontia the involved teeth are smaller than normal. As with macrodontia, microdontia may involve all the teeth or be limited to a single tooth or group of teeth. Relative microdontia can also occur. In this condition normal-sized teeth develop in an individual with large jaws. Generalized microdontia is extremely rare, although it does occur in some patients with pituitary dwarfism. Supernumerary teeth are frequently microdont. Also the lateral incisors and third molars, which often are developmentally missing, may be small.

Clinical features.   The involved teeth are noticeably small and may have altered morphology. Microdont molars may have altered shape—from five to four cusps in mandibular molars and from four to three in upper molars (Fig. 17-10). Microdont lateral incisors are also smaller and peg-shaped (Fig. 17-11).

Radiographic features.   The shape of these small teeth may be normal, but more frequently they are malformed.

Differential diagnosis.   The recognition of small teeth indicates the diagnosis. The number and distribution of microdonts may also suggest consideration of syndromes (e.g., congenital heart disease, progeria).

Management.   Restorative or prosthetic treatment may be considered to create a more normal-appearing tooth, especially when considering esthetic concerns in the anterior dentition.

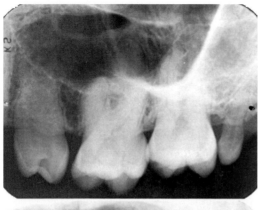

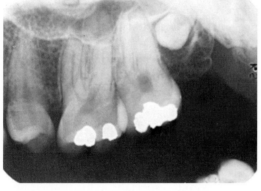

FIG. **17-10** Microdontia of the maxillary third molars, showing reduction in both the size and number of cusps.

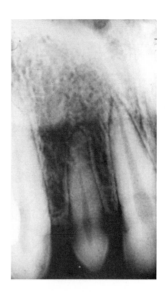

FIG. **17-11** Microdontia of the maxillary lateral incisor results in a characteristic peg-shaped deformity.

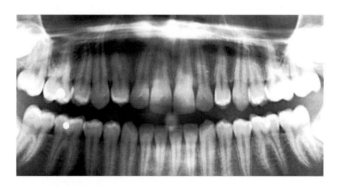

FIG. **17-12** A cropped panoramic image demonstrating bilateral transposition of the maxillary canines and first bicuspids.

ERUPTION OF TEETH

Transposition

Definition. Transposition is the condition in which two teeth have exchanged positions.

Clinical features. The most frequently transposed teeth are the permanent canine and first premolar (more often than the lateral incisor). Second premolars infrequently lie between first and second molars. The transposition of central and lateral incisors is rare. Transposition in the primary dentition has not been reported. It can occur with hypodontia, supernumerary teeth, or the persistence of a deciduous predecessor.

Radiographic features. Radiographs reveal transposition when the teeth are not in their usual sequence in the dental arch (Fig. 17-12).

Differential diagnosis. Transposed teeth are usually easily recognized.

Management. Transposed teeth are frequently altered prosthetically to improve function and esthetics.

ALTERED MORPHOLOGY OF TEETH

Fusion

Synonym. *Synodontia*

Definition. Fusion of teeth results from the combining of adjacent tooth germs, resulting in union of the developing teeth. Some authors believe that fusion results when two tooth germs develop so close together that as they grow, they contact and fuse before calcification. Others contend that a physical force or pressure generated during development causes contact of adjacent tooth buds. The genetic basis for the anomaly is probably autosomal dominant with reduced penetrance. Males and females experience fusion in equal numbers, and the incidence is higher in Asians and Native Americans.

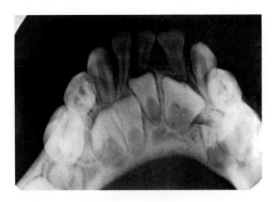

FIG. **17-13** Fusion of the central and lateral incisors in both the primary and the permanent dentition. Note the reduction in number of teeth and the increased width of the fused tooth mass.

Clinical features. Fusion usually causes a reduced number of teeth in the arch. It occurs in deciduous and permanent dentitions, although it is more common between deciduous teeth. When a deciduous canine and lateral incisor fuse, the corresponding permanent lateral incisor may be absent. Fusion is more common in anterior teeth of both the permanent and deciduous dentition (Fig. 17-13). Fusion may be total or partial depending on the stage of odontogenesis and the proximity of the developing teeth. The result can vary from a single tooth of about normal size to a tooth of nearly twice the normal size. A bifid crown may exist, or two recognizable teeth may be joined by dentin or enamel. The crowns of fused teeth usually appear to be large and single, or an inciso-cervical groove of varying depth or a bifid crown occurs.

Radiographic features. Radiographs disclose the unusual shape or size of the entire tooth. The true nature and extent of the union are frequently more evident on the radiograph than can be determined by clinical examination. Fused teeth may show an unusual configuration of the pulp chamber, root canal, or crown.

Differential diagnosis. The differential diagnosis for fused teeth includes gemination and macrodontia. Fusion may be differentiated from gemination due to the reduced number of teeth, except in an unusual case, in which the fusion is between a supernumerary tooth and a normal tooth. The differentiation is usually academic because little difference exists in the treatment provided.

Management. The management of a case of fusion depends on which teeth are involved, the degree of fusion, and the morphologic result. If the affected teeth are de-

ciduous, they may be retained as they are. If the clinician contemplates extraction, it is important first to determine whether the succedaneous teeth are present. In the case of fused secondary teeth, the fused crowns may be reshaped with a restoration that mimics two independent crowns. The morphology of fused teeth requires radiographic evaluation before they are reshaped. Endodontic therapy may be necessary and perhaps may be difficult or impossible if the root canals are of unusual shape. In some cases it is most prudent to leave the teeth as they are.

Concrescence

Definition. Concrescence occurs when the roots of two or more teeth are united by cementum. It may involve either primary or secondary teeth. Although its cause is unknown, many authorities suspect that space restriction during development, local trauma, excessive occlusal force, or local infection after development plays an important role. If the condition occurs during development, it is called *true concrescence;* if later, it is *acquired concrescence.*

Clinical features. Maxillary molars are the teeth most frequently involved, especially a third molar and a supernumerary tooth. Involved teeth may fail to erupt or may erupt incompletely. The sexes are equally affected.

Radiographic features. A radiographic examination may not always distinguish between concrescence and teeth that are in close contact or are simply superimposed (Fig. 17-14). When the condition is suspected on a radiograph and extraction of one of the teeth is being considered, additional projections at different angles may be obtained to better delineate the condition.

Differential diagnosis. It is usually impossible to determine radiographically with certainty whether the teeth whose root images are superimposed are actually joined. Is the periodontal membrane space continuous around each root? If the roots are joined, it may not be possible to tell whether the union is by cementum or by dentin (fusion).

Management. Concrescence affects treatment only when the decision is made to remove one or both of the involved teeth. This condition complicates the extraction. The clinician should warn the patient that an effort to remove one may result in the unintended and simultaneous removal of the other.

Gemination
Synonym. *Twinning*

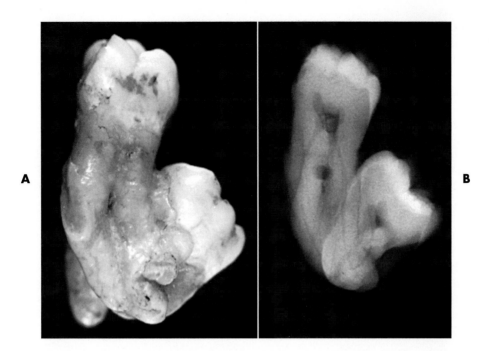

FIG. **17-14** **A,** Concrescence occurs when two teeth are joined by a mass of cementum. **B,** Extraction of one tooth may result in the unintended removal of the second because cementum is often not well visualized radiographically. (Courtesy R. Kienholz, DDS, Dallas, Tex.)

Definition. Gemination is a rare anomaly that arises when the tooth bud of a single tooth attempts to divide. The result may be an invagination of the crown, with partial division, or in rare cases complete division throughout the crown and root, producing identical structures. Complete twinning results in a normal tooth plus a supernumerary tooth in the arch. Its cause is unknown, but some evidence exists that it is familial.

Clinical features. Gemination more frequently affects the primary teeth, but it may occur in both dentitions, usually in the incisor region. It can be detected clinically after the anomalous tooth erupts. The occurrence in males and females is about equal. The enamel or dentin of geminated teeth may be hypoplastic or hypocalcified.

Radiographic features. Radiographs reveal the altered shape of the hard tissue and pulp chamber of the germinated tooth. Radiopaque enamel outlines the clefts in the crowns and invaginations and thus accentuates them. The pulp chamber is usually single and enlarged and may be partially divided (Fig. 17-15). In the rare case of premolar gemination the tooth image suggests a molar with an enlarged crown and two roots.

Differential diagnosis. The differential diagnosis of gemination includes fusion. If the malformed tooth is

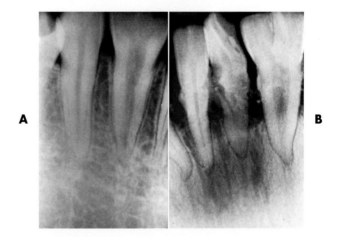

FIG. **17-15** **A,** Gemination of a mandibular lateral incisor showing bifurcation of the crown with a single enlarged pulp chamber. **B,** Gemination of a mandibular central incisor with two crowns and a common root.

counted as one, individuals with gemination have a normal tooth count, whereas those with fusion are seen to be missing a tooth.

Management. A geminated tooth in the anterior region may compromise arch esthetics. Areas of hypoplasia and invagination lines or areas of coronal separation represent caries-susceptible sites that may in time result in pulpal infection. Affected teeth can cause malocclusion and lead to periodontal disease. Consequently the affected tooth may be removed (especially if it is deciduous), the crown(s) may be restored or reshaped, or the tooth may be left untreated and periodically examined to preclude the development of complications. Before treatment is initiated on primary teeth, the status of the succedaneous teeth and configuration of their root canals should be determined radiographically.

Taurodontism

Definition. Taurodont teeth have longitudinally enlarged pulp chambers. The crown is of normal shape and size, but the body is elongated and the roots are short. The pulp chamber extends from a normal position in the crown throughout the length of the extended body, leading to an increased distance between the cementoenamel junction and the furcation. Tau-

rodontism may occur in either the permanent or primary dentition (or both). Although some evidence of the trait can be seen in any tooth, it is usually fully expressed in the molars and less often in the premolars. Single or multiple teeth may show taurodont features, unilaterally or bilaterally and in any combination of teeth or quadrants.

Clinical features. Because the body and roots of taurodont teeth lie below the alveolar margin, the distinguishing features of these teeth are not recognizable clinically.

Radiographic features. The distinctive morphology of taurodont teeth is quite apparent on radiographs. The peculiar feature is an extension of the rectangular pulp chamber into the elongated body of the tooth (Fig. 17-16). The shortened roots and root canals are a function of the long body and normal length of the tooth. The size of the crown is normal.

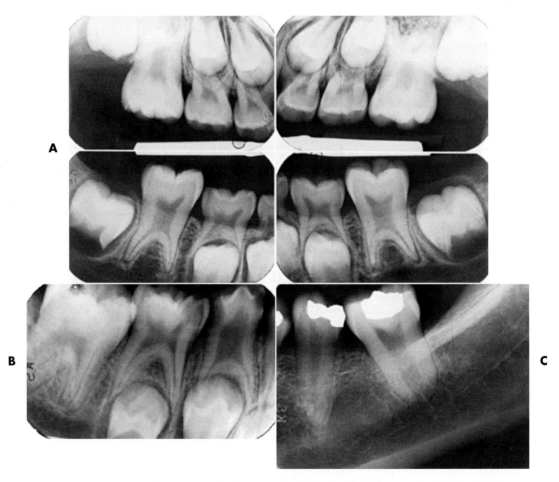

FIG. **17-16** Taurodontia, revealed as an enlarged pulp chamber, in all permanent first molars, **A,** in a primary first molar, **B,** and in a permanent first molar, **C.**

Differential diagnosis. The image of the taurodont tooth is characteristic and easily recognized radiographically. The developing molar may appear similar; however, the identification of the wide apical foramina and incompletely formed roots helps in the differential diagnosis. Taurodontism has been reported with greater frequency in trisomy 21 syndrome.

Management. Taurodont teeth do not require treatment.

Dilaceration

Definition. Dilaceration is a disturbance in tooth formation that produces a sharp bend or curve in the tooth. One of the oldest concepts is that it is probably the result of mechanical trauma to the calcified portion of a partially formed tooth. Although this may occur, especially to the maxillary incisors, most are likely to be a true developmental anomaly. The angular distortion may occur anywhere in the crown or root.

Clinical features. Most cases of radicular dilaceration are not recognized clinically. If the dilaceration is so pronounced that the tooth does not erupt, the only clinical indication of the defect is a missing tooth. If the defect is in the crown of an erupted tooth, it may be readily recognized as an angular distortion (Fig. 17-17).

Radiographic features. Radiographs provide the best means of detecting a radicular dilaceration. The condition occurs most often in permanent maxillary premo-

lars. One or more teeth may be affected. If the roots bend mesially or distally, the condition is clearly apparent on a periapical radiograph (Fig. 17-18). When the roots are bent buccally (labially) or lingually, the central ray passes approximately parallel with the deflected portion of the root. The dilacerated portion then appears at the apical end of the unaltered root as a rounded opaque area with a dark shadow in its central region cast by the apical foramen and root canal (an appearance like a bull's-eye). The periodontal ligament (PDL) space around this dilacerated portion may be seen as a radiolucent halo (Fig. 17-19), and the radiopacity of this segment of root is greater than the rest of the root. In some cases, especially in the maxilla, the geometry of the projections may preclude the recognition of a dilaceration.

Differential diagnosis. Occasionally dilacerated roots are difficult to differentiate from fused roots, condensing osteitis, or a dense bone island. They can usually be

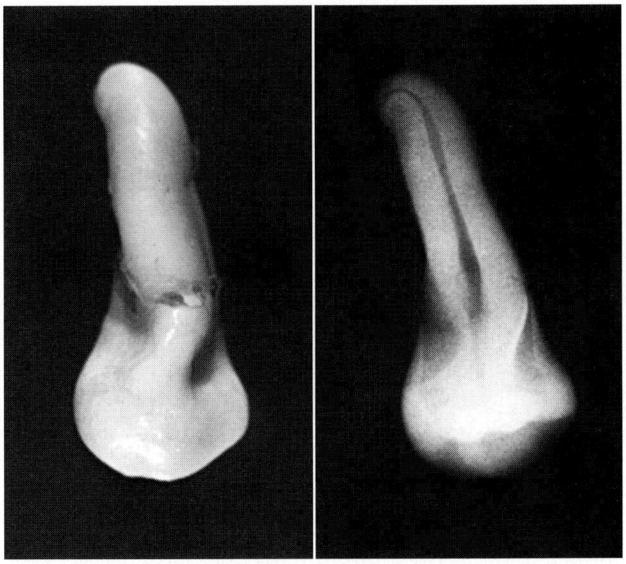

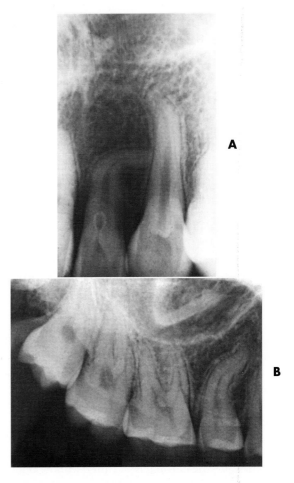

FIG. **17-17** **A,** Dilaceration of the crown may be readily recognized clinically. **B,** Radiograph of the specimen in **A.** (Courtesy Dr. R. Kienholz, Dallas, Tex.)

FIG. **17-18** **A,** Dilaceration of the root of a maxillary lateral incisor (note the coincidental dens in dente), and **B,** dilaceration of the root of a maxillary second premolar.

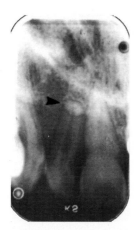

FIG. **17-19** *Dilacerated root.* The apical portion of the root is bent buccally or lingually into the plane of the central ray. Note the halo in the apical region, produced by the PDL space *(arrow).*

identified, however, by obtaining radiographs exposed from different angles.

Management. The dilacerated root generally does not require treatment because it provides adequate support. If it must be extracted for some other reason, its removal can be complicated, especially if the surgeon is not prepared with a preoperative radiograph. In contrast, dilacerated crowns are frequently restored with a crown to improve esthetics and function.

Dens in Dente

Synonym. *Dens invaginatus, dilated odontome,* and *gestant odontome*

Definition. Dens in dente results from an infolding of the outer surface into the interior of a tooth. This can occur in either the crown or the root during tooth development and may involve the pulp chamber or root canal, resulting in deformity of either the crown or the root. These anomalies are seen most often in tooth crowns. Coronal invaginations usually originate from an anomalous infolding of the enamel organ into the dental papilla. In a mature tooth the result is a fold of hard tissue within the tooth characterized by enamel lining the fold (Fig. 17-20). The most extreme form of this anomaly is referred to as the *dilated odontome.*

When dens in dente involves a root (radicular dens invaginatus), it appears to be the result of an invagination of Hertwig's epithelial root sheath. This results in an accentuation of the normal longitudinal root groove. In contrast to the coronal type (lined with enamel), the radicular-type defect is lined with cementum. If the invagination retracts and is cut off, it leaves a longitudinal structure of cementum, bone, and remnants of PDL within the pulp canal. The structure often extends for

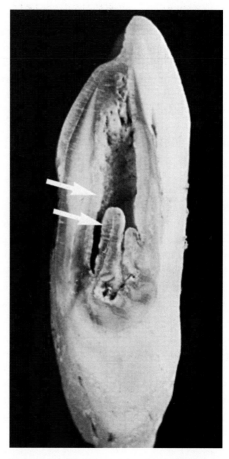

FIG. **17-20** Dens in dente is characterized by an infolding of enamel into the tooth. This sectioned canine with a dens in dente shows enamel *(arrows)* folded into the tooth's interior.

most of the root length. In other cases the root sheath may bud off a saclike invagination that produces a circumscribed cementum defect in the root. Mandibular first premolars and second molars are especially prone to develop the radicular variety of this invagination anomaly.

Little difference in the frequency of occurrence exists among white and Asian people. If all grades of expression of invagination, mild to severe, are included, the condition is found in approximately 5% of these two racial groups. The condition appears to be rare in blacks. No sexual predilection exists. Although specific mode of inheritance seems to fit all the data, a high degree of inheritability seems to exist.

Clinical features. Coronal dens in dente may be identified clinically as a pit at the incisal edge or the cingulum. The pit in the cingulum may be particularly broad and deep, especially when these features occur in the lateral incisor. Often the lingual marginal ridges or cingula are prominent. In most cases, however, the dens in dente is not large, and crown morphology appears nor-

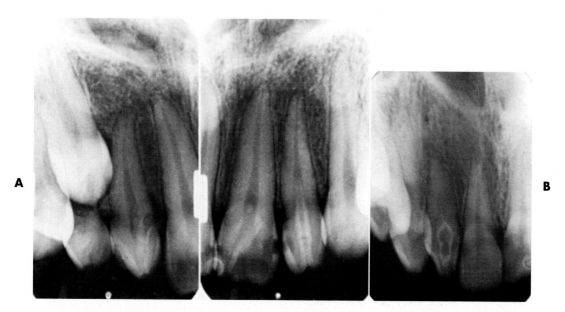

FIG. **17-21** *Dens in dente is seen radiographically as a radiopaque infolding of enamel into the tooth's pulp chamber.* **A,** Involvement of both maxillary lateral incisors. **B,** Altered coronal morphology.

mal. Dens in dente occurs most frequently in the permanent maxillary lateral incisors, followed by (in decreasing frequency) the maxillary central incisors, premolars, and canines and less often in the posterior teeth. Invagination is rare in the crowns of mandibular teeth and in deciduous teeth. It occurs symmetrically in about half the cases. Concomitant involvement of the central and lateral incisors may occur.

The clinical importance of dens invaginatus results from the risk of pulpal disease. Although enamel lines the coronal defect, it is frequently thin, often of poor quality, and even missing in some areas. Furthermore, the cavity is usually separated from the pulp chamber by a relatively thin wall and opens into the oral environment through a narrow constriction. The pit is often difficult to keep clean, and consequently it offers conditions favorable for the development of caries. Such carious lesions are difficult to detect clinically and will rapidly involve the pulp. In addition, sometimes fine canals extend between the invagination and the pulp chamber, resulting in pulpal disease even in the absence of caries.

Radiographic features. Most cases of dens in dente are discovered radiographically. The infolding of the enamel lining is more radiopaque than the surrounding tooth structure and can easily be identified (Fig. 17-21). Less frequently the radicular invaginations appear as poorly defined, slightly radiolucent structures running longitudinally within the root. The defects, especially the coronal variety, may vary in size and shape from

small and superficial to large and deep. If a coronal invagination is extensive, the crown is almost invariably malformed; and when the crown is malformed, the apical foramen is usually wide (Fig. 17-22). A frequent cause of an open apical foramen is the cessation of root development that occurs as a result of death of the pulpal tissue. In the most severe form (dilated odontome) the tooth is severely deformed, having a circular or oval shape with a radiolucent interior (Fig. 17-23). Dens in dente can be identified in the radiographic image even before the tooth erupts.

Differential diagnosis. The appearance and usual occurrence in incisors are so characteristic that, once recognized, little probability exists that the anomaly will be confused with another condition.

Management. Although it is important to evaluate every case individually, the placement of a prophylactic restoration in the defect is typically the treatment of choice and should ensure a normal life span for the tooth. Failure of early identification and hence treatment may result in premature tooth loss or the requirement for root canal therapy.

Dens Invaginatus
Synonym. *Leong's premolar*

Definition. In contrast to the dens in dente, dens invaginatus is the result of an outfolding of the enamel organ. The result is an enamel-covered tubercle, usually

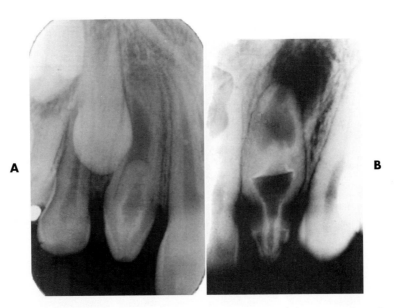

FIG. **17-22**   Severe malformations of dens in dente may result in open apices, **A,** and often is associated with periapical inflammatory lesions, **B.**

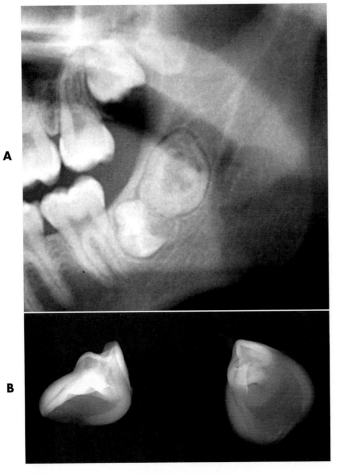

FIG. **17-23**   **A,** A dilated odontome is positioned just posterior to the developing mandibular third molar in this panoramic film. **B,** The specimen radiographs represent two views of a dilated odontome.

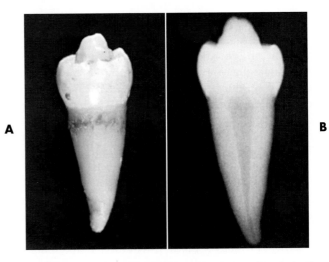

FIG. **17-24**   **A,** Dens invaginatus, seen as a tubercle in the mandibular premolar. **B,** Radiograph of the specimen. (Courtesy Dr. R. Kienholz, Dallas, Tex.)

in or near the middle of the occlusal surface of a premolar or occasionally a molar (Fig. 17-24). Canines are rarely affected. The frequency of occurrence of dens invaginatus is highest in Asians and Native Americans.

Clinical features.   Clinically, dens invaginatus appears as a tubercle of enamel on the occlusal surface of the affected tooth. A polyp-like protuberance exists in the central groove or lingual ridge of a buccal cusp. Dens invaginatus may occur bilaterally and usually in the mandible. The tubercle often has a dentin core, and a very slender pulp horn frequently extends into the invagination. After the tubercle is worn by the opposing teeth, it appears as a small circular facet with a small black pit in the center. Wear, fracture, or indiscriminate surgical removal of this tubercle may precipitate a pulpal infection. In rare cases a microscopic direct communication may occur between the pulp and the oral cavity through this tubercle. In these instances the pulp may become infected shortly after eruption.

Radiographic features. The radiographic image shows an extension of a dentin tubercle on the occlusal surface unless the tubercle is already worn down. The dentin core is usually covered with opaque enamel. A fine pulp horn may extend into the tubercle, but this may not be visible radiographically. If the tubercle has been worn to the point of pulpal exposure or has fractured, pulpal necrosis may result (Fig. 17-25). This is indicated by an open apical foramen and periapical radiolucency.

Differential diagnosis. The clinical and radiographic appearance may be characteristic or may be difficult to visualize if the tubercle has been worn down to the occlusal surface.

Management. If the tubercle causes any occlusal interference or shows evidence of marked abrasion, it should probably be removed under aseptic conditions and the pulp capped, if necessary. Such a precaution may preclude pulpal exposure and infection as the result of accidental fracture or advanced abrasion.

Amelogenesis Imperfecta

Definition. Amelogenesis imperfecta is a developmental disturbance that interferes with normal enamel formation. It leads to marked changes in the enamel of all or nearly all the teeth in both dentitions. Most forms are autosomal dominant or recessive, but two types are X-linked. It is not related to any time or period of enamel development or any clinically demonstrable alteration (disease or dietary abnormality) in other tissues. The enamel may lack the normal prismatic structure, being laminated throughout its thickness or at the periphery. As a result these teeth are more resistant to decay. The dentin and root form are usually normal. Eruption of the affected teeth is often delayed, and a tendency for impaction exists. Although at least 14 variants of the condition have been described, four general types have characteristic clinical or radiographic appearances: a hypoplastic type, a hypomaturation type, a hypocalcified type, and a hypomaturation-hypocalcified type associated with taurodontism.

Clinical features

Hypoplasia. As a result of some defect in ameloblasts, the enamel of the affected teeth fails to develop to its

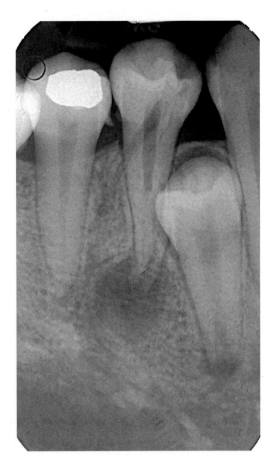

FIG. **17-25** A mandibular first bicuspid with a dens invaginatus and apical rarefying osteitis.

normal thickness. It is so thin that the dentin shows through and imparts a yellowish-brown color to the tooth. In the various hypoplastic forms the enamel may be pitted, rough, or smooth and glossy. The crowns of the teeth may not have the usual contour of enamel but rather have a roughly square shape. The reduced enamel thickness also causes the teeth to be undersized, with lack of contact between adjacent teeth (Fig. 17-26). The occlusal surfaces of the posterior teeth are relatively flat with low cusps. This is a result of the attrition of cusp tips that were initially low and not fully formed. An anterior open bite may be noted.

Hypomaturation. In the hypomaturation form of amelogenesis imperfecta the enamel has a normal thickness but a mottled appearance. It is softer than normal (density comparable to dentin) and may crack away from the crown. Its color may range from clear to cloudy white, yellow, or brown. In one form of hypomaturation the teeth appear to be snow capped (with white opaque enamel).

Hypocalcification. Hypocalcification of teeth is more common than the hypoplastic variety of amelogenesis imperfecta. The crowns of the teeth are normal in size and shape when they erupt because the

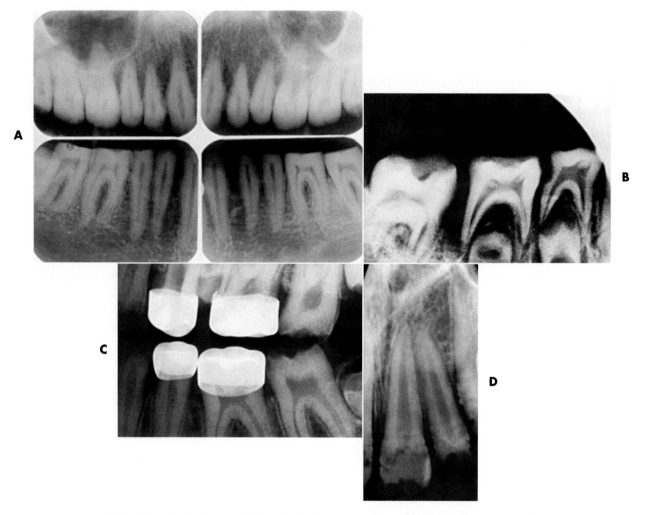

FIG. **17-26**   **A,** Amelogenesis imperfecta (generalized hypoplastic form) recognized by the complete absence of enamel. **B,** Primary and permanent dentition with amelogenesis imperfecta. **C** and **D,** Severe mottling of the enamel surface.

enamel is of regular thickness (Fig. 17-27). However, because the enamel is poorly mineralized (less dense than dentin), it starts to fracture away shortly after it comes into function. This creates clinically recognizable defects. The soft enamel abrades rapidly and the softer dentin also wears down rapidly, resulting in a grossly worn tooth, sometimes to the level of the gingiva. An explorer point under pressure can penetrate the soft enamel. Yet caries in these worn teeth is unusual. The hypocalcified enamel has increased permeability and becomes stained and darkened. The teeth of a young person with generalized hypomineralization of the enamel are frequently dark brown from food stains.

Hypomaturation/hypocalcification. This classification indicates a combination of hypomaturation and hypocalcification that involves both the permanent and deciduous dentition. If the dominant defect is hypo-

maturation, then the term *hypomaturation-hypocalcification* is used. The enamel is usually mottled and discolored (yellow and brown). The enamel has the same radiopacity as the dentin. When the dominant defect is hypocalcification, the term *hypocalcification-hypomaturation* is used. The appearance of the teeth is similar but the enamel is thin.

Radiographic features. Identification of amelogenesis imperfecta is made primarily by clinical examination. Although this condition manifests radiographically, the radiographic features substantiate the clinical impression. The radiographic signs of *hypoplastic* amelogenesis imperfecta include a square shape of the crown, a relatively thin opaque layer of enamel, and low or absent cusps. The density of the enamel is normal. Pitted enamel appears as sharply localized areas of mottled density, quite different from the image cast by a tooth that is

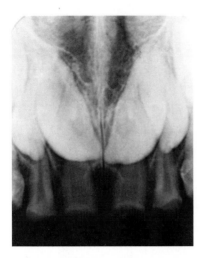

FIG. **17-27** Amelogenesis imperfecta (generalized hypomineralized form). Note the reduced enamel density and the rapid abrasion of the crowns of primary teeth.

normal in shape and density. The *hypomaturation* form demonstrates a normal thickness of the enamel, but its density is the same as that of dentin. In the *hypocalcified* forms the enamel thickness is normal but its density is even less (more radiolucent) than that of dentin. With advanced abrasion, obliteration of the pulp chambers may complicate recognition of the radiographic picture.

Differential diagnosis. If advanced abrasion is present and secondary dentin obliterates the pulp chambers, the radiographic picture of the amelogenesis imperfecta appears similar to that of dentinogenesis imperfecta. However, the presence of bulbous crowns and narrow roots, the relatively normal density of any remaining enamel, and the obliteration of pulp chambers and root canals, in the absence of marked attrition, are characteristic of dentinogenesis imperfecta (see the following section) and should distinguish it from amelogenesis imperfecta.

Management. Appropriate treatment for amelogenesis imperfecta is restoration of the esthetics and function of the affected teeth.

Dentinogenesis Imperfecta
Synonym. *Hereditary opalescent dentin**

---

*Although the terms *dentinogenesis imperfecta* and *hereditary opalescent dentin* have been used interchangeably for more than 40 years, evidence suggests they are two distinct entities. Dentinogenesis imperfecta is the dental defect that accompanies osteogenesis imperfecta, whereas hereditary opalescent dentin is an isolated defect. Because these conditions share common clinical, radiographic, and dental features, the author refers to the defect for convenience as dentinogenesis imperfecta, which is the term that most dentists associate with this condition.

Definition. Dentinogenesis imperfecta is a developmental disturbance primarily of the dentin. Enamel may be thinner than normal in this condition. Dentinogenesis imperfecta is an autosomal dominant disturbance of high penetrance and occurs with equal frequency in both sexes. Both the deciduous and permanent dentition may show this defect. It usually affects whites.

Two types of dentinogenesis imperfecta exist. *type I* is associated with osteogenesis imperfecta (see following description). The tooth roots and pulp chambers are generally small and underdeveloped. The lesion affects the primary dentition more severely than the permanent teeth. *type II* lesions are similar to type I lesions but affect only the dentin without any skeletal defects. The expression of type II lesions is variable, and occasionally individuals show enlarged pulp chambers in the primary teeth.

Clinical features. The appearance of the teeth with dentinogenesis imperfecta is characteristic. They show a high degree of amberlike translucency and a variety of colors from yellow to blue-gray. The colors change according to whether the teeth are observed by transmitted light or reflected light. The enamel easily fractures from the teeth and the crowns wear readily. In adults they may frequently wear down to the gingiva. The exposed dentin becomes stained. The color of the abraded teeth may change to dark brown or even black. Some patients demonstrate an anterior open bite.

Radiographic features. The images of the crowns in patients with dentinogenesis imperfecta are usually of normal size, but a constriction of the cervical portion of the tooth gives the crown a bulbous appearance. Radiographs may reveal slight to marked attrition of the occlusal surface. The roots are usually short and slender. Types I and II show partial or complete obliteration of the pulp chambers. Early in development, the teeth may appear to have large pulp chambers, but these are quickly obliterated by the formation of dentin. Ultimately the root canals may be absent or threadlike (Fig. 17-28). Occasional periapical radiolucencies are seen in association with sound teeth without evidence of pulpal involvement, which may occur from microscopic communication between residual pulp and the oral cavity. These lesions do not occur as frequently as in dentin dysplasia. The architecture of the bone in the maxilla and mandible is normal.

Differential diagnosis. See the following section on the differential diagnosis of dentin dysplasia.

Management. The placement of prosthetic crowns on the affected teeth is usually unsuccessful unless they have good root support. The teeth should not be ex-

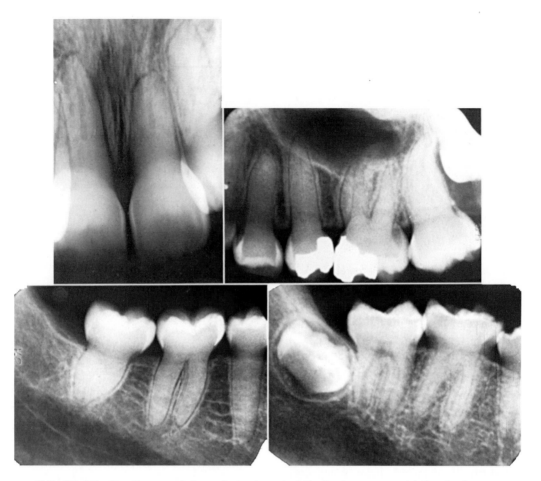

FIG. **17-28**   Dentinogenesis imperfecta characteristically shows a constriction in the cervical portion of the root, a bulbous crown, short roots, and a reduced size of the pulp chamber and root canals.

tracted from patients 5 to 15 years of age. It is generally preferable to place full overdentures on the teeth to prevent alveolar resorption. In adults extraction of the teeth and their replacement can be recommended. Alveolectomy may be required in these latter cases.

Osteogenesis Imperfecta

Osteogenesis imperfecta is a hereditary disorder characterized by osseous fractures. The pathogenesis is believed to be an inborn error in the synthesis of type I collagen, which results in brittle bones. It is usually transmitted as an autosomal dominant trait. Patients may have blue sclera, wormian bones (bones in skull sutures), skeletal deformities, and progressive osteopenia. Dentinogenesis imperfecta is found in approximately 25% of cases. In addition, oral findings may include class III malocclusions and an increased incidence of impacted first and second molars.

Dentin Dysplasia

Definition.   Dentin dysplasia is an autosomal dominant trait that resembles opalescent dentin. It is rarer than

dentinogenesis imperfecta (1:100,000 compared with 1:8000). Two types have been described, type I (radicular) and type II (coronal) dentin dysplasia. In type I disease, the most marked alterations are found in the appearance of the roots. In type II disease, changes in the crown are most clearly seen in the altered shape of the pulp chambers.

Clinical features.   Clinically, teeth with dentin dysplasia have characteristic features. In the radicular pattern (type I) the teeth have mostly normal color and shape in both dentitions. Occasionally a slight bluish-brown translucency is apparent. Teeth in patients with the type I defect are often malaligned in the arch, and patients may describe drifting and state that the teeth exfoliate with little or no trauma. In the coronal pattern (type II) the crowns of primary teeth appear to be of the same color, size, and contour as those in dentinogenesis imperfecta. The permanent teeth are normal in these respects. Apparently no other distinctive clinical features exist. Although not universally accepted, reports exist that primary teeth rapidly abrade.

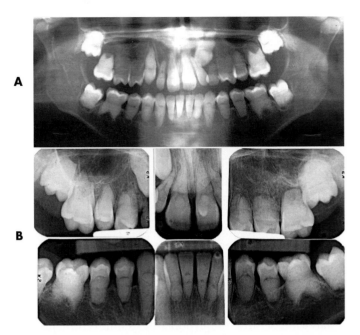

FIG. **17-29** A panoramic film, **A,** and periapical f ms, **B,** of the same case show the short and poorly developed roots, obliterated pulp chambers and root canals, and periapical inflammatory lesions associated with dentin dysplasia, type I (radicular).

Radiographic features. In *type I* (radicular dentin dysplasia) the roots of all teeth, primary and permanent, are either short or abnormally shaped (Fig. 17-29). The roots of primary teeth may be only spicules. The pulp chambers and root canals completely fill in before eruption. The extent of obliteration of the pulp chambers and canals is variable. In addition, about 20% of teeth with type I disease have periapical radiolucencies, which are described as either cysts or granulomas. This is likely the result of microscopic communication between the residual pulp and the oral cavity. Association of these periapical radiolucencies with noncarious teeth is an important feature for recognition of this particular entity.

In *type II* (coronal dentin dysplasia), obliteration of the pulp chamber (Fig. 17-30) and reduction in the caliber of the root canals occurs after eruption (at least by 5 or 6 years). These changes are not seen before eruption. As the chambers of the molars are being filled with hypertrophic dentin, the pulp chambers may become flame shaped and may have multiple pulp stones. Occasionally the anterior teeth and premolars develop a pulp chamber that is thistle-tube in shape because of its extension into the root. The roots of the coronal variety are normal in shape and proportions.

Differential diagnosis. The differential diagnosis for dentin dysplasia may include only one other entity, dentinogenesis imperfecta. Because these two condi-

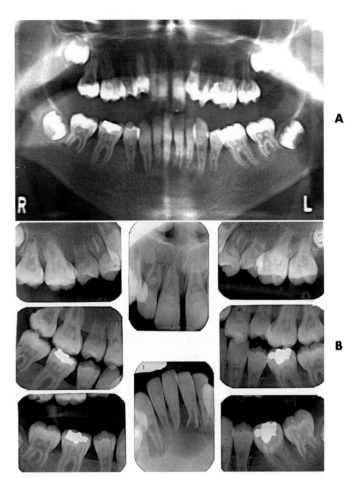

FIG. **17-30** A panoramic film, **A,** and periapical f ms, **B,** of the same case show obliteration of the pulp chamber, reduction in the caliber of root canals, and pulp stones obscuring the flame-shaped pulp chambers associated with dentin dysplasia, type II (coronal dentin dysplasia). Periapical inflammatory lesions are associated with some of the mandibular anterior teeth.

tions seem to form a continuum, their differentiation may be difficult at first. Both entities can produce altered color and occluded pulp chambers. In type II dentin dysplasia, however, the pulp chambers do not fill in before eruption. Also, finding a thistle-tube–shaped pulp chamber in a single-rooted tooth strengthens the probability of dentin dysplasia. In addition, crown size can help distinguish between the two: the teeth in dentinogenesis imperfecta have typical bell-shaped crowns with a constriction in the cervical region, whereas the crowns in dentin dysplasia are usually of normal shape, size, and proportions. If the roots are short and narrow, the condition is likely to be dentinogenesis imperfecta. On the other hand, normal-appearing roots or practically no roots at all should suggest dentin dysplasia. Periapical rarefying osteitis in association with noncarious teeth are more commonly seen in dentin dysplasia.

Management. Teeth with type I dentin dysplasia have such poor root support that prosthetic replacement is about the only practical treatment. On the other hand, teeth that are of normal shape, size, and support (type II) can be crowned if they seem to be rapidly abrading. At the same time the esthetics of discolored anterior teeth can be improved by prosthetic treatment.

Regional Odontodysplasia

Synonyms. *Odontogenesis imperfecta*

Definition. Regional odontodysplasia is a relatively rare condition in which both enamel and dentin are hypoplastic and hypocalcified. The result is localized arrest in tooth development. Typically, regional odontodysplasia affects only a few adjacent teeth in a quad-

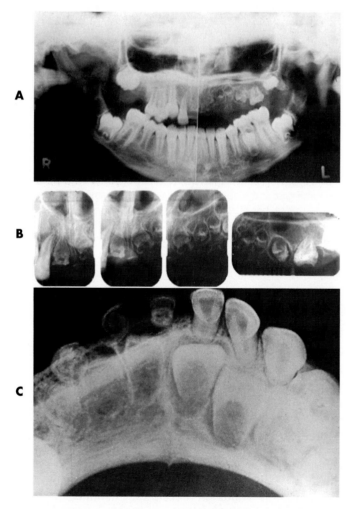

FIG. 17-31 *Odontodysplasia revealing poor mineralization of both enamel and dentin.* **A** and **B,** Note the involvement of the left maxilla. **C,** Involvement of the primary and secondary dentitions also is evident.

rant. They may be either primary or permanent teeth. If the primary teeth are affected, their successors are usually involved. Although many theories exist regarding the etiology of this condition, its cause is unknown.

Clinical features. Teeth affected with regional odontodysplasia are small and mottled brown as a result of staining of the hypocalcified hypoplastic enamel. They are especially susceptible to caries, are brittle, and are subject to fracture and pulpal infection. Central incisors are most often affected, with lateral incisors and canines also occasionally showing the defect (most often in the maxilla). Eruption of the defective teeth is often delayed and in severe cases they may not erupt.

Radiographic features. The radiographic images of teeth with regional odontodysplasia have a ghostlike appearance. The pulp chambers are large and the root canals wide because the hypoplastic dentin is thin, just serving to outline the image of the root (Fig. 17-31). The poorly outlined roots are short. The enamel is, likewise, thin and less dense than usual, sometimes so thin and poorly mineralized that it may not be evident on the radiograph. The tooth is little more than a thin shell of hypoplastic enamel and dentin. Teeth that do not erupt are so hypomineralized and hypoplastic that they appear to be resorbing.

Differential diagnosis. The malformed teeth occasionally seen in one of the expressions of dentinogenesis imperfecta may occasionally be confused with those in regional odontodysplasia. The fact that the dentinogenesis imperfecta trait usually carries a history of familial involvement, however, in contrast to odontodysplasia (which is not hereditary), is an important distinguishing feature. Also the enamel in regional odontodysplasia is obviously hypoplastic, which is not the case in dentinogenesis imperfecta. Finally, only a few teeth of either dentition in an isolated segment of the arch are affected in regional odontodysplasia, whereas the type of dentinogenesis imperfecta that resembles regional odontodysplasia involves all primary teeth.

Management. With the advent of newer restorative materials, it is recommended to retain and restore the affected teeth as much as possible. Uneruptedteeth should be retained during the period of skeletal growth. Severely damaged permanent teeth that become pulpally involved may require removal and replacement.

Enamel Pearl

Synonyms. *Enamel drop, enamel nodule,* and *enameloma*

Definition. The enamel pearl is a small globule of enamel 1 to 3 mm in diameter that occurs on the roots of molars (Fig. 17-32). It is found in about 3% of the population, probably formed by Hertwig's epithelial root sheath before the epithelium loses its enamel-forming potential. Usually only one pearl develops, but occasionally more develop. Enamel pearls may have a core of dentin and rarely a pulp horn extending from the chamber of the host tooth.

Clinical features. Most enamel pearls form below the crest of the gingiva and are not detected during a clinical examination. However, they develop at the trifurcation of a maxillary molar (usually third molar) or the bifurcation of a mandibular molar. Some lie at or just apical to the cementoenamel junction. Those that form on the maxillary molars are usually at the mesial or distal aspect, in contrast to those on the mandibular molars, which are most often buccal or lingual. Usually no clinical symptoms are associated with their presence, although they may predispose to periodontal pocket formation and subsequent periodontal disease.

Radiographic features. The enamel pearl appears smooth, round, and comparable in degree of radiopacity

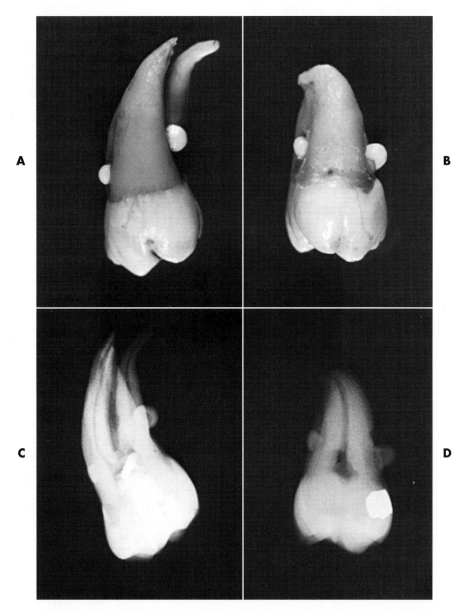

FIG. **17-32**   **A** and **B,** Enamel pearls are small outgrowths of enamel and dentin seen in the furcation area of a tooth. **C** and **D,** Radiographs of these teeth. (**A** to **D** courtesy Dr. R. Kienholz, Dallas, Tex.)

to the enamel covering the crown. Occasionally the dentine casts a small, round, radiolucent shadow in the center of the radiopaque sphere of enamel. If projected over the crown, it may be obscured.

Differential diagnosis. It is possible to mistake an enamel pearl for an isolated piece of calculus or a pulp stone. The differentiation between a pulp stone and an enamel pearl can be made by increasing the vertical angle of projection to move the image of the enamel pearl away from the pulp chamber. If the opacity is calculus, it is usually clinically detectable. Occasionally oblique views of maxillary or mandibular molars may cause superimposition of a portion of the roots in the region of the furcation, producing a density that appears similar to an enamel pearl. In this case, producing another image at a slightly different horizontal angle eliminates this radiopaque region.

Management. As a rule, the recognition that a radiopaque mass superimposed on the tooth is an enamel pearl precludes the necessity for treatment. The clinician can remove the mass if its location at the cementoenamel junction predisposes to periodontal disease. The possibility must always be considered that it may contain a pulp horn.

Talon Cusp

Definition. The talon cusp is an anomalous hyperplasia of the cingulum of a maxillary or mandibular incisor. It results in the formation of a supernumerary cusp. Normal enamel covers the cusp and fuses with the lingual aspect of the tooth. Any developmental grooves that are present may become caries-susceptible areas. The cusp may or may not contain an extension (horn) of the pulp. No apparent racial association exists.

Clinical features. The talon cusp is infrequently encountered. It may be found in either sex and on both primary and permanent incisors. It varies in size from that of a prominent cingulum to that of a cusplike structure extending to the level of the incisal edge. When viewed from its incisal edge, an incisor bearing the cusp is T-shaped with the top of the T representing the incisal edge. Although it usually occurs as an isolated entity, its incidence has been reported to be increased in teeth related to cleft palate syndromes and in association with other anomalies.

Radiographic features. The radiopaque image of a talon cusp is superimposed on that of the crown of the involved incisor (Fig. 17-33). Its outline is smooth, and a layer of normal-appearing enamel is generally distin-

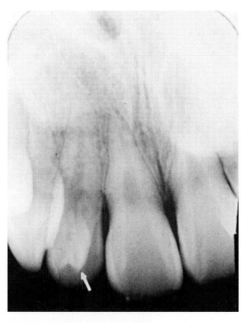

FIG. 17-33 Maxillary lateral incisor bearing a talon cusp *(arrow)*. Note that the tooth also has two enamel invaginations. (Courtesy Dr. R. A. Cederberg, Dallas, Tex.)

guishable. The radiograph may not reveal a pulp horn. The cusp is often apparent radiographically before eruption and may simulate the presence of a supernumerary tooth.

Differential diagnosis. The appearance of a talon cusp is quite distinctive. Although it may not be distinguishable from a supernumerary tooth with a single film, using a second image with either the parallax or the buccal object technique can demonstrate a connection to the tooth.

Management. If developmental grooves are present where the cusp fuses with the lingual surface of the incisor, treatment may be required to prevent the development of decay. If the cusp is large, it may pose an esthetic or occlusal problem. Slowly removing the cusp over a long period may stimulate the formation of secondary dentin and prevent exposure of a pulp horn.

Turner's Hypoplasia
Synonym. *Turner's tooth*

Definition. *Turner's hypoplasia* is a term used to describe a permanent tooth with a local hypoplastic defect in its crown. This defect may have been caused by the extension of a periapical infection from its deciduous prede-

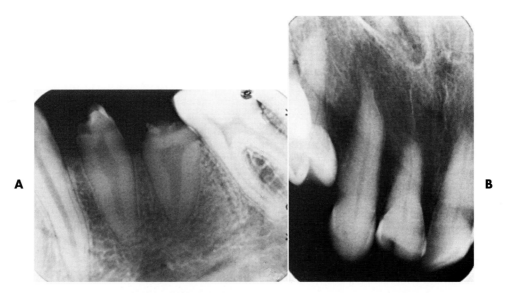

FIG. **17-34** **A,** Turner's hypoplasia, demonstrated as an extensive malformation and hypomineralization of the crowns of both premolars. **B,** Defect in the incisal edge of the lateral incisor after trauma to the primary dentition. (**B** courtesy W. Brown, DDS, Dallas, Tex.)

cessor or by mechanical trauma transmitted through the deciduous tooth. If the trauma (whether infectious or mechanical) takes place while the crown is forming, it may adversely affect the ameloblasts of the developing tooth and result in some degree of enamel hypoplasia or hypomineralization.

Clinical features. Turner's hypoplasia most often affects the mandibular premolars, generally because of the relative susceptibility of the deciduous molars to caries, their proximity to the developing premolars, and their relative time of mineralization. The severity of the defect depends on the severity of the infection or mechanical trauma and on the stage of development of the permanent tooth. It may disturb matrix formation or calcification, in which case the result varies from a hypoplastic defect to a hypomineralization spot in the enamel. The hypomineralized area may become stained, and the tooth usually shows a brownish spot on the crown. If the insult is severe enough to cause hypoplasia, the morphology of the crown may show pitting or a more pronounced defect.

Radiographic features. The enamel irregularities associated with Turner's hypoplasia that alter the normal contours of the affected tooth are apparent on a radiograph (Fig. 17-34). The involved region of the crown may appear as an ill-defined radiolucent region. A stained hypomineralized spot is not apparent because a sufficient difference does not exist in the degree of radiopacity between the spot and the crown of the tooth. Also, the hypomineralized areas may become remineralized by continued contact with saliva.

Differential diagnosis. Other conditions that result in deformation of the tooth crown, such as the delivery of high doses of therapeutic radiation, should be considered. Small defects may simulate the appearance of carious lesions but can be easily differentiated with clinical inspection.

Management. If a radiograph of a tooth affected by Turner's hypoplasia shows that the tooth has good root support, the esthetics and function of the deformed crown can be restored.

Congenital Syphilis
Definition. About 30% of people with congenital syphilis develop dental hypoplasia that involves the permanent incisors and first molars. Development of primary teeth is seldom disturbed. The affected incisors are called *Hutchinson's teeth* and the molars *mulberry molars.* The changes characteristic of the condition seem to result from a direct infection of the developing tooth because the spirochete of syphilis has been identified in the tooth germ.

Clinical features. The affected incisor has a characteristic screwdriver-shaped crown, with the mesial and distal

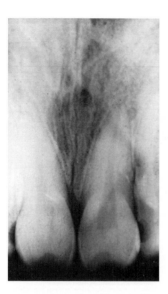

FIG. **17-35** Congenital syphilis may induce a developmental malformation of the maxillary central incisors characterized by tapering of the mesial and distal surfaces toward the incisal edge with notching of the incisal edge.

surfaces tapering from the middle of the crown to the incisal edge (Fig. 17-35). The effect is that the edge may be no wider than the cervical area of the tooth. The incisal edge is also frequently notched. Although maxillary central incisors usually demonstrate these syphilitic changes, the maxillary lateral and mandibular central incisors may also be involved.

As with incisor crowns, the crowns of affected first molars are quite characteristic, being usually smaller than normal and maybe even smaller than second molar crowns. The most distinctive feature is the constricted occlusal third of the crown, with the occlusal surface no wider than the cervical portion of the tooth. The cusps of these molars are also reduced in size and poorly formed. The enamel over the occlusal surface is hypoplastic, unevenly formed in irregular globules, like the surface of a mulberry.

Radiographic features. The characteristic shapes of the affected incisor and molar crowns can be identified in the radiographic image. Because the crowns of these teeth form at about 1 year of age, radiographs may reveal the dental features of congenital syphilis 4 to 5 years before the teeth erupt.

Management. Hutchinson's teeth and mulberry molars often do not require dental treatment. Esthetic restorations may be used to correct the hypoplastic defects as indicated clinically.

Acquired Abnormalities

Acquired changes of the dentition, those that are initiated after development of the tooth, range in severity from changes that have no clinical significance to those that cause tooth loss. In the latter case early detection and treatment is required to preserve the tooth.

ACQUIRED PATHOLOGIC CONDITIONS

Attrition
Definition. Attrition is the physiologic wearing away of the dentition resulting from occlusal contacts between the maxillary and mandibular teeth. It occurs on the incisal, occlusal, and interproximal surfaces. Interproximal wear causes the contact points to become flattened into interproximal surfaces. Attrition occurs in more than 90% of young adults and is generally more severe in men than women. Its extent depends on the abrasiveness of the diet, salivary factors, mineralization of the teeth, and emotional tension. Physiologic attrition is a component of the aging process. When the loss of dental tissue becomes excessive, however, as from bruxism, the attrition becomes pathologic.

Clinical features. The tooth wear patterns from attrition are characteristic. Wear facets first appear on cusps and marginal oblique and transverse ridges. The incisal edges of the maxillary and mandibular incisors show evidence of broadening. The wear facets on the occlusal surfaces of molars become more pronounced, with the lingual cusps of maxillary teeth and the buccal cusps of mandibular posteriors showing the most wear. When the dentin is exposed, it usually becomes stained and the color contrast between stained dentin and enamel highlights the areas of attrition. The incisal edges of mandibular incisors tend to become pitted because the dentin wears more rapidly than its surrounding enamel. In the case of pathologic attrition the patterns of wear are generally not as uniformly progressive as those described for physiologic attrition. The wear facets develop at a faster rate. It is important to emphasize, however, that *physiologic attrition* is a relative term and its clinical manifestations vary with the customs (dietary and otherwise) of the population in question.

Radiographic features. The radiographic appearance of attrition results in a change in the normal outline of the tooth structure, altering the normal curved surfaces into flat planes. The crown is shortened and is bereft of the incisal or occlusal surface enamel (Fig. 17-36). Often a

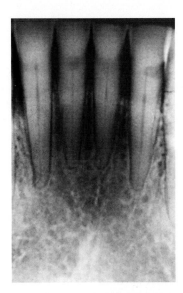

FIG. **17-36** Attrition is the physiologic wearing away of tooth structure. Note the wearing of incisal edges of these lower incisors plus the reduction in the size of the pulp chambers.

number of adjacent teeth in each arch show this wear pattern. Reduction in the size of the pulp chambers and canals may occur because attrition stimulates the deposition of secondary dentin. This may result in complete obliteration of the pulp chamber and canals. A simultaneous widening of the PDL space frequently occurs if the tooth is mobile. Occasionally evidence of hypercementosis is present.

Differential diagnosis. Recognition of physiologic attrition is usually not difficult given the characteristic history, location, and extent of wear. The general pattern is predictable and familiar.

Management. Physiologic attrition does not require treatment.

ABRASION

Abrasion is the nonphysiologic wearing away of teeth by contact with foreign substances. It results from friction induced by factitious habits or occupational hazards. A clinical examination usually readily reveals it. Although many causes exist, two occur with moderate frequency and can usually be eliminated: that from improper tooth brushing and that from dental floss. Other causes include pipe smoking, opening hairpins with the teeth, improper use of toothpicks, and cutting thread with the teeth.

Toothbrush Injury
Clinical features. Toothbrush abrasion is probably the most frequently observed type of injury and is usually the result of improper technique, most frequently a back-and-forth movement of the brush with heavy pressure. This causes the bristles to assume a wedge-shaped arrangement between the crowns and the gingiva. The brushing wears a V-shaped groove into the cervical area of the tooth, usually involving enamel and the softer root surface.

Abraded teeth may become sensitive as the dentin is exposed. The abraded areas are usually most severe at the cementoenamel junction on the labiobuccal surfaces of maxillary premolars, canines, and incisors, in approximately that order. The enamel generally limits the coronal extension of abrasion. The lesions are more common and more pronounced on the left side for a right-handed person, and vice versa. The deposition of secondary dentin opposite the abraded areas usually keeps pace with the destruction at the surface, so pulpal exposure is rarely a complication.

Radiographic features. The radiographic appearance of toothbrush abrasion is radiolucent defects at the cervical level of teeth. These defects have well-defined semilunar shapes with borders of increasing radiopacity. The pulp chambers of the more seriously involved teeth are frequently partially or completely obliterated. The most common location of this injury is the premolar areas, usually in the upper arch.

Dental Floss Injury
Clinical features. Excessive and improper use of dental floss, particularly in conjunction with toothpaste, may result in abrasion of the dentition (Fig. 17-37). The most frequent site is the cervical portion of the proximal surfaces just above the gingiva.

Radiographic features. The radiographic appearance of dental floss abrasion is narrow semilunar radiolucency in the interproximal surfaces cervical area. Most often the radiolucent grooves on the distal surfaces of the teeth are deeper than those on the mesial surfaces, probably because it is easier to exert more pressure in a forward direction by pulling than by pushing the floss backward into the mouth.

Differential diagnosis. Dental floss abrasion is readily identified by its clinical and radiographic appearance. Its location provides some evidence regarding the nature of the cause. This can be verified by the patient history. On occasion the radiolucencies simulate carious lesions located at the cervical region of the tooth.

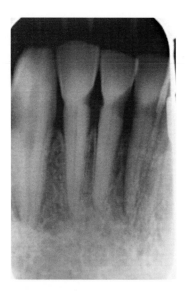

FIG. **17-37**   Abrasion of the cervical portion of these teeth is evident from excessive (and improper) use of dental floss. Note the obliteration of the pulp chambers and reduction in size of the root canals.

The differential diagnosis is accomplished with clinical inspection.

Management. The primary treatment recommended for abrasion is elimination of the causative agents or habits. Extensively abraded areas can be restored.

OTHER ACQUIRED PATHOLOGIES

Erosion

Definition. Erosion of teeth results from a chemical action not involving bacteria. Although in many cases the cause is not apparent, in others it is obviously the contact of acid with teeth. The source of the acid may be (1) chronic vomiting or acid reflux from gastrointestinal disorders or (2) a diet in which the individual consumes large amounts of acidic foods, citrus fruits, or carbonated beverages. Some occupations involve contact with acids that can induce dental erosion. The location of the erosion, the pattern of eroded areas, and the appearance of the lesion usually provide clues as to the origin of the decalcifying agent. Regurgitated acids attack lingual surfaces; dietary acids primarily demineralize labial surfaces. All surfaces are affected by industrial dental erosion.

Clinical features. Dental erosion is usually found on incisors, often involving multiple teeth. The lesions are generally smooth, glistening depressions in the enamel surface, frequently near the gingiva. Erosion may result

in so much loss of enamel that a pink spot shows through the remaining enamel.

Radiographic features. Areas of erosion appear as radiolucent defects on the crown. Their margins may be either well defined or diffuse. A clinical examination usually resolves any questionable lesions.

Differential diagnosis. The diagnosis of erosion is based on the recognition of dished-out or V-shaped defects in the buccal and labial enamel and dentinal surfaces. The margins of a restoration may project above the remaining tooth surface. The edges of lesions caused by erosion are usually more rounded off than those caused by abrasion.

Management. As with abrasion, erosion is managed with identification and removal of the causative agent. If the cause is chronic vomiting from a psychologic disorder, then a daily fluoride rinse should be prescribed during counseling therapy. If the cause is unknown, management depends solely on restoration of the defect. This prevents additional damage, possible pulp exposure, and objectionable esthetic appearance.

Resorption

Resorption is the removal of tooth structure by osteoclasts, referred to as *odontoclasts* when they are resorbing tooth structure. Resorption is classified as internal or external on the basis of the surface of the tooth being resorbed. External resorption affects the outer tooth surface, and internal resorption affects the inner surface of the pulp chamber and canal. These two types differ in their radiographic appearance and treatment. The resorption discussed here is not that associated with the normal loss of deciduous teeth. Although the etiology of most resorptive lesions remains unknown, at least presumptive evidence exists that some lesions are the sequelae of chronic infection (inflammation), excessive pressure and function, or factors associated with local tumors and cysts.

Internal resorption

Definition. Internal resorption occurs within the pulp chamber or canal and involves resorption of the surrounding dentin. This results in enlargement of the size of the pulp space at the expense of tooth structure. This condition may be transient and self-limiting or progressive. The etiology of the recruitment and activation of odontoclasts is unknown but may be related to inflammation of the pulpal tissues. Internal resorption has been reported to be initiated by acute trauma to the tooth, direct and indirect pulp capping, pulpotomy, and enamel invagination.

Clinical features. Internal resorption may affect any tooth in either the primary or secondary dentition. It occurs most frequently in permanent teeth, usually in central incisors and first and second molars. The resorption most commonly begins during the fourth and fifth decades and is more common in males. When the lesion is in the pulp chamber of the crown, it may enlarge until the crown has a dark shadow. If the enlarging pulp perforates the dentin and involves the enamel, it may appear as a pink spot. If the condition is not intercepted, it may perforate the crown, with hemorrhagic tissue projecting from the perforation, and lead to infectious pulpitis. When the lesion occurs in the root of a tooth, it is for the most part clinically silent. If the resorption is extensive, it may weaken the tooth and result in a fracture. It is also possible that the pulp may expand into the periodontal ligament and communicate with a deep periodontal pocket or the gingival sulcus, also leading to pulpal infection.

Radiographic features. Radiographs can reveal symptomless early lesions of internal resorption. The lesions are radiolucent and round, oval, or elongated within the root or crown and continuous with the image of the pulp chamber or canal. The outline is sharply defined and smooth or slightly scalloped. The result is an irregular widening of the pulp chamber or canal (Fig. 17-38). It is characteristically homogeneous, without bony trabeculation or pulp stones. However, the internal structure may seem to be apparent, if the surface of the resorbed tooth structure is very irregular and has a scalloped texture. In some cases virtually the whole pulp may enlarge within a tooth, although more commonly the lesion remains localized.

Differential diagnosis. The most common lesions to be confused with internal root resorption are dental caries on the buccal or lingual surface of a tooth and external root resorption. Carious lesions have more diffuse margins than lesions caused by internal root resorption. Clinical inspection quickly reveals caries on the buccal or lingual surface of a tooth. Also, the mesial and distal surfaces of the pulp chamber and canal may usually be separated from the borders of the carious lesion. With internal root resorption, however, the image of the resorption cannot be separated from the pulp chamber or canal by altering the horizontal angulation of the x-ray beam.

Management. The treatment for internal resorption depends on the condition of the tooth. If the process has not led to a serious weakening defect in the structure, filling the root canal halts the resorption. If the expanding pulp has not structurally compromised the tooth but a perforation of the root has occurred, the perforated surface can be surgically exposed and retrofilled. If the tooth has been badly excavated and weakened by the resorption, extraction may be the only alternative.

External resorption

Definition. In external resorption odontoclasts resorb the outer surface of the tooth. This most commonly involves the root surface but may also involve the crown of an unerupted tooth. The resorption may involve cementum and dentine and in some cases gradually extends to the pulp. Because odontoclasts require an intact blood supply, only sections of the tooth with soft tissue coverage are susceptible to this resorption. This resorption may occur to a single tooth, multiple teeth, or, in rare cases, all of the dentition. In many cases the etiology is unknown but in others causes can be attributed to localized inflammatory lesions, reimplanted teeth, tumors and cysts, excessive mechanical (orthodontic) and occlusal forces, and impacted teeth.

Clinical features. External resorption is usually not recognized because often no characteristic signs or symptoms exist. Even when considerable loss of tooth structure occurs, the tooth in question is frequently firm and immobile in the dental arch. In advanced resorption, some nonspecific pain or fracture of the resorbed root occurs.

External resorption may appear at the apex of the tooth or on the lateral root surface, although it most commonly occurs in the apical and cervical regions. It is slightly more prevalent in mandibular teeth than in maxillary teeth and involves primarily the central incisors, canines, and premolars. External root resorption is common. One study of 18- to 25-year-old men and women found that all patients exhibited some degree of external root resorption in four or more teeth.

Radiographic features. Common sites for external root resorption are the apical and cervical regions. When the lesion begins at the apex, it generally causes a smooth resorption of the tooth structure resulting in blunting of the root apex (Fig. 17-39). Almost always the bone and lamina dura follow the resorbing root and present a normal appearance around this shortened structure. When external root resorption occurs as the result of a periapical inflammatory lesion, the lamina dura is lost around the apex. After normal apexification (constriction of the walls of the pulp canal at the apex) of the pulp canal, it is very difficult or impossible to see the canal exit the apex of the tooth. However, if resorption of the apical region has occurred, the pulp canal is visible and is abnormally wide at the apex.

Occasionally external root resorption involves the lateral aspects of roots (Fig. 17-40). Such lesions tend to be irregular, may involve one side more than the other, and occur in any tooth. A common cause of external resorption on the side of a root is the presence of an unerupted adjacent tooth. Examples of such include resorption of the distal aspect of the roots of an upper second molar by the crown of the adjacent third molar and

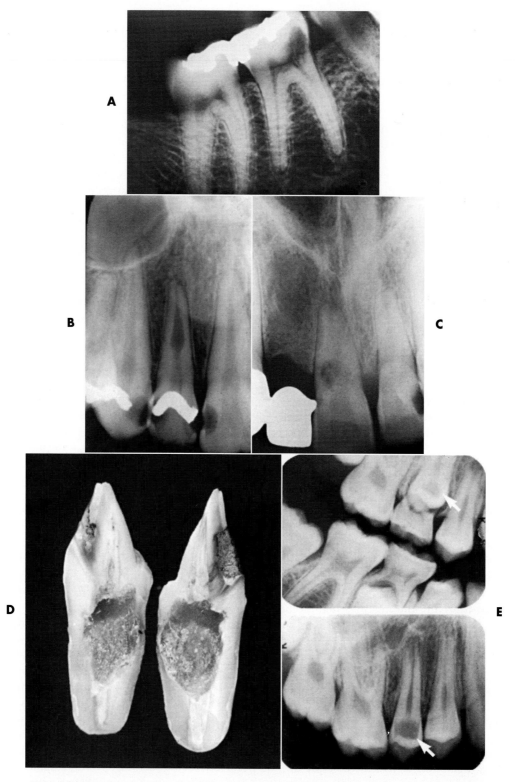

FIG. **17-38**   Internal root resorption may be seen in the crown, **A,** as a widening of the pulp chamber or in the root, **B** and **C,** as widening of the pulp canal. In a sectioned incisor (after crown reduction), **D,** note the large area of internal root resorption. Internal resorption can also be seen in the crown of a second premolar, **E,** before eruption. (**D** courtesy Dr. R. Kienholz, Dallas, Tex.)

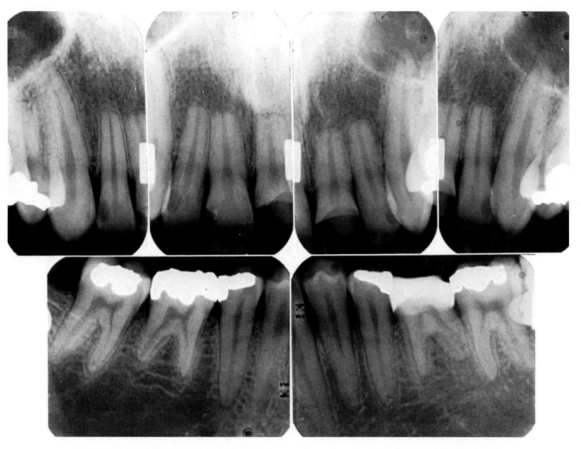

FIG. **17-39**   External root resorption results in a loss of tooth structure from the apex. Note the wide openings of the pulp canals and the intact lamina dura.

resorption of the root of a permanent central or lateral incisor, or both, by an unerupted maxillary canine. External resorption of an entire tooth can occur when the tooth is unerupted and completely embedded in bone (Fig. 17-41), usually involving the maxillary canine or third molar. In such instances the entire tooth, including the root and crown, may undergo resorption.

Differential diagnosis.   External root resorption on the apex or lateral surface of a root is radiographically self-evident. When the lesion lies on the buccal or lingual surface of a root and above the level of the adjacent bone, the differential diagnosis includes caries and internal resorption. Internal resorption characteristically appears as an expansion of the pulp chamber or canal. In the case of external resorption the image of the normal intact pulp chamber or canal may be traced through the radiolucent area of external resorption. Also, projections made at different angles can be compared. The location of the radiolucency caused by external root resorption moves with respect to the pulp canal, whereas the image of internal resorption remains fixed to the canal.

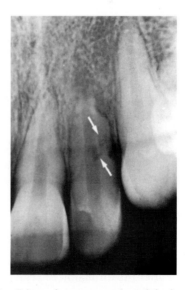

FIG. **17-40**   *External root resorption of the lateral root surface.* Note the irregular radiolucent defects *(arrows)* associated with resorption on the buccal or palatal surface as well as at the apex.

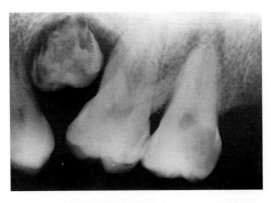

FIG. **17-41**   External root resorption of an unerupted tooth, showing loss of enamel and dentin.

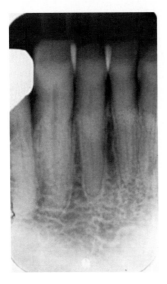

FIG. **17-42**   Secondary dentin formation may cause apparent obliteration of the pulp canal and chamber.

Management. When the cause of external root resorption is known, the treatment is usually to remove the etiologic factors. This may mean cessation of excessive mechanical forces, removal of an adjacent impacted tooth, or eradication of a cyst, tumor, or source of inflammation. If the area of resorption is broad and on an accessible surface of the root (such as at the cervical location), curettage of the defect and the placement of a restoration usually stops the process.

Secondary Dentin
Definition. Secondary dentin is that deposited in the pulp chamber after the formation of primary dentin has been completed. This is a normal aging process and results from such stimuli as chewing or slight trauma. Secondary dentin also develops after chronic trauma from such pathologic conditions as moderately progressive caries, trauma, erosion, attrition, abrasion, or a dental restorative procedure. This specific stimulus promotes a more rapid and localized coronal response than that seen as a result of normal aging. The term *tertiary dentin* has been suggested to identify dentin specifically initiated by stimuli other than the normal aging response and normal biologic function.

Clinical features. The response of odontoblasts in producing secondary dentin reduces the sensitivity of teeth to stimuli from the external environment. In elderly individuals with extensive secondary dentin formation, this reduced sensitivity may be especially pronounced. Similarly, the formation of an additional layer of dentin between the pulp and a region of insult reduces the sensitivity often experienced by individuals with recent dental restorations or coronal fractures.

Radiographic features. Radiographically, secondary dentin is indistinguishable from primary dentin. It is visible as a reduction in size of the normal pulp chamber and canals (Fig. 17-42). When secondary dentin formation results from the normal aging process, the result is a generalized reduction in pulp chamber and canal size, maintaining a relatively normal shape. Often there remains only a thin, narrow pulp chamber and canal. The pulp horns usually disappear relatively early, followed by a reduction in size of the pulp chamber and narrowing of the canals. When more specific stimuli initiate secondary dentin formation, it begins in the region adjacent to the source of stimuli and alters the normal shape of the pulp chamber. Although formation of secondary dentin may continue until the pulp appears to be completely obliterated, histologic studies show that even in these extreme cases a small thread of viable pulp tissue remains.

Differential diagnosis. Secondary dentin is recognized indirectly by the reduction in size of the pulp chamber. This appearance differs from the pulp stone. The pulp stone (see the following description) simply occupies some pulp chamber or canal space, but it has a round to oval shape (conforming to the chamber).

Management. Secondary dentin per se does not require treatment. The precipitating cause is removed if possible and the tooth restored when appropriate.

Pulp Stones
Definition. Pulp stones are foci of calcification in the dental pulp. They are probably apparent microscopically in more than half the teeth from young people and in almost all the teeth from people older than 50 years of age. Although most are microscopic, they vary in size,

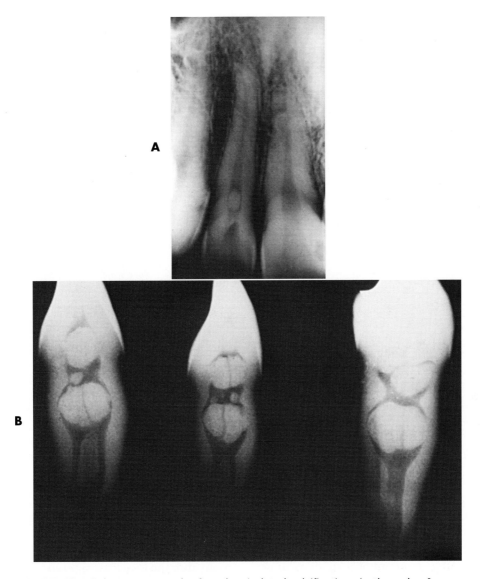

FIG. **17-43** Pulp stones may be found as isolated calcifications in the pulp, **A,** or may cause deformation of pulp chamber and canals, **B.**

with some as large as 2 or 3 mm in diameter, almost filling the pulp chamber. Only these larger concretions are radiographically apparent. Although the larger masses represent only 15% to 25% of pulpal calcification, they are a common radiographic finding and may appear in a single tooth or several teeth. Their cause is unknown, and no firm evidence exists that they are associated with any systemic or pulpal disturbance.

Clinical features. Pulp stones are not clinically discernible.

Radiographic features. The radiographic appearance of pulp stones is quite variable; they may be seen as radiopaque structures within pulp chambers or root canals or extending from the pulp chamber into the root canals (Fig. 17-43). No uniform shape or number exists. They may be round or oval; and some, occupying most of the pulp chamber, will conform to its shape. In rare instances the canal remodels and increases its girth to accommodate a large stone. Also, pulp stones may occur as a single dense mass or as several small radiopacities. Their outline, likewise, varies from sharply defined to a more diffuse margin. They occur in all tooth types but most commonly in molars.

Differential diagnosis. Although pulp stones are variable in size and form, their recognition is usually not dif-

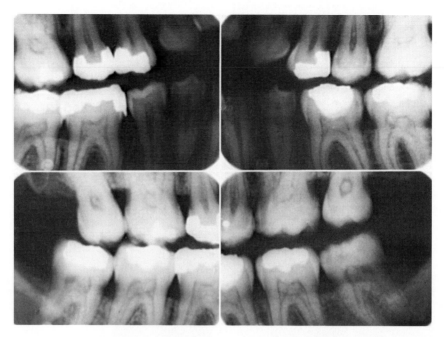

FIG. **17-44**   Pulpal sclerosis is seen as diffuse calcification of the pulp chamber and canals.

ficult. However, in some cases differentiation from pulpal sclerosis is difficult.

Management. Pulp stones do not require treatment.

Pulpal Sclerosis

Definition. Pulpal sclerosis is another form of calcification in the pulp chamber and canals of teeth. In contrast to pulp stones, pulpal sclerosis is a diffuse process. Its specific cause is unknown, although its appearance correlates strongly with age. About 66% of all teeth in individuals between the ages of 10 and 20 years, and 90% of all teeth in individuals between the ages of 50 and 70 years, show histologic evidence of pulpal sclerosis. Histologically the pattern of calcification is amorphous and unorganized, being evident as linear strands or columns of calcified material paralleling blood vessels and nerves in the pulp.

Clinical features. Pulpal sclerosis is a clinically silent process without clinical manifestation.

Radiographic features. Early pulpal sclerosis, a degenerative process, is not radiographically demonstrable. Diffuse pulpal sclerosis produces a generalized, ill-defined collection of fine radiopacities throughout large areas of the pulp chamber and pulp canals (Fig. 17-44).

Differential diagnosis. The differential diagnosis includes small pulp stones, but this differentiation is academic because neither condition requires treatment.

Management. Pulpal sclerosis does not require treatment. As with pulp stones, its only importance may be that it can cause difficulty in the performance of endodontic therapy when such a procedure is indicated for other reasons.

Hypercementosis

Definition. Hypercementosis is excessive deposition of cementum on the tooth roots. In most cases its cause is unknown. Occasionally it appears on a supraerupted tooth after the loss of an opposing tooth. Another cause of hypercementosis is inflammation, usually resulting from periapical inflammatory lesions. In this condition, cementum is deposited on the root surface adjacent to the apex. Occasionally hypercementosis has been associated with teeth that are in hyperocclusion or that have been fractured. Finally, hypercementosis occurs in patients with Paget's disease of bone (see Chapter 22) and with hyperpituitarism (gigantism and acromegaly).

Clinical features. Hypercementosis does not cause any clinical signs or symptoms.

Radiographic features. Hypercementosis is evident radiographically as an excessive buildup of cementum around all or part of a root (Fig. 17-45). The outline is usually smooth but on occasion may be seen as an irregular enlargement of the root. It is most evident at the apical end and is usually seen as a mildly irregular accumulation of cementum. This cementum is slightly more radiolucent than dentin. Of importance is the

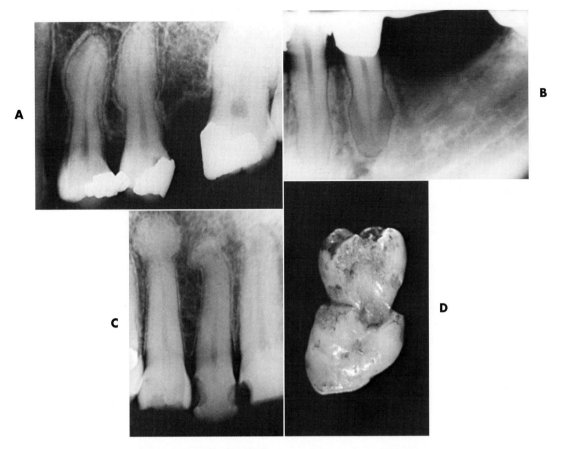

FIG. **17-45** **A** through **C,** Hypercementosis is evident as a buildup of cementum on the root surface of teeth. Note the continuity of the lamina dura and the PDL space that encompasses the extra cementum. **D,** Extracted molar, showing extensive hypercementosis. (**D** courtesy Dr. R. Kienholz, Dallas, Tex.)

fact that the lamina dura and PDL space encompass the extra dentin. In the case of Paget's disease the hypercementosis is usually very exuberant and irregular in outline.

Differential diagnosis. The differential diagnosis may include any radiopaque structure that is seen within the vicinity of the root such as enostosis or mature cemental dysplasia. The differentiating characteristic is the presence of the periodontal membrane space around the hypercementosis. There may be a resemblance to a small benign cementoblastoma. Occasionally a severely dilacerated root may have the appearance of hypercementosis.

Management. Hypercementosis itself requires no treatment. If a related condition such as a periapical inflammatory lesion exists, treatment may be necessary. Perhaps the primary significance of hypercementosis relates to the difficulty that the root configuration can pose if extraction is indicated.

SUGGESTED READINGS

DEVELOPMENTAL ABNORMALITIES

Bergsma D, editor: *Birth defects compendium,* ed 2, New York, 1979, Alan R Liss.

Dixon GH, Stewart RE: Genetic aspects of anomalous tooth development. In Steward RE, Prescott GH, editors: *Oral facial genetics,* St Louis, 1976, Mosby.

Pindborg JJ: Pathology of the dental hard tissues, *N Engl J Med* 301:13, 1979.

Schulze C: Developmental abnormalities of the teeth and jaws. In Gorlin RJ, Goldman HM, editors: *Thoma's oral pathology,* ed 6, vol 1, St Louis, 1970, Mosby.

Witkop CJ Jr, Rao S: Inherited defects in tooth structure. In Bergsma D, editor: *Birth defects. XI. Orofacial structures,* vol 7, no 7, Baltimore, 1971, Williams & Wilkins.

Worth HM: *Principles and practice of oral radiologic interpretation,* Chicago, 1963, Year Book Medical Publishers.

SUPERNUMERARY TEETH

Grahnen H, Lindahl B: Supernumerary teeth in the permanent dentition: a frequency study, *Odontol Rev* 12:290, 1961.

Grimanis GA, Kyriakides AT, Spyropoulos ND: A survey on supernumerary molars, *Quintess Int* 22:989, 1991.

Niswander JD: Effects of heredity and environment on development of the dentition, *J Dent Res* 42:1288, 1963.

Rao SR: Supernumerary teeth. In Bergsma D, editor: *Birth defects compendium,* ed 2, New York, 1979, Alan R Liss.

Yusof WZ: Non-syndrome multiple supernumerary teeth: literature review, *J Can Dent Assoc* 56:147, 1990.

DEVELOPMENTALLY MISSING TEETH

al-Emran S: Prevalence of hypodontia and developmental malformation of permanent teeth in Saudi Arabian school children, *Br J Orthod* 17:115, 1990.

Garn SM, Lewis AB: The relationship between third molar agenesis and reduction in tooth number, *Angle Orthod* 32:14, 1962.

Keene HJ: The relationship between third molar agenesis and the morphologic variability of the molar teeth, *Angle Orthod* 35:289, 1965.

Levin LS: Dental and oral abnormalities in selected ectodermal dysplasia syndromes, *Birth Defects* 24:205, 1988.

O'Dowling IB, McNamara TG: Congenital absence of permanent teeth among Irish school-children, *J Ir Dent Assoc* 36:136, 1990.

MACRODONTIA

Garn SM, Lewis AB, Kerewsky BS: The magnitude and implications of the relationship between tooth size and body size, *Arch Oral Biol* 13:129, 1968.

TRANSPOSITION

Schacter H: A treated case of transposed upper canine, *Dent Res* 71:105, 1951.

FUSION

Hagman FT: Anomalies of form and number, fused primary teeth, a correlation of the dentitions, *J Dent Child* 55:359, 1988.

Sperber GH: Genetic mechanisms and anomalies in odontogenesis, *J Can Dent Assoc* 33:433, 1967.

GEMINATION

Tannenbaum KA, Alling EE: Anomalous tooth development: case report of gemination and twinning, *Oral Surg* 16:883, 1963.

TAURODONTISM

Bixler D: Heritable disorders affecting dentin. In Steward RE, Prescott GA, editors: *Oral facial genetics,* St Louis, 1976, Mosby.

DENS IN DENTE

Oehlers FAC: The radicular variety of dens invaginatus, *Oral Surg* 11:1251, 1958.

Rushton MA: A collection of dilated composite odontomes, *Br Dent J* 63:65, 1937.

Soames JV, Kuyebi TA: A radicular dens invaginatus, *Br Dent J* 152:308, 1982.

DENS INVAGINATUS

Oehlers FA, Lee KW, Lee EC: Dens invaginatus (invaginated odontome), *Dent Pract* 17:239, 1967.

Sykaras SN: Occlusal anomalous tubercle on premolars of a Greek girl, *Oral Surg* 38:88, 1974.

Yip WW: The prevalence of dens invaginatus, *Oral Surg* 38:80, 1974.

AMELOGENESIS IMPERFECTA

Crawford PJ, Aldred MJ: X-linked amelogenesis imperfecta: presentation of two kindreds and a review of the literature, *Oral Surg* 73:449, 1992.

Toller PA: A clinical report of six cases of amelogenesis imperfecta, *Oral Surg* 12:325, 1959.

Witkop CJ Jr: Amelogenesis imperfecta, dentinogenesis imperfecta and dentin dysplasia revisited: problems in classification, *J Oral Pathol* 17:547, 1988.

Witkop CJ Jr, Saulk JJ: Heritable defects of enamel. In Stewart RE, Prescott GA, editors: *Oral facial genetics,* St Louis, 1976, Mosby.

DENTINOGENESIS IMPERFECTA

Schwartz S, Tsipouras P: Oral findings in osteogenesis imperfecta, *Oral Surg* 57:161, 1984.

Winter GB: Hereditary and idiopathic anomalies of tooth number, structure, and form, *Dent Clin North Am* 13:355, 1969.

Witkop CJ Jr: Hereditary defects in enamel and dentin. Proceedings of the First International Congress on Human Genetics, *Acta Genet Stat Med* 7:236, 1957.

DENTIN DYSPLASIA

O'Carroll MK, Duncan WK, Perkins TM: Dentin dysplasia: review of the literature and a proposed subclassification based on radiographic findings, *Oral Surg* 72:119, 1991.

Richardson AS, Fantin TD: Occlusal anomalous dysplasia of dentin: report of a case, *J Can Dent Assoc* 36:189, 1970.

Shields EP, Bixler D, El-Kafraevy AM: A proposed classification for heritable human dentin defects with a description of a new entity, *Arch Oral Biol* 18:543, 1973.

Witkop CJ Jr: Hereditary defects of dentin, *Dent Clin North Am* 19:25, 1975.

REGIONAL ODONTODYSPLASIA

Crawford PJ, Aldred MJ: Regional odontodysplasia: a bibliography, *J Oral Pathol Med* 18:251, 1989.

ENAMEL PEARL

Moskow BS, Canut PM: Studies on root enamel. II. Enamel pearls: a review of their morphology, localization, nomenclature, occurrence, classification, histogenesis, and incidence, *J Clin Periodontol* 17:275, 1990.

TALON CUSP

Meskin LH, Gorlin RJ: Agenesis and peg-shaped permanent lateral incisors, *J Dent Res* 42:1476, 1963.

Natkin E, Pitts DL, Worthington P: A case of talon cusp associated with other odontogenic abnormalities, *J Endod* 9:491, 1983.

TURNER'S HYPOPLASIA

Via WF Jr: Enamel defects induced by trauma during tooth formation, *Oral Surg* 25:49, 1968.

CONGENITAL SYPHILIS

Bradlaw RV: Dental stigmata of prenatal syphilis, *Oral Surg* 6:147, 1953.

Putkonen P: Dental changes in congenital syphilis, *Acta Derm Venereol* 42:44, 1962.

Sarnat BG, Shaw NG: Dental development in congenital syphilis, *Am J Orthod* 29:270, 1943.

ACQUIRED ABNORMALITIES

Baden E: Environmental pathology of the teeth. In Gorlin RJ, Goodman HM, editors: *Thoma's oral pathology*, ed 6, vol 1, St Louis, 1970, Mosby.

Mitchell DF, Standish SM, Fast TB: *Oral diagnosis/oral medicine*, Philadelphia, 1978, Lea & Febiger.

Pindborg JJ: *Pathology of the dental hard tissues*, Philadelphia, 1970, WB Saunders.

Shafer WG, Hine MK, Levy BM: *Oral pathology*, ed 4, Philadelphia, 1983, WB Saunders.

ATTRITION

Johnson GK, Sivers JE: Attrition, abrasion, and erosion: diagnosis and therapy, *Clin Prev Dent* 9:12, 1987.

Murphy TR: Reduction of the dental arch by approximal attrition: quantitative assessment, *Br Dent J* 116:483, 1964.

Russell MD: The distinction between physiological and pathological attrition: a review, *J Ir Dent Assoc* 33:23, 1987.

Seligman DA, Pullinger AG, Solberg WK: The prevalence of dental attrition and its association with factors of age, gender, occlusion, and TMJ symptomatology, *J Dent Res* 67:1323, 1988.

ABRASION

Bull WH et al: The abrasion and cleaning properties of dentifrices, *Br Dent J* 125:331, 1968.

Erwin JC, Buchner CM: Prevalence of tooth root exposure and abrasion among dental patients, *Dent Items Interest* 66:760, 1944.

EROSION

Bruggen ten Cate JH: Dental erosion in industry, *Br J Industr Med* 25:249, 1968.

Stafne EC, Lovestedt SA: Dissolution of tooth substance by lemon juice, acid beverages, and acid from some other sources, *J Am Dent Assoc* 34:586, 1949.

RESORPTION

Bakland LK: Root resorption, *Dent Clin North Am* 36:491, 1992.

Bennett TG, Paleway SA: Internal resorption, post-pulpotomy type, *Oral Surg* 17:228, 1964.

Goldman HM: Spontaneous intermittent resorption of teeth, *J Am Dent Assoc* 49:522, 1954.

Massler M, Perreault JG: Root resorption in the permanent teeth of young adults, *J Dent Child* 21:158, 1954.

Phillips JR: Apical root resorption under orthodontic therapy, *Angle Orthod* 20:1, 1955.

Simpson HE: Internal resorption, *J Can Dent Assoc* 30:355, 1964.

Solomon CS, Notaro PJ, Kellert M: External root resorption: fact or fancy, *J Endod* 15:219, 1989.

Stafne EC, Austin LT: Resorption of embedded teeth, *J Am Dent Assoc* 32:1003, 1945.

Tronstad L: Root resorption: etiology, terminology, and clinical manifestations, *Endod Dent Traumatol* 4:241, 1988.

SECONDARY DENTIN

Kuttler Y: Classification of dentin into primary, secondary and tertiary, *Oral Surg* 12:966, 1959.

PULP STONES

Moss-Salentijn L, Hendricks-Klyvert M: Calcified structures in human dental pulps, *J Endod* 14:184, 1988.

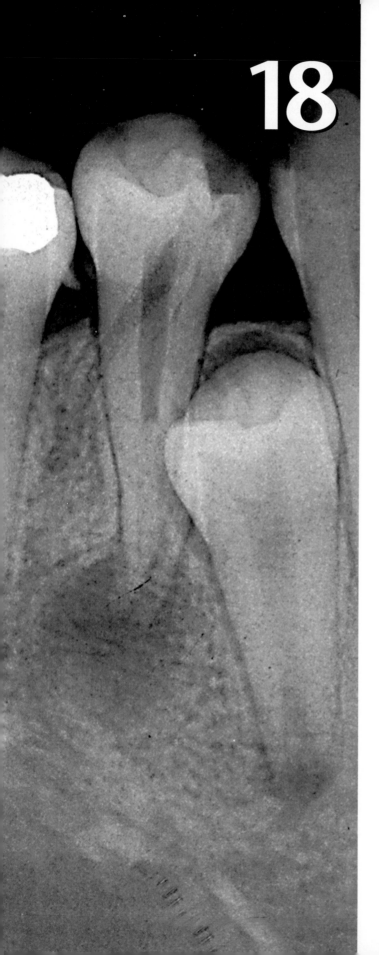

18 Inflammatory Lesions of the Jaws

LINDA LEE

Inflammatory lesions are by far the most common pathologic condition of the jaws. The jaws are unique from other bones of the body in that the presence of teeth creates a direct pathway for infectious and inflammatory agents to invade bone by means of caries and periodontal disease. The body responds to chemical, physical, or microbiologic injury with inflammation. The inflammatory response destroys or walls off the injurious stimulus and sets up an environment for repair of the damaged tissue.

Under normal conditions, bone metabolism represents a balance of osteoclastic bone resorption and osteoblastic bone production. This is a complex, interdependent relationship in which osteoblasts mediate the resorptive activity of the osteoclasts. Mediators of inflammation (cytokines, prostaglandins, and many growth factors) tip this balance to favor either bone resorption or bone formation. For the purposes of this chapter, all inflammatory conditions of bone, regardless of the specific etiology, are considered to represent a spectrum or continuum of conditions with different clinical features (e.g., site, severity, duration).

When the initial source of inflammation is a necrotic pulp and the bony lesion is restricted to the region of the tooth, the condition is called a *periapical inflammatory lesion*. When the infection spreads in the bone marrow and is no longer contained, it is called *osteomyelitis*. Another type of inflammatory lesion in bone is characterized by extension of inflammation into the overlying soft tissues; this type of lesion includes periodontal lesions (see Chapter 16) and pericoronitis, an inflammation that arises in the tissues surrounding the crown of a partially erupted tooth. It must be emphasized that the names of the various inflammatory lesions tend to describe their clinical and radiologic presentations and behavior; however, all have the same underlying disease mechanism.

General Clinical Features

The four cardinal signs of inflammation—redness, swelling, heat, and pain—may be observed in varying degrees with inflammation of the jaws. Acute lesions are those of recent onset. The onset typically is rapid, and these lesions cause pronounced pain, often accompanied by fever and swelling. Chronic lesions have a prolonged course. Also, the onset tends to be more insidious, and the pain is less intense. Fever may be intermittent and low grade, and swelling may occur gradually. In fact, some chronic, low-grade infections may not produce any significant clinical symptoms.

General Radiographic Features

LOCATION

With periapical inflammatory lesions, which are pathologic conditions of the pulp, the epicenter typically is located at the apex of a tooth. However, lesions of pulpal origin also may be located cervically because of accessory canals or perforations caused by root canal therapy or root fractures. Periodontal lesions are centered about the alveolar crest. If periodontal bone loss is severe, the epicenter may be located more apically at the root furcation level or even at the root apex. Osteomyelitis, a diffuse, uncontained inflammation of the bone, most commonly is found in the posterior mandible. The maxilla rarely is involved.

PERIPHERY

Most often the periphery is ill defined, and the normal trabecular pattern gradually changes into an internal sclerotic pattern or into an internal radiolucent region.

INTERNAL STRUCTURE

The internal structure of inflammatory lesions presents a spectrum of appearances. Cancellous bone may respond to an insult by tipping the metabolic balance either in favor of resorption (giving the area a radiolucent appearance) or toward bone formation (resulting in a radiopaque or sclerotic appearance). Usually a combination of the two reactions results. The radiolucent regions may show no evidence of previous trabeculation or a very faint pattern of trabeculation. The increased radiopacity is caused by an increase in bone formation on existing trabeculae. Radiographically these trabeculae appear thicker and more numerous, replacing marrow spaces. In acute disease, resorption typically predominates; with a chronic disease, excessive bone formation leads to an overall radiopaque, sclerotic appearance. In cases of osteomyelitis, careful examination of the x-ray films may reveal sequestra, which appear as ill-defined areas of radiolucency containing a radiopaque island of nonvital bone.

EFFECTS ON SURROUNDING STRUCTURES

The effects of inflammation on surrounding cancellous bone include stimulation of bone formation, resulting in a sclerotic pattern, or bone resorption, resulting in radiolucency. The periodontal ligament space involved in the lesion will be widened; this widening is greatest at the source of the inflammation. For example, with periapical lesions the widening is greatest around the apical region of the root; in periodontal disease the widening is greatest at the alveolar crest. With chronic infections, root resorption may occur and cortical boundaries may be resorbed. The periosteal component of bone, whether on the surface of the jaws or lining the floor of the maxillary sinus, also responds to inflammation. The periosteum contains a layer of pluripotential lining cells that, under the right conditions, differentiate into osteoblasts and lay down new bone. Inflammatory exudate from infection within the bone can penetrate the cortex, lift up the periosteum from the surface of the bone, and stimulate the periosteum to produce new bone. Because inflammatory exudate is a fluid, the periosteum is lifted from the surface of bone in a manner that positions the periosteum almost parallel to the surface of the bone; thus the layer of new bone is almost parallel to the bone surface.

PERIAPICAL INFLAMMATORY LESIONS

Synonyms

Periapical inflammatory lesions have been called *acute apical periodontitis, chronic apical periodontitis, periapical abscess,* and *periapical granuloma.* Radiolucent presentations have been called *rarefying osteitis,* whereas radiopaque presentations have been called *sclerosing osteitis, condensing osteitis,* and *focal sclerosing osteitis.* Chapter 19

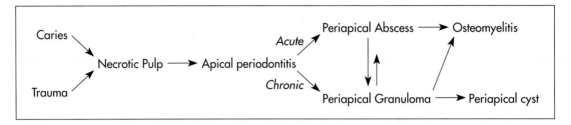

FIG. **18-1**   Interrelationship of possible results of periapical inflammation.

presents a discussion of periapical cysts of inflammatory origin (radicular cysts).

Definition

A *periapical inflammatory lesion* is defined as a local response of the bone around the apex of a tooth that occurs secondary to necrosis of the pulp or through destruction of the periapical tissues by extensive periodontal disease (Fig. 18-1). The pulpal necrosis may occur secondary to pulpal invasion of bacteria through caries or trauma. In the case shown in the figure, the periapical inflammatory lesion is characterized by apical periodontitis, a periapical abscess, and a periapical granuloma. Toxic metabolites from the necrotic pulp exit the root apex to incite an inflammatory reaction in the periapical periodontal ligament and surrounding bone *(apical periodontitis)*. This reaction is characterized histologically by an inflammatory infiltrate composed predominantly of lymphocytes mixed with polymorphonuclear neutrophils. Depending on the severity of the response, the neutrophils may collect to form pus, resulting in an *apical abscess*. This result is categorized as acute inflammation. Alternatively, in an attempt to heal from apical periodontitis, the body stimulates the formation of granulation tissue mixed with a chronic inflammatory infiltrate composed predominantly of lymphocytes, plasma cells, and histiocytes, giving rise to *periapical granuloma*. Entrapped epithelium (the rests of Malassez) may proliferate to form a radicular or apical cyst. Acute exacerbations of the chronic lesions may occur intermittently.

If the surrounding bone marrow becomes involved with the inflammatory reaction through the spread of pyogenic organisms, the localized periapical abscess may transform into osteomyelitis. The exact point at which a periapical inflammatory lesion becomes osteomyelitis is not easily determined or defined. The size of the area of inflammation is not as important as the severity of the reaction. However, considering the size of the lesion as one factor, periapical inflammatory lesions usually involve only the local bone adjacent to the apex of the tooth, and osteomyelitis involves a larger area of bone. Periapical lesions occasionally may be large, but the epicenter of the lesion remains in the vicinity of the tooth apex. If the periapical lesion extends farther, so that the

lesion no longer is centered on the tooth apex, osteomyelitis may be considered as a possible diagnosis. The distinction between periapical inflammation and osteomyelitis can be made if sequestra are detected radiographically. Progression from periapical inflammation to osteomyelitis is relatively rare, and other factors play a role in its development, such as host defenses and the virulence of pathogenic microorganisms.

Clinical Features

The symptoms of periapical inflammatory lesions can range across a broad spectrum, from being asymptomatic, to an occasional toothache, to severe pain with or without facial swelling, fever, and lymphadenopathy. A periapical abscess usually manifests with severe pain, mobility and sometimes elevation of the involved tooth, swelling, and tenderness to percussion. Palpation of the apical region elicits pain. Spontaneous drainage into the oral cavity through a fistula (parulis) may relieve the acute pain. In rare cases a dental abscess may manifest with systemic symptoms (e.g., fever, facial swelling, lymphadenopathy) along with the pain. The acute lesion may evolve into a chronic one (periapical granuloma or cyst), which may be asymptomatic except for intermittent flare-ups of "toothache" pain, which mark the acute exacerbation of the chronic lesion. Patients often give a history of intermittent pain. The associated tooth may be asymptomatic, or it may be sensitive to percussion and mobile. More often, however, the periapical lesion arises in the chronic form *de novo;* in this case it may be asymptomatic. It is important to understand that the clinical presentation does not necessarily correlate with the histologic or radiographic findings.

Radiographic Features

The radiographic features of periapical inflammatory lesions vary depending on the time course of the lesion. Because very early lesions may not show any radiographic changes, diagnosis of these lesions relies solely on the clinical symptoms (Fig. 18-2). More chronic lesions may show lytic or sclerotic changes, or both.

Location. In most cases the epicenter of periapical inflammatory lesions is found at the apex of the involved

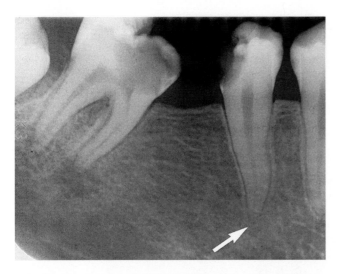

FIG. **18-2** A very early lesion involving the pulp of the second bicuspid without significant change in the periapical bone *(arrow)*. In contrast, note the loss of the lamina dura and periapical bone at the apex of the mesial root of the second molar. Also note the subtle halo of sclerotic bone reaction around this apical radiolucency.

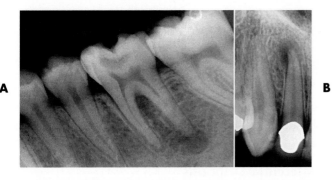

A | B

FIG. **18-3** Periapical inflammatory lesions associated with a mandibular first molar **(A)** and a maxillary lateral incisor **(B)**. Note that in both cases the epicenter of bone destruction is located at the apex of the root.

tooth (Fig. 18-3). The lesion usually starts within the apical portion of the periodontal ligament space. Less often, such lesions are centered cervically up the tooth root. This may occur because of accessory pulpal canals, perforation of the root structure from instrumentation of the pulp canal, and root fracture.

Periphery. In most instances the periphery of periapical inflammatory lesions is ill defined, showing a gradual transition from the surrounding normal trabecular pattern into the abnormal bone pattern of the lesion (Figs. 18-1 and 18-4). Occasionally the periphery may be well defined, with a sharp transition zone and an appearance suggesting a cortical boundary.

Internal structure. Early periapical inflammatory lesions may show no radiographic change in the normal bone pattern. The earliest detectable change is loss of bone density, which usually results in widening of the periodontal ligament space at the apex of the tooth and later involves a larger diameter of surrounding bone. At this early stage no evidence may be seen of a sclerotic bone reaction (see Fig. 18-1). Later in the evolution of the disease, a mixture of sclerosis and rarefaction (loss of bone giving a radiolucent appearance) of normal bone occurs (see Fig. 18-4). The percentage of these two bone reactions varies. When most of the lesion consists of increased bone formation, the term *periapical sclerosing osteitis* is used (Fig. 18-5), and when most of the lesion is undergoing bone resorption, the term *periapical rarefying osteitis* is used. The area of greatest bone destruction usually is centered around the apex of the tooth, with the sclerotic pattern located at the periphery. The radiolucent regions may be bereft of any bone structure or may have a faint outline of trabeculae. Close inspection of sclerotic regions reveals thicker than normal trabeculae and sometimes an increase in the number of trabeculae per unit area. In chronic cases the new bone formation may result in a very dense sclerotic region of bone, obscuring individual trabeculae. Occasionally the lesion may appear to be composed entirely of sclerotic bone (sclerosing osteitis), but usually some evidence exists of widening of the apical portion of the periodontal membrane space (see Fig. 18-5).

Effects on surrounding structures. As mentioned previously, periapical inflammatory lesions may stimulate either the resorption of bone or the manufacture of new bone. The lamina dura around the apex of the tooth usually is lost. The sclerotic reaction of the cancellous bone may be limited to a small region around the tooth apex or in some cases may be extensive. In rare instances in the mandible the sclerotic reaction may extend to the inferior cortex. In chronic cases external resorption of the apical region of the root may occur. If the lesion is long-standing, the pulp canal may appear wider than adjacent teeth. This is a result of the death of odontoblasts and subsequent cessation of the formation of secondary dentin, which occurs naturally with time to diminish the caliber of the pulp canal slowly.

Nearby cortical boundaries may be destroyed, such as a segment of the floor of the maxillary antrum, the floor of the nasal fossa, or the buccal or lingual plates of the alveolar process immediately adjacent to the root apex. These lesions are capable of producing an inflammatory periosteal reaction, most notably in the adjacent floor of the maxillary antrum. This usually results in a thin layer of new bone within the maxillary antrum, sometimes referred to as a "halo shadow" (Fig. 18-6). A regional mucositis may be present within the adjacent segment of the

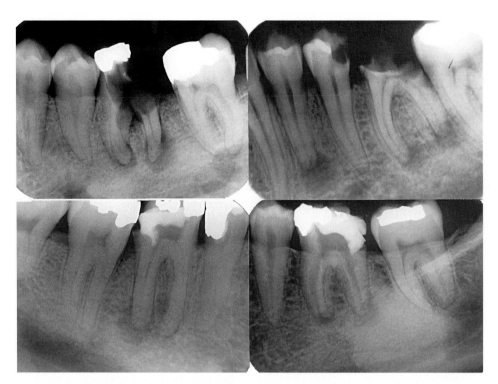

FIG. **18-4** *Several examples of a mixture of rarefying and sclerosing osteitis.* Note the similarity of the pattern, composed of a radiolucent region at the apex of the tooth surrounded by a radiopaque reaction of sclerotic dense bone. Also note that most often a gradual transition occurs from the sclerotic bone reaction to the more normal surrounding bone pattern.

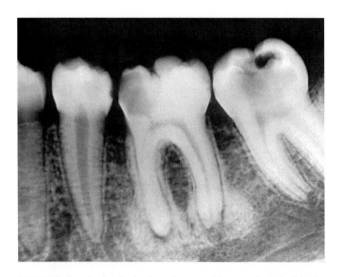

FIG. **18-5** *Periapical sclerosing osteitis associated with the first molar.* This is called a *sclerosing lesion* because most of the lesion is bone formation, resulting in a very radiopaque density. Note, however, the small region of bone loss next to the root apex and the widening of the periodontal membrane space.

maxillary antrum. Periosteal reaction may also occur on the buccal or lingual surfaces of the alveolar process and in rare cases on the inferior aspect of the mandible.

Differential Diagnosis

The two types of lesions that most often must be differentiated from periapical inflammatory lesions are periapical cemental dysplasia (PCD) and an enostosis (dense bone island, osteosclerosis) at the apex of a tooth. In the early radiolucent phase of PCD, the radiographic characteristics may not reliably differentiate this lesion from a periapical inflammatory lesion (Fig. 18-7). The differential diagnosis may rely solely on the clinical examination, including a test of tooth vitality. With long-standing periapical inflammatory lesions, the pulp chamber of the involved tooth may be wider than the adjacent teeth. More mature PCD lesions may show evidence of a dense, radiopaque structure within the radiolucency, which helps in the differential diagnosis. Also, a common site for PCD is the mandibular anterior teeth. External root resorption is more common with inflammatory lesions than with PCD. When enostosis is centered around the root apex, it may mimic an inflamma-

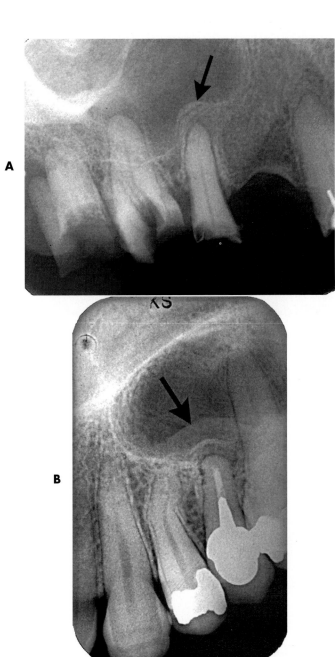

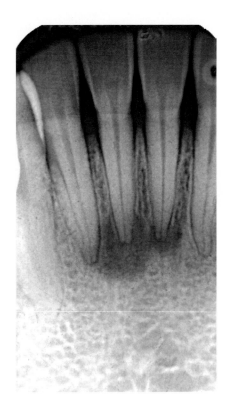

FIG. **18-7** Two early lesions of PCD related to the apical region of the mandibular central incisors.

FIG. **18-6** *Periostitis emanating from the floor of the maxillary antrum that arises secondary to apical inflammatory lesions.* **A,** Laminated type of periostitis *(arrow).* **B,** Periostitis and mucositis. The mucositis is characterized by a slight radiopaque band *(arrow).*

tory lesion. However, the periodontal ligament space around the apex of the tooth has a normal uniform width (Fig. 18-8). Also, the periphery of an enostosis usually is well defined.

Small, radiolucent periapical lesions with a well-defined periphery simulating a cortex may be either peri-

apical granulomas or cysts (radicular cysts). Differentiation may not be possible unless other characteristics of a cyst are present such as displacement of adjacent structures and expansion of the outer cortical boundaries of the jaw. Lesions larger than 1 cm in diameter usually are radicular cysts. If the patient has had endodontic treatment or apical surgery, a periapical radiolucency may remain that may look like periapical rarefying osteitis (Fig. 18-9). In either case the destroyed bone may not be replaced with normal bone but with scar tissue. The differential diagnosis cannot be made on radiologic grounds alone, thus the clinical signs and symptoms must take precedence.

In rare cases metastatic lesions and malignancies such as leukemia may grow in the periapical segment of the periodontal membrane space. Close inspection of the surrounding bone may reveal other small regions of malignant bone destruction.

Management

Standard dental treatment of periapical lesions includes root canal therapy or extraction with the intention of eliminating the necrotic material in the root canal and hence the source of inflammation. If left untreated, the tooth may become asymptomatic because of drainage

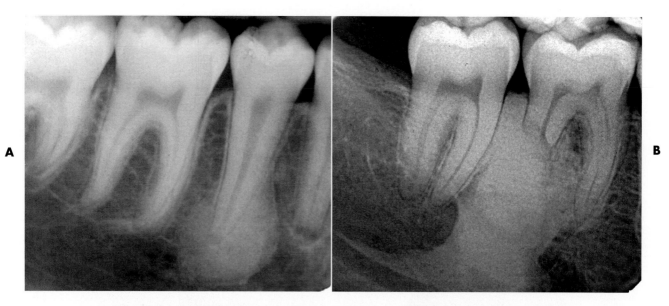

FIG. **18-8** *Enostosis (dense bone island) in periapical positions.* **A,** Enostosis around the apex of a second bicuspid. Note that the periodontal membrane space is uniform in width. **B,** Enostosis associated with apical root resorption of a vital tooth. The most common site of enostosis and root resorption is the mesial or distal root of mandibular first molars.

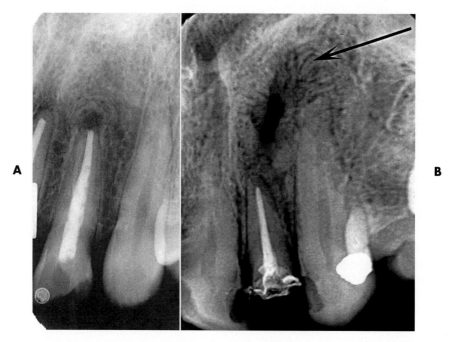

FIG. **18-9** **A,** Radiolucent apical scar left after successful endodontic treatment. **B,** Healing periapical inflammatory lesion associated with the apical region of a maxillary lateral incisor. Note the radiating, spokelike pattern of new bone forming from the periphery of the lesion.

established through the carious lesion or a parulis. However, the possibility always exists that the lesion will spread to involve a larger area of bone, resulting in osteomyelitis or into the surrounding soft tissue, which may result in a space infection or cellulitis.

PERICORONITIS

Synonym
Operculitis

Definition
The term *pericoronitis* refers to inflammation of the tissues surrounding the crown of a partially erupted tooth. It is most often seen in association with the mandibular third molars in young adults. The gingiva surrounding the erupted portion of the crown becomes inflamed when food or microbial debris becomes trapped under the soft tissue. The gingiva subsequently becomes swollen and may become secondarily traumatized by the opposing occlusion. This inflammation may extend into the bone surrounding the crown of the tooth.

Clinical Features
Patients with pericoronitis typically complain of pain and swelling. Trismus is a common presentation when the partially erupted tooth is a lower third molar, and usually pain is felt on occlusion. An ulcerated operculum is usually the source of the pain. Pericoronitis can affect patients of any age or gender but is most commonly seen during the time of eruption of the third molars in young adults.

Radiographic Features
The radiologic signs of pericoronitis can range from no changes when the inflammatory lesion is confined to the soft tissues, to localized rarefaction and sclerosis, to osteomyelitis in the most severe cases.

Location. When bone changes are associated with pericoronitis, they are centered around the follicular space or the portion of the crown still embedded in bone or in close proximity to bone. The mandibular third molar region is the most common location.

Periphery. The periphery of pericoronitis is ill defined, with a gradual transition of the normal trabecular pattern into a sclerotic region.

Internal structure. The internal structure of bone adjacent to the pericoronitis most often is sclerotic with thick trabeculae. An area of bone loss or radiolucency immediately adjacent to the crown may be seen that enlarges the follicular space (Fig. 18-10). If this lesion

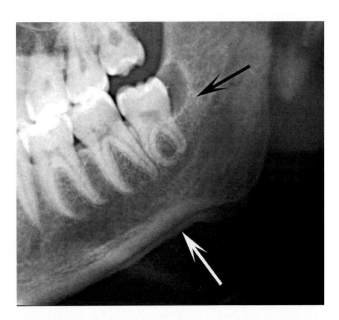

FIG. **18-10** *Panoramic view of a case of pericoronitis related to a partially erupted third molar.* Note the sclerotic bone reaction adjacent to the follicular cortex *(black arrow)* and the periosteal reaction *(white arrow)*.

spreads considerably, the internal pattern becomes consistent with osteomyelitis (see the next section).

Effects on surrounding structures. As with the periapical inflammatory lesions, pericoronitis may cause the typical changes of sclerosis and rarefaction of surrounding bone. In extensive cases evidence of periosteal new bone formation may be seen at the inferior cortex, the posterior border of the ramus, and along the coronoid notch of the mandible.

Differential Diagnosis
The differential diagnosis of pericoronitis includes other mixed density or sclerotic lesions that can exist adjacent to the crown of a partially erupted third molar. These include enostosis and fibrous dysplasia. The clinical symptoms indicative of an inflammatory lesion usually exclude these conditions. Neoplasms to be considered include the sclerotic form of osteosarcoma and, in older patients, squamous cell carcinoma. The occurrence of squamous cell carcinoma in the midst of a preexisting inflammatory lesion may be difficult to identify. Features characteristic of malignant neoplasia, such as profound cortical bone destruction and invasion, help with the diagnosis.

Management
The aim of treatment of pericoronitis is removal of the partially erupted tooth. However, in the acute phase, when trismus may prevent adequate access, antibiotic

therapy and reduction in occlusion of the opposing tooth should relieve the symptoms until definitive treatment is provided.

OSTEOMYELITIS

Definition

Osteomyelitis is an inflammation of bone. The inflammatory process may spread through the bone to involve the marrow, cortex, cancellous portion, and periosteum. In the jaws osteomyelitis usually is caused by pyogenic organisms that reach the bone marrow from abscessed teeth or postsurgical infection. However, in some instances no source of infection can be identified, and hematogenous spread is presumed to be the origin. In some patients no infectious organisms can be identified, possibly because of previous antibiotic therapy or inadequate methods of bacterial isolation. Bacterial colonies also may be present in small, isolated pockets of bone that may be missed during sampling.

In patients with osteomyelitis, the bacteria and their products stimulate an inflammatory reaction in bone, causing destruction of the endosteal surface of the cortical bone. This destruction may progress through the cortical bone to the outer periosteum. In young patients, in whom the periosteum is more loosely attached to the outer cortex of bone than it is in adults, the periosteum is lifted up by inflammatory exudate, and new bone is laid down. This periosteal reaction is a characteristic but not pathognomonic feature of osteomyelitis. The hallmark of osteomyelitis is the development of sequestra. A sequestrum is a segment of bone that has become necrotic because of ischemic injury caused by the inflammatory process.

Numerous forms of osteomyelitis have been described. For the sake of simplicity, we group them into two major categories, acute and chronic, recognizing that these represent two ends of a continuum in the process of bone inflammation. Other forms of osteomyelitis have been described as separate and distinct clinicopathologic entities with unique radiographic features. These are Garré's osteomyelitis and diffuse sclerosing osteomyelitis. We consider them as part of the same continuum. Garré's osteomyelitis is an exuberant periosteal response to inflammation. Diffuse sclerosing osteomyelitis is a chronic form of osteomyelitis with a pronounced sclerotic response. It is important to understand that all these variations of osteomyelitis have the same underlying process of bone's response to inflammation. The features expressed by each subtype represent only variations in the type and degree of bone reaction.

Osteomyelitis may resolve spontaneously or with appropriate antibiotic intervention. However, if the condition is not treated or is treated inadequately, the infection may persist and become chronic in about 20% of patients. Some chronic systemic diseases, immunosuppressive states, and disorders of decreased vascularity may predispose an individual to the development of osteomyelitis. For example, osteopetrosis, sickle cell anemia, and acquired immunodeficiency syndrome (AIDS) have been documented as underlying factors in the development of osteomyelitis.

ACUTE OSTEOMYELITIS

Synonyms

Acute suppurative osteomyelitis, pyogenic osteomyelitis, subacute suppurative osteomyelitis, Garré's osteomyelitis, proliferative periostitis, periostitis ossificans

Definition

Acute osteomyelitis is caused by infection that has spread to the bone marrow. With this condition, the medullary spaces of the bone contain an inflammatory infiltrate consisting predominantly of neutrophils and, to a lesser extent, mononuclear cells. In the jaws the most common source of infection is a periapical lesion from a nonvital tooth. Infection also can occur as a result of trauma or hematogenous spread.

Garré's osteomyelitis may accompany acute osteomyelitis. It is believed that the inflammatory exudate spreads subperiosteally, elevating the periosteum and stimulating formation of new bone. This condition is more common in younger people because in these individuals the periosteum is loosely attached to the bone surface and has greater osteogenic potential.

Clinical Features

Acute osteomyelitis can affect people of all ages, and it has a strong male predilection. It is much more common in the mandible than in the maxilla, possibly because of the poorer vascular supply to the mandible. The typical signs and symptoms of acute osteomyelitis are rapid onset, pain, swelling of the adjacent soft tissues, fever, lymphadenopathy, and leukocytosis. The associated teeth may be mobile and sensitive to percussion. Purulent drainage also may be present. Paresthesia of the lower lip in the third division of the fifth cranial nerve distribution is not uncommon.

Radiographic Features

Very early in the disease, no radiographic changes may be identifiable. The bone may be filled with inflammatory exudate and inflammatory cells and may show no radiographic change.

Location. The most common location is the posterior body of the mandible. The maxilla is a rare site.

Periphery. Acute osteomyelitis most often presents an ill-defined periphery with a gradual transition to normal trabeculae.

Internal structure. The first radiographic evidence of acute osteomyelitis is a slight decrease in the density of the involved bone, with a loss of sharpness of the existing trabeculae. In time the bone destruction becomes more profound, resulting in an area of radiolucency in one focal area or in scattered regions throughout the involved bone (Fig. 18-11). Later, the appearance of scle-rotic regions becomes apparent. Sequestra may be present but usually are more numerous in chronic forms. Sequestra can be identified by closely inspecting a region of bone destruction (radiolucency) for an island of bone. This island of nonvital bone may vary in size from a small dot (smaller sequestra usually are seen in young patients) to larger segments of radiopaque bone (Fig. 18-12).

Effects on surrounding structures. Acute osteomyelitis can stimulate either bone resorption or bone formation.

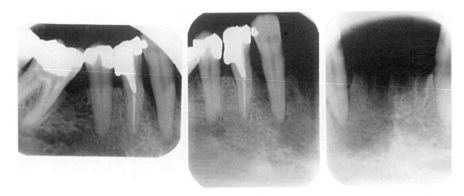

FIG. **18-11** Acute osteomyelitis involving the body of the right mandible, with initial blur-ring of bony trabeculae.

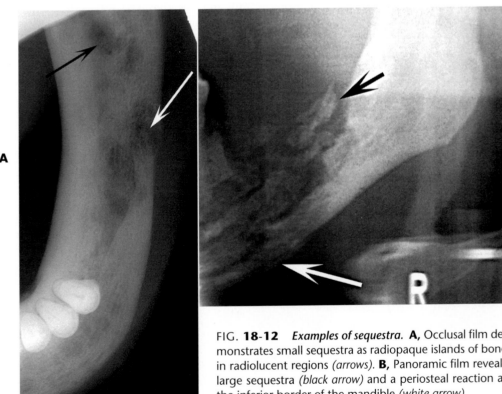

FIG. **18-12** *Examples of sequestra.* **A,** Occlusal film demonstrates small sequestra as radiopaque islands of bone in radiolucent regions *(arrows).* **B,** Panoramic film reveals large sequestra *(black arrow)* and a periosteal reaction at the inferior border of the mandible *(white arrow).*

Portions of cortical bone may be resorbed. An inflammatory exudate can lift the periosteum and stimulate bone formation. Radiographically, this appears as a thin, faint, radiopaque line adjacent to and almost parallel or slightly convex to the surface of the bone. A radiolucent band separates this periosteal new bone from the bone surface (Fig. 18-13). As the lesion develops into a more chronic phase, cyclic and periodic acute exacerbations may produce more inflammatory exudate, which again lifts the periosteum from the bone surface and stimulates the periosteum to form a second layer of bone.

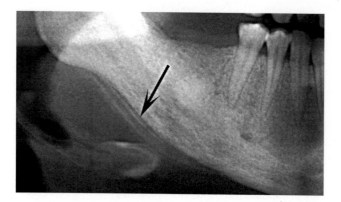

FIG. **18-13** *Osteomyelitis of the mandible with a periosteal reaction located at the inferior cortex.* Note the radiolucent line *(arrow)* between the inferior cortex of the mandible and the first layer of periosteal new bone. A second radiolucent line separates the second layer of new bone from the first layer.

This is detected radiographically as a second radiopaque line almost parallel to the first and separated from it by a radiolucent band. This process may continue and may result in several lines (an onion-skin appearance), and eventually a massive amount of new bone may be formed. This is referred to as *proliferative periostitis* and is seen more often in children (Fig. 18-14). The effects on the teeth and lamina dura may be the same as those described for periapical inflammatory lesions.

Additional Imaging

A two-phase nuclear medicine study composed of a technetium bone scan followed by a gallium citrate scan may help to confirm the diagnosis. With inflammatory lesions, a positive result on the technetium scan indicates increased bone metabolic activity, and a positive result on the gallium scan in the same location indicates an inflammatory cell infiltrate. Computed tomography (CT) is the imaging method of choice. CT reveals more bone surface for detecting periosteal new bone and is the best imaging method for detecting sequestra (Fig. 18-15).

Differential Diagnosis

The differential diagnosis of acute osteomyelitis may include fibrous dysplasia, especially in children. Aside from the clinical signs of acute infection, the most useful radiographic characteristic to distinguish osteomyelitis from fibrous dysplasia is the way the enlargement of the bone occurs. The new bone that enlarges the jaws in osteomyelitis is laid down by the periosteum and therefore

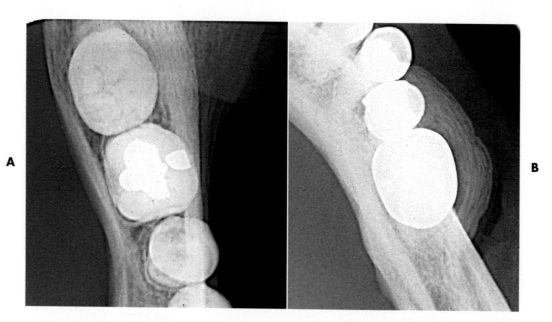

FIG. **18-14** **A** and **B,** Proliferative periostitis resulting from inflammatory lesions. Note the multiple layers of new bone, resulting in an onion-skin appearance.

is on the outside of the outer cortical plate. In fibrous dysplasia the new bone is manufactured on the inside of the mandible; thus the outer cortex, which may be thinned, is on the outside and contains the lesion. This point of differentiation is important because the histologic appearance of a biopsy of new periosteal bone in osteomyelitis may be similar to that of fibrous dysplasia, and the condition may be reported as such.

Malignant neoplasia (e.g., osteosarcoma, squamous cell carcinoma) that invades the mandible at times may be difficult to differentiate from acute osteomyelitis, especially if the malignancy has been secondarily infected via an oral ulcer; this may result in a mixture of inflammatory and malignant radiographic characteristics. If part of the inflammatory periosteal bone has been destroyed, the possibility of a malignant neoplasm should be considered. The differential diagnosis may include other lesions that can cause bone destruction and may stimulate a periosteal reaction that is similar to that seen in inflammatory lesions. Langerhans' cell histiocytosis causes lytic ill-defined bone destruction and often results in the formation of periosteal reactive new bone. This lesion rarely stimulates a sclerotic bone reaction such as that seen in osteomyelitis. Leukemia and lymphoma may stimulate a similar periosteal reaction.

Management

As with all inflammatory lesions of the jaws, removal of the source of inflammation is the primary goal of therapy. Antimicrobial treatment is the mainstay of treatment of acute osteomyelitis, along with establishing drainage.

This may entail removal of a tooth, root canal therapy, or surgical incision and drainage.

CHRONIC OSTEOMYELITIS

Synonyms

Chronic diffuse sclerosing osteomyelitis, chronic nonsuppurative osteomyelitis, chronic osteomyelitis with proliferative periostitis, Garré's chronic nonsuppurative sclerosing osteitis

Definition

Chronic osteomyelitis may be a sequela of inadequately treated acute osteomyelitis, or it may arise *de novo*. *Diffuse sclerosing osteomyelitis* refers to chronic osteomyelitis in which the balance in bone metabolism is tipped toward increased bone formation, producing a subsequent sclerotic radiographic appearance. The symptoms of chronic osteomyelitis generally are less severe and have a longer history than those of acute osteomyelitis. They include intermittent, recurrent episodes of swelling, pain, fever, and lymphadenopathy. As with the acute form, paresthesia and drainage with sinus formation also may occur. In some cases pain may be limited to the advancing front of the osteomyelitis, or the patient may have little or no pain. Histologically, a chronic inflammatory infiltrate may be seen within the medullary spaces of bone; however, this may be quite sparse, with only fibrosis of the marrow seen with scattered regions of inflammation. At this stage of the disease, the offending etiologic agent rarely is found because culture results

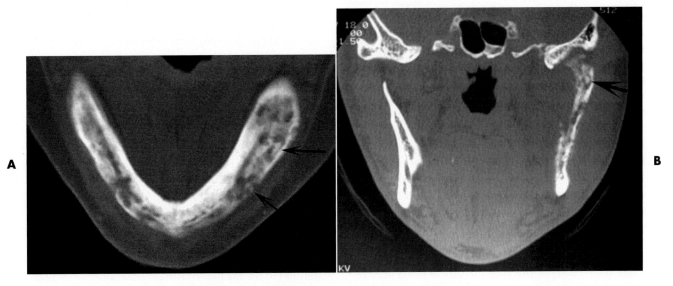

FIG. **18-15** *CT image of multiple sequestra.* **A,** An axial scan (bone window) revealing multiple sequestra *(arrows),* and **B,** a coronal scan (bone window) demonstrating a sequestrum *(arrow).*

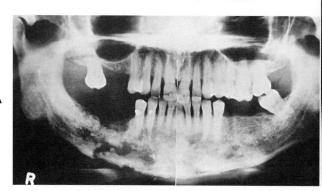
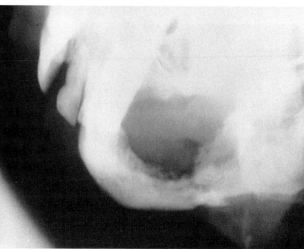

FIG. **18-16** *Chronic osteomyelitis.* **A,** Note the scattered areas of bone destruction surrounded by extremely dense bone and the presence of small islands of bone, or sequestra. **B,** Note the extreme radiopaque bone pattern.

usually are negative. If left untreated, osteomyelitis can spread and involve both sides of the mandible. Further spread into the temporomandibular joint may cause a septic arthritis, and ear infections and infection of the mastoid air cells also may develop.

Radiographic Features

Location. As in acute osteomyelitis, the most common site is the posterior mandible.

Periphery. The periphery may be better defined than in acute osteomyelitis, but it is still difficult to determine the exact extent of chronic osteomyelitis. Usually a gradual transition is seen between the normal surrounding trabecular pattern and the dense granular pattern characteristic of this disease. When the disease is active and is spreading through bone, the periphery may be more radiolucent and have poorly defined borders.

Internal structure. The internal structure comprises regions of greater and lesser radiopacity compared with surrounding normal bone (Fig. 18-16). Most of the lesion usually is composed of the more radiopaque or sclerotic bone pattern (Fig. 18-17). In older, chronic lesions the internal bone density can be exceedingly radiopaque and equivalent to cortical bone (see Fig. 18-16, *B*). In these cases no obvious regions of radiolucency may be seen. In other cases, small regions of radiolucency may be scattered throughout the radiopaque bone. A close inspection of the radiolucent regions may reveal an island of bone or sequestrum within the center. Often the sequestrum appears more radiopaque than the surrounding bone. Detection may require illumina-

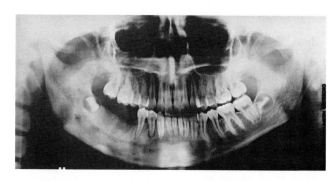

FIG. **18-17** *Chronic diffuse sclerosing osteomyelitis.* Most of the body and ramus of the right mandible is involved. Note the predominance of the sclerotic bone pattern with small regions of radiolucency and the slight enlargement of the mandible, resulting from previous periostitis and consolidation of this periosteal bone with the body of the mandible. (Courtesy L. Hollender, DDS, Seattle, Wash.)

tion of the radiolucent regions of the film with an intense light source. CT is superior for revealing the internal structure and sequestra, especially in cases with very dense sclerotic bone. The bone pattern usually is very granular, obscuring individual bone trabeculae.

Effects on surrounding structures. Chronic osteomyelitis often stimulates the formation of periosteal new bone, which is seen radiographically as a single radiopaque line or a series of radiopaque lines (similar to onion skin) parallel to the surface of the cortical bone. Over time the radiolucent strip that separates this new bone from the outer cortical bone surface may be filled in with granular sclerotic bone. When this occurs, it may not be possible

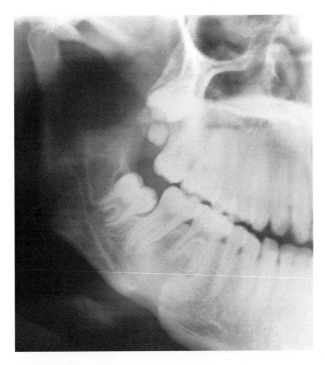

FIG. **18-18** A fistulous tract extending inferiorly from the apex of the first molar to the inferior cortex of the mandible.

to identify the original cortex, which makes it difficult to determine whether the new bone is derived from the periosteum. After a considerable amount of time the outer contour of the mandible also may be altered, assuming an abnormal shape, and the girth of the mandible may be much larger than on the unaffected side. The roots of teeth may undergo external resorption, and the lamina dura may become less apparent as it blends with the surrounding granular sclerotic bone. If a tooth is nonvital, the periodontal ligament space usually is enlarged in the apical region. In patients with extensive chronic osteomyelitis, the disease may slowly spread to the mandibular condyle and into the joint, resulting in a septic arthritis. Further spread may involve the inner ear and mastoid air cells. Chronic lesions may develop a draining fistula, which may appear as a well-defined break in the outer cortex or in the periosteal new bone (Fig 18-18).

Differential Diagnosis

Very sclerotic, radiopaque chronic lesions of osteomyelitis may be difficult to differentiate from fibrous dysplasia, Paget's disease, and osteosarcoma. In children, osteomyelitis with a proliferative periosteal response may be misinterpreted as fibrous dysplasia (see the section Differential Diagnosis under Acute Osteomyelitis). Differentiation of chronic osteomyelitis may be even more difficult if considerable remodeling and loss of a

distinct original cortex have occurred. In these cases, inspection of the bone surface at the periphery of the lesion may reveal subtle evidence of periosteal new bone formation. The presence of sequestra indicates osteomyelitis. Paget's disease affects the entire mandible, which is rare in osteomyelitis. Periosteal new bone formation and sequestra are not seen in Paget's disease. Dense, granular bone may be seen in some forms of osteosarcoma, but usually evidence of bone destruction is found. A characteristic spiculated (sunray-like) periosteal response also may be seen. As mentioned in the section on acute osteomyelitis, other entities such as Langerhans' cell histiocytosis, leukemia, and lymphoma may stimulate a similar periosteal response, but these usually produce evidence of bone destruction.

The imaging method of choice for aiding in the differential diagnosis is CT because of its ability to reveal sequestra and periosteal new bone. Also, CT allows accurate staging of the disease, which is important for future assessment of healing. Scintigraphy using bone scans, gallium, or labeled white blood cells is not particularly useful for differential diagnosis. Bone scans indicate increased bone formation, which is nonspecific, and often gallium scans (which highlight inflammatory cells) are not supportive.

Management

Chronic osteomyelitis tends to be more difficult to eradicate than the acute form. In cases involving an extreme osteoblastic response (very sclerotic mandible), the subsequent lack of a good blood supply may work against healing. Hyperbaric oxygen therapy and creative modes of long-term antibiotic delivery have been used with limited success. Surgical intervention, which may include sequestrectomy, decortication, or resection, often is necessary. The probability of successful treatment, especially when using long-term antibiotic therapy with decortication, is greater in the first two decades of life.

DIAGNOSTIC IMAGING OF SOFT TISSUE INFECTIONS

Diagnostic imaging may be used to confirm the presence and extent of soft tissue infections. Magnetic resonance imaging (MRI) and CT may be used to differentiate soft tissue neoplasia from inflammatory lesions. CT usually is used with intravenous contrast. The CT image characteristics that suggest the presence of a soft tissue inflammation include abnormal fascial planes, thickening of the overlying skin and adjacent muscles, streaking of the fat planes, and abnormal collections of gas in the soft tissue (Fig. 18-19). Over time the contrast between soft tissue planes may disappear, and the presence of an abscess may become evident as a well-defined

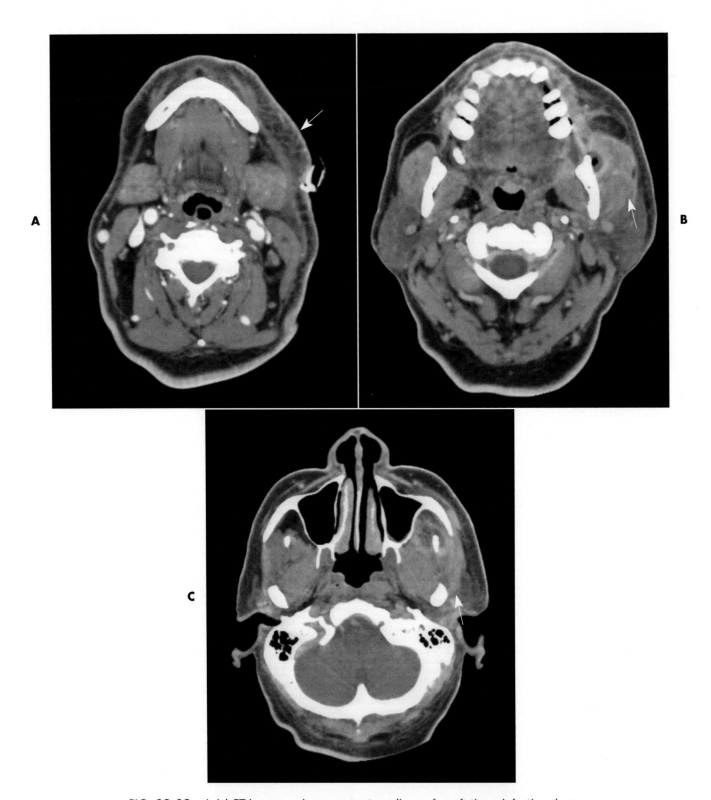

FIG. **18-19**   Axial CT images, using a contrast medium, of a soft tissue infection demonstrating streaking of the fat planes and thickening of the skin *(arrow)* **(A);** thickening of the masseter muscle and radiolucent pockets of gas *(arrow)* **(B);** and loss of soft tissue planes (individual muscles are difficult to distinguish compared with the other side) *(arrow)* **(C).** (Courtesy Stuart White, DDS, Los Angeles, Calif.)

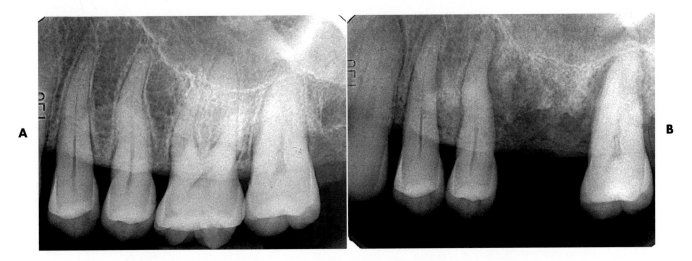

FIG. **18-20** *Osteoradionecrosis of the maxilla.* This periapical film was taken before radiotherapy, **A,** and within 6 months of receiving the radiation, **B.** Note the combination of bone sclerosis and profound bone destruction around the teeth and alveolar crest.

region of low density surrounded by a wide border of contrast-enhanced (more radiopaque) tissue.

OSTEORADIONECROSIS

Definition

Osteoradionecrosis refers to an inflammatory condition of bone (osteomyelitis) that occurs after the bone has been exposed to therapeutic doses of radiation. Doses above 50 Gy usually are required to cause this irreversible damage. Osteoradionecrosis is believed to be a result of radiation damage to bone, with consequent hypoxia, hypocellularity, and hypovascularity. Although infection may be a contributing factor, it is not necessarily the primary insult after the radiation damage has occurred. The result is delayed healing or lack of healing. Secondary infection is common, further fomenting the inflammatory reaction. Because of the difficulty of management, this serious complication of radiation therapy carries a high morbidity.

Clinical Features

The mandible is the most commonly involved bone, possibly because of the microanatomy and reduced vasculature of this bone. The posterior mandible is affected more often than the anterior portion, probably because the field of radiation therapy often is located in this region, which is a common location of malignant lesions, and because these lesions involve the lymph nodes of the neck. Loss of epithelial covering and exposure of bone is a common characteristic of osteoradionecrosis. This may occur spontaneously or after dental extractions or denture ulceration. Pathologic fracture also may occur. The exposed bone becomes necrotic as a result of loss of vascularity from the periosteum and subsequently sequestrates, often leading to exposure of more bone. Pain may or may not be present; intense pain often occurs, with intermittent swelling and drainage extraorally, but many patients experience no pain with bone exposure.

Radiographic Features

The radiographic features of osteoradionecrosis have many similarities to those of chronic osteomyelitis, and the reader is referred to that section for a detailed description. The following is a description of the radiographic changes seen in bone that has received a considerable amount of therapeutic radiation. The presence of osteoradionecrosis cannot always be diagnosed radiographically.

Location. The mandible, especially the posterior mandible, is the most common location for osteoradionecrosis. The maxilla may be involved in some cases.

Periphery. The periphery is ill defined and similar to that in osteomyelitis. If the lesion reaches the inferior border of the mandible, irregular resorption of this bony cortex often occurs.

Internal structure. A range of bone formation to bone destruction occurs, with the balance heavily toward more bone formation, giving the affected bone an overall sclerotic or radiopaque appearance. This is very similar to chronic osteomyelitis. The bone pattern is granular. Scattered regions of radiolucency may be seen, with and without central sequestra. The affected maxillary bone may also be very sclerotic and have areas of bone resorption (Fig. 18-20).

Effects on surrounding structures. Inflammatory new bone formation is uncommon, possibly because of the deleterious effects of radiation on potential osteoblasts in the periosteum. In very rare cases the periosteum appears to have been stimulated to produce bone, resulting in new bone formation on the outer cortex in an unusual shape. Radiation exposure may also stimulate the resorption of bone, especially in the maxilla, which may be similar in appearance to bone destruction caused by a malignant neoplasm. The most common effect on the surrounding bone is the stimulation of sclerosis.

Differential Diagnosis

Bone resorption, stimulated by high levels of irradiation, may simulate bone destruction from a malignant neoplasm, especially in the maxilla. For this reason, the detection of a recurrence of the malignant neoplasm (usually squamous cell carcinoma) in the presence of osteoradionecrosis may be very difficult. If recurrence is suspected, CT and MRI scanning may be used to detect an associated soft tissue mass. Differentiation from other sclerotic lesions, as in chronic osteomyelitis, is less difficult because of the history of radiation therapy.

Management

The treatment of osteoradionecrosis currently is unsatisfactory. Decortication with sequestrectomy and hyperbaric oxygen with antibiotics have been used with limited success. Fortunately, the incidence of osteoradionecrosis has declined because preventive therapy has proved quite effective. Removal of borderline teeth before radiation treatment and excellent oral and denture hygiene are the mainstays of preventive treatment.

BIBLIOGRAPHY

PERIAPICAL INFLAMMATORY LESIONS

Heersche JNM: Bone cells and bone turnover: the basis for pathogenesis. In Tam CS et al, editors: *Metabolic bone disease: cellular and tissue mechanisms,* Boca Raton, Fla., 1989, CRC Press.

Shafer WG et al: *A textbook of oral pathology,* Philadelphia, 1983, WB Saunders.

Stern MH et al: Quantitative analysis of cellular composition of human periapical granuloma, *J Endocrinol* 7:117, 1981.

PERICORONITIS

Blakey GH et al: Clinical/biological outcomes of treatment for pericoronitis, *J Oral Maxillofac Surg* 54:1150, 1996.

OSTEOMYELITIS

Cotran RS et al: *Pathologic basis of disease,* ed 4, Philadelphia, 1989, WB Saunders.

Harel-Raviv M et al: Oral osteomyelitis: pre-AIDS manifestation or strange coincidence? *Dental Update* 23:26, 1996.

Lawoyin DO et al: Osteomyelitis of the mandible associated with osteopetrosis: report of a case, *Br J Oral Maxillofac Surg* 26:330, 1988.

Nordin U et al: Antibody response in patients with osteomyelitis of the mandible, *Oral Surg Oral Med Oral Pathol* 79:429, 1995.

Olaitan AA et al: Osteomyelitis of the mandible in sickle cell disease, *Br J Oral Maxillofac Surg* 35:190, 1997.

Orpe E et al: Radiographic features of osteomyelitis of the jaws, *Dentomaxillofac Radiol* 25:125, 1996.

Petrikowski CG et al: Radiographic differentiation of osteogenic sarcoma, osteomyelitis, and fibrous dysplasia of the jaws, *Oral Surg Oral Med Oral Pathol* 80:747, 1995.

Van Merkesteyn JPR et al: Diffuse sclerosing osteomyelitis of the mandible: clinical radiographic and histologic findings in twenty-seven patients, *J Oral Maxillofac Surg* 46:825, 1988.

Wannfors K: *Chronic osteomyelitis of the jaws,* Stockholm, 1990, Gotab (thesis).

Wannfors K, Hammarstrom L: Infectious foci in chronic osteomyelitis of the jaws, *Int J Oral Surg* 14:493, 1985.

Wood RE et al: Periostitis ossificans versus Garré's osteomyelitis. I. What did Garré really say? *Oral Surg Oral Med Oral Pathol* 65:773, 1988.

OSTERADIONECROSIS

Curi MM, Dib LL: Osteoradionecrosis of the jaws: a retrospective study of the background factors and treatment in 104 cases, *J Oral Maxillofac Surg* 55:540, 1997.

Hermans R et al: CT findings in osteoradionecrosis of the mandible, *Skeletal Radiol* 25:31, 1996.

Marx RE: Osteoradionecrosis: a new concept of its pathophysiology, *J Oral Maxillofac Surg* 41:283, 1983.

Wong JK et al: Conservative management of osteoradionecrosis, *Oral Surg Oral Med Oral Pathol* 84:16, 1997.

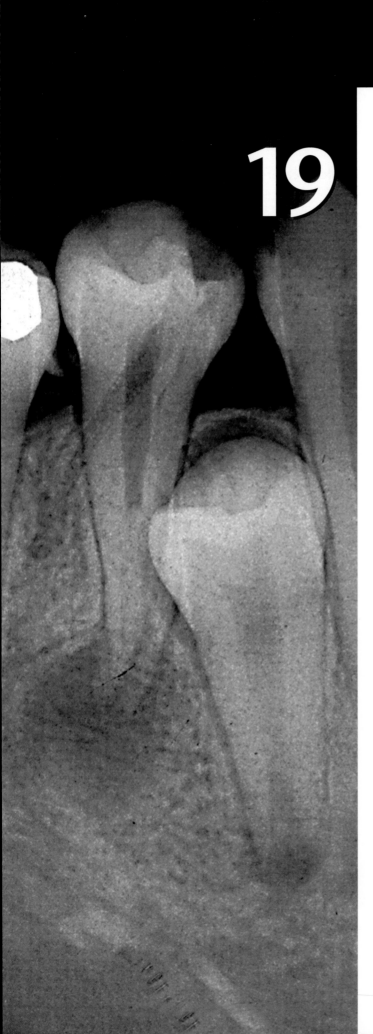

19

Cysts of the Jaws

A *cyst is a pathologic cavity filled with fluid,* lined by epithelium, and surrounded by a definite connective tissue wall. The cystic fluid either is secreted by the cells lining the cavity or derives from the surrounding tissue fluid.

Clinical Features

Cysts occur more often in the jaws than in any other bone because most cysts originate from the numerous rests of odontogenic epithelium that remain after tooth formation. Cysts are radiolucent lesions, and the prevalent clinical features are swelling, lack of pain (unless the cyst becomes secondarily infected or is related to a nonvital tooth), and missing teeth, especially third molars.

Radiographic Features

LOCATION

Cysts may occur centrally in any location in the maxilla or mandible but are rare in the condyle and coronoid process. Cysts are found most often in the tooth-bearing region. In the mandible, they occur most often above the inferior alveolar nerve canal. Odontogenic cysts may grow into the maxillary antrum. Some nonodontogenic cysts also originate within the antrum (see Chapter 25). A few cysts arise in the soft tissues of the orofacial region.

PERIPHERY

Central cysts usually have a periphery that is well defined and corticated (characterized by a fairly uniform, thin, radiopaque line). However, a secondary infection or a chronic state can change this radiographic picture. In such cases the thin corticated line may change into a thick sclerotic boundary.

SHAPE

Cysts usually are round or oval, resembling a balloon. Some cysts may have a scalloped boundary.

INTERNAL STRUCTURE

Cysts often are radiolucent. However, long-standing cysts may have dystrophic calcification, which can give the internal aspect a sparse, particulate appearance on x-rays. Some cysts have septa, which are multiple loculations separated by bony walls. Cysts that have a scalloped periphery may appear to have internal septa.

EFFECTS ON SURROUNDING STRUCTURES

Cysts grow slowly, sometimes causing displacement and resorption of teeth. The area of tooth resorption often has a sharp, curved shape. Cysts can expand the mandible, usually in a smooth, curved manner, and change the buccal or lingual cortical plate into a thin cortical boundary. Cysts may displace the inferior alveolar nerve canal in an inferior direction or invaginate the maxillary antrum, maintaining a thin layer of bone that separates the internal aspect of the cyst from the antrum.

Odontogenic Cysts

RADICULAR CYST

Synonyms
Periapical cyst, apical periodontal cyst, or *dental cyst*

Definition
A radicular cyst is a cyst that most likely results when rests of epithelial cells in the periodontal ligament are stimulated by inflammatory products from a nonvital tooth.

Clinical Features
Radicular cysts are the most common type of cyst in the jaws. They arise from nonvital teeth (i.e., teeth that have lost vitality because of extensive caries, large restorations, or previous trauma). Often radicular cysts produce no symptoms unless secondary infection occurs. A cyst that becomes large may cause swelling. On palpation the swelling may feel bony and hard if the cortex is intact, crepitant as the bone thins, and rubbery and fluctuant if bone destruction has occurred. The incidence of radicular cysts is greater in the third to sixth decades and shows a slight male predominance.

Radiographic Features
Location. In most cases the epicenter of a radicular cyst is located approximately at the apex of a nonvital tooth (Fig. 19-1). Occasionally it appears on the mesial or distal surface of a tooth root, at the opening of an accessory canal, or infrequently in a deep periodontal pocket. Most radicular cysts (60%) are found in the maxilla, especially around incisors and canines. Because of the distal inclination of the root, cysts that arise from the maxillary lateral incisor may invaginate the antrum. Radicular cysts may also form in relation to a nonvital deciduous molar and be positioned buccal to the developing bicuspid.

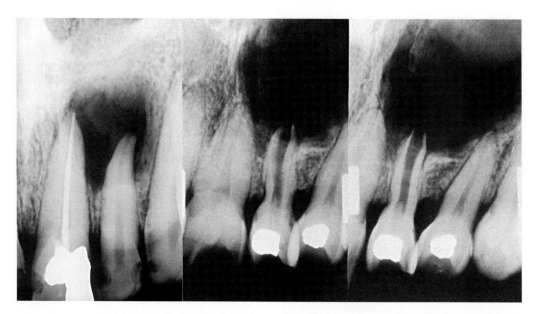

FIG. **19-1** *Radicular cysts.* Note that the epicenter of the lesion is in the vicinity of the periapical region of the involved tooth. Also, the caliber of the pulp chamber of the nonvital tooth is larger than normal.

Periphery and shape. The periphery usually has a well-defined cortical border (Fig. 19-2). If the cyst becomes secondarily infected, the inflammatory reaction of the surrounding bone may result in destruction of the cortex or alteration of the cortex into a more sclerotic border. The outline of a radicular cyst usually is curved or circular unless it is influenced by surrounding structures such as cortical boundaries.

Internal structure. In most cases the internal structure of radicular cysts is radiolucent. Occasionally, dystrophic calcification may develop in long-standing cysts, appearing as sparsely distributed, small particulate radiopacities.

Effects on surrounding structures. If a radicular cyst is large, displacement and resorption of the roots of adjacent teeth may occur. The resorption pattern may have a curved outline. In rare cases the cyst may resorb the roots of the related nonvital tooth. The cyst may invaginate the antrum, but evidence should be seen of a cortical boundary between the contents of the cyst and the internal structure of the antrum. The outer cortical plates of the maxilla or mandible may expand in a curved or circular shape (Fig. 19-3). Cysts may displace the mandibular alveolar nerve canal in an inferior direction.

Differential Diagnosis
Differentiation of a small radicular cyst from an apical granuloma may be difficult and in some cases impossible. A round shape, a well-defined cortical border, and a size greater than 2 cm in diameter are more characteristic of a cyst. Other periapical radiolucencies to consider are an apical scar or a surgical defect because in such cases normal bone may never fill in the defect completely. The patient's history helps with the differentiation. Radicular cysts that originate from the maxillary lateral incisor and are positioned between the roots of the lateral incisor and the cuspid may be difficult to differentiate from an odontogenic keratocyst or a lateral periodontal cyst. The vitality of the involved tooth should be tested. A nonvital tooth may have a larger pulp chamber than neighboring teeth because of the lack of secondary dentin, which normally forms with time in the pulp chamber and canal of a vital tooth (see Fig. 19-1).

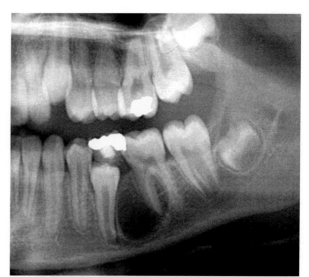

A

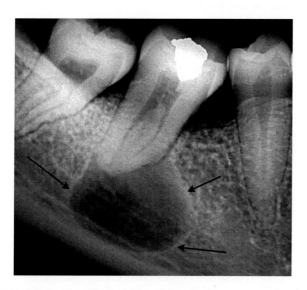

FIG. **19-2** A periapical film of a radicular cyst reveals a lesion with a well-defined cortical boundary *(arrows).* Note that the presence of the inferior cortex of the mandible has influenced the circular shape of the cyst.

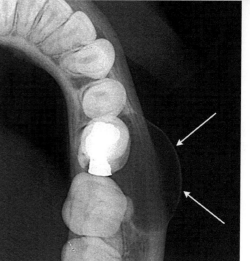

B

FIG. **19-3** **A** and **B,** Two images of a radicular cyst originating from a nonvital deciduous second molar show expansion of the buccal cortical plate to a circular or hydraulic shape *(arrows)* and displacement of the adjacent permanent teeth.

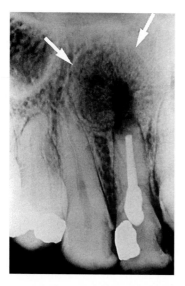

FIG. **19-4** A radicular cyst that is healing after endodontic treatment. Arrows show the original outline of the cyst; note that the new bone grows toward the center from the periphery.

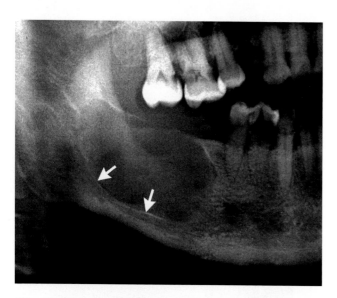

FIG. **19-5** The epicenter of this infected residual cyst is above the inferior alveolar nerve canal and has displaced the canal in an inferior direction (arrows). Note that the cortical boundary is not continuous around the whole cyst.

A large radicular cyst that has invaginated the antrum may collapse and start filling in with new bone. With biopsy, the histologic analysis may result in an erroneous diagnosis of ossifying fibroma or a benign fibroosseous lesion. Radiographically, the important feature is that the new bone always forms first at the periphery of the cyst wall as the cyst shrinks; this is a different pattern of bone formation than that which occurs with a benign fibroosseous lesion.

Management

Treatment of a tooth with a radicular cyst may include extraction, endodontic therapy, and apical surgery. Treatment of a large radicular cyst usually involves surgical removal or marsupialization. The radiographic appearance of the periapical area of an endodontically treated tooth should be checked periodically to make sure that normal healing is occurring (Fig. 19-4). Characteristically, new bone grows into the defect from the periphery, sometimes resulting in a radiating pattern resembling the spokes of a wheel. However, in a few cases normal bone may not fill the defect, especially if a secondary infection or a considerable amount of bone destruction occurred. Recurrence of a radicular cyst is unlikely if it has been removed completely.

RESIDUAL CYST

Definition

A residual cyst is a cyst that develops after incomplete removal of the original cyst. The term *residual* is used most often for a radicular cyst that may be left behind or that develops after extraction of a tooth.

Clinical Features

A residual cyst usually is asymptomatic and often is discovered on radiographic examination of an edentulous area. However, there may be some expansion of the jaw or pain in the case of secondary infection.

Radiographic Features

Location. Residual cysts occur in both jaws, although they develop slightly more often in the mandible. The epicenter is found in a periapical location if the teeth are still present. In the mandible the epicenter is always above the inferior alveolar nerve canal (Fig. 19-5).

Periphery and shape. A residual cyst has a cortical margin unless it becomes secondarily infected. Its shape is oval or circular.

Internal structure. The internal aspect of a residual cyst typically is radiolucent. Dystrophic calcifications may be present in long-standing cysts.

Effects on surrounding structures. Residual cysts can cause tooth displacement or resorption. The outer cortical plates of the jaws may expand. The cyst may invaginate the maxillary antrum or depress the inferior alveolar nerve canal.

Differential Diagnosis

Without the patient's history and previous radiographs, the clinician may have difficulty determining if a solitary cyst in the jaws is a residual cyst. Other examples of common solitary cysts include odontogenic keratocysts. A residual cyst has greater potential for expansion compared with an odontogenic keratocyst. The epicenter of a Stafne developmental salivary gland defect is located below the mandibular canal (and thus is unlikely to be odontogenic in nature).

Management

The treatment for residual cysts is surgical removal or marsupialization, or both, if the cyst is large.

DENTIGEROUS CYST

Synonym

Follicular cyst

Definition

A dentigerous cyst is a cyst that forms around the crown of an unerupted tooth. It begins when fluid accumulates in the layers of reduced enamel epithelium or between the epithelium and the crown of the unerupted tooth. An eruption cyst is the soft tissue counterpart of a dentigerous cyst.

Clinical Features

Dentigerous cysts are the second most common type of cyst in the jaws. They develop around the crown of an unerupted or supernumerary tooth. The clinical examination reveals a missing tooth or teeth and possibly a hard swelling, occasionally resulting in facial asymmetry. The patient typically has no pain or discomfort. About 4% of individuals with at least one unerupted tooth have a dentigerous cyst. Dentigerous cysts around supernumerary teeth account for about 5% of all dentigerous cysts, most developing around a mesiodens in the anterior maxilla.

Radiographic Features

Location. The epicenter of a dentigerous cyst is found just above the crown of the involved tooth, which usually is the mandibular third molar or the maxillary canine, the teeth most commonly affected (Fig. 19-6). An important diagnostic point is that this cyst attaches at the cementoenamel junction. Some dentigerous cysts are eccentric, developing from the lateral aspect of the follicle so that they occupy an area beside the crown instead of above the crown (see Fig. 19-6, *D*). Cysts related to maxillary third molars often grow into the maxillary antrum and may become quite large before they are dis-

covered. Cysts attached to the crown of mandibular molars may extend a considerable distance into the ramus.

Periphery and shape. Dentigerous cysts typically have a well-defined cortex with a curved or circular outline. If infection is present, the cortex may be missing.

Internal structure. The internal aspect is completely radiolucent except for the crown of the involved tooth.

Effects on surrounding structures. A dentigerous cyst has a propensity to displace and resorb adjacent teeth (Fig. 19-7). It commonly displaces the associated tooth in an apical direction. The degree of displacement may be considerable. For instance, maxillary third molars or cuspids may be pushed to the floor of the orbit (see Fig. 19-7), and mandibular third molars may be moved to the condylar or coronoid regions or to the inferior cortex of the mandible (Fig. 19-8). The floor of the maxillary antrum may be displaced as the cyst invaginates the antrum, and the cyst may displace the inferior alveolar nerve canal in an inferior direction. This slow-growing cyst often expands the outer cortical boundary of the involved jaw.

Differential Diagnosis

Because the histopathologic appearance of the lining epithelium is not specific, the diagnosis relies on the radiographic and surgical observation of the attachment of the cyst to the cementoenamel junction. A histopathologic examination must be done to eliminate other possible lesions in this location.

One of the most difficult differential diagnoses to make is between a small dentigerous cyst and a hyperplastic follicle. A cyst should be considered with any evidence of tooth displacement or considerable expansion of the involved bone. The size of the normal follicular space is 2 to 3 mm. If the follicular space exceeds 5 mm, a dentigerous cyst is more likely. If uncertainty remains, the region should be reexamined in 4 to 6 months to detect any increase in size or any influence on surrounding structures characteristic of cysts.

The differential diagnosis also may include an odontogenic keratocyst, an ameloblastic fibroma, and a cystic ameloblastoma. An odontogenic keratocyst does not expand the bone to the same degree as a dentigerous cyst, is less likely to resorb teeth, and may not attach precisely at the cementoenamel junction. It may not be possible to differentiate a small ameloblastic fibroma or cystic ameloblastoma from a dentigerous cyst if there is no internal structure. Other rare lesions that may have a similar pericoronal appearance are adenomatoid odontogenic tumors and calcified odontogenic cysts, both of

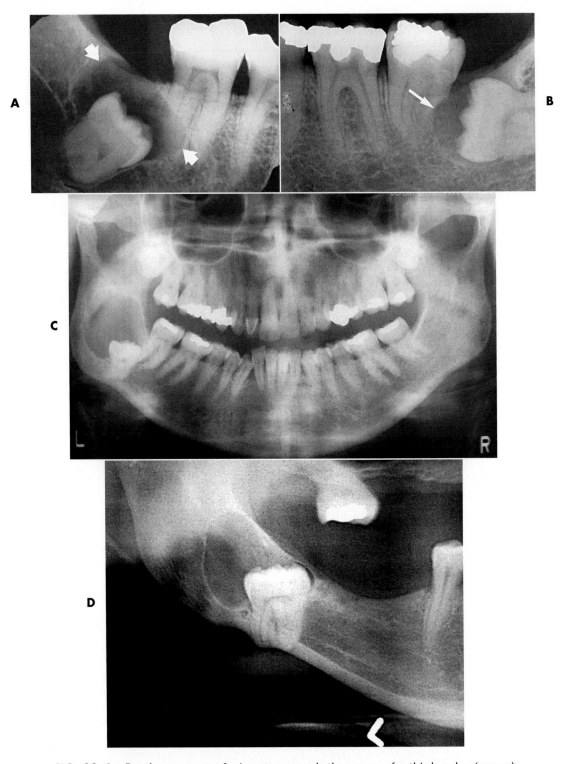

FIG. **19-6** *Dentigerous cysts.* **A,** A cyst surrounds the crown of a third molar *(arrows);* note the resorption of the distal root of the second molar *(arrow)* **(B). C,** A cyst that involves the ramus of the mandible. **D,** A dentigerous cyst that is expanding distally from the involved third molar.

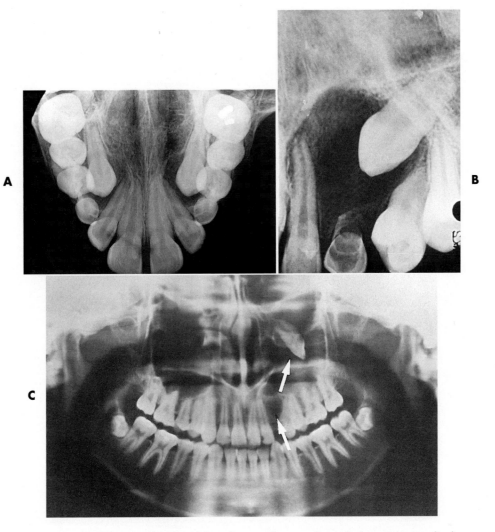

FIG. **19-7** *Dentigerous cysts involving the maxillary canines.* **A,** A cyst causes displacement toward the midline, impeding eruption **(B). C,** Displacement of the cuspid into the space occupied by the maxillary antrum and displacement of the lateral incisor and the first premolar.

which can surround the crown and root of the involved tooth. Evidence of a radiopaque internal structure should be sought in these two lesions. Occasionally a radicular cyst at the apex of a primary tooth surrounds the crown of the permanent tooth that is developing apical to it, giving the false impression that a dentigerous cyst exists involving the permanent tooth. This occurs most often with the mandibular deciduous molars and the developing bicuspids. In these cases the clinician should look for deep caries or extensive restorations in a primary tooth that would indicate a radicular cyst.

Management

Dentigerous cysts are treated by surgical removal, which may include the tooth as well. Large cysts may be treated by marsupialization before removal. The cyst lining should be submitted for histologic examination because ameloblastomas have been reported to occur in the cyst lining. In addition, squamous cell carcinoma has been reported to arise from the cyst lining that may develop in chronically infected cysts. Mucoepidermoid carcinoma also has been reported.

BUCCAL BIFURCATION CYST

Synonyms
Mandibular infected buccal cyst, paradental cyst, or *inflammatory collateral dental cyst*

Definition
The source of epithelium probably is the epithelial cell rests in the periodontium of the buccal bifurcation of

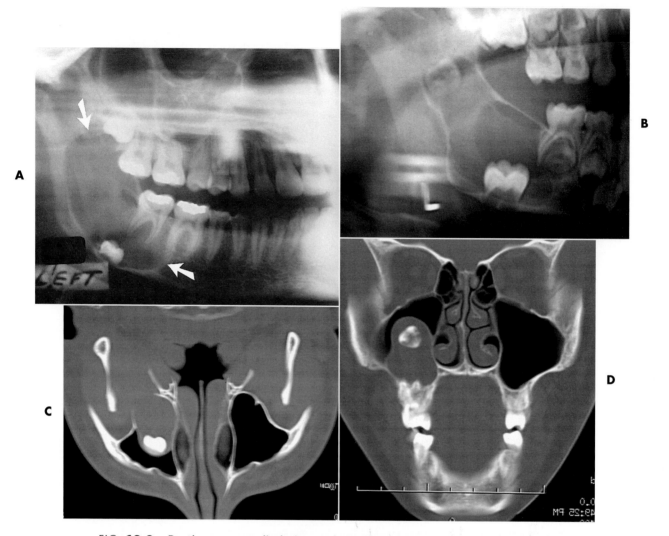

FIG. **19-8** *Dentigerous cysts displacing teeth.* **A,** The third molar has been displaced to the inferior cortex. **B,** The second molar has been displaced into the ramus by a cyst associated with the first molar. Axial **(C)** and coronal **(D)** CT images using bone algorithm reveal a maxillary third molar displaced into the space occupied by the maxillary antrum.

mandibular molars. The histopathologic characteristics of the lining are not distinctive. The etiology of proliferation is unknown; one theory holds that inflammation is the stimulus, but inflammation is not always present. The World Health Organization includes these cysts under inflammatory cysts.

It is unclear whether the paradental cyst of the third molar and the buccal bifurcation cyst (associated with first and second molars) are the same entity. The buccal bifurcation cyst (BBC) is certainly a distinct *clinical* entity. An associated enamel extension into the furcation region of third molars with paradental cysts has not been documented with molars involved in a BBC. Also,

the inflammatory component associated with paradental cysts is not always present with BBCs.

Clinical Features

A common sign is the lack of or a delay in eruption of a mandibular first or second molar. On clinical examination the molar may be missing or the lingual cusp tips may be abnormally protruding through the mucosa, higher than the position of the buccal cusps. The first molar is involved more frequently than the second molar. The teeth are always vital. A hard swelling may be present buccal to the involved molar, and if it is secondarily infected, the patient has pain. The age of detec-

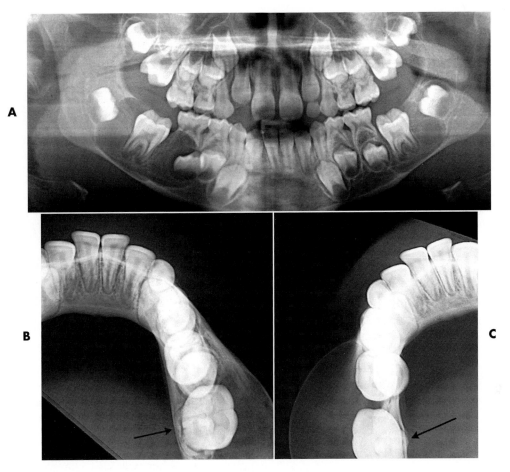

FIG. **19-9** *Bilateral buccal bifurcation cysts.* **A,** A panoramic image showing cysts related to the mandibular first molars. Note that the occlusal surface of each tooth has been tipped in relation to the other teeth and that adjacent teeth have been displaced. **B** and **C,** Occlusal films of the same case. Note the circular expansion of the buccal cortex and the displacement of the roots of the first molars into the lingual cortical plate *(arrows).*

tion is younger: within the first two decades for a BBC and in the third decade for a paradental cyst of the third molar.

Radiographic Features

Location. The mandibular first molar is the most common location of a BBC, followed by the second molar. The cyst occasionally is bilateral. It is always located in the buccal furcation of the affected molar (Fig. 19-9). On periapical and panoramic films the lesion may appear to be centered a little distal to the furcation of the involved tooth.

Periphery and shape. In some cases the periphery is not readily apparent, and the lesion may be a very subtle radiolucent region superimposed over the image of the roots of the molar. In other cases the lesion has a circu-

lar shape with a well-defined cortical border. Some cysts can become quite large before they are detected.

Internal structure. The internal structure is radiolucent.

Effects on surrounding structures. The most striking diagnostic characteristic of a BBC is the tipping of the involved molar so that the root tips are pushed into the lingual cortical plate of the mandible (see Fig. 19-9, *B* and *C*) and the occlusal surface is tipped toward the buccal aspect of the mandible (see Fig. 19-9, *A*). This accounts for the lingual cusp tips being positioned higher than the buccal tips. This tipping may be detected in a panoramic or periapical film if the image of the occlusal surface of the affected tooth is apparent whereas the unaffected teeth are not. The best diagnostic film is the cross-sectional (standard) mandibular occlusal projection, which demonstrates the abnormal position of the root apex. If the cyst is large enough, it may displace and resorb the adjacent teeth and cause a considerable amount of smooth expansion of the buccal cortical plate. If the cyst is secondarily infected, periosteal new bone formation is seen on the buccal cortex adjacent to the involved tooth.

Differential Diagnosis

Diagnosis of a BBC relies entirely on clinical and radiographic information. The major differential diagnosis includes lesions that could elicit an inflammatory periosteal response on the buccal aspect of mandibular molars such as a periodontal abscess or Langerhans' cell histiocytosis. The fact that only a BBC tilts the molar as described helps to differentiate it from other lesions. Also in the differential diagnosis is the dentigerous cyst. However, the epicenter of a dentigerous cyst is different because a BBC starts near the bifurcation region of the tooth and does not surround the crown, as does a dentigerous cyst.

Management

A BBC usually is removed by conservative curettage, although some cases have resolved without intervention. The involved molar should not be removed. BBCs do not recur.

ODONTOGENIC KERATOCYST

Synonym

It is a commonly held view that primordial cysts are odontogenic keratocysts. However, this view is not universally accepted.

Definition

An odontogenic keratocyst (OKC) is a noninflammatory odontogenic cyst that arises from the dental lamina. Unlike other cysts, which are thought to grow solely by osmotic pressure, the epithelium in an OKC appears to have innate growth potential, much as in a benign tumor. This difference in the mechanism of growth gives OKCs a different radiographic appearance. The epithelial lining is distinctive because it is keratinized (hence the name) and thin (4 to 8 cells thick). Occasionally budlike proliferations of epithelium grow from the basal layer into the adjacent connective tissue wall. Also, islands of epithelium in the wall may give rise to satellite microcysts. The inside of the cyst often contains a viscous or cheesy material derived from the epithelial lining.

Clinical Features

OKCs account for about one tenth of all cysts in the jaws. They occur in a wide age range, but most develop during the second and third decades, with a slight male

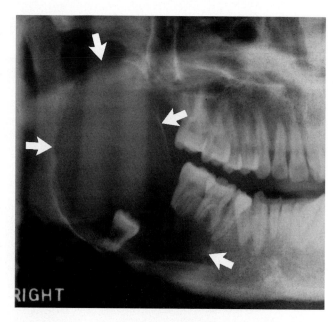

FIG. 19-10 OKC occupying most of the right mandibular ramus. (Courtesy B. Gratt, DDS, Los Angeles, Calif.)

predominance. The cysts sometimes form around an unerupted tooth. OKCs usually have no symptoms, although mild swelling may occur. Pain may occur with secondary infection. Aspiration may reveal a thick, yellow, cheesy material (keratin). It is important to note that, unlike other cysts, OKCs have a high propensity for recurrence, possibly because of small satellite cysts or fragments of epithelium left behind after surgical removal of the cyst.

Radiographic Features

Location. The most common location of an OKC is the posterior body of the mandible (90% occur posterior to the canines) and ramus (more than 50%) (Fig. 19-10). The epicenter is located superior to the inferior alveolar nerve canal. This type of cyst occasionally has the same pericoronal position as and is indistinguishable from a dentigerous cyst (Fig. 19-11).

Periphery and shape. As with other cysts, OKCs usually show evidence of a cortical border unless they have become secondarily infected. The cyst may have a smooth round or oval shape identical to that of other cysts, or it may have a scalloped outline (a series of contiguous arcs) (see Fig. 19-11, *B*).

Internal structure. The internal structure most commonly is radiolucent. The presence of internal keratin does not increase the radiopacity. In some cases curved internal septa may be present, giving the lesion a multilocular appearance (see Fig. 19-11, *C*).

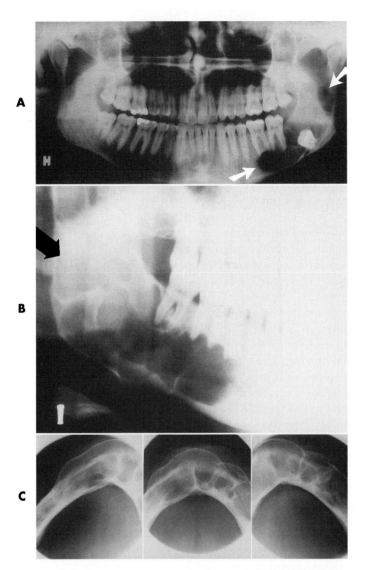

FIG. **19-11** OKCs **(A)** *(arrows)* can become quite large before they are detected, partly because the involved bone expands only slightly. **B,** The superior margin of this cyst has a scalloped periphery. **C,** This cyst occupies all of the anterior of the mandible and shows only a small amount of buccal-lingual expansion compared with extension along the body of the mandible. (Courtesy L. Hollender, DDS, Seattle, Wash.)

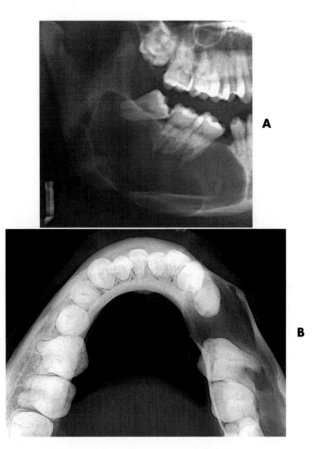

FIG. **19-12** A large keratocyst occupying most of the right body and ramus of the mandible. **A,** Note that, despite the cyst's size, the buccal and lingual cortical plates of the mandible have expanded only slightly, as can be seen in the occlusal film **(B).**

Effects on surrounding structures. An important characteristic of the OKC is its propensity to grow along the internal aspect of the jaws, causing minimal expansion (Fig. 19-12). This occurs throughout the mandible except for the upper ramus and coronoid process, where considerable expansion may occur. Occasionally the expansion of large cysts may exceed the ability of the periosteum to form new bone, thus allowing the cyst wall to contact soft tissue peripheral to the outer cortex of the mandible (Fig. 19-13). The relatively slight expansion common with these cysts probably contributes to their late detection, which occasionally allows them to reach a large size. OKCs can displace and resorb teeth but to a slightly lesser degree than dentigerous cysts. The inferior alveolar nerve canal may be displaced inferiorly. In the maxilla this cyst can invaginate and occupy the entire maxillary antrum.

Differential Diagnosis

When in a pericoronal position, an OKC may be indistinguishable from a dentigerous cyst. The cyst is likely to be an OKC if the cyst is connected to the tooth at a point apical to the cementoenamel junction or if no expansion of the cortical plates has occurred. The typical scalloped margin and multilocular appearance of the OKC may resemble an ameloblastoma, but the latter has a greater propensity to expand. An OKC may show some similarity to an odontogenic myxoma, especially in the characteristics of mild expansion and multilocular appearance. A simple bone cyst often has a scalloped margin and

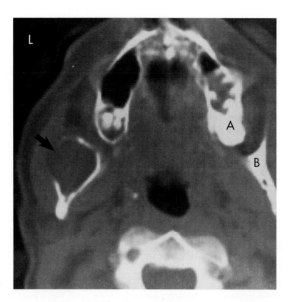

FIG. **19-13**   An axial CT image slice at the level of the mandibular ramus shows perforation of the lateral cortical plate of the ramus and extension into the adjacent masseter muscle *(arrow)*. *A,* Maxillary alveolus. *B,* Ramus on the normal side. (From Frame JW, Wake MJC: *Br Dent J* 153:93, 1982.)

minimal bone expansion, as with an OKC; however, the margins of a simple bone cyst usually are more delicate and often difficult to detect. If several OKCs are found (which occurs in 4% to 5% of cases), these cysts may constitute part of a basal cell nevus syndrome.

Management

If an OKC is suspected, referral to a radiologist for a complete radiologic examination is advisable. Because this cyst has a propensity to recur, an accurate determination of the extent and location of any cortical perforations with soft tissue extension is best achieved with computed tomography. In the case of multiple cysts and the possibility of basal cell nevus syndrome, a thorough radiologic examination is required. This allows accurate determination of the number of cysts and other osseous characteristics that confirm the diagnosis.

Surgical treatment may vary and can include resection, curettage, or marsupialization to reduce the size of large cysts before surgical excision. More attention usually is devoted to complete removal of the walls of the cyst to reduce the chance of recurrence. After surgical treatment, it is important to make periodic post-treatment clinical and radiographic examinations to detect any recurrence. Recurrent lesions usually develop within the first 5 years but may be delayed as long as 10 years.

BASAL CELL NEVUS SYNDROME

Synonyms

Nevoid basal cell carcinoma syndrome or *Gorlin-Goltz syndrome*

Definition

The term *basal cell nevus syndrome* comprises a number of abnormalities such as multiple nevoid basal cell carcinomas of the skin, skeletal abnormalities, central nervous system abnormalities, eye abnormalities, and multiple OKCs. It is inherited as an autosomal dominant trait with variable expressivity.

Clinical Features

Basal cell nevus syndrome starts to appear early in life, usually after 5 years of age and before 30 years of age, with the development of jaw cysts and skin basal cell carcinomas. The lesions occur as multiple OKCs of the jaws, usually appearing in multiple quadrants and earlier in life than solitary OKCs. The recurrence rate of OKCs in this syndrome appears to be higher than with the solitary variety. The skin lesions are small, flattened, flesh-colored or brown papules that can occur anywhere on the body but are especially prominent on the face, neck, and trunk. Occasionally basal cell carcinomas form later in life than the jaw cysts or not at all. Skeletal anomalies include bifid rib (most common) and other costal abnormalities such as agenesis, deformity, and synostosis of the ribs, kyphoscoliosis, vertebral fusion, polydactyly, shortening of the metacarpals, temporal and temporoparietal bossing, minor hypertelorism, and mild prognathism. Calcification of the falx cerebri and other parts of the dura occur early in life.

Radiographic Features

Location. The location is the same as that of solitary OKCs, as described previously. The multiple keratocysts may develop bilaterally and can vary in size from 1 mm to several centimeters in diameter (Fig. 19-14).

Other radiographic features. See the preceding radiographic description of OKCs. In addition, a radiopaque line of the calcified falx cerebri may be prominent on the posteroanterior skull projection. Occasionally this calcification may appear laminated.

Differential Diagnosis

The presence of a cortical boundary and other cystic characteristics differentiate basal cell nevus syndrome from other abnormalities characterized by multiple radiolucencies (e.g., multiple myeloma). Cherubism appears as bilateral multilocular lesions but usually has significant jaw expansion, which is not characteristic of

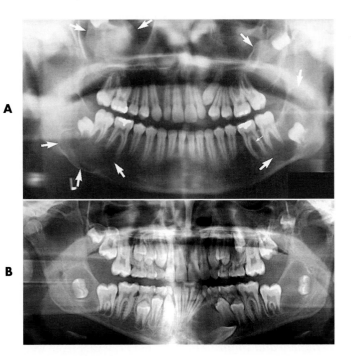

FIG. 19-14 Multiple OKCs associated with nevoid basal cell carcinoma syndrome. **A,** The upper arrows point to opacified maxillary antra; the smaller arrow indicates the extension of one of the mandibular cysts *(lower arrows)* into the bifurcation region of a mandibular molar. **B,** Five cysts are present, which are related to the mandibular third molars and left cuspid and to the maxillary left second premolar and third molar.

basal cell nevus syndrome. Also, cherubism pushes posterior teeth in an anterior direction, a distinctive characteristic. Occasionally patients with multiple dentigerous cysts may show some similarities, but dentigerous cysts are more expansile.

Management

The keratocysts are treated more aggressively than other solitary OKCs because there appears to be an even greater propensity for recurrence. It is reasonable to examine the patient yearly for new and recurrent cysts. A panoramic film serves as an adequate screening film. Referral for genetic counseling may be appropriate.

LATERAL PERIODONTAL CYST

Definition

Lateral periodontal cysts are thought to arise from epithelial rests in periodontium lateral to the tooth root. This condition usually is unicystic, but it may appear as a cluster of small cysts, a condition referred to as *botryoid*

odontogenic cysts. It is important to differentiate a lateral periodontal cyst from an inflammatory (radicular) cyst, which occasionally forms in this location. It has been postulated that the lateral periodontal cyst is the intrabony counterpart of the gingival cyst in the adult.

Clinical Features

The lesions usually are asymptomatic and less than 1 cm in diameter. The disorder has no apparent sexual predilection, and the age distribution extends from the second to the ninth decades (the mean age is about 50 years). If these cysts become secondarily infected, they will mimic a lateral periodontal abscess.

Radiographic Features

Location. Fifty percent to 75% of lateral periodontal cysts develop in the mandible, mostly in a region extending from the lateral incisor to the second premolar (Fig. 19-15). Occasionally these cysts appear in the maxilla, especially between the lateral incisor and the cuspid.

Periphery and shape. A lateral periodontal cyst appears as a well-defined radiolucency with a prominent cortical boundary and a round or oval shape. Rare large cysts have a more irregular shape.

Internal structure. The internal aspect usually is radiolucent. The botryoid variety has a multilocular appearance.

Effects on surrounding structures. Small cysts may efface the lamina dura of the adjacent root. Large cysts can displace adjacent teeth and cause expansion.

Differential Diagnosis

Because the location and radiographic appearance of a lateral periodontal cyst are similar in other conditions, the following lesions should be included in the differential diagnosis: a small OKC, small mental foramen, or small neurofibroma or a radicular cyst at the foramen of a lateral (accessory) pulp canal. The multiple (botryoid) cysts with a multilocular appearance may resemble a small ameloblastoma.

Management

Lateral periodontal cysts usually do not require sophisticated imaging because of their small size. Excisional biopsy or simple enucleation is the treatment of choice, since these cysts do not tend to recur.

CALCIFYING ODONTOGENIC CYST

Synonyms

Calcifying epithelial odontogenic cyst or *Gorlin cyst*

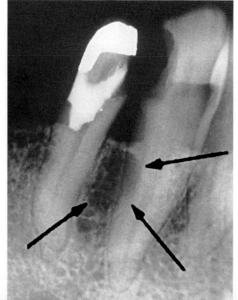

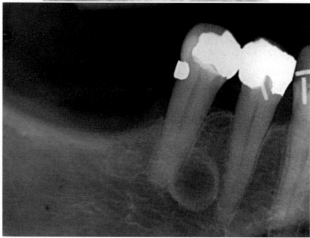

FIG. **19-15** Lateral periodontal cysts in the mandibular premolar region. Note the well-defined, corticated periphery.

Definition

Calcifying odontogenic cysts are uncommon, slow-growing, benign lesions. They occupy a spectrum ranging from a cyst to an odontogenic tumor, with characteristics of a cyst alone or sometimes those of a solid neoplasm (epithelial proliferation and a tendency to continue growing). The World Health Organization now categorizes calcifying odontogenic cysts as benign tumors. This lesion may manufacture calcified tissue identified as dysplastic dentin, and in some instances the lesion is associated with an odontoma. This lesion also sometimes contains a more solid component that gives it an appearance resembling an ameloblastoma, although it does not behave like one.

Clinical Features

Calcifying odontogenic cysts have a wide age distribution that peaks at 10 to 19 years of age, with a mean age of 36 years. A second incidence peak occurs during the seventh decade. Clinically, the lesion usually appears as a slow-growing, painless swelling of the jaw. Occasionally the patient complains of pain. In some cases the expanding lesion may destroy the cortical plate, and the cystic mass may become palpable as it extends into the soft tissue. The patient may report a discharge from such advanced lesions. Aspiration often yields a viscous, granular, yellow fluid.

Radiographic Features

Location. At least 75% of calcifying odontogenic cysts occur in bone, with a nearly equal distribution between the jaws. Most (75%) occur anterior to the first molar, especially associated with cuspids and incisors, where the cyst sometimes manifests as a pericoronal radiolucency.

Periphery and shape. The periphery can vary from well defined and corticated with a curved, cystlike shape to ill defined and irregular.

Internal structure. The internal aspect can vary in appearance. It may be completely radiolucent; it may show evidence of small foci of calcified material that appear as white flecks; or it may show even larger, solid, amorphous masses (Fig. 19-16). In rare cases the lesion may appear multilocular.

Effects on surrounding structures. Occasionally (20% to 50% of cases) the cyst is associated with a tooth (most commonly a cuspid) and impedes its eruption. Displacement of teeth and resorption of roots may occur. Perforation of the cortical plate may be seen radiographically with enlarging lesions.

Differential Diagnosis

When no internal calcifications are evident and this lesion has a pericoronal position, it may be indistinguishable from a follicular cyst. Of the other lesions that may have a cyst shape and internal calcifications, the ameloblastic fibroodontoma resembles this lesion the most. Other calcifying lesions to be considered include an adenomatoid odontogenic tumor, calcifying epithelial odontogenic tumor, and ossifying fibroma. Finally, longstanding cysts may have dystrophic calcification, giving a similar appearance.

Management

Although this cyst does have some neoplastic characteristics, such as a tendency for continued growth, the treatment should be enucleation and curettage. Because

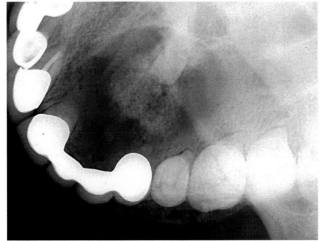

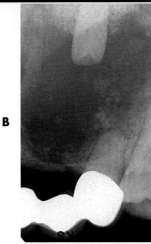

FIG. 19-16 A and **B,** A calcifying odontogenic cyst related to the lateral incisor. Note the well-defined, corticated border, internal calcifications, and resorption of part of the root of the central incisor.

clinicians generally have little experience with the more solid neoplastic variants, it is wise to follow treatment with periodic radiographic evaluation for recurrence.

Nonodontogenic Cysts

NASOPALATINE DUCT CYST

Synonyms
Nasopalatine canal cyst, incisive canal cyst, nasopalatine cyst, median palatine cyst, or *median anterior maxillary cyst*

Definition
The nasopalatine canal usually contains remnants of the nasopalatine duct, a primitive organ of smell, as well as the nasopalatine vessels and nerves. Occasionally a cyst forms in the nasopalatine canal when these embryonic epithelial remnants of the nasopalatine duct undergo proliferation and cystic degeneration.

Clinical Features
Nasopalatine duct cysts account for about 10% of jaw cysts. The age distribution is broad, with most cases being discovered in the fourth through sixth decades. The incidence is three times higher in males. Most of these cysts are asymptomatic or cause such minor symptoms that they are tolerated for long periods. The most frequent complaint is a small, well-defined swelling just posterior to the palatine papilla. This swelling usually is fluctuant and blue if the cyst is near the surface. The deeper nasopalatine duct cyst is covered by normal-appearing mucosa unless it is ulcerated from masticatory trauma. If the cyst expands, it may penetrate the labial plate and produce a swelling below the maxillary labial frenum or to one side. The lesion also may bulge into the nasal cavity and distort the nasal septum. Pressure from the cyst on the adjacent nasopalatine nerves that occupy the same canal may cause a burning sensation or numbness over the palatal mucosa. In some cases cystic fluid may drain into the oral cavity through a sinus tract or a remnant of the nasopalatine duct. The patient usually detects the fluid and reports a salty taste.

Radiographic Features
Location. Most nasopalatine duct cysts are found in the nasopalatine foramen or canal. However, if this cyst extends posteriorly to involve the hard palate (Fig. 19-17), it often is referred to as a *median palatal cyst.* If it expands anteriorly between the central incisors, destroying or expanding the labial plate of bone and causing the teeth to diverge, it sometimes is referred to as a *median anterior maxillary cyst.* This cyst may not always be positioned symmetrically.

Periphery and shape. The periphery usually is well defined and corticated and is circular or oval in shape. The shadow of the nasal spine sometimes is superimposed on the cyst, giving it a heart shape.

Internal structure. Most nasopalatine duct cysts are totally radiolucent. Some rare cysts may have internal dystrophic calcifications, which may appear as ill-defined, amorphous, scattered radiopacities.

Effects on surrounding structures. Most commonly this cyst causes the roots of the central incisors to diverge, and occasionally root resorption occurs (Fig. 19-18). Seen from a lateral perspective, the cyst may expand the labial cortex as well as the palatal cortex (Fig. 19-19). The floor of the nasal fossa may be displaced in a superior direction.

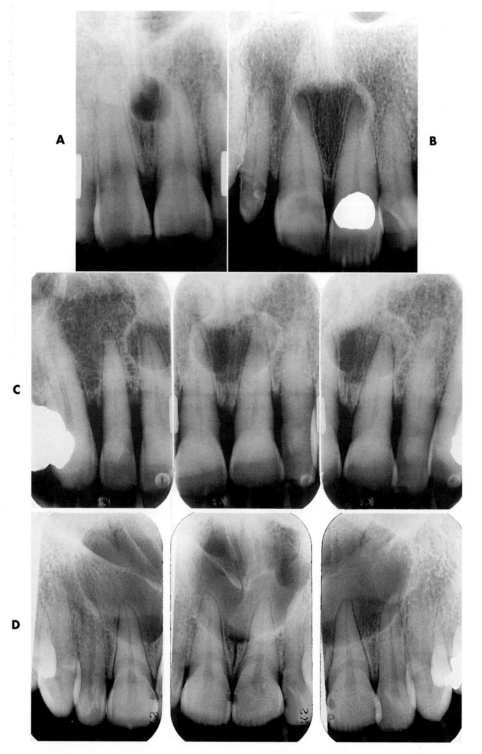

FIG. **19-17**   *Nasopalatine duct cysts.* Note the intact lamina dura around all the apices. **A** through **D** show variations in size. The differential diagnosis of a smaller cyst with a normal nasopalatine foramen may be difficult.

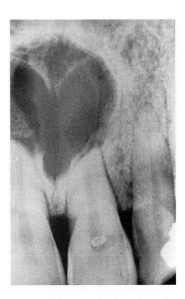

FIG. **19-18** A nasopalatine canal cyst causing external root resorption of a maxillary central incisor.

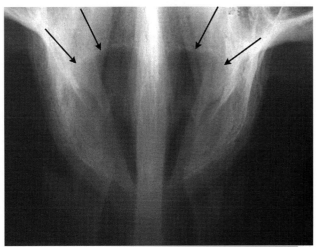

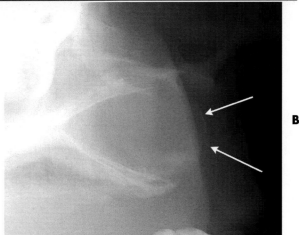

FIG. **19-19** A nasopalatine canal cyst viewed from two perspectives: **(A)** a standard occlusal view and **(B)** from the lateral aspect, which is created by placing the film outside the mouth against the cheek and directing the x-ray beam at a tangent to the labial surface of the central incisors.

Differential Diagnosis

The most common differential diagnosis is a large incisive foramen. A foramen larger than 6 mm may simulate the appearance of a cyst. However, a clinical examination should reveal the expansion characteristic of a cyst and other changes that occur with a space-occupying lesion, such as displacement of teeth. A lateral view of the anterior maxilla, using an occlusal film held outside the mouth and against the cheek, also can help in making the differential diagnosis, as can a cross-sectional (standard) occlusal view. If doubt still exists, comparison with previous images may be useful, or aspiration may be attempted, or another image may be made in 6 months to 1 year to assess any change in size. A radicular cyst or granuloma associated with a central incisor is similar in appearance to an asymmetric nasopalatine cyst. The presence or absence of the lamina dura and enlargement of the periodontal ligament space around the apex of the central incisor indicate an inflammatory lesion. A vitality test of the central incisor may be useful. A second periapical view taken at a different horizontal angulation should show an altered position of the image of a nasopalatine duct cyst, whereas a radicular cyst should remain centered about the apex of the central incisor.

Management

The appropriate treatment for a nasopalatine cyst is enucleation, preferably from the palate to avoid the nasopalatine nerve. If the cyst is large and the danger exists of devitalizing the tooth or creating a nasooral or antrooral fistula, the surgeon may elect to marsupialize the cyst.

NASOLABIAL CYST

Synonym

Nasoalveolar cyst

Definition

The exact origin of nasoalveolar cysts is unknown. They may be fissural cysts arising from the epithelial rests in fusion lines of the globular, lateral nasal, and maxillary processes. Alternatively, the source of the epithelium may be from the embryonic nasolacrimal duct, which initially lies on the bone surface.

Clinical Features

When this rare lesion is small, it may produce a very subtle, unilateral swelling of the nasolabial fold and may elicit pain or discomfort. When large, it may bulge into

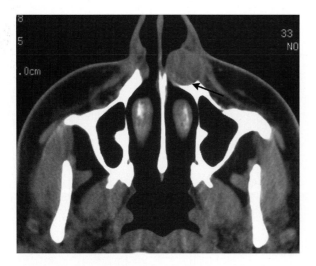

FIG. **19-20**   A nasolabial cyst shown in an axial CT image using a soft tissue algorithm. Note the well-defined periphery and the erosion of the labial aspect of the alveolar process *(arrow).*

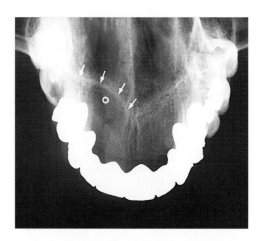

FIG. **19-21**   *An occlusal view of a nasolabial cyst.* The radiograph shows erosion of the alveolar bone *(o)* and elevation of the floor of the nasal fossa *(arrows).* (From Montenegro Chineallato LE, Demante JH: *Oral Surg* 58:729, 1984.)

the floor of the nasal cavity, causing some obstruction, flaring of the alae, distortion of the nostrils, and fullness of the upper lip. If infected, it may drain into the nasal cavity. It usually is unilateral, but bilateral lesions have occurred. The age of detection ranges from 12 to 75 years, with a mean age of 44 years. About 75% of these lesions occur in females.

Radiographic Features
Location. Nasolabial cysts are primarily soft tissue lesions located adjacent to the alveolar process above the apices of the incisors. Because this is a soft tissue lesion, plain radiographs may not show any detectable changes. The investigation could include either computed tomography (CT) or magnetic resonance imaging (MRI), both of which can provide an image of soft tissues (Fig. 19-20).

Periphery and shape. Thin axial CT images using the soft tissue algorithm with contrast reveal a circular or oval lesion with slight soft tissue enhancement of the periphery.

Internal structure. In CT images using the soft tissue algorithm the internal aspect appears homogeneous and relatively radiolucent compared with the surrounding soft tissues.

Effects on surrounding structures. Occasionally a cyst causes erosion of the underlying bone (Fig. 19-21), producing an increased radiolucency of the alveolar process beneath the cyst and apical to the incisors. Also, the

usual outline of the inferior border of the nasal fossa may become distorted, resulting in a posterior bowing of this margin.

Differential Diagnosis
The swelling caused by an infected nasolabial cyst may simulate an acute dentoalveolar abscess. It is important to establish the vitality of the adjacent teeth. This cyst may also resemble a nasal furuncle if it pushes upward into the floor of the nasal cavity. A large mucous extravasation cyst or a cystic salivary adenoma should also be considered in the differential diagnosis of an uninfected nasolabial cyst.

Management
The nasolabial cyst should be excised through an intraoral approach. These cysts do not tend to recur.

DERMOID CYST
Definition
Dermoid cysts are a cystic form of a teratoma thought to be derived from trapped embryonic cells that are totipotential. The resulting cysts are lined with epidermis and cutaneous appendages and filled with keratin or sebaceous material (and in rare cases with bone, teeth, muscle, or hair, in which case they are properly called *teratomas*).

Clinical Features
Dermoid cysts may develop in the soft tissues at any time from birth, but they usually become clinically apparent

between 12 and 25 years of age, about equally distributed between the sexes. The swelling, which is slow and painless, can grow to several centimeters in diameter, and when located in the neck or tongue, it may interfere with breathing, speaking, and eating. Depending on how deep the cyst is positioned in the neck, it can deform the submental area. On palpation these cysts may be fluctuant or doughy, according to their contents. Because they usually are in the midline, they do not affect the teeth.

Radiographic Features

Because dermoid cysts are soft tissue cysts, diagnostic imaging is best accomplished by CT or MRI.

Location. A dermoid cyst is a rare developmental anomaly that may occur anywhere in the body. About 10% or fewer arise in the head and neck, and only 1% to 2% develop in the oral cavity. Of these, about 25% occur in the floor of the mouth and on the tongue. They may be midline or lateral in location.

Periphery and shape. The periphery of the lesion usually is well defined by more radiopaque soft tissue of this cyst compared with surrounding soft tissue, as seen in CT scans.

Internal structure. Dermoid cysts seldom have any internal mineralized structures when they occur in the oral cavity; therefore they are radiolucent on conventional radiographs. However, a CT scan of the area may reveal a soft tissue multilocular appearance (Fig. 19-22). If teeth or bone form in the cyst, their radiopaque images, with characteristic shapes and densities, are apparent on the radiograph.

Differential Diagnosis

Lesions that are clinically similar to dermoid cysts are ranula (unilateral or bilateral blockage of Wharton's ducts), thyroglossal duct cysts, cystic hygromas, branchial cleft cysts, cellulitis, tumors (lipoma and liposarcoma), and normal fat masses in the submental area.

Management

Dermoid cysts do not recur after surgical removal.

FORMER CYSTS

In recent years it has become clear that some names used to describe distinct entities are no longer valid. These names include *primordial cysts* (now recognized largely to be OKCs), *median palatal cysts* (now recognized as a variant of the nasopalatine duct cyst), and *median mandibular and globulomaxillary cysts* (because the

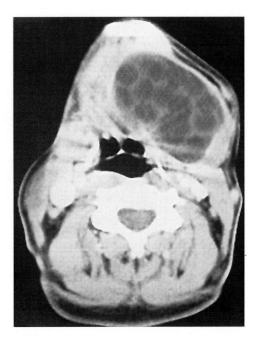

FIG. **19-22** A CT scan of a dermoid cyst, showing an encapsulated mass on the left and several soft tissue loculations. (From Hunter TB et al: *Am J Roentgenol* 141:1229, 1983.)

entrapment of epithelium theory is no longer accepted). Globulomaxillary cysts are now recognized to be radicular or lateral periodontal cysts or OKCs.

Cystlike Lesions

Simple bone cysts are included in this chapter because of their historic classification and because the characteristics and behavior seen in diagnostic imaging are cystic in nature. However, it is important to remember that these lesions are not true cysts.

SIMPLE BONE CYST

Synonyms
Traumatic bone cyst, hemorrhagic bone cyst, extravasation cyst, progressive bone cavity, solitary bone cyst, or *unicameral bone cyst*

Definition
A simple bone cyst (SBC) is a cavity within bone that is lined with connective tissue. It may be empty, or it may contain fluid. However, because it has no epithelial lining, it is not a true cyst. The etiology of SBCs is unknown, although they may be a localized aberration in normal bone remodeling or metabolism. This theory is supported indirectly by the fact that these bony cavities often occur inside lesions of cementoosseous dysplasia

A   **B**   **C**

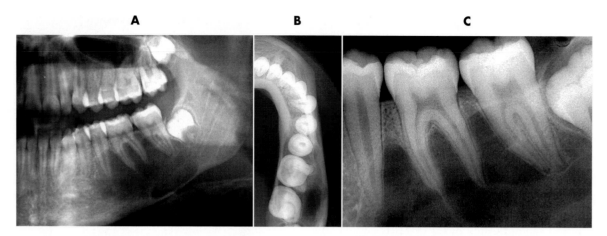

FIG. **19-23**   A simple bone cyst radiographed with a panoramic film **(A)**, a periapical film **(B)**, and an occlusal film **(C)**. Note that, except for the superior border, the borders are ill defined and that the lesion has scalloped around the teeth and thinned the inferior border of the mandible. The occlusal film shows that no expansion has occurred in the buccal or lingual cortical plates.

A   **B**   **C**

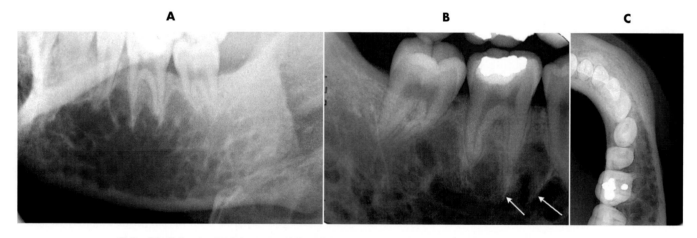

FIG. **19-24**   An SBC has a multilocular appearance in this lateral oblique view of the mandible **(A)**. The periapical view **(B)** appears to show internal septa because of the scalloping of the endosteal surface of the cortical plates, as is seen in the inferior cortex in **A** and in the buccal cortex of the occlusal view **(C)**.

and fibrous dysplasia. No evidence exists to support a traumatic cause.

Clinical Features
SBCs are very common lesions. Most occur in the first two decades of life, with a mean age of 17 years. The lesion shows a male predominance of approximately 2:1. Multiple SBCs can develop, especially when the disorder occurs with cementoosseous dysplasia. The occurrence of SBCs in cementoosseous dysplasia is seen in an older population, with a mean age of 42 years, and with a female predominance of 4:1. SBCs are asymptomatic in most cases, but occasionally pain or tenderness may

be present, especially if the cyst has become secondarily infected. Expansion of the mandible or tooth movement is possible but unusual. The teeth in the affected region usually are vital. Most SBCs are discovered only by chance, during radiographic examinations, and for this reason they can become quite large. There is no significant incidence of pathologic fractures. When aspiration is productive, usually only a few milliliters of straw-colored or serosanguineous fluid are obtained.

Radiographic Features
Location. Almost all SBCs are found in the mandible; in rare cases they develop in the maxilla (Fig. 19-23). The

lesion can occur anywhere in the mandible but is seen most often in the ramus and posterior mandible in older patients. SBCs also frequently occur with cementoosseous and fibrous dysplasia.

Periphery and shape. The margin may vary from a well-defined, delicate cortex to an ill-defined border that blends into the surrounding bone. The boundary usually is better defined in the alveolar process around the teeth than in the inferior aspect of the body of the mandible. The shape most often is smooth and curved, like a cyst, with an oval or scalloped border. The lesion often scallops between the roots of the teeth (see Fig. 19-23).

Internal structure. The internal structure is totally radiolucent, but occasionally it may appear multilocular, although the lesion does not contain true septa. This appearance is the result of pronounced scalloping of the endosteal surface of either the buccal or lingual plates (Fig. 19-24). The ridges of bone produced by the scalloping give the appearance of septa on a lateral view of the mandible.

Effects on surrounding structures. In most cases these lesions have no effect on the surrounding teeth, although rare cases of tooth displacement and resorption have been documented. Often the lesion involves all the bone around the roots of the teeth but leaves the lamina dura intact or only partly disrupted (Fig. 19-25). Similarly, the sparing of the cortical boundary of the crypt around a developing tooth is characteristic. As previously mentioned, these lesions have a propensity to scallop the endosteal surface of the outer cortex of the mandible. SBCs also have a tendency to grow along the long axis of the bone, causing minimal expansion (Fig. 19-26). However, expansion of the involved bone can occur and is more common with larger lesions (Fig. 19-27).

Differential Diagnosis

An SBC may have an appearance similar to that of a true cyst, especially an OKC. This is because OKCs tend to grow along bone with very little expansion and often have scalloped borders similar to those of an SBC. However, OKCs usually have a more definite cortical boundary, resorb and displace teeth, and occur in an older age group. Because the SBC may remove bone around teeth without affecting the teeth, there may be a tendency to include a malignant lesion in the differential. However, maintenance of some lamina dura and the lack of an invasive periphery and bone destruction should be enough to remove this category of diseases from consideration.

The diagnosis relies primarily on radiographic and surgical observations because the histopathologic as-

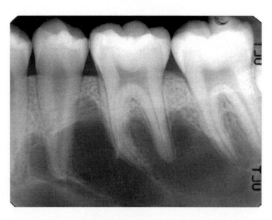

FIG. **19-25** An SBC in which the lamina dura is maintained on most root surfaces involved with the lesion except for the mesial surface of the distal root tip of the first molar.

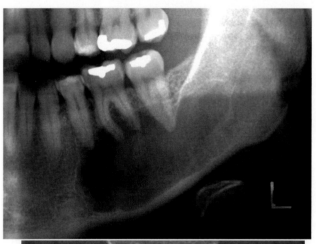

A

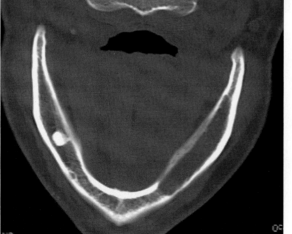

B

FIG. **19-26** **A** and **B,** An SBC extending from the first bicuspid posteriorly to the base of the ramus and occupying most of the mandible. Considering the extent of the lesion, very little expansion of the buccal or lingual cortical plates has occurred, as can be seen in the axial CT image **(B)** using bone algorithm.

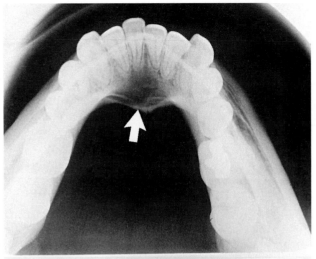

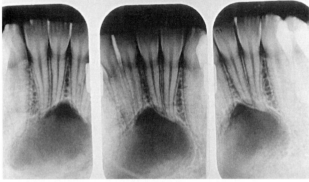

FIG. **19-27**   An SBC *(arrow)* positioned in the anterior of the mandible. Note that the superior aspect of the peripheral cortex is better defined than the inferior border and that evidence exists of some expansion of the mandible's lingual cortex.

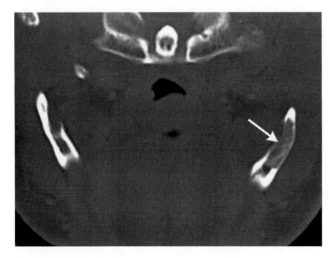

FIG. **19-28**   An axial CT image using a bone algorithm displaying a small SBC in the process of healing *(arrow)*. Note the fine internal granular bone and very slight expansion of the ramus.

pects are not characteristic. These lesions occasionally heal spontaneously. A biopsy and analysis of a healing cyst may falsely indicate the presence of an ossifying fibroma or fibrous dysplasia because of the formation of new immature bone (Fig. 19-28).

Management

The customary treatment is a conservative opening into the lesion and careful curettage of the lining; this usually initiates bleeding and subsequent healing. Spontaneous healing has been reported. Periodic follow-up radiographic examinations are advisable, especially if the patient declines treatment. These lesions rarely recur.

SUGGESTED READINGS

Shear M: Cysts of the jaws: recent advances, *J Oral Pathol* 14:43, 1985.

Shear M: Developmental odontogenic cysts: an update, *J Oral Pathol Med* 23:1, 1994.

ODONTOGENIC CYSTS

Radicular cyst

Stockdale CR, Chandler NP: The nature of the periapical lesion: a review of 1108 cases, *J Dent* 16(3):123, 1988.

Syrjauanen S et al: Radiological interpretation of the periapical cysts and granulomas, *Dentomaxillofac Radiol* 11:89, 1982.

Toller PA: Origin and growth of cysts of the jaws, *Ann R Coll Surg Engl* 40:306, 1967.

Wood RE et al: Radicular cysts of primary teeth mimicking premolar dentigerous cysts: report of three cases, *ASDC J Dent Child* 55(4):288, 1988.

Residual cyst

High AS, Hirschmann PN: Age changes in residual cysts, *J Oral Pathol* 15:524, 1986.

Schwimmer AM et al: Squamous cell carcinoma arising in residual odontogenic cyst: report of a case and review of literature, *Oral Surg* 72(2):218, 1991.

Dentigerous cyst

Daley TD, Wysocki GP: The small dentigerous cyst, *Oral Surg Oral Med Oral Pathol Oral Radiol Endod* 79:77, 1995.

Lustmann J, Bodner L: Dentigerous cysts associated with supernumerary teeth, *Int J Oral Maxillofac Surg* 17(2):100, 1988.

Main DMG: Follicular cysts of mandibular third molar teeth: radiological evaluation of enlargement, *Dentomaxillofac Radiol* 18:156, 1989.

Maxymiw WG, Wood RE: Carcinoma arising in a dentigerous cyst: a case report and review of the literature, *J Oral Maxillofac Surg* 49(6):639, 1991.

Buccal bifurcation cyst

Bohay RN, Weinberg S: The paradental cyst of the mandibular permanent first molar: report of a bilateral case, *J Dent Child* Sept-Oct:361, 1992.

Fowler CB, Brannon RB: The paradental cyst: a clinicopathologic study of six new cases and review of the literature, *J Oral Maxillofac Surg* 47:243, 1989.

Packota GV et al: Paradental cysts on mandibular first molars in children: report of five cases, *Dentomaxillofac Radiol* 19:126, 1990.

Shear M: *Cysts of the oral regions,* Bristol, UK, 1976, John Wright & Sons.

Stoneman DW, Worth HM: The mandibular infected buccal cyst—molar area, *Dent Radiogr Photogr* 56:1, 1983.

Odontogenic keratocyst

Brannon RB: The odontogenic keratocyst: a clinicopathological study of 312 cases. I. Clinical features, *Oral Surg* 42:54, 1976.

Browne RM: *Investigative pathology of the odontogenic cysts,* Boca Raton, Fla, 1991, CRC Press.

Browne RM: The odontokeratocyst: clinical aspects, *Br Dent J* 128:225, 1970.

Frame JW, Wake MJC: Computerized axial tomography in the assessment of mandibular keratocysts, *Br Dent J* 153:93, 1982.

Kakarantza-Angelopoulou E, Nicolatou O: Odontogenic keratocysts: clinicopathologic study of 87 cases, *J Oral Maxillofac Surg* 48(6):593, 1990.

Kondell PA, Wiberg J: Odontogenic keratocysts: a follow-up study of 29 cases, *Swed Dent J* 12(1-2):57, 1988.

Partridge M, Towers JF: The primordial cyst (odontogenic keratocyst): its tumor-like characteristics and behavior, *Br J Oral Maxillofac Surg* 25:271, 1987.

Basal cell nevus syndrome

Angelopoulou E, Angelopoulos AP: Lateral periodontal cyst: review of the literature and report of a case, *J Periodontol* 61(2):126, 1990.

Donatsky O et al: Clinical, radiographic, and histologic features of the basal cell nevus syndrome, *Int J Oral Surg* 5:19, 1976.

Evans DC et al: The incidence of Gorlin syndrome in 173 consecutive cases of medulloblastoma, *Br J Cancer* 64(5):959, 1991.

Gorlin RJ: Nevoid basal cell carcinoma syndrome, *Medicine* 66(2):98, 1987.

Lateral periodontal cyst

Regezi JA et al: The pathology of head and neck tumors: cysts of the jaw. XII, *Head Neck Surg* 4:48, 1981.

Shear M, Pindborg JJ: Microscopic features of the lateral periodontal cyst, *Scand J Dent Res* 83:103, 1975.

Weathers DR, Waldron CA: Unusual multilocular cysts of the jaws (botryoid odontogenic cysts), *J Periodontol* 41:249, 1970.

Wysocki GP et al: Histogenesis of the lateral periodontal cyst and the gingival cyst of the adult, *Oral Surg* 50:327, 1980.

Calcifying odontogenic cyst

Altini M, Farman AG: The calcifying odontogenic cyst: eight new cases and a review of the literature, *Oral Surg* 20:751, 1975.

Fejerskov O, Krough J: The calcifying ghost cell odontogenic tumor or the calcifying odontogenic cyst, *J Oral Pathol* 1:272, 1972.

Freedman PD et al: Calcifying odontogenic cyst, *Oral Surg* 40:93, 1975.

Hirshberg A et al: Calcifying odontogenic cyst associated with odontoma, *J Oral Maxillofac Surg* 52:555, 1994.

Saito I et al: Calcifying odontogenic cyst: case reports, variations, and tumorous potential, *J Nihon Univ Sch Dent* 24:69, 1982.

NONODONTOGENIC CYSTS
Nasopalatine duct cyst

Abrams AM et al: Nasopalatine cysts, *Oral Surg* 16:306, 1963.

Allard RHB et al: Nasopalatine duct cyst, *Int J Oral Surg* 10:447, 1981.

Hartziotis J: Median palatine cyst: report of a case, *J Oral Surg* 24:343, 1966.

Nortjé CJ, Farman AG: Nasopalatine duct cyst: an aggressive condition in adolescent Negroes from South Africa? *Int J Oral Surg* 7:65, 1978.

Nasolabial cyst

Roed-Petersen B: Nasolabial cysts, *Br J Oral Surg* 7:85, 1970.

Seward GR: Nasolabial cysts and their radiology, *Dent Pract* 12:154, 1962.

Walsh-Waring GP: Nasoalveolar cysts: aetiology, presentation, and treatment, *J Laryngol Otol* 81:263, 1967.

Dermoid cyst

Seward GR: Dermoid cysts of the floor of the mouth, *Br J Oral Surg* 3:36, 1965.

CYSTLIKE LESIONS
Simple bone cyst

Feinberg S et al: Recurrent "traumatic" bone cysts of the mandible, *Oral Surg* 57:418, 1984.

Kaugars GE, Cale AE: Traumatic bone cyst, *Oral Surg Oral Med Oral Pathol* 63:318, 1987.

Saito Y et al: Simple bone cyst: a clinical and histopathologic study of fifteen cases, *Oral Surg Oral Med Oral Pathol* 74:487, 1992.

Sapp PJ, Stark ML: Self-healing traumatic bone cysts, *Oral Surg Oral Med Oral Pathol* 69:597, 1990.

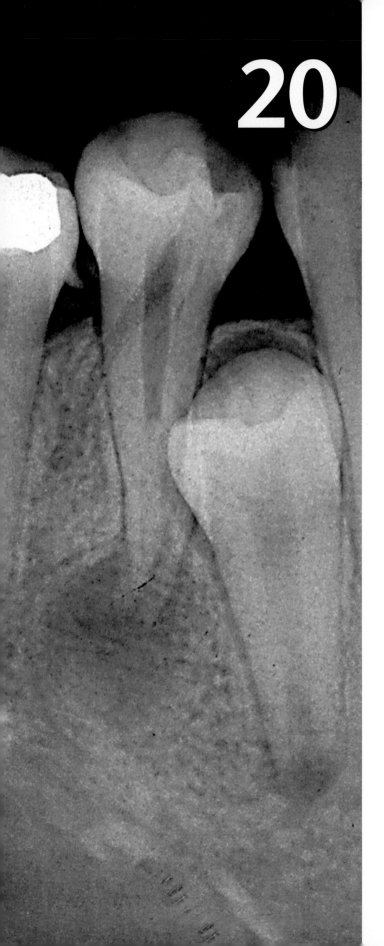

20 Benign Tumors of the Jaws

STEPHEN R. MATTESON

A *benign tumor is a new growth* that resembles the tissue of origin. For example, a benign odontogenic tumor may consist of normal enamel, dentin, or pulpal tissue, but it forms abnormally into a growing mass instead of a tooth. Benign tumors usually are true *neoplasms;* that is, they continue to grow until treated. However, several types of benign tumors, called *hamartomas,* are not actually neoplasms but rather atypical growths of normal tissue caused by abnormal growth and development. Hamartomas are not considered true neoplasms because they do not grow indefinitely. An odontoma is a good example of this type of growth; it develops from components of the dental follicle but stops growing at approximately the same time normal odontogenic tissues complete their growth. *Hyperplasias* are lesions formed by an increase in the number of cells of a tissue in a normal arrangement. Hyperplasias are slow growing and have limited growth potential, although they may continue to increase in size for varying periods before undergoing spontaneous arrest.

Clinical Features

Benign tumors typically have an insidious onset and grow slowly. These tumors usually are painless, do not metastasize, and are not life threatening unless they interfere with a vital organ by direct extension.

Benign tumors may be detected clinically if the dentist notes enlargement of a facial bone or finds a lesion radiographically. When a tumor is detected, thorough clinical and radiographic examinations are performed to determine the extent of the lesion and to identify its specific characteristics.

Radiographic Examination

The radiographic examination provides information for analysis. That information includes the tumor's location, the three-dimensional anatomic relationships, and the radiodensity and architecture of the tumor tissue, as well as the lesion's size, its shape and the configuration of its borders, and its effect on adjacent structures (e.g., bony cortex, teeth, periosteum). Tentative identification of the lesion as benign, aggressive benign, or malignant early in the diagnostic workup is important. Such a designation leads to a set of well-planned diagnostic and therapeutic steps.

The number and type of radiographs needed to examine a tumor varies according to the location, size, and three-dimensional aspects of the lesion. The radiographic examination should include all the margins of the lesion, and orthogonal views should be made when expansion or perforation of the bony cortex is likely. Panoramic, intraoral, and occlusal radiographs are excellent films to use for this purpose. Computed tomography (CT) or magnetic resonance imaging (MRI) also may be needed for large lesions and for those that threaten vital structures.

Thoughtful examination of radiographic images of a tumor may yield important information about the nature and destructive potential of the lesion. The radiographic signs associated with lesions are examined and may indicate the type of tumor and may provide a specific diagnosis. For example, the appearance of periapical cemental dysplasia and odontomas are so characteristic that a specific diagnosis can be made from radiographs alone. Other benign tumors at times resemble one another radiographically and therefore can be categorized only as benign and aggressive or nonaggressive in nature. For these lesions a histopathologic examination is required. Even then, diagnosis may require consideration of all appropriate clinical, radiologic, histopathologic, and laboratory data.

Radiographic Features

The following general features suggest the presence of a benign neoplasm.

LOCATION

Because many tumors have a specific anatomic predilection, the location of a particular neoplasm is extremely important in establishing the differential diagnosis. For example, odontogenic lesions occur naturally in the alveolar processes above the inferior alveolar nerve canal, where tooth formation occurs. Vascular and neural lesions may originate inside the mandibular canal, arising from the neurovascular tissues. Cartilaginous tumors occur in jaw locations where residual cartilaginous cells lie, such as around the mandibular condyle.

PERIPHERY AND SHAPE

Benign tumors typically have a smooth, round, or oval periphery. The bony margin usually is regular, corticated, and well defined. Often, benign lesions are encapsulated in connective tissue and therefore show a radiolucent band separating the lesion from the surrounding bone. Benign tumors enlarge gradually by formation of additional internal tissue. Because of this, the radiographic borders of benign tumors appear relatively smooth, well defined, and sometimes corticated.

INTERNAL STRUCTURE

The radiodensity of lesions is an important feature that lends evidence to their clinical behavior. Benign tumors may be radiolucent, mixed radiolucent and radiopaque, or radiopaque. Because both benign and malignant tumors may be radiolucent, they must be differentiated by other radiographic features. Lesions with internal calcification in the form of calcified flecks, septa, or patterned compartments usually are benign. This is true because of the time required for residual trabeculae to remodel into septa and because some benign lesions are capable of producing calcified tissue. Similarly, radiopaque lesions usually are benign because of the presence of bone (osteoma) or dental tissues (odontoma).

EFFECTS ON SURROUNDING STRUCTURES

The manner in which a tumor affects adjacent tissues may also signal that it is benign. A benign tumor exerts pressure on neighboring structures, resulting in the displacement of teeth or bony cortices. For example, as a slowly expanding benign tumor mass extends to the inferior cortex of the mandible, the cortex is displaced or bows outward (Fig. 20-1). This is caused by simultaneous resorp-

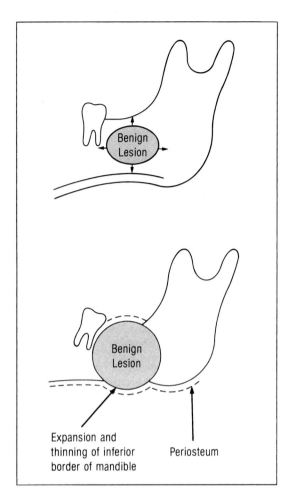

FIG. **20-1**   Benign lesions growing in bone tend to be round or oval. They grow by displacing adjacent tissues. (From Matteson SR et al: *Dent Radiogr Photogr* 57:35, 1985.)

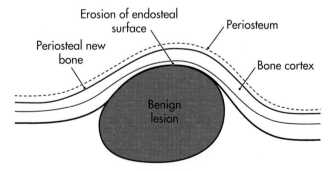

FIG. **20-2**   The host bone of a benign tumor may expand as a result of outward remodeling of its cortical borders. As the benign tumor extends toward the periphery of the bone, the periosteum lays down new bone along the outer cortex, thereby maintaining the integrity of the cortex.

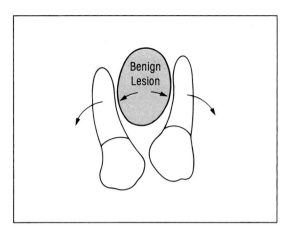

FIG. **20-3**   A benign lesion usually grows slowly, causing displacement of adjacent teeth. (From Matteson SR et al: *Dent Radiogr Photogr* 57:35, 1985.)

tion of bone along the inner edge of the cortex and de-position of bone along the outer cortical surface by the periosteum (Fig. 20-2). Through this remodeling process, the cortex maintains its integrity and resists perforation. Benign tumors may also cause bodily displacement of nearby teeth (Fig. 20-3). The movement of teeth adjacent to benign tumors is slow because these lesions grow slowly.

The roots of teeth may be resorbed by both benign and malignant tumors, but root resorption more commonly is associated with benign processes. The benign tumors especially likely to resorb roots are ameloblastomas, ossifying fibromas, and central giant cell granulomas. Benign tumors tend to resorb the adjacent root surfaces in a smooth fashion, and the resorption occurs in a position on the root surface adjacent to the tumor. Fibroosseous lesions do not usually resorb teeth. In certain rare tumors, such as carcinoma of the maxillary sinus, the root surfaces of the maxillary molars may be surrounded by the lesion and resorbed in a global fashion. This process results in a narrowing of the root structure, sometimes described as a "spiked root."

The following discussion considers bony hyperplasias separately from tumors because bony hyperplasias are more functional in origin and behavior (with perhaps a genetic component) than are neoplasias. The benign neoplasias are separated into odontogenic tumors (lesions of tooth germ origin) and nonodontogenic tumors.

Hyperplasias

Bony hyperplasias are growths of normal new bone that occur in characteristic locations on the skull and facial skeleton. Some examples are the relatively common tori and other forms of exostoses. Hyperplasias never seem

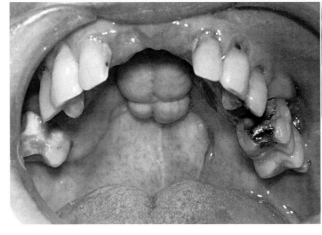

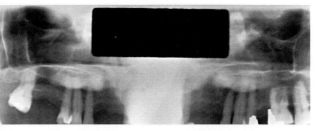

FIG. **20-4** **A,** A clinical photograph of torus palatinus. **B,** A panoramic radiograph shows the radiopaque shadow of torus palatinus above the maxillary premolars and canine. (Courtesy Ronald Baker, DDS, Chapel Hill, N.C.)

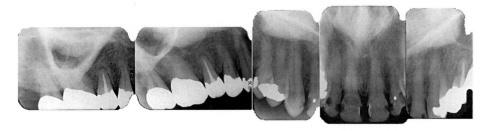

FIG. **20-5** Maxillary periapical radiographs show a radiopaque area with the well-defined borders of torus palatinus.

to regress in size. Tori are examples of exostoses that are located in specific locations on the jaws.

TORUS PALATINUS

Synonym
Palatine torus

Definition
Torus palatinus is a bony protuberance in the midline of the hard palate usually found in the middle third.

Clinical Features
Torus palatinus, the most common of the exostoses, occurs in about 20% of the population, although various studies have shown marked differences in racial groups. It develops about twice as often in women as in men and more often in Native Americans, Eskimos, and Norwegians. Although it may be discovered at any age, it is rare in children. It usually begins developing in young adults before 30 years of age and is thought to arise through an interplay of genetic and environmental factors. The base of the bony nodule extends along the central portion of the hard palate, and the bulk reaches downward into the oral cavity. The size and shape of a torus palatinus can vary, and these le-

sions have been described as flat, spindled, nodular, or mushroomlike (Fig. 20-4, *A*). Normal mucosa covers the bony mass and may appear pale and sometimes ulcerated when traumatized. Patients often are unaware of the lesion, and those who do discover it may insist that it occurred suddenly and has been growing rapidly.

Radiographic Features
Location. On maxillary periapical or panoramic radiographs, a torus palatinus appears as a dense radiopaque shadow below and attached to the hard palate. It may be superimposed over the apical areas of the maxillary teeth, especially if the torus has developed in the middle or anterior regions of the palate. The image of a palatal torus projecting over the roots of the maxillary molars may resemble that of a zygoma (Fig. 20-4, *B*).

Periphery and shape. The border of the opaque shadow usually is well defined because the surface of the torus is compact bone (Fig. 20-5). The occlusal radiograph shown in Fig. 20-6 provides a good example of a palatal torus. Its image is oval, and both the radiopaque border of compact bone and the less dense interior area of medullary bone are apparent.

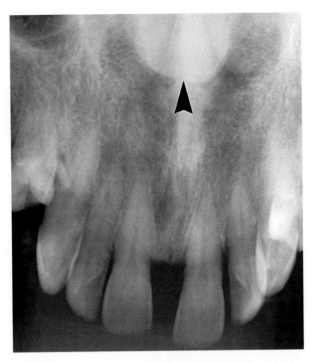

FIG. **20-6**   An occlusal radiograph of torus palatinus (*arrowhead*).

Internal structure. The internal aspect is homogeneously radiopaque.

Treatment

A torus palatinus usually does not require treatment, although removal may be necessary if a maxillary denture is to be made.

TORUS MANDIBULARIS

Synonym
Mandibular torus

Definition
Torus mandibularis is an exostosis that protrudes from the lingual aspect of the mandible, usually near the premolar teeth.

Clinical Features
Tori occur less often on the lingual surface of the mandible than on the palate, with the former occurring in about 8% of the population. These tori develop singly or multiply, unilaterally or bilaterally (usually bilaterally), and most often in the premolar region. The size also varies, ranging from an outgrowth that is just palpable to one that contacts a torus on the opposite side. In contrast to torus palatinus, torus mandibularis develops later, being first discovered in middle-aged adults. However, it has the same gender predilection as torus

palatinus. In women the occurrence of torus mandibularis correlates with that of torus palatinus, but this apparently is not the case in men. As with torus palatinus, torus mandibularis may occur more often in those of Mongoloid ancestry.

Genetic and environmental factors seem to be involved in the development of torus mandibularis, but masticatory stress is reported as an essential factor underlying its formation. The high prevalence among Eskimos and other subarctic peoples who make extraordinary chewing demands on their teeth seems to support this suggestion. Also, a patient with a torus mandibularis has, on average, more teeth present than a patient without a torus.

Radiographic Features
Location. Recognition of mandibular tori relies on their appearance and location. Their presence bilaterally reinforces this impression. On mandibular periapical radiographs, a torus mandibularis appears as a radiopaque shadow, usually superimposed on the roots of premolars and molars and occasionally over a canine or incisor. It usually lies over about three teeth.

Periphery. The images of these overgrowths usually are not as well defined from the adjacent normal bone as are those of the palatal variety. Also, the distinction between cortical bone and cancellous bone is not as apparent as with palatine tori. Mandibular tori are sharply demarcated anteriorly on periapical films and are less dense and less well defined as they extend posteriorly (Fig. 20-7).

Internal structure. On occlusal radiographs a mandibular torus appears as a radiopaque, homogeneous, knobby protuberance from the lingual surface of the mandible. The border between it and the bone is not sharp but somewhat continuous, suggesting that the exostosis is not a growth on the bone but part of the bone (Fig. 20-8).

Treatment
A torus mandibularis usually does not require treatment, although removal may be necessary if a mandibular denture is planned.

EXOSTOSES

Synonym
Hyperostoses

Definition
Exostoses are small regions of osseous hyperplasia of cortical bone and occasionally cancellous bone on the surface of the alveolar process.

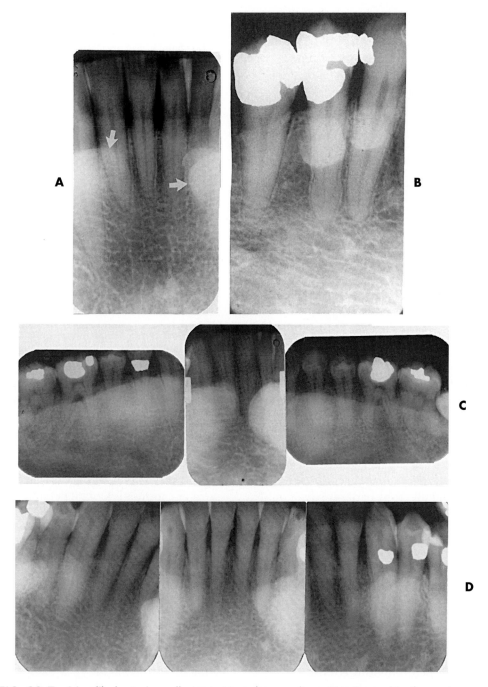

FIG. **20-7** Mandibular tori usually are seen as dense radiopacities *(arrows)* in the canine region **(A)** and the premolar region **(B). C,** Large mandibular tori are seen from the molar region to the midline. **D,** Note the common appearance of mandibular tori on these anterior periapical radiographs.

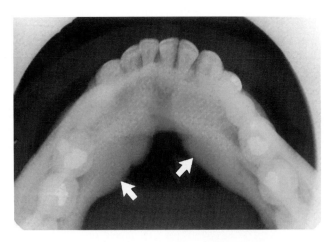

FIG. **20-8**   An occlusal radiograph shows bilateral mandibular tori (arrows).

Clinical Features

Small exostoses may develop on the facial surface of the maxillary alveolar process at the border between the attached gingiva and the vestibular mucosa, usually in the canine or molar area. They are less common than mandibular or palatine tori, seldom attain a large size, and may be solitary or multiple. They are nodular, pedunculated, or flat prominences on the surface of the bone, and because of their small size they seldom are clinically significant while teeth are present. They are covered with a normal mucosa and are bony hard on palpation. No published data indicate their actual incidence or if they occur more often in one gender. As with the exostoses described previously, they appear to be more prevalent in Native Americans.

Radiographic Features

Location. The maxillary alveolar process is the most common location.

Periphery. Radiographically, an exostosis generally appears as a circumscribed, smoothly contoured, somewhat rounded radiopaque mass (Fig. 20-9). However, some may have poorly defined borders that blend radiographically into the surrounding normal bone.

Internal structure. The internal aspect of an exostosis usually is homogeneous and radiopaque. Although large exostoses can show interior medullary bone, they most often consist only of cortical bone.

Treatment

Exostoses usually do not require treatment.

ENOSTOSES

Synonyms
Dense bone island and *periapical idiopathic osteosclerosis*

Definition
Enostoses are the internal counterparts of exostoses. They are localized growths of compact bone that extend from the inner surface of cortical bone into the cancellous bone.

Clinical Features
Enostoses are asymptomatic.

Radiographic Features
Location. Enostoses are more common in the mandible than in the maxilla. They occur most often in the premolar-molar area (Fig. 20-10), although their existence does not correlate with the presence or absence of teeth.

Periphery. The radiographic image of an enostosis is a single, isolated radiopacity with borders that usually are diffuse but that may be well defined. The trabeculae blend with those of the adjacent normal bone. No trace of a radiolucent margin or capsule lies in the sclerotic area.

Internal structure. The internal aspect of an enostosis shows varying degrees of radiopacity.

Effects on surrounding structures. In rare instances an area of enostosis is located periapical to a tooth root and is associated with external root resorption. The tooth most often involved is the mandibular first molar.

Differential Diagnosis
Several radiopaque lesions must be considered in forming a differential diagnosis. Periapical cemental dysplasia has a lucent margin. Hypercementosis and cementoblastoma both develop around the roots of teeth, and osteosarcoma and chondrosarcoma show evidence of a radiolucent component, as do osteoblastoma and metastatic osteoblastic (prostatic) carcinoma. When an area of enostosis is located at the root apex and especially when it is associated with root resorption, the differential diagnosis should include periapical sclerosing osteitis. However, this inflammatory lesion should cause an associated widening of the periapical segment of the periodontal membrane space, which the enostosis does not. Also, an inflammatory lesion may have an apparent etiology such as a large restoration or carious lesion. If several areas of enostosis (five or more) are present, multiple polyposis syndromes (e.g., Gardner's syndrome) should be considered.

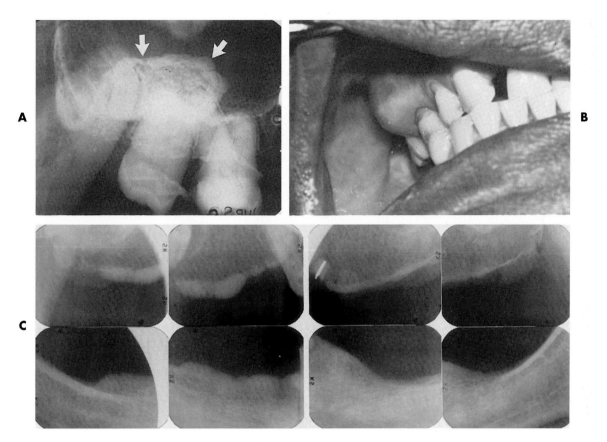

FIG. **20-9** *An exostosis.* **A,** A periapical film shows a radiopaque bony exostosis on the buccal alveolar ridge superimposed on the molar teeth. **B,** A clinical photograph of an alveolar exostosis in another patient. **C,** An alveolar exostosis in the molar regions along the alveolar crests. (**A** courtesy A. Shawkat, DDS, Radcliff, Ky.; **B** courtesy R. Langlais, DDS, San Antonio, Tex.; **C** courtesy B. Glass, DDS, San Antonio, Tex.)

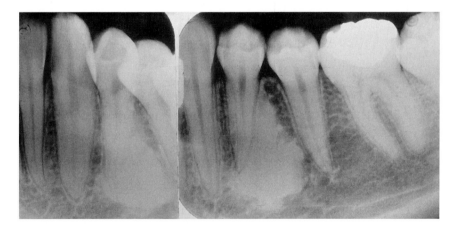

FIG. **20-10** A radiopaque area between the mandibular premolars indicates an area of enostosis (dense bone island). Note the normal appearance of the periodontal membrane.

Treatment

Most cases of enostosis go unrecognized and are not clinically important. If a lesion is suspected of being one of the serious osteoblastic diseases listed in the differential diagnosis, it should be examined periodically for evidence of growth. If the increasing size of a lesion arouses suspicion, the tissue in question must be excised for microscopic examination.

Odontogenic Tumors

Odontogenic tumors arise in the tissues of the odontogenic apparatus. These tumors consist of two main groups, ectodermal (epithelial) odontogenic tumors and mesodermal (connective tissue) odontogenic tumors. Tumors that consist of both epithelium and connective tissue make up another group, known as *mixed* or *composite (ectodermal-mesodermal) odontogenic tumors.* Odontogenic tumors account for 1 in 50,000 tumors and for 1.3% to 15% of all oral tumors. The following discussion presents benign jaw tumors according to their tissues of origin. This format should assist the reader in learning to correlate the radiographic appearance of tumors with the underlying pathologic basis of the disease process.

EPITHELIAL TUMORS

Ameloblastoma

Synonyms. *Adamantinoma, adamantoblastoma, adontomes embryolastiques* and *epithelial odontoma. Ameloblastoma* is considered a more appropriate term than *adamantinoma* because the term *adamantinoma* implies production of mineralized enamel, and enamel or other calcified tissues are not present in this tumor.

Definition. The ameloblastoma, a true neoplasm of odontogenic epithelium, is a persistent and locally invasive tumor, but almost invariably benign in its growth characteristics. The ameloblastoma represents about 1% of all oral ectodermal tumors and 11% of odontogenic tumors. It is an aggressive neoplasm that arises from remnants of the dental lamina and dental organ (odontogenic epithelium). Its histologic appearance is similar to that of the early cap-stage ameloblastic elements of developing without complete differentiation to the stage of enamel formation. An untreated tumor may grow to great size yet usually remains localized. As it develops, this tumor causes bony expansion and possibly erosion of adjacent cortical plates. Local invasion of the adjacent soft tissues may follow, and lesions have been known to spread to the cranial base by local extension. Malignant forms of this neoplasm do exist and are discussed in

Chapter 21. Occasionally an ameloblastoma forms from the epithelial lining of a dentigerous cyst and this is called a *mural* (within the wall) *ameloblastoma* (Fig. 20-11). The existence of peripheral (soft tissue location) forms of this neoplasm is well documented.

Clinical features. There is a slight predilection for this lesion to occur in men, and it develops more often in blacks. Although it may be found in the young (3 years) and in individuals older than 80 years, most patients are between 20 and 50 years, with the average age at discovery about 40 years. The tumor is frequently discovered during a routine dental examination.

Ameloblastomas grow slowly, and few, if any, symptoms occur in the early stages. Usually the patient eventually notices gradually increasing facial asymmetry. Swelling of the cheek, gingiva, or hard palate has been reported as the chief complaint in 95% of untreated maxillary ameloblastomas. The mucosa over the mass is normal, but teeth in the involved region may be displaced and become mobile. Generally patients with ameloblastomas do not have pain, paresthesia, fistula, ulcer formation, or tooth mobility, but these features have been described. As the tumor enlarges, palpation may elicit a bony hard sensation or crepitus as the bone thins. If the lesion destroys overlying bone, the swelling may feel firm or fluctuant. Tumors that develop in the maxilla may extend into the paranasal sinuses, orbit, nasopharynx, or vital structures at the base of the skull. Recurrence rates are higher in older patients and in those with multilocular lesions. As seen with other jaw tumors, local recurrence, whether detected radiographically or histologically, may have a more aggressive character than the original tumor. Nasal obstruction and epistaxis occur primarily in previously treated patients.

Radiographic features. The radiographic appearance of the ameloblastoma varies according to the stage of its development and whether it has perforated a cortical border and extended into adjacent soft tissues.

Location. Most ameloblastomas (80%) develop in the molar-ramus region of the mandible, but they may extend to the symphyseal area. Most lesions that occur in the maxilla are in the third molar area, followed by the maxillary sinus and nasal floor.

Periphery. The ameloblastoma is usually well defined and frequently delineated by a cortical or hyperostotic border. The periphery of lesions in the maxilla may be ill defined.

Internal structure. In its early stage of development the ameloblastoma may appear as a unilocular radiolucency with no internal structure (Fig. 20-12). Advanced cases tend to be larger and also to develop internal compartments that are separated by distinct septa reaching into

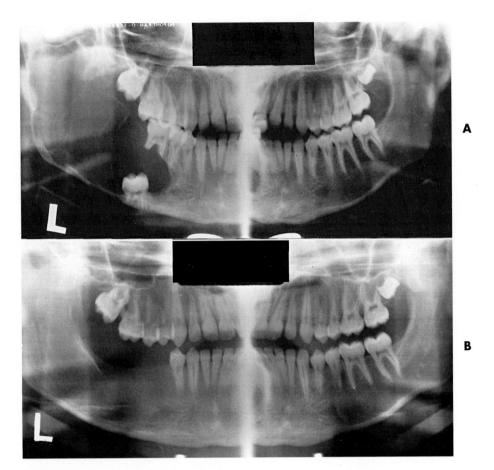

FIG. **20-11** *A mural ameloblastoma.* **A,** A cystic lesion shows expansion of the mandibular body and ramus to the sigmoid notch and condylar neck, as well as inferior displacement of the mandibular second molar and root resorption of the alveolar left first molar. **B,** The appearance of the area after surgical treatment and healing. (Courtesy E.J. Burkes, DDS, Chapel Hill, N.C.)

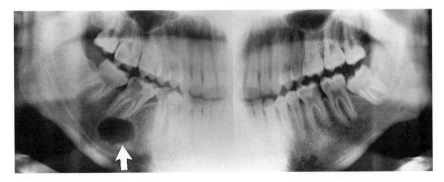

FIG. **20-12** A panoramic radiograph of a monolocular ameloblastoma *(arrow)* in the body of the right mandible. The lesion, which has a well-defined, corticated border, has caused apical root resorption of the mesial root of tooth no. 31. This lesion easily could be misdiagnosed as a radicular cyst. (Courtesy E.J. Burkes, DDS, Chapel Hill, N.C.)

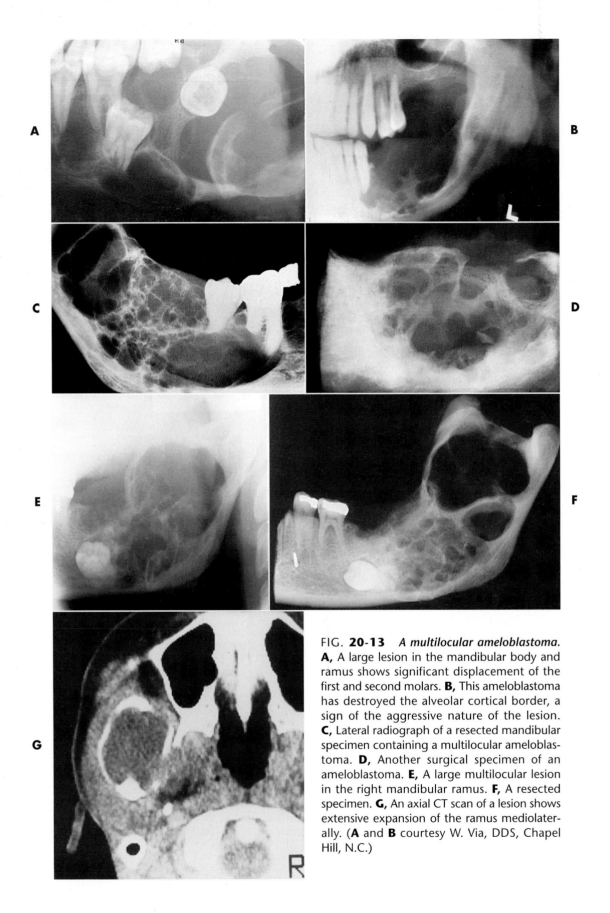

FIG. **20-13**   *A multilocular ameloblastoma.*
A, A large lesion in the mandibular body and ramus shows significant displacement of the first and second molars. **B,** This ameloblastoma has destroyed the alveolar cortical border, a sign of the aggressive nature of the lesion. **C,** Lateral radiograph of a resected mandibular specimen containing a multilocular ameloblastoma. **D,** Another surgical specimen of an ameloblastoma. **E,** A large multilocular lesion in the right mandibular ramus. **F,** A resected specimen. **G,** An axial CT scan of a lesion shows extensive expansion of the ramus mediolaterally. (**A** and **B** courtesy W. Via, DDS, Chapel Hill, N.C.)

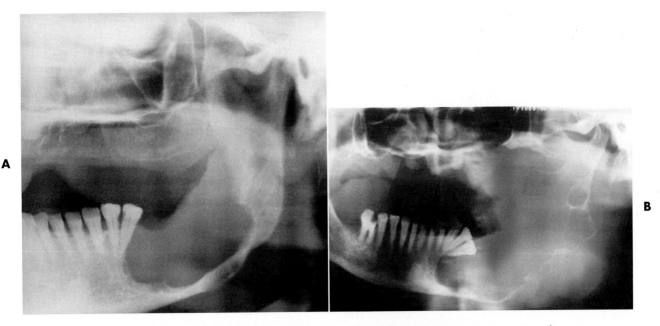

FIG. **20-14** *A massive ameloblastoma of the right mandibular body.* **A,** A portion of a panoramic radiograph made on the patient's first visit. **B,** A panoramic radiograph of the same patient 2 years later. The patient had refused treatment, and the lesion has doubled in size. The inferior border of the mandible has thinned, the crest of the alveolar ridge has been destroyed, and the premolar teeth have been significantly displaced mesially. (Courtesy B. Gratt, DDS, Los Angeles, Calif.)

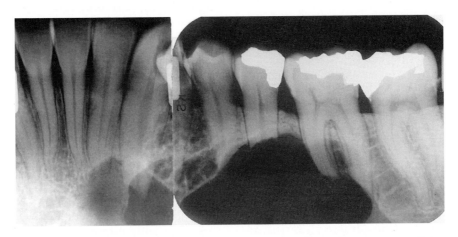

FIG. **20-15** Root resorption of the premolars and canine adjacent to a radiolucent ameloblastoma in the left mandible.

the radiolucent area (Fig. 20-13, *A*). These septa are usually coarse and curved. In some cases the number and arrangement of septa may give the area a honeycomb (numerous small compartments or loculations) or soap bubble (larger compartments of variable size) appearance (Fig. 20-13, *B* through *G*). Generally the loculations are larger in the posterior mandible and smaller in the anterior mandible. Massive ameloblastomas have been reported (Fig. 20-14).

Effects on surrounding structures. A more pronounced tendency exists for an ameloblastoma to cause extensive root resorption than is observed with other lesions (Fig. 20-15). Tooth displacement is common. Because a common point of origin is above the occlusal region of a tooth, some teeth are displaced apically. An occlusal radiograph may demonstrate expansion and thinning of an adjacent cortical plate, but, notably, a thin "eggshell" of bone usually persists. Actual perfora-

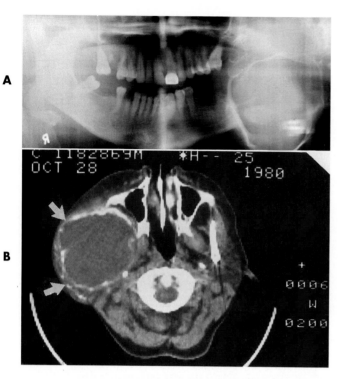

FIG. 20-16 *A CT scan of a large ameloblastoma in the left mandibular ramus.* **A,** A panoramic radiograph shows that the lesion extends beyond the mandibular border inferiorly and that it has well-corticated borders. **B,** A CT scan shows the extensive expansion of the ramus mediolaterally and confirms that the tumor margins are corticated *(arrows).* Note the normal maxillary sinuses and the contralateral mandibular ramus.

tion of bone is a late feature of ameloblastoma. Unicystic types of ameloblastoma may cause extreme expansion of the mandibular ramus.

Additional imaging. CT and MRI are useful modalities for the examination of ameloblastoma. CT not only suggests the diagnosis but also demonstrates the anatomic location and detects encroachment into such vital regions as the floor of the mouth, infratemporal fossa, and submandibular region (Fig. 20-16). CT imaging is also useful in detecting perforation of the mandibular cortical plates caused by rapid enlargement of the tumor. MRI helps to clarify evaluation of the interface between the tumor and normal soft tissue. MRI is superior to CT in the assessment of recurrent disease and is a useful supplement to CT in the presurgical and follow-up assessment of ameloblastoma.

Differential diagnosis. Early ameloblastomas usually develop in the mandible of a younger patient. These lesions may suggest a dentigerous cyst if they occur

as a radiolucency surrounding the crown of an unerupted tooth. Likewise, a monolocular tumor that has involved the roots of a functioning tooth may resemble a radicular cyst (Fig. 20-17). Ameloblastomas may share common radiographic characteristics with other lesions as well, such as residual cysts, traumatic bone cysts, lateral periodontal cysts, giant cell granulomas, and odontogenic myxomas. All these lesions, except residual cysts and lateral periodontal cysts, tend to occur in people in their mid-twenties or younger; ameloblastomas, however, usually develop in older patients. Giant cell granulomas generally occur anterior to the molars and have more granular or ill-defined septa. Lateral periodontal cysts occur in the incisor-canine-premolar region of the mandible, and ameloblastomas occur in the molar region. More advanced ameloblastomas may have a dense, multilocular appearance similar to that of an odontogenic myxoma. Odontogenic myxomas are extremely rare. Also, the septa dividing the image of a myxoma usually are finer than those in an ameloblastoma, and close inspection often reveals a few straight septa.

Treatment. Whatever surgical procedures are used to treat an ameloblastoma, the surgeon must consider the tendency of the neoplasm to invade adjacent bone beyond its apparent margins. CT and MRI are useful in determining the location of tumor margins. If the ameloblastoma is relatively small, it may be removed completely by an intraoral approach and without a full-thickness resection of the jaw. The maxilla is the most dangerous primary location for ameloblastomas, and these lesions often go undetected for years, allowing considerable growth. If the lesion is extensive, excision may require en bloc resection of the jaw. Although megavoltage radiotherapy can reduce the size of an ameloblastoma (primarily the part that has expanded the jaw or broken into the soft tissues), it does not appear to be an appropriate treatment for operable ameloblastomas. Radiation therapy is used mainly for inoperable tumors, especially those in the posterior maxilla.

Adenomatoid Odontogenic Tumor
Synonyms. *Adenoameloblastoma* and *ameloblastic adenomatoid tumor*

Definition. Adenomatoid odontogenic tumors are uncommon, nonaggressive tumors of odontogenic epithelium. This lesion, first reported by Stafne, has distinctive clinical and microscopic features and behavior patterns that sharply differ from ameloblastomas. The origin of adenomatoid odontogenic tumors is still in doubt. Although the lesion is classified as an odontogenic ep-

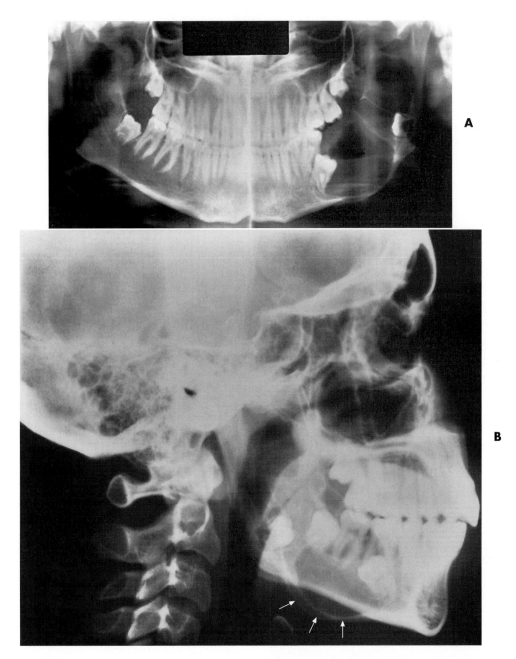

FIG. **20-17** *A mural ameloblastoma.* **A,** A panoramic radiograph of a large ameloblastoma in the left mandibular body and ramus. The second and third molars have been displaced inferiorly. Several vertical septa are present within the lesion, and the tumor has expanded the mandible. **B,** A lateral cephalometric radiograph shows the inferior extent of the lesion and that the border is corticated and intact *(arrows).* (Courtesy J. Miller, DDS, Hickory, N.C.)

ithelial tumor, many experts believe that it is most likely a hamartoma and not a neoplasm. Adenomatoid odontogenic tumors account for 3% of oral tumors. Central and peripheral ameloblastic odontogenic tumors occur. The two types of central lesions are the follicular type (those associated with an embedded tooth) and the extrafollicular type (those with no embedded tooth). Approximately 73% of central lesions are the follicular type.

Clinical features. Adenomatoid odontogenic tumors appear in the age range of 5 to 50 years; however, about 70% occur in the second decade, with an average age of 16 years. The tumor has a 2:1 female predilection. The follicular type is diagnosed somewhat earlier than the extrafollicular type, probably because the failure of the associated tooth to erupt is noted. The tumor is slow growing, and as it enlarges, a gradually enlarging, pain-

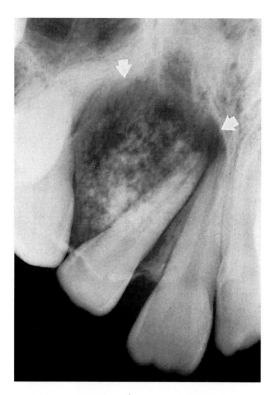

FIG. **20-18**   An adenomatoid odontogenic tumor in the region of the right maxillary canine and lateral incisor. Calcification is present within the tumor mass, and the canine and lateral incisor have been displaced by the lesion. (Courtesy R. Howell, DDS, Morgantown, W.V.)

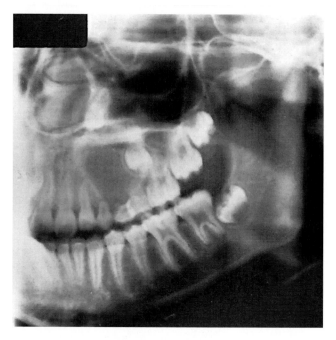

FIG. **20-20**   *An adenomatoid odontogenic tumor.* A portion of a panoramic radiograph of a lesion in the anterior left maxilla. The maxillary left canine and premolar have been displaced superiorly by the tumor. One premolar is absent. (Courtesy E.J. Burkes, DDS, Chapel Hill, N.C.)

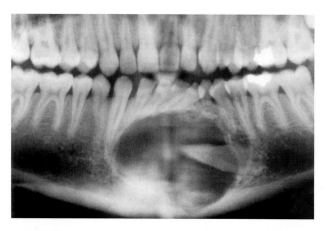

FIG. **20-19**   *A mandibular adenomatoid odontogenic tumor.* The mandibular left canine is engulfed by the lesion and has been displaced inferiorly.

less swelling or asymmetry is noticed, often associated with a missing tooth.

Radiographic features

Location. At least 75% of adenomatoid odontogenic tumors occur in the maxilla (Fig. 20-18). The incisor-canine-premolar region is the usual area involved in both jaws (more than 90% occur in the incisor region). A common and notable feature of this lesion is that the tumor surrounds the entire tooth, most often a canine, especially when it occurs in the mandible (Fig. 20-19).

Periphery. The usual radiographic appearance is a well-defined corticated or sclerotic border.

Internal structure. Radiographically, radiopacities develop in about two thirds of cases (see Fig. 20-18). One tumor may be completely radiolucent, another may contain faint radiopaque foci (Fig. 20-20), and some may show dense clusters of radiopacities, sometimes appearing as small pebbles (Fig. 20-21). Intraoral radiographs may be required to demonstrate the calcifications within the lesion, which may not be seen on panoramic radiographs. Microscopic studies have verified that the size, number, and density of small radiopacities in the central radiolucency of the lesion vary from tumor to tumor and seem to increase with age.

Effects on surrounding structures. As the tumor enlarges, adjacent teeth are displaced. Root resorption is rare. This lesion also may inhibit eruption of an involved tooth. Although some expansion of the jaw may occur, the outer cortex is maintained.

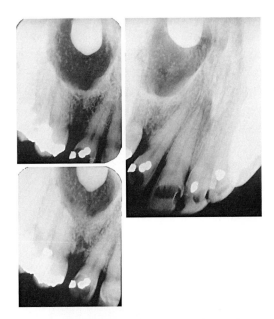

FIG. **20-21** *Periapical radiographs of an adenomatoid odontogenic tumor in the right maxilla.* The maxillary right canine is impacted. The lesion is associated with the crown of the canine. (Courtesy L. Hollender, DDS, Seattle, Wash.)

Differential diagnosis. The differential diagnosis for an adenomatoid odontogenic tumor should include the pericoronal radiolucencies: dentigerous cysts, ameloblastomas, and ameloblastic fibromas. The combination of a relatively early age of occurrence, a predilection for the anterior region of the jaws, and a tendency to surround more than just the crown of the unerupted tooth with which it generally is associated suggests adenomatoid odontogenic tumor. The follicular type of this tumor mimics a follicular cyst and the peripheral type, a gingival cyst. Other radiolucent lesions with small foci of calcifications should be considered, including ameloblastic fibroodontomes and calcifying odontogenic cysts.

Treatment. Conservative surgical excision is adequate because the tumor is not locally invasive, is well encapsulated, and is separated easily from the bone. The theory that adenomatoid odontogenic tumors are hamartomas is supported by the innocuous behavior of the lesion because, as with odontomas, adenomatoid odontogenic tumors stop developing about the time tooth structures complete their growth. Repair of maxillary lesions using guided tissue regeneration has been reported. The recurrence rate is 0.2%.

Calcifying Epithelial Odontogenic Tumor
Synonyms. *Pindborg tumor* and *ameloblastoma of unusual type with calcification*

Definition. Calcifying epithelial odontogenic tumors are rare neoplasms of the tooth-producing apparatus. They account for about 1% of odontogenic tumors. These tumors usually are located within bone, produce a mineralized substance, and are often amyloid. Calcifying epithelial odontogenic tumors have a distinctive microscopic appearance that may arise from the stratum intermedium of the enamel organ.

Clinical features. A calcifying epithelial odontogenic tumor (CEOT) behaves much like an ameloblastoma; it also is locally invasive, has a high recurrence rate, and is found in about the same age group. This similarity extends even to the occurrence of rare extraosseous lesions. The neoplasm is somewhat more common in men, and patients range in age from 8 to 92 years, with an average age of about 42 years (considerably younger in men and somewhat older in women). Jaw expansion is a regular feature and about the only symptom, although one case was reported of a patient who described an associated mild paresthesia. Palpation of the swelling reveals a hard tumor that may be quite well defined or diffuse. Maxillary cases occur more often with swelling.

Radiographic features
Location. As with ameloblastomas, calcifying epithelial odontogenic tumors have a definite predilection for the mandible, with a ratio of at least 2:1, and most develop in the premolar-molar area, with a 52% association with an unerupted or impacted tooth. In about half of cases, radiographs taken early in the development of these tumors reveal a radiolucent area around the crown of a mature, unerupted tooth.

Periphery. The radiolucent, cystlike area may be well delineated (Fig. 20-22). In some tumors the boundary may change from well defined to diffuse.

Internal structure. The radiograph of a mature lesion reveals a unilocular or multilocular cystic lesion with numerous scattered, radiopaque foci of varying size and density. The most characteristic and diagnostic finding is the appearance of radiopacities close to the crown of the embedded tooth. In addition, small, thin, opaque trabeculae may cross the radiolucency in many directions.

Effects on surrounding structures. Calcifying epithelial odontogenic tumors may displace a developing tooth or prevent its eruption. Associated expansion of the jaw with maintenance of a cortical boundary may also occur.

Differential diagnosis. Early lesions may mimic dentigerous cysts or even ameloblastomas. Although all radiolucent lesions with radiopaque foci should be considered in the differential diagnosis, the radiographic

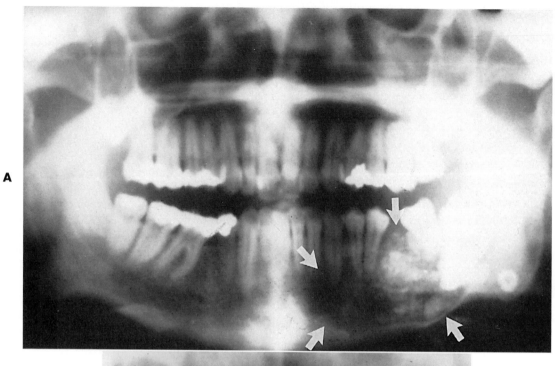

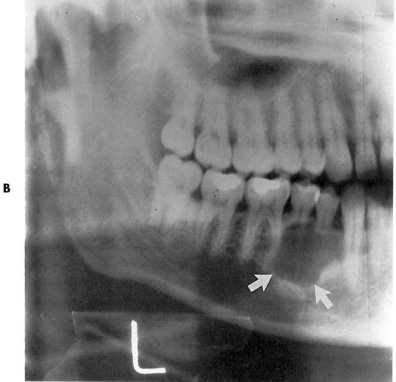

FIG. **20-22** *A calcifying odontogenic tumor, or Pindborg tumor (arrows).* **A,** The tumor appears as a mixed radiolucent-radiopaque lesion associated with an unerupted tooth *(arrows).* **B,** The tumor has caused resorption of the mandibular premolar roots. (**A** courtesy M. Gornitsky, DDS, Montreal, Canada; **B** courtesy J.R. Jacoway, DDS, Chapel Hill, N.C.)

features of the CEOT most closely resemble those of central odontogenic fibromas, calcifying odontogenic cysts, odontomas (intermediate stage), and adenomatoid odontogenic tumors. These other lesions can be differentiated from calcifying epithelial odontogenic tumors by their clinical features.

Treatment. Because a CEOT tumor behaves clinically like an ameloblastoma, it should be treated as one.

MIXED TUMORS (ECTODERMAL-MESODERMAL)

Odontoma

Synonyms. *Compound odontoma, compound composite odontoma, complex odontoma, complex composite odontoma, odontogenic hamartoma, calcified mixed odontoma,* and *cystic odontoma*

Definition. The term *odontoma* is used to identify a tumor that is radiographically and histologically characterized by the production of mature enamel, dentin, cementum, and pulp tissue. These components are seen in various states of histodifferentiation and morphodifferentiation. Although any tumor that arises from the odontogenic apparatus may be considered by precise definition to be an odontoma, the limited and sluggish growth potential of this lesion distinguishes it from other neoplastic odontogenic tumors. In fact, some authorities consider an odontoma to be a hamartoma rather than a neoplasm and refer to it as an *odontogenic hamartoma.*

The structural relationship of the component tissues may vary from nondescript masses of dental tissue (complex odontoma) to multiple well-formed teeth (compound odontoma). A third, even less common, variety, the ameloblastic fibroodontoma, can be identified histologically. In one series of more than 700 odontogenic tumors, 67% of the lesions were compound or complex odontomas and fewer than 4% were ameloblastic fibroodontomas.

Clinical features. Odontomas are the most common odontogenic tumor. They often interfere with the eruption of permanent teeth (Fig. 20-23). The lesion shows no gender predilection, and most begin forming while the normal dentition is developing (Fig. 20-24). Odontomas develop and mature while the corresponding teeth are forming and cease development when the associated teeth complete development. Most odontomas occur in the second decade of life. In rare cases odontomas form with primary teeth. They persist if left untreated and may be discovered throughout life. Compound odontomas are about twice as common as the complex type. Although the compound variety forms equally between men and women, 60% of complex odontomas occur in women. Compound odontomas seldom cause bony expansion or exceed a normal tooth crown in size; most are 1 to 3 cm in diameter. Most odontomas are discovered before 20 years of age and many times are found during investigation of delayed eruption of adjacent teeth or retained primary teeth. In rare circumstances a compound odontoma may erupt into the oral cavity of a child.

Radiographic features

Location. More of the compound variety of odontomas (62%) occur in the anterior maxilla in association with the crown of an unerupted canine. In contrast, 70% of complex odontomas are found in the mandibular first and second molar area.

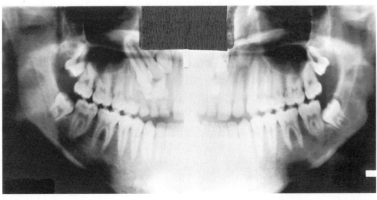

A

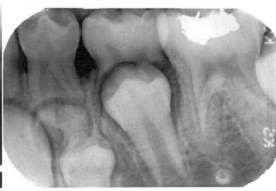

B

FIG. **20-23** *A compound odontoma.* **A,** A panoramic radiograph of a compound odontoma in the right maxillary anterior region. The lesion has prevented eruption of the right maxillary canine and the lateral incisor and central incisors. **B,** Another compound odontoma in the mandibular premolar region. Eruption of the mandibular left first premolar has been impeded by the odontoma. (From Matteson SR et al: *Semin Adv Oral Radiol Dent Radiol Photogr* 57(1-4):1, 1985.)

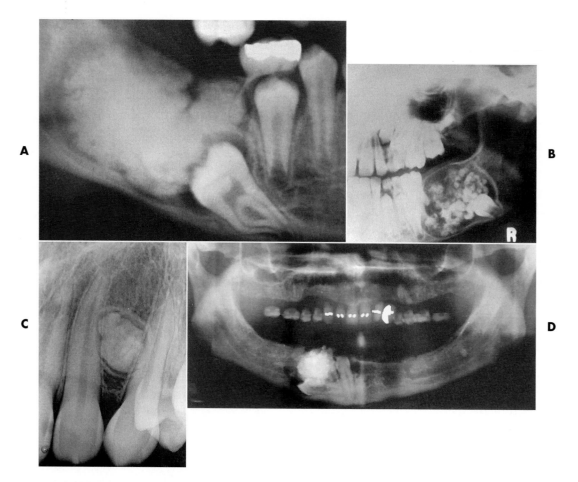

FIG. **20-24** *Complex odontomas.* **A,** Note the thin radiolucent space around the calcified mass. **B** and **C,** A peripheral cortical margin is evident around a calcified mass. **D,** A complex odontoma in the anterior mandible. (**C** courtesy A.G. Farman, DDS, Louisville, Ky.; C.J. Nortje, DDS, Tygerberg, Cape Province, South Africa; and R.E. Wood, DDS, Toronto, Canada.)

Periphery. The borders of odontomas are well defined and may be smooth or irregular. Most have a hyperostotic or cortical border. Immediately inside and adjacent to the cortical border is a soft tissue capsule.

Internal structure. The contents of these lesions are largely radiopaque. Compound odontomas have a number of toothlike structures (Fig. 20-25). Complex odontomas contain an irregular mass of calcified tissue (Fig. 20-26). The degree of radiopacity is equivalent to or exceeds adjacent tooth structure. The extent to which the radiopaque structures occupy the radiolucent area and their variations in radiographic density vary from tumor to tumor. These variations are caused by the unique distribution of enamel and dentin in each lesion. A dilated odontome has a single internal calcified structure that may take the form of a donut with a more radiolucent central portion.

Effects on surrounding structures. Most odontomas (70%) are associated with abnormalities such as impaction, malpositioning, diastema, aplasia, malforma-

tion, and devitalization of adjacent teeth. Large complex odontomes may cause expansion of the jaw with maintenance of the cortical boundary.

Differential diagnosis. A toothlike appearance of the radiopaque structures within a well-defined lesion leads to easy recognition of a compound odontoma. Complex odontomas differ from cementoossifying fibromas by their tendency to associate with unerupted molar teeth and because they usually are more radiopaque than fibromas. Odontomas may also develop in much younger patients than cementoossifying fibromas. Adenomatoid odontogenic tumors rarely are as opaque as complex odontomas and usually form with the maxillary canines. Periapical cemental dysplasia usually is a smaller lesion than a complex odontoma and occurs most often in the periapical location in the mandibular anterior region of middle-aged adults. However, when a region of cemental dysplasia occurs in the posterior mandible, it may be differentiated by

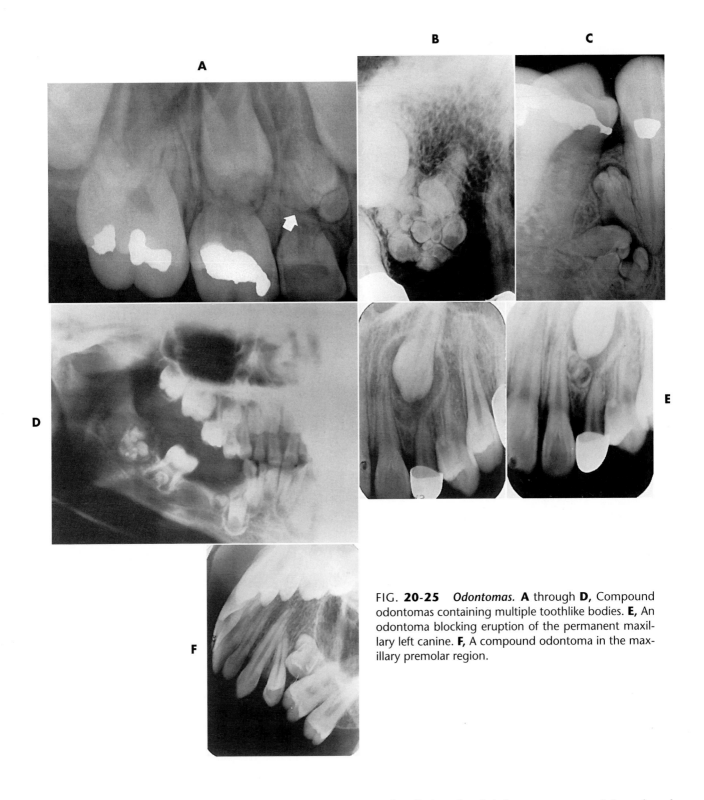

FIG. **20-25** *Odontomas.* **A** through **D**, Compound odontomas containing multiple toothlike bodies. **E,** An odontoma blocking eruption of the permanent maxillary left canine. **F,** A compound odontoma in the maxillary premolar region.

its lack of a well-defined cortical border and its more diffuse sclerotic periphery. Areas of enostosis, although radiopaque, do not have a soft tissue capsule, as is seen with odontomes.

Treatment. Complex and compound odontomas are removed by simple excision. They do not recur and are

not locally invasive. It is important not to injure the adjacent periodontium during surgical removal.

Ameloblastic Fibroodontoma

A related but extremely rare lesion, the ameloblastic fibroodontoma, also known as a *soft and calcified odontoma* or *odontoblastoma,* consists of elements of ameloblastic fi-

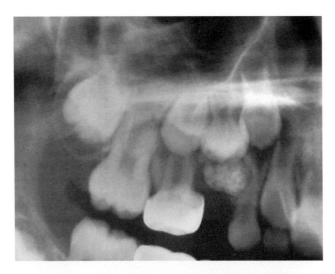

FIG. **20-26**   A complex odontoma in the maxillary right premolar area of a child with mixed dentition. The odontoma is impeding eruption of a permanent premolar.

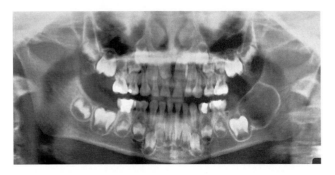

FIG. **20-27**   An ameloblastic fibroodontoma in the left second and third molar area of a child with early mixed dentition. (Courtesy Karl Kliner, DDS, Columbia, S.C.)

broma with small segments of enamel and dentin. Radiographically the amount of radiolucent internal structure exceeds the radiopaque structure. Small lesions may appear as enlarged follicles with only one or two small, discrete radiopacities. Larger lesions may have a more extensive calcified internal structure (Fig. 20-27). Most often an associated impacted tooth is present. The treatment is conservative enucleation, and recurrence has been reported.

Ameloblastic Fibroma

Synonyms. *Soft odontoma, soft mixed odontoma, mixed odontogenic tumor, fibroadamantoblastoma,* and *granular cell ameloblastic fibroma*

Definition. Ameloblastic fibromas are benign, mixed odontogenic tumors. They are characterized by neo-

plastic proliferation of maturing and early functional ameloblasts as well as the primitive mesenchymal components of the dental papilla. Enamel, dentin, and cementum are not formed in this tumor.

Clinical features. The behavior of ameloblastic fibromas is completely benign. Complete agreement has not been reached regarding sex predilection. Most of these tumors occur between 5 and 20 years of age, during the period of tooth formation, with an average age of about 15 years. They usually produce a painless, slow-growing expansion and displacement of the involved teeth (Fig. 20-28). Although the most common symptom is swelling or occlusal pain, the tumor may be discovered on a routine dental radiograph. It may be associated with a missing tooth.

Radiographic features
Location. Ameloblastic fibromas usually develop in the premolar-molar area of the mandible. In some cases the tumor may involve the ramus and extend forward to the premolar-molar area. It may be associated with an unerupted tooth (located occlusal to the tooth), or it may arise in an area where a tooth failed to develop.

Periphery. The borders of an ameloblastic fibroma are well defined and often corticated in a manner similar to that of a cyst.

Internal structure. An ameloblastic fibroma may be either unilocular or multilocular (Fig. 20-29).

Effects on surrounding structures. An expanded, intact cortical plate often can be seen on the radiograph. The associated tooth or teeth may be inhibited from normal eruption or may be displaced in an apical direction.

Differential diagnosis. An ameloblastic fibroma may appear as a unilocular or multilocular lesion, usually in teenagers, and may be similar to an ameloblastoma. The differential diagnosis includes central giant cell granuloma, aneurysmal bone cyst, odontogenic myxoma, central hemangioma, keratocyst (from a supernumerary tooth), and ameloblastoma. Distinguishing features that help differentiate an ameloblastic fibroma are as follows: giant cell granulomas, odontogenic myxomas, and central hemangiomas have a finer trabeculation with a honeycomb pattern or one suggesting the strings of a tennis racket, and none of these three necessarily are associated with a tooth. Giant cell granulomas tend to occur in the anterior jaw. Central hemangiomas also may show local gingival bleeding and rebound mobility of adjacent teeth (i.e., when depressed into their sockets, the teeth rebound to their original position within several minutes because of the pressure of the vascular network below the tooth). Furthermore, ameloblastomas usually develop in a much older age group. In

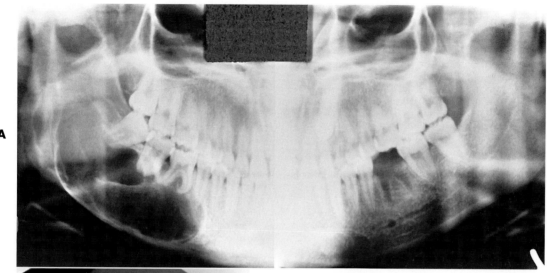

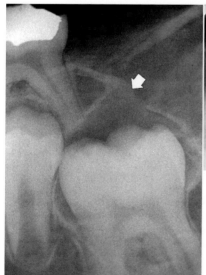

FIG. **20-28** *An ameloblastic fibroma in the body and ramus of the right mandible.* **A,** A panoramic radiograph. **B,** An occlusal radiograph showing mediolateral expansion of the mandible adjacent to the lesion.

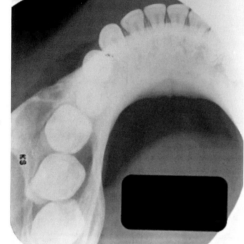

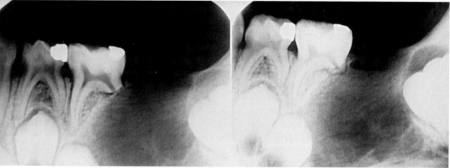

FIG. **20-29** *An ameloblastic fibroma.* **A,** An ameloblastic fibroma appearing as a unilocular outgrowth of the follicle of the unerupted first permanent molar. **B,** An ameloblastic fibroma with a radiolucent appearance. The permanent second premolar is being displaced inferiorly, and the distal root of the second primary molar has been resorbed. (**A** courtesy R. White, DDS, Chapel Hill, N.C.; **B** courtesy L. Hollender, DDS, Seattle, Wash.)

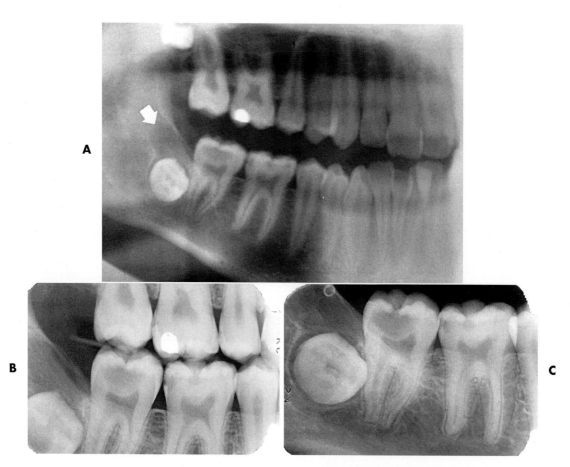

FIG. **20-30** *An ameloblastic fibroma.* **A,** An ameloblastic fibroma seen as a radiolucency above the unerupted third molar *(arrow).* **B,** A bitewing radiograph of the same lesion. **C,** A periapical radiograph. (Courtesy G. Sanders, DDS, LaCrosse, Wisc.)

some cases ameloblastic fibromas have a tendency to appear as outgrowths from the dental follicle (Fig. 20-30) rather than as symmetric enlargements encompassing the crown, which is characteristic of a dentigerous cyst.

Treatment. Ameloblastic fibromas are benign, and the rate of recurrence is low. A conservative surgical approach, including enucleation and mechanical curettage of the surrounding bone, is reported to be successful for these cases.

MESODERMAL TUMORS

Odontogenic Myxoma
Synonyms. *Myxoma, myxofibroma and fibromyxoma*

Definition. Odontogenic myxomas are uncommon, accounting for only 3% to 6% of odontogenic tumors. They are benign, intraosseous neoplasms that arise from the mesenchymal portion of the dental papilla. These myxomas are locally aggressive but nonmetastasizing neoplasms. They have a loose, gelatinous consistency and

show microscopic characteristics similar to those of soft tissue myxomas of the extremities. Odontogenic myxomas develop only in the bones of the facial skeleton. The theory that this lesion develops from odontogenic rather than nonodontogenic mesenchyme is supported by the fact that it appears only in the jaws, it affects young people, it occasionally is related to a tooth that failed to erupt or is missing, and in some cases odontogenic epithelium can be detected microscopically.

Clinical features. If odontogenic myxomas have a gender predilection, they slightly favor females. Although the lesion can occur at any age, more than half arise in individuals between 10 and 30 years; it rarely occurs before age 10 or after age 50. This tumor often is associated with a congenitally missing or unerupted tooth. It grows slowly and may or may not cause pain. Eventually it causes expansion and may grow quite large if left untreated. It may also invade the maxillary sinus and cause exophthalmos. Recurrence rates as high as 25% have been reported. This high rate may be explained by the lack of encapsulation of the tumor, its poorly defined boundaries, and the extension of nests or pockets of myxoid (jellylike) tumor into trabecular spaces, where they are difficult to detect and remove surgically.

Radiographic features

Location. Myxomas more commonly affect the mandible by a margin of 3:1. In the mandible these tumors occur in the premolar and molar areas and only rarely in the ramus and condyle (non–tooth-bearing areas). Myxomas in the maxilla rarely affect the anterior area and usually involve the alveolar process in the premolar and molar regions and the zygomatic process of the maxilla.

Periphery. The lesion usually is well defined, and it often has a corticated margin. However, the outline of some lesions, especially those in the maxilla, is poorly defined (Fig. 20-31).

Internal structure. When it occurs pericoronally with an impacted tooth, an odontogenic myxoma is most likely to have a cystlike, unilocular outline, although it may have a mixed radiolucent-radiopaque image. Therefore this lesion may be either unilocular or multilocular, although some describe it as typically multilocular, especially after it has enlarged. Although the locules usually are small and uniform with a typical honeycomb pattern, the arrangement of the trabeculae may also show a tennis racket pattern (Fig. 20-32). However, this classic description is rare, and only one or two fine, straight septa may be found. Often exceptionally fine septa cross the radiolucent areas, producing a wispy, soap bubble appearance.

Effects on surrounding structures. When the tumor expands in a tooth-bearing area, it displaces and loosens teeth, but root resorption is rare. The lesion also frequently scallops between the roots of adjacent teeth, and in rare cases the roots may show resorption.

Additional imaging.
CT and MRI enhance visualization of the anatomic extent of the lesion and better define the tumor–normal tissue interface. Recurrent tumors can be detected by their high signal in T2-weighted MRI scans. These advanced imaging procedures may aid in the planning of surgical treatment (Fig. 20-33).

Differential diagnosis.
Because the radiographic image of most odontogenic myxomas is a multilocular radiolucency, the differential diagnosis should include all lesions that may produce such a pattern, including ameloblastomas, central giant cell granulomas, cherubism, aneurysmal bone cysts, and central hemangiomas.

Treatment.
Odontogenic myxomas are treated by resection with a generous amount of surrounding bone to ensure removal of myxomatous tumor that infiltrates the adjacent marrow spaces. With appropriate treatment, the prognosis is good.

Benign Cementoblastoma
Synonyms. *Cementoblastoma* and *true cementoma*

Definition.
Benign cementoblastomas are slow-growing, mesenchymal neoplasms composed principally of cementum. The tumor manifests as a bulbous growth around and attached to the apex of a tooth root. Its histologic characteristics are similar to those of osteoblastomas, and it is composed of cementoblasts that arise from the mesenchyme of the periodontal ligament. The tumor most often develops with permanent teeth but in rare cases occurs with primary teeth.

Clinical features.
Although statistical data suggest that benign cementoblastomas are uncommon, many believe that they occur more often than published accounts indicate. The lesion is more common in males than females, and the ages of reported patients range from 12 to 65 years, although most patients are relatively young. There is no racial predilection. The tumor usually is a solitary lesion that is slow growing but that may eventually displace teeth. The involved tooth is vital and often painful. The pain seems to vary from patient to patient and can be relieved by antiinflammatory drugs. In many cases endodontic treatment has been performed in an attempt to treat the pain associated with these tumors. In some cases the lesion may cause expansion of the jaw.

Radiographic features

Location. Benign cementoblastomas occur more often in the mandible (78%) and form most commonly on a premolar or first molar (90%).

Periphery. The lesion is a well-defined radiopacity with a radiolucent halo surrounding the calcified mass. The outer boundary consists of a cortical border adjacent to the radiolucent layer.

Internal structure. Benign cementoblastomas are mixed radiolucent-radiopaque lesions that may be amorphous or may have a wheel spoke pattern (Fig. 20-34). The density of the cemental mass usually obscures the outline of the enveloped root.

Effects on surrounding structures. If the root outline is apparent, in most cases some external resorption has occurred. An occlusal radiograph can show expansion of the cortex of the mandible.

Differential diagnosis.
The differential diagnosis for benign cementoblastoma should include periapical cemental dysplasia, periapical sclerosing osteitis (osteosclerosis), enostosis, and hypercementosis. However, the clinical and radiographic features usually allow differentiation of benign cementoblastomas from these other periapical radiopacities. Distinguishing features of cementoblastoma include its intimate association with a tooth root, root resorption, a larger size than hyperce-

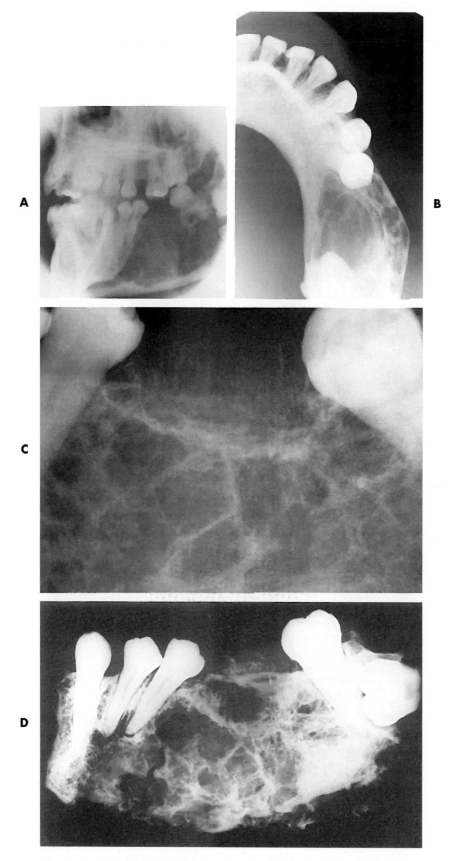

FIG. **20-31**   *An odontogenic myxoma.* **A,** A large myxoma in the body of the mandible. **B,** An occlusal view shows buccal expansion of the lesion. **C,** A periapical view shows an angular trabecular pattern. **D,** A lateral radiograph of a surgical specimen from the same patient.

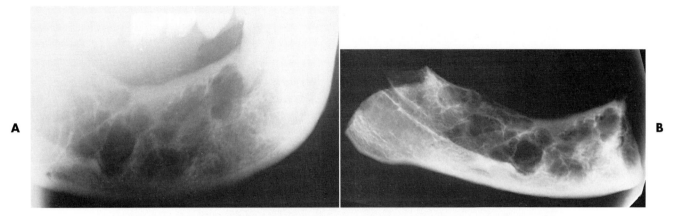

FIG. **20-32** *An odontogenic myxoma with ill-defined borders.* **A,** A lateral oblique radiograph. **B,** A lateral radiograph of the surgical specimen.

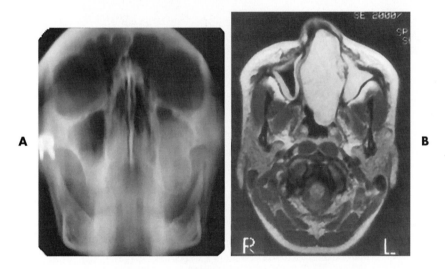

FIG. **20-33** *A myxoma in the left maxilla.* **A,** A coronal tomogram shows clouding of the left maxillary sinus, with expansion of the sinus borders laterally and inferiorly. **B,** An MRI in the axial plane through the maxillary sinuses shows a high-signal area in the right sinus representing the myxoma. (Courtesy A.G. Farman, DDS, Louisville, Ky.; C.J. Nortje, DDS, Tygerberg, Cape Province, South Africa; and R.E. Wood, DDS, Toronto, Canada.)

mentosis, and separation from the surrounding bone by a radiolucent rim. Also, this neoplasm can expand the jaw. The histologic appearance may be identical to that of a benign osteoblastoma.

Treatment. Benign cementoblastomas are apparently self-limiting and rarely recur after enucleation. Simple excision and extraction of the associated tooth are sufficient treatment. In some cases the tumor may be amputated from the tooth, which is then treated endodontically.

Central Odontogenic Fibroma
Synonyms. *Simple odontogenic fibroma* and *odontogenic fibroma (World Health Organization [WHO] type)*

Definition. Central odontogenic fibromas are rare neoplasms that sometimes are divided into two types according to histologic appearance: the simple type contains mature fibrous tissue with sparsely scattered odontogenic epithelial rests; the WHO type, which is more cellular, has more epithelial rests and may contain calcifications that resemble dysplastic dentin, cementum, or osteoid. One theory is that these types merely represent a spectrum and that odontogenic myxoma may be a part of this range.

Clinical features. Most cases of central odontogenic fibromas occur between the ages of 11 and 39 years. The neoplasm shows a definite female preponderance, with a reported ratio of 2.2:1. Affected patients may be asymptomatic or may have swelling and mobility of the teeth.

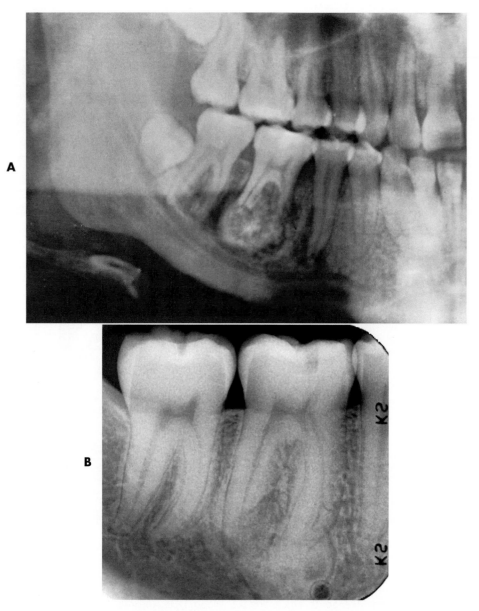

FIG. **20-34**   *A cementoblastoma.* **A,** A portion of a panoramic radiograph showing a large, bulbous, radiopaque mass associated with the apical portion of the mandibular right first molar. A radiolucent band can be seen surrounding the mass, and root resorption of the molar roots has occurred. **B,** A periapical radiograph of the same lesion. (Courtesy M. Pharoah, DDS, Toronto, Canada.)

Radiographic features

Location. Central odontogenic fibromas occur slightly more often in the mandible. The prevalent site in the mandible is the molar-premolar region, and in the maxilla it is the anterior region.

Periphery. The periphery usually is well defined.

Internal structure. Smaller lesions usually are unilocular, and larger lesions have a multilocular pattern. The internal septa may be fine and straight, as in odontogenic myxomas, or it may be granular, resembling those seen in giant cell granulomas. Some lesions are totally

radiolucent, whereas unorganized internal calcification has been reported in others.

Effects on surrounding structures. A central odontogenic fibroma may cause expansion with maintenance of a thin cortical boundary. Tooth displacement is common, and root resorption has been reported.

Differential diagnosis. The histologic features may resemble those of desmoplastic fibroma if no epithelial rests are apparent. Desmoplastic fibromas tend to invade surrounding tissue and thus are not well defined. They also commonly break through the cortical boundaries and invade surrounding soft tissue. If thin, straight septa can be seen in the odontogenic fibroma, it may not be possible to differentiate this neoplasm from an odontogenic myxoma on radiographic criteria alone. If granular septa are present, the radiographic appearance may be identical to that of a giant cell granuloma.

Treatment. Central odontogenic fibromas are treated with simple excision. These lesions have a very low recurrence rate.

Nonodontogenic Tumors

Ectodermal and mixed ectodermal-mesodermal benign nonodontogenic tumors are tumors of neural tissue. Benign intraosseous nerve tumors arise from nerve sheaths and nerve fibers in combination with their supporting tissues. These are the neuromas, neurofibromas, and neurilemomas. Although they are rare, most occur in the jaws, especially in the body and ramus of the mandible. Most nerve sheath tumors may occur in the mandible because the mandibular canal conveys a larger neurovascular bundle for a longer distance than does any other bony canal in the body.

ECTODERMAL TUMORS

Neurilemoma
Synonym. *Schwannoma*

Definition. A central neurilemoma is a tumor of neuroectodermal origin, arising from the Schwann cells that make up the inner layer covering the peripheral nerves. Although rare, it is the most common intraosseous nerve tumor. This tumor has practically no potential for malignant transformation.

Clinical features. Neurilemomas grow slowly, can occur at any age (but most commonly arise in the second and third decades), and occur with equal frequency in both males and females. The mandible and sacrum are the most common sites. These lesions cause few symptoms other than those related to the location and size of the tumor. The usual complaint is a "lump in the jaw." The tumors usually occur singly, and jaw expansion may lead to perforation of a cortical border and a mass that is firm to palpation. Because they are solid tumor tissue, they are nonproductive on aspiration. Although pain is uncommon unless the tumor encroaches on adjacent nerves, paresthesia may arise with these bony lesions. Pain, when present, usually develops at the site of the tumor; if paresthesia occurs, it is felt anterior to the tumor.

Radiographic features

Location. Neurilemomas most often involve the mandible, with fewer than 1 in 10 cases occurring in the maxilla. The tumor most often is located within an expanded inferior alveolar nerve canal posterior to the mental foramen.

Periphery. In keeping with its slow growth rate, the margins of these tumors are well defined, cystlike, and often surrounded by a sclerotic rim or cortex.

Internal structure. Neurilemomas usually are seen as round or oval radiolucent areas of bone destruction. Loculations or areas of cortical erosion may suggest a multilocular structure, causing the lesion to resemble an ameloblastoma.

Effects on surrounding structures. If the tumor protrudes from the mental foramen, an erosive lesion may develop on the surface of the jawbone from pressure caused by the overlying tumor. The expanding tumor may cause root resorption of adjacent teeth. Depending on its size, this neoplasm may expand the inferior alveolar canal, the mental foramen, the mandibular foramen, and the mandible while maintaining cortical boundaries.

Differential diagnosis. Because neurilemomas, like other nerve sheath tumors, have a solitary or multilocular radiographic image, the differential diagnosis includes cysts, ameloblastomas, and vascular lesions. The neural nature of the lesion is suggested when the lesion is small and confined to a clear expansion of the inferior alveolar dental canal. Odontogenic lesions occur above the canal. It is imperative that vascular lesions be considered and ruled out in these cases. The expansion of the canal caused by a neural neoplasm is more concentric, creating a fusiform shape, whereas vascular lesions increase the girth of the canal down the entire length and often alter the shape into a serpiginous form.

Treatment. Excision is usually the treatment of choice. These lesions generally do not recur if completely removed. A capsule usually is present, facilitating surgical removal, although occasionally preservation of the nerve may not be possible. However, periodic examination is indicated to check for recurrence.

Neuroma
Synonyms. *Amputation neuroma* and *traumatic neuroma*

Definition. Despite its name, a neuroma is not a neoplasm. Rather, it is an overgrowth of severed nerve fibers attempting to regenerate when scar tissue or malalignment of a fractured nutrient canal blocks the distal end. As a result, the proliferating nerve forms a disorganized collection of nerve fibers composed of varying proportions of axons, perineural connective tissue, Schwann cells, and scar tissue. The original nerve damage may be the result of mechanical or chemical irritation of the nerve caused by fracture, orthognathic surgery, removal of a tumor or cyst, extrusion of endodontic cement, dental implants, or tooth extraction.

Clinical features. Central neuromas are slow-growing, reactive hyperplasias that seldom become large, rarely exceeding 1 cm in diameter. They may cause a variety of symptoms, including severe pain resulting from pressure applied as the tangled mass enlarges in its bony cavity or as the result of external trauma. The patient may have reflex neuralgia, with pain referred to the eyes, face, and head.

Radiographic features. The radiographic features of a neuroma relate to the extent and shape of the proliferating mass of neural tissue.

Location. The most common location is the mental foramen, then the anterior maxilla and the posterior mandible.

Periphery. Neuromas usually have well-defined, corticated borders. They may occur in various shapes, depending on the amount of resistance to expansion offered by the surrounding bone. In the mandible the tumor usually forms in the mandibular canal, which helps distinguish it from a cyst.

Internal structure. When the mass grows larger than the trabecular spaces, it appears as a radiolucent area in bone with well-defined borders.

Effects on surrounding structures. Some expansion of the inferior alveolar nerve canal may occur.

Differential diagnosis. The presence of a painful or extremely sensitive cystlike radiolucency in the bone and a history of fracture or surgery in the same region suggest a neuroma.

Treatment. Treatment is recommended because neuromas tend to continue to enlarge. They also may cause pain. Regardless of the type of injury that precipitates development of the neuroma, recurrence is uncommon after simple excision.

MIXED TUMORS (ECTODERMAL-MESODERMAL)

Neurofibroma
Synonym. Neurinoma

Definition. Neurofibromas are moderately firm, benign, well-circumscribed tumors caused by proliferation of Schwann cells in a disorderly pattern that includes portions of nerve fibers, such as peripheral nerves, axons,

and connective tissue of the sheath of Schwann. As neurofibromas grow, they incorporate axons. In contrast, neurilemomas are composed entirely of Schwann cells and grow by displacing axons.

Clinical features. The central lesion of a neurofibroma is the same as the multiple lesions that develop in von Recklinghausen's disease. Central lesions also may occur in that syndrome but are rare. Neurofibromas can occur at any age but usually are found in young patients. Their distribution in both jaws tends to be more proximal than that of neurilemomas, and neurofibromas have a high potential for malignant change. Central lesions may also be multiple lesions, occurring in both jaws simultaneously and expanding and filling the maxillary sinus. Solitary central lesions and brown spots on the skin may be early signs of the syndrome. Neurofibromas associated with the mandibular nerve are most likely to produce pain or paresthesia, but fortunately this type of neurofibroma is rare. Neurofibromas also may expand and perforate the cortex, causing swelling that is hard or firm to palpation.

Radiographic features

Location. Central neurofibromas may occur in the mandibular canal, in the cancellous bone, and below the periosteum.

Periphery. As with neurilemomas, the margins of the radiolucency in neurofibromas usually are sharply defined and may be corticated. However, despite the benign nature and slow growth of the neurofibroma, some of these lesions have indistinct margins.

Internal structure. The tumors usually appear unilocular, but a multilocular lesion may occur.

Effects on surrounding structures. A neurofibroma of the inferior dental nerve shows a fusiform enlargement of the canal (Fig. 20-35).

Differential diagnosis. Lesions localized to the mandibular canal suggest early nerve tumors. Changes in the canal from neural lesions are more localized and have a fusiform enlargement, whereas vascular lesions enlarge the whole canal and alter its path. Vascular lesions should also be considered when lesions involving the mandibular canal expand beyond the confines of the canal.

Treatment. Solitary central lesions that have been excised seldom recur. However, it is wise to reexamine the area periodically because these tumors are not encapsulated, and some undergo malignant change.

Neurofibromatosis
Synonym. von Recklinghausen's disease

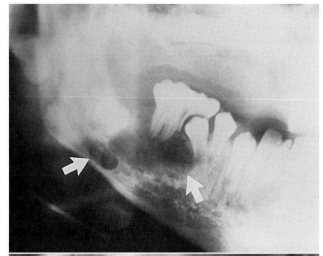

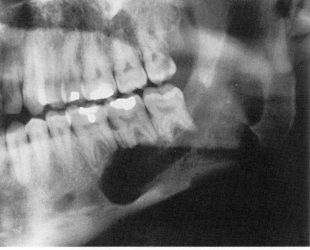

FIG. 20-35 *A neurofibroma.* **A,** A portion of a panoramic radiograph showing a neurofibroma *(arrow)* in an 11-year-old boy with von Recklinghausen's disease. **B,** A portion of a panoramic radiograph showing a neurofibroma forming in the mandibular body along the path of the mandibular canal. (**A** courtesy P. Boyne, DDS, Loma Linda, Calif. **B** courtesy M. Pharoah, DDS, Toronto, Canada.)

Definition. Neurofibromatosis is a syndrome consisting of café au lait spots on the skin, multiple peripheral nerve tumors, and a variety of other dysplastic abnormalities of the skin, nervous system, bones, endocrine organs, and blood vessels. The two major classifications are NF-1, a generalized form, and NF-2, a central form. Oral lesions may occur as part of NF-1 or may be solitary and are called *segmental* or *forme fruste manifestations.* Recent observations of abnormal fat tissue in close association with changes in the osseous structure of the mandible support the theory that a mesodermal dysplasia is part of the spectrum of changes that may be observed in NF-1 lesions.

Clinical features. Neurofibromatosis is one of the most common genetic diseases, occurring in 1 in every 3000 births and present in about 30 people per 10,000 population. The peripheral nerve tumors are of two types, schwannomas and neurofibromas. Some manifestations are congenital, but most appear gradually during childhood and adult life. Café-au-lait spots become larger and more numerous with age; most patients eventually have more than six spots larger than 1.5 cm in diameter. Other skin lesions include freckles; soft, pedunculated, cutaneous neurofibromas; and firm, subcutaneous neurofibromas.

Radiographic features. The radiographic changes in the jaws with neurofibromatosis can be characteristic. These changes include the following alterations in the shape of the mandible: enlargement of the coronoid notch in either or both the horizontal and vertical dimensions; an obtuse angle between the body and the ramus; deformity of the condylar head; lengthening of the condylar neck; and lateral bowing and thinning of the ramus, as seen in basal skull views. Other radiographic changes include enlargement of the mandibular canal and mental and mandibular foramina and an increased incidence of branched mandibular canal. Erosive changes to the outer contour of the mandible and interference with normal eruption of the molars also may occur. Abnormal accumulations of fatty tissue within deformities of the mandible have been observed in images produced by computed tomography (CT).

Treatment. Most patients live a normal life with few or no symptoms. Small cutaneous and subcutaneous neurofibromas can be removed if they are painful, but large plexiform neurofibromas should be left alone. Malignant conversion of these lesions has occurred in rare cases.

MESODERMAL TUMORS

Osteoma
Definition. Osteomas usually form from membranous bones of the skull and face. The cause of the slowly growing osteoma is obscure, but the tumor may arise from cartilage or embryonal periosteum. It is not clear whether osteomas are benign neoplasms or hamartomas. The lesion may occur on more than one bone or with more than one osteoma on a single bone. This tumor may be located in a periosteal or endosteal position. The periosteal type may occur either externally or within the paranasal sinuses. It is more common in the frontal and ethmoid sinuses than in the maxillary sinuses (see Chapter 25). Structurally, osteomas can be divided into three types: those composed of compact bone, those composed of cancellous bone, and those

composed of a combination of compact and cancellous bone.

Clinical features. Osteomas can occur at any age but most frequently are found in individuals older than 40 years. The only symptom of a developing osteoma is the asymmetry caused by a bony, hard swelling on the jaw. Because these tumors have a surface of cortical bone, the osteoma is bony hard to palpation. The swelling is painless until its size or position interferes with function. The osteoma may be attached to the cortex of the jaw by a pedicle or along a wide base. The mucosa covering the tumor is normal in color and freely movable. The compact or ivory type consists of cortical bone, whereas many cancellous osteomas consist of both cortical and medullary bone. Cortical lesions develop more often in men, whereas women have the highest incidence of the cancellous type. Although most osteomas are small, some may become large enough to cause severe damage, especially those that develop in the frontoethmoid region (Fig. 20-36).

Radiographic features

Location. The usual location of an osteoma of the jaw is on the mandible. It is found most frequently on the lingual side of the ramus or on the inferior mandibular border below the molars (Fig. 20-37). Other locations include the condylar and coronoid regions. The mandibular lesion may be exophytic, extending outward into adjacent soft tissue spaces that can be observed on panoramic, periapical, or extraoral radiographs. The lesions also occur in the paranasal sinuses, especially the frontal sinus.

Periphery. Osteomas have well-defined borders.

Internal structure. Osteomas composed solely of compact bone are uniformly radiopaque; those containing cancellous bone show evidence of internal trabecular structure.

Effects on surrounding structures. Large lesions can displace adjacent soft tissues, such as muscles, and cause dysfunction.

Additional imaging. CT scans of osteomas reveal the three-dimensional topography of the lesions. Figure 20-38 shows osteomas that are affixed to the lingual side of the mandibular ramus and the lateral side of the condylar neck.

Differential diagnosis. The clinical appearance and location of a characteristic bony enlargement of anticipated size and shape, coupled with the radiographic image of a dense radiopaque mass, indicates an osteoma. However, a mature ossifying fibroma, early (small) osteogenic sarcoma, or small chondrosarcoma occasion-

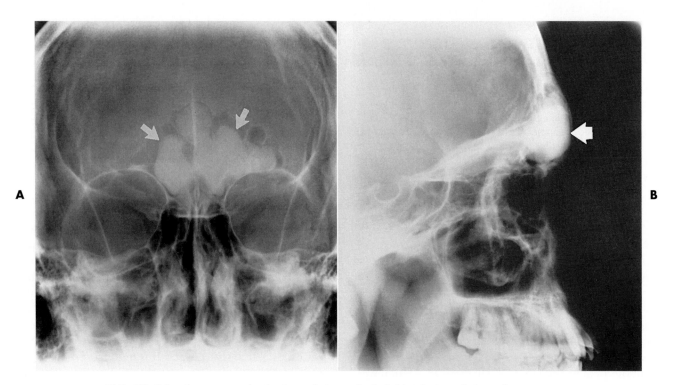

FIG. **20-36** *An osteoma in the frontal sinus.* **A,** A Caldwell view shows a large, amorphous mass in the frontal sinus *(arrows).* **B,** A lateral view shows an osteoma occupying most of the space in the sinus *(arrow).* (Courtesy G. Himadi, DDS, Chapel Hill, N.C.)

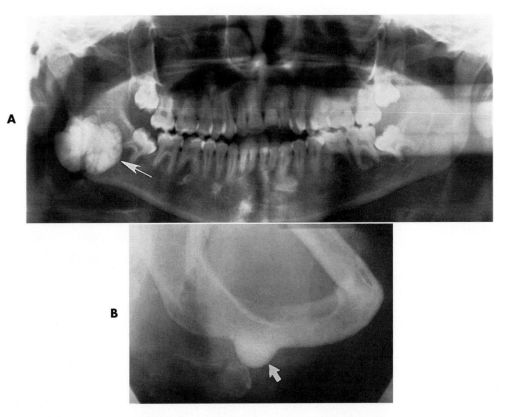

FIG. **20-37** *An osteoma.* **A,** A panoramic radiograph shows an osteoma in the right mandibular angle region *(arrow).* **B,** An oblique lateral jaw radiograph shows a solid radiopaque osteoma attached to the inferior border of the mandible *(arrow).* (**A** from Matteson SR et al: *Semin Adv Oral Radiol Dent Radiol Photogr* 57(1-4):1, 1985.)

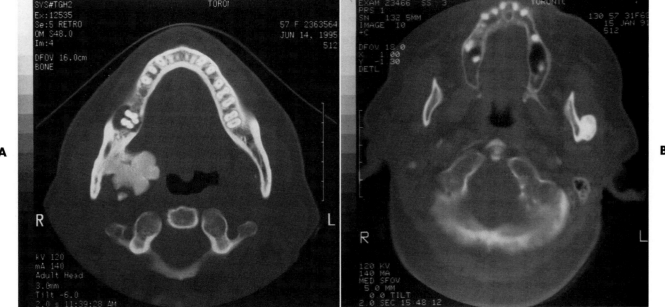

FIG. **20-38** *CT scans of osteomas.* **A,** An osteoma on the lingual side of the mandibular ramus. **B,** An osteoma on the lateral side of the mandibular ramus. (Courtesy M. Pharoah, DDS, Toronto, Canada.)

ally may resemble an osteoma. In the condylar region the differential diagnosis includes an osteochondroma, condylar hyperplasia, or an osteophyte.

Treatment. Resection of osteomas generally is successful. The surrounding capsule clearly delineates the periphery of the lesion surgically, and therefore its removal usually is unremarkable. Recurrence is rare. Treatment of these lesions may be postponed unless they are causing some undesirable phonetic effect or interfere with the construction or function of a prosthetic device. Ex-

ternal osteomas of the mandible may require removal for cosmetic reasons.

Gardner's Syndrome

Gardner's syndrome is a hereditary condition characterized by multiple osteomas, cutaneous sebaceous cysts, subcutaneous fibromas, and multiple polyps of the small and large intestine. The associated osteomas appear during the second decade. They are most common in the frontal bone, mandible, maxilla, and sphenoid bones. A significant feature of Gardner's syndrome is the predilection of

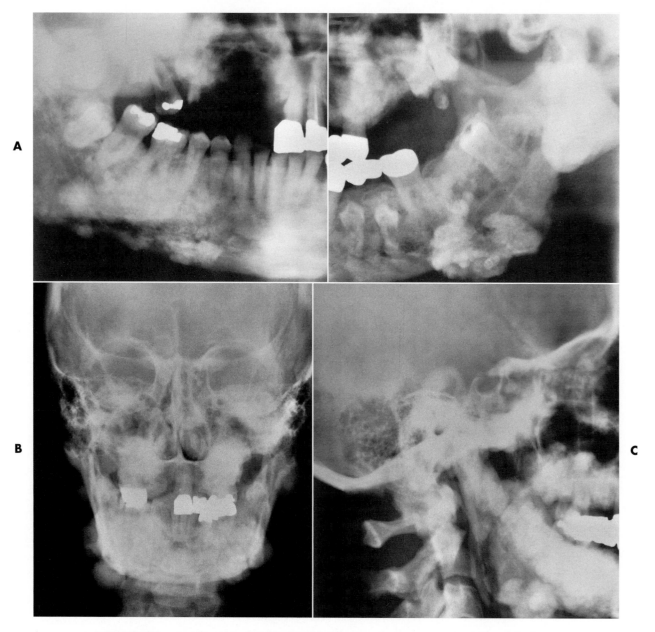

FIG. **20-39** *An osteoma with Gardner's syndrome.* **A,** A panoramic radiograph shows several osteomas and enostoses throughout both jaws. Note the impacted mandibular left second premolars. **B,** A posteroanterior radiograph shows numerous osteomas. **C,** A lateral cephalometric radiograph of the same patient.

the intestinal polyps to undergo malignant conversion, making early detection of the syndrome important. Because the osteomas often develop before the intestinal polyps, early recognition of the syndrome may be a life-saving event. Multiple unerupted supernumerary and permanent teeth in both jaws also occur with Gardner's syndrome (Fig. 20-39). Multiple osteomas also may occur on the mandible (Fig. 20-40) and in the frontal and maxillary sinuses as isolated findings in the absence of the diseases associated with Gardner's syndrome.

Nuclear medicine bone scanning is used to demonstrate the physiologic activity of the skeletal osteomas in Gardner's syndrome and to assess for thyroid carcinoma and skeletal metastasis when colon carcinoma is present (Fig. 20-41). CT also is reported to be useful for examining maxillary osteomas and displaying internal wavy cortical thickening in the mandible.

Treatment. The removal of osteomas is not generally necessary unless the tumors are symptomatic. However, if one of these bony growths is causing masticatory trauma or an intraosseous osteoma is close to the surface in an intended denture-bearing area, surgical removal should be undertaken. The important concern is to refer any patient suspected of having Gardner's syndrome for proctosigmoidoscopy to check for intestinal polyposis. Osteomas of the sinus walls carry a low but dangerous potential for intracranial complications.

Central Hemangioma

Definition. A hemangioma is a congenital anomaly in which proliferation of blood vessels leads to a mass that resembles a neoplasm. Hemangiomas can occur anywhere in the body but are most frequently noticed in the skin and subcutaneous tissues. The central type most often is found in the vertebrae and skull. It rarely develops in the jaws. Fewer than 50 mandibular heman-

giomas and an even smaller number of maxillary lesions have been reported. The lesions may be developmental or traumatic in origin.

Clinical features. Hemangiomas are more prevalent in females than males, the ratio being 2:1. Although they occur in individuals of all ages, at least 50% form before and during the teen years. Enlargement is slow, producing a nontender expansion of the jaw that occurs over several months or years. The swelling may or may not be painful, is not tender, and usually is bony hard. Pain, if present, probably is the throbbing type. Some tumors may be compressible or pulsate, and a bruit may be detected on auscultation. Anesthesia of the skin supplied by the mental nerve may occur. The lesion may cause loosening and migration of teeth in the affected area. Bleeding may occur from the gingiva around the neck of the affected teeth. These teeth may demonstrate rebound mobility; that is, when depressed into their sockets, they rebound to their original position within several minutes because of the pressure of the vascular network below the tooth. Aspiration produces arterial blood that may be under pressure and detected through the syringe plunger.

Radiographic features. A hemangioma of bone appears radiographically as an osteolytic defect that may take many forms, especially in the mandible.

Location. Hemangiomas affect the mandible about twice as often as the maxilla. Those that occur in the mandible form predominantly in the body and ramus. In the mandible they often are located within the inferior alveolar canal.

Periphery. In some instances the periphery is well defined and corticated, and in other cases it may be ill defined, as is seen with malignant tumors. This variation probably is related to the amount of residual bone present.

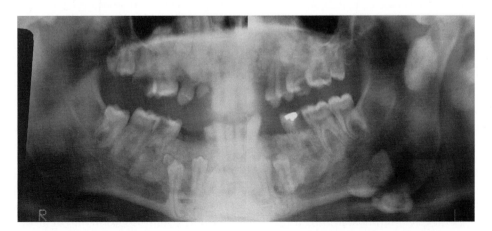

FIG. **20-40** *An osteoma with Gardner's syndrome.* A posterior portion of a panoramic radiograph of this patient shows multiple osteomas in the mandible. Note the impacted mandibular premolars.

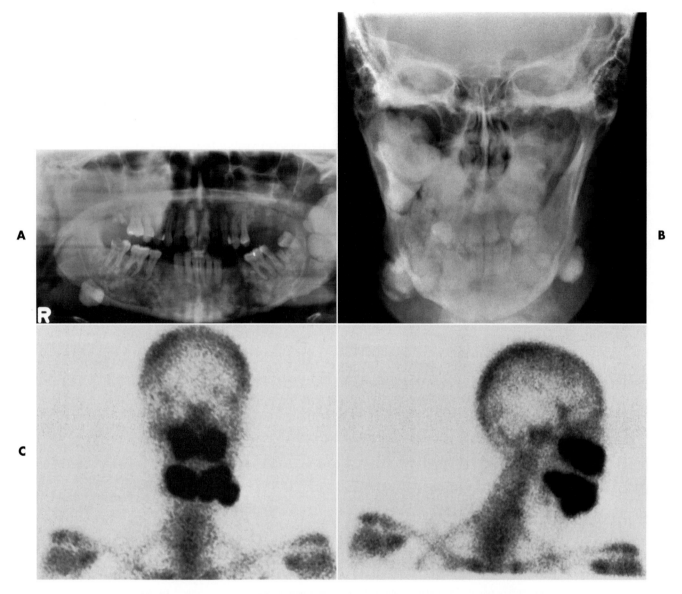

FIG. **20-41**   *An osteoma with Gardner's syndrome.* **A,** A panoramic radiograph shows a large osteoma in the left mandibular ramus and a smaller one in the posterior area of the right mandibular body. Several small internal osteomas can be seen throughout the mandible and maxilla. **B,** Posteroanterior radiograph shows several osteomas. **C,** An anterior bone nuclear scan *(left)* and lateral scan *(right)* show areas of increased accumulation of radiopharmaceutical in both jaws, caused by the increased metabolic activity and bone mass in the osteomas. (Courtesy R. Blumhardt, MD, San Antonio, Tex.)

Internal structure. The locules formed in the maxilla by a central hemangioma resemble enlarged trabecular spaces, and the trabeculae are coarse, dense, and well defined (Fig. 20-42). The radiolucencies most often observed are multicystic and often have a soap bubble or honeycomb appearance that results from a fine trabeculation within the locules. A multilocular appearance may also result from the serpiginous deformity of the inferior alveolar canal. The corticated, cystlike spaces may

be visible because the vessel is oriented in the direction of the x-ray beam. Other lesions may present linear trabeculations or may be radiolucent (Fig. 20-43). In addition, a projection that demonstrates the expanding lesion in profile may show a sunray or sunburst image. Phleboliths (small areas of calcification or concretions found in a vein) occasionally occur within surrounding soft tissues (Fig. 20-44) and are caused by slowing of peripheral blood flow. They develop from thrombi that be-

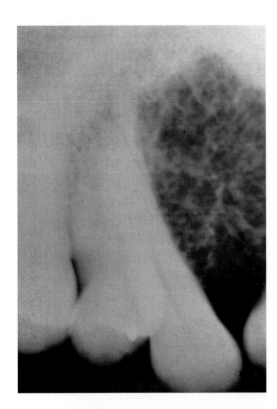

FIG. **20-42** A hemangioma in the anterior maxilla shows a coarse trabecular pattern. (Courtesy E.J. Burkes, DDS, Chapel Hill, N.C.)

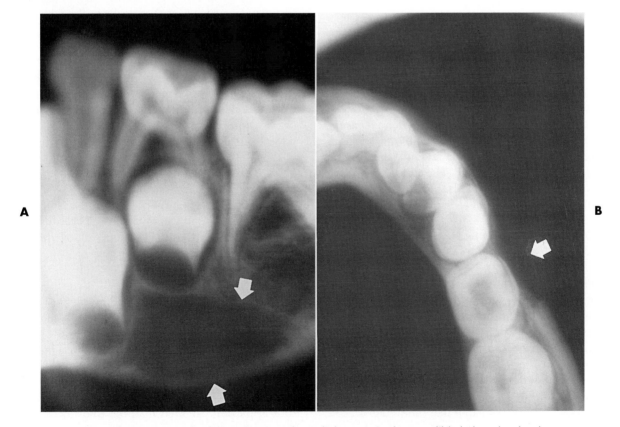

A

B

FIG. **20-43** *A vascular lesion.* **A,** Note the radiolucency in the mandible below the developing first premolars *(arrows).* **B,** An occlusal radiograph shows expansion of the mandible with loss of the buccal cortical border *(arrow).* (Courtesy R. White, DDS, Chapel Hill, N.C.)

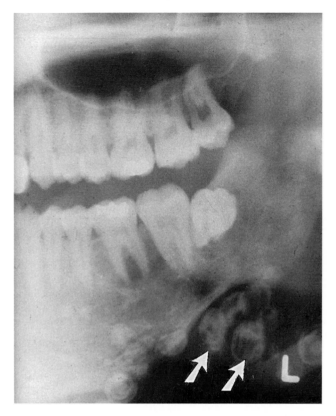

FIG. **20-44**   A soft tissue hemangioma with phleboliths *(arrows).*

come organized and mineralized and consist of calcium phosphate and calcium carbonate.

Effects on surrounding structures. The roots of teeth in the invaded area often are resorbed. When the lesion involves the inferior alveolar nerve canal, the canal can be enlarged along its entire length and its shape may be changed to a serpiginous path. The mandibular and mental foramen may be enlarged. Hemangiomas can influence the growth of bone and teeth. The involved bone may be enlarged and have coarse, internal trabeculae. Also, developing teeth may be larger and erupt earlier when in an intimate relationship with a hemangioma.

Differential diagnosis. The dentist must regard any multilocular, radiolucent lesion in the jaws as a potentially dangerous lesion and must try to eliminate the possibility of a central hemangioma. Aspiration of the lesion can determine whether the radiolucency in question is a vascular tumor. If it is not, multilocular lesions in general should be in the differential diagnosis. Coarsely multilocular regions of rarefaction that accompany cortex expansion to the thickness of paper may mimic a giant cell tumor of the jaws. However, some investigators believe that the loculations produced by a hemangioma are smaller and are interspersed with a fine fibrillar net-

work. It is important to examine carefully the relationship of the lesions to the inferior alveolar canal to help with the differential diagnosis. In most cases, soft tissue signs suggest a vascular lesion. Traumatic bone cysts and keratocysts generally are more radiolucent and have better-defined borders.

Treatment. Central hemangiomas should be treated without delay because trauma that disrupts the integrity of the affected jaw may result in lethal exsanguination. Specifically, embolization (introduction of inert materials into the lesion by a vascular route), surgery (en bloc resection with ligation of the external carotid artery), and sclerosing techniques have been used singly or together.

Arteriovenous Fistula

Synonyms. *A-V defect, A-V shunt, A-V aneurysm,* and *A-V malformation*

Definition. An arteriovenous (A-V) fistula, an uncommon lesion, is a direct communication between an artery and a vein that bypasses the intervening capillary bed. It usually results from trauma but in rare instances may be a developmental anomaly. An arteriovenous shunt can occur anywhere in the body, in soft tissue, in the alveolar process, and centrally in the jaw. The head and neck are the most common sites.

Clinical features. The clinical appearance of a central arteriovenous shunt can vary considerably, depending on the extent of bone or soft tissue involvement. The lesion may expand bone, and a mass may be present in the extraosseous soft tissue. The soft tissue swelling may have a purple discoloration. Palpation or auscultation of the swelling may reveal a pulse. On the other hand, neither the bone nor the soft tissue may be expanded, and no pulse may be clinically apparent. Aspiration produces blood. Recognition of the hemorrhagic nature of these lesions is of utmost importance because extraction of an associated tooth may be immediately followed by life-threatening bleeding.

Radiographic features
Location. These lesions most commonly develop in the ramus and retromolar area of the mandible and involve the mandibular canal.

Periphery. The margins usually are well defined and corticated.

Internal structure. The central lesions may be multilocular. The wall of the shunt may contain radiographically apparent, calcified material that may suggest the nature of the lesion.

Effects on surrounding structures. Both central lesions and those in the soft tissue that erode bony surfaces

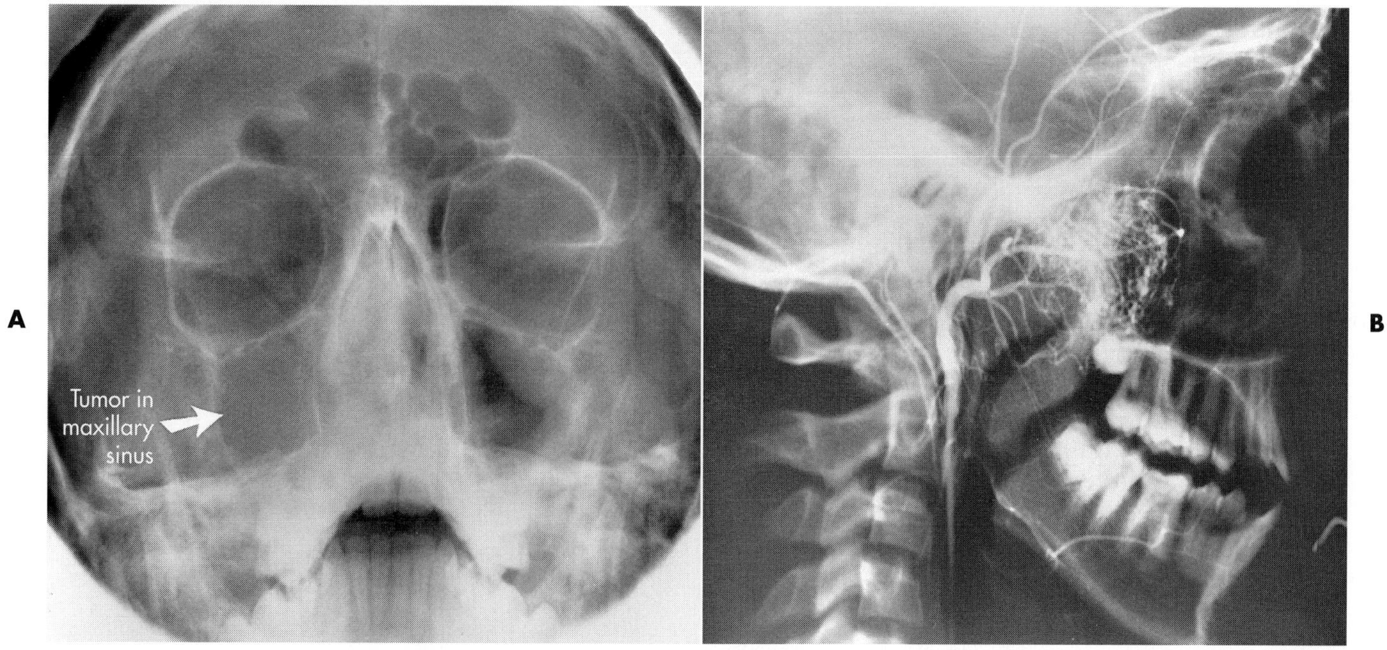

FIG. **20-45** *A vascular lesion in the right maxillary sinus.* **A,** A Waters' radiograph shows the opacified maxillary antrum *(arrow).* **B,** Note the tumor vascularization in this angiogram. A radiopaque dye has been injected into the vasculature to enhance visualization. (Courtesy G. Himadi, DDS, Chapel Hill, N.C.)

cause well-defined (cystlike), resorptive lesions in the bone. Changes in the inferior alveolar canal may occur, as described in the preceding section on hemangiomas.

Additional imaging. CT with contrast injection is a useful method for aiding the differential diagnosis of any vascular lesion and other neoplasms of the jaws. Angiography, a radiographic procedure performed by injecting radiopaque dye into vessels and making radiographs, is useful for demonstrating the size and extent of a vascular tumor of the jaw. It displays an abnormal collection of vessels in the suspected area, with many vessels feeding and draining the lesion (Fig. 20-45). Angiography demonstrates the nature of the vascular derangement, its relationship to the bony defect, and associated abnormal arterial and venous vasculature (Fig. 20-46).

Differential diagnosis. Occasionally the radiographic appearance is not specific for the A-V fistula. The differential diagnosis should include the multilocular lesions that occur, with hemangiomas and ameloblastomas assigned a relatively high priority. In addition, radicular and dentigerous cysts should be considered. As with hemangiomas, the relationship of the lesion to the inferior alveolar canal is examined. The soft tissue hemangioma usually does not involve bone, which may help to distinguish it.

Treatment. An A-V fistula is treated surgically.

Osteoblastoma
Synonym. *Giant osteoid osteoma*

Definition. An osteoblastoma is an uncommon, benign tumor of osteoblasts with areas of osteoid and calcific tissue. This tumor occurs most often in the spine of a young person. Agreement apparently is increasing that if osteoblastomas and osteoid osteomas are different lesions, they differ only in size and minor morphologic and histologic features. For example, the osteoid trabeculae in an osteoblastoma generally are larger (broader and longer, with wider trabecular spaces than those in an osteoid osteoma). An osteoblastoma also is usually more vascular and less painful, and it has more osteoclasts. In addition, benign osteoblastomas are considered more aggressive lesions. On the level of their ultrastructures, the two lesions essentially are similar or at least closely related.

Clinical features. Both osteoblastomas and osteoid osteomas are rare in the jaws. The male-to-female ratio is 2:1, and the average age of occurrence is 17 years, with most lesions occurring in the second and third decades of life. Clinically, patients often report pain and swelling of the affected region.

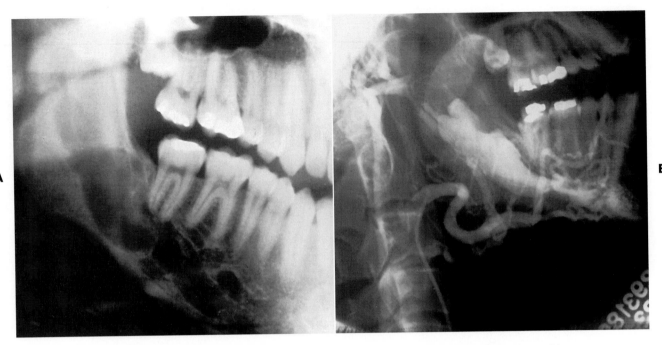

FIG. **20-46** *An arteriovenous malformation in the right posterior mandible.* **A,** In this segment from a panoramic radiograph, note the multilocular radiolucency along the course of the mandibular neurovascular canal. **B,** An external carotid angiogram. A radiopaque dye is distributed throughout the lesion. (From Kelly DE et al: *J Oral Surg* 35:387, 1977.)

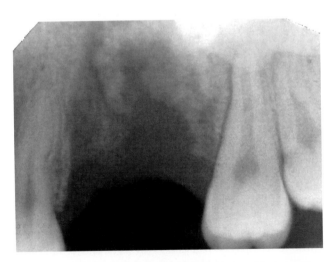

FIG. **20-47** An osteoblastoma in a 21-year-old man with a history of pain for 3 months. Note the evidence of bone formation and the diffuse margins of the lesion. (Courtesy B. Gratt, DDS, Los Angeles, Calif.)

Radiographic features. The radiographic appearance of an osteoblastoma can vary considerably.

Location. Osteoblatomas are found both in the tooth-bearing regions and around the temporomandibular joint (within the condyle or the temporal bone).

Periphery. The borders may be diffuse or may show some sign of a cortex. Mandibular lesions have been reported that contain a radiolucent halo within the outer cortical boundary.

Internal structure. The tumor may be entirely radiolucent (Fig. 20-47) or may show varying degrees of calcification. The internal calcification may take the form of a sunray pattern or fine granular bone trabeculae.

Effects on surrounding structures. Osteoblastomas may expand bone, but usually a thin outer cortex is maintained. This lesion may invaginate the maxillary sinus or the middle cranial fossa.

Differential diagnosis. If the radiographic appearance of an osteoblastoma is lucent with ill-defined borders, infection or malignancy may be present. Osteoid osteomas can be differentiated from benign osteoblastomas by their sclerotic borders. The sclerotic border is given more weight than the size of the lesion because a sclerotic lesion indicates osteoid osteoma, even if it is larger than 1 cm. Symptoms are not a specific aid for diagnosis. The benign radiographic appearance can help with the differentiation of an osteogenic sarcoma, which at times may have a similar histologic appearance.

Treatment. Osteoblastomas are treated with curettage or local excision, which relieves the pain. Recurrences have been described, and a few are suspected of becoming sarcomas or at least of being initially unrecognized low-grade osteosarcomas.

Osteoid Osteoma

Definition. An osteoid osteoma is a benign tumor that is rare in the jaws. Its true nature is not known, but some investigators think it is a variant of osteoblastoma. The tumor has an oval or round, tumorlike core usually only about 1 cm in diameter, although some may reach 5 or 6 cm. This core consists of osteoid and newly formed trabeculae within highly vascularized, osteogenic connective tissue. The tumor may develop within the cancellous bone or near or within the cortex; it is usually intracortical. In the spongiosa, a thin rim of sclerotic bone develops around the core, but when the lesion is intracortical, the cortex becomes dense, thickened, and hard for a considerable distance beyond the core.

Clinical features. Osteoid osteomas occur most often in young people, usually males between the ages of 10 and 25 years. They seldom occur before 4 years or after 40 years. This condition affects at least twice as many males as females. Most of the lesions occur in the femur and tibia; the jaws are rarely involved. Severe pain in the bone that can be relieved by antiinflammatory drugs is characteristic. In addition, the soft tissue over the involved bony area may be swollen and tender.

Radiographic features

Location. The lesion is most common in the cortex of the limb bones. In those that do occur in the jaws, somewhat more develop in the body of the mandible.

Periphery. The margins are well defined by a rim of sclerotic bone (Fig. 20-48).

Internal structure. The internal aspect is composed of a small ovoid or round radiolucent area (core). The central radiolucency may have some radiopaque foci.

Effects on surrounding structures. In an occlusal projection, the overlying cortex is thickened by new bone being formed subperiosteally (see Fig. 20-48).

Differential diagnosis. Osteoid osteomas are rare in the jaws. A clinician who suspects that a sclerotic lesion is an osteoid osteoma should also consider sclerosing osteitis, ossifying fibroma, monostatic fibrous dysplasia, benign cementoblastoma, and periapical cemental dysplasia. The presence of a central radiolucency usually eliminates enostosis or osteosclerosis. If a diagnosis cannot be made with confidence at this point, further effort should be made to rule out other rare entities that may share features with osteoid osteoma, including osteogenic sarcoma, chondroblastoma, ameloblastoma, cementifying fibroma, and benign osteoblastoma. The

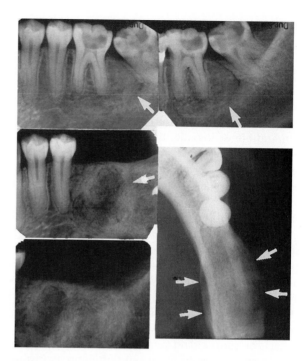

FIG. **20-48** An osteoid osteoma *(arrow)* appears as a mixed radiolucent-radiopaque lesion in the molar region; the lesion has caused expansion of the buccal and lingual cortex of the mandible *(arrows)*. (Courtesy A. Shawkat, DDS, Radcliff, Ky.)

presence of tooth images superimposed over the lesion and the possibility of associated idiopathic osteosclerosis can complicate the interpretation of radiographs of cases that develop in the jaws, compared with the images seen in other bones.

Treatment. Complete excision currently is the recommended treatment because it often relieves the pain and cures the disease. Although spontaneous remission can occur in some cases, the data are insufficient for identifying such cases in advance.

Desmoplastic Fibroma of Bone

Synonym. *Aggressive fibromatosis* (usually reserved for tumors that originate in soft tissue)

Definition. A desmoplastic fibroma of bone is an aggressive, infiltrative neoplasm that produces abundant collagen fibers. It is poorly cellular and has fibroblast-like cells that have ovoid or elongated nuclei. The lack of pleomorphism of the cells is important.

Clinical features. Patients usually complain of facial swelling, pain (in rare cases), and sometimes dysfunction, especially when the neoplasm is close to the joint. The lesion occurs most often in the first two decades of life, with a mean reported age of 14 years. Although it originates in bone, the tumor may invade the surrounding soft tissue extensively. It also may occur as part of Gardner's syndrome.

Radiographic features

Location. Desmoplastic fibromas of bone may occur in the mandible or maxilla; but the most common site is the ramus and posterior mandible.

Periphery. The periphery most often is ill defined and has an invasive characteristic commonly seen in malignant tumors.

Internal structure. The internal aspect may be totally radiolucent, especially when the lesion is small. Larger lesions appear to be multilocular with very coarse, thick septa. These septa may be straight or may have an irregular shape. In T1-weighted MRI scans the internal structure has a low signal, which helps in determining intraosseous extent because of the contrast with the high signal from the bone marrow.

Effects on surrounding structures. Desmoplastic fibromas of bone can expand bone and often break through the outer cortex, invading the surrounding soft tissue. Usually CT or MRI is required to determine the exact soft tissue extent of the lesion.

Differential diagnosis. Distinguishing this neoplasm from a fibrosarcoma may be difficult during the histologic examination. The radiographic appearance may not be helpful because a desmoplastic fibroma often has the appearance of a malignant neoplasm. However, the presence of coarse, irregular, and sometimes straight septa may help support the correct diagnosis. The appearance of these septa also helps differentiate the lesion from other multilocular tumors. Very small lesions may resemble simple bone cysts.

Treatment. Resection of this neoplasm with adequate margins is recommended because of its high recurrence rate. Patients who have been treated for the condition should be followed closely with frequent radiologic examinations.

BIBLIOGRAPHY

Daley TD et al: Relative incidence of odontogenic tumors and oral and jaw cysts in a Canadian population, *Oral Surg Oral Med Oral Pathol* 77:276, 1994.

Gorlin RJ et al: Odontogenic tumors: clinical behavior in man and domesticated animals, *Cancer* 14:73, 1961.

Hoffman S et al: *Intraosseous and parosteal tumors of the jaws, atlas of tumor pathology,* series 2, fascicle 24, Washington, DC, 1987, Armed Forces Institute of Pathology.

Krishnan Unni K: *Dahlin's bone tumors: general aspects and data on 11,087 cases,* ed 5, Philadelphia, 1996, Lippincott-Raven.

Pindborg J, Kramer IRA: *Histological typing of odontogenic tumours, jaw cysts, and allied lesions, International Histological Classification of Tumors,* no 5, Geneva, 1971, World Health Organization.

Regezi JA et al: Odontogenic tumors: an analysis of 706 cases, *J Oral Surg* 36:771, 1978.

SUGGESTED READINGS

TORUS PALATINUS

Eggan S et al: Variation in torus palatinus prevalence in Norway, *Scand J Dent Res* 102:54, 1994.

Gorsky M et al: Prevalence of torus palatinus in a population of young and old Israelis, *Arch Oral Biol* 41:623, 1996.

Haugen LK: Palatine and mandibular tori; a morphologic study in the current Norwegian population, *Acta Odontol Scand* 50:65, 1992.

TORUS MANDIBULARIS

Eggen S, Natvig B: Concurrence of torus mandibularis and torus palatinus, *Scand J Dent Res* 102:60, 1994.

ENOSTOSIS

McDonnel D: Dense bone island: a review of 107 patients, *Oral Surg Oral Med Oral Pathol* 76:124, 1993.

Petrikowski GC, Peters E: Longitudinal radiographic assessment of dense bone islands of the jaws, *Oral Surg Oral Med Oral Pathol Oral Radiol Endod* 83:627, 1997.

AMELOBLASTOMA

Atkinson CH et al: Ameloblastoma of the jaw: a reappraisal of the role of megavoltage irradiation, *Cancer* 53:869, 1984.

Heffez L et al: The role of magnetic resonance imaging in the diagnosis and management of ameloblastoma, *Oral Surg Oral Med Oral Pathol* 65:212, 1988.

Ueta E et al: Intraosseous carcinoma arising from mandibular ameloblastoma with progressive invasion and pulmonary metastasis, *Int J Oral Maxillofac Surg* 25:370, 1996.

Weissman JL et al: Ameloblastoma of the maxilla: CT and MR appearance, *Am J Neuroradiol* 14:223, 1993.

ADENOMATOID ODONTOGENIC TUMOR

Dare A et al: Limitation of panoramic radiography in diagnosing adenomatoid odontogenic tumors, *Oral Surg Oral Med Oral Pathol* 77:662, 1994.

Giansanti JS et al: Odontogenic adenomatoid tumor (adenoameloblastoma), *Oral Surg Oral Med Oral Pathol* 30:69, 1969.

Hicks MJ et al: Pathology consultation: adenomatoid and calcifying epithelial odontogenic tumors, *Ann Otol Rhinol Laryngol* 102:159, 1993.

Philipsen HP et al: Adenomatoid odontogenic tumor: biologic profile based on 499 cases, *J Oral Pathol Med* 20:149, 1991.

Stafne EC: Epithelial tumors associated with developmental cysts of the maxilla, *Oral Surg* 1:887, 1948.

Vitkus R, Meltzer JA: Repair of defect following the removal of a maxillary adenomatoid odontogenic tumor using guided tissue regeneration: a case report, *J Periodontol* 67:46, 1996.

CALCIFYING EPITHELIAL ODONTOGENIC TUMOR

Franklin CD, Pindborg JJ: The calcifying epithelial odontogenic tumor: a review and analysis of 113 cases, *Oral Surg Oral Med Oral Pathol* 42:753, 1976.

Pindborg JJ: The calcifying epithelial odontogenic tumor: review of literature and report of extraosseous case, *Acta Odontol Scand* 24:419, 1966.

Vap OR et al: Pindborg tumor: the so-called calcifying epithelial odontogenic tumor, *Cancer* 25:629, 1970.

COMPOUND ODONTOMA

Haishima K et al: Compound odontomes associated with impacted maxillary primary central incisors: report of 2 cases, *Int J Pediatr Dent* 4:251, 1994.

Kaugars GE et al: Odontomas, *Oral Surg Oral Med Oral Pathol* 67:172, 1989.

Nik-Hussein NN, Majid ZA: Erupted compound odontoma, *Ann Dent* 52:8, 1993.

AMELOBLASTIC FIBROMA

Dallera P et al: Ameloblastic fibroma: a follow-up of six cases, *Int J Oral Maxillofac Surg* 25:199, 1996.

Trodahl JN: Ameloblastic fibroma: a survey of cases from the Armed Forces Institute of Pathology, *Oral Surg Oral Med Oral Pathol* 33:547, 1972.

ODONTOGENIC MYXOMA

Cohen MA, Mendelsohn DB: CT and MR imaging of myxofibroma of the jaws, *J Comput Assist Tomogr* 14:281, 1990.

Peltola J et al: Odontogenic myxoma: a radiographic study of 21 tumours, *Br J Oral Maxillofac Surg* 32:298, 1994.

Zachariades N, Papanicolaou S: Treatment of odontogenic myxoma, *Ann Dent* 6:34, 1987.

BENIGN CEMENTOBLASTOMA

Berwick JE et al: Benign cementoblastoma, *J Oral Maxillofac Surg* 48:208, 1990.

Jelic JS et al: Benign cementoblastoma: report of an unusual case and analysis of 14 additional cases, *J Oral Maxillofac Surg* 51:1037, 1993.

Ruprecht A, Ross AS: Benign cementoblastoma (true cementoblastoma), *Dentomaxillofac Radiol* 12:31, 1983.

Ulmansky M et al: Benign cementoblastoma: a review and five new cases, *Oral Surg Oral Med Oral Pathol* 77:48, 1994.

CENTRAL ODONTOGENIC FIBROMA

Gardner DG: Central odontogenic fibroma: current concepts, *J Oral Pathol Med* 25:556, 1996.

Handlers JP et al: Central odontogenic fibroma: clinicopathologic features of 19 cases and review of the literature, *J Oral Maxillofac Surg* 49:46, 1991.

Kaffe I, Buchner A: Radiologic features of central odontogenic fibroma, *Oral Surg Oral Med Oral Pathol* 78:811, 1994.

HEMANGIOMA

Lund BA, Dahlin DC: Hemangiomas of the mandible and maxilla, *J Oral Surg* 22:234, 1964.

OSTEOMA

Earwaker J: Paranasal osteomas: a review of 46 cases, *Skeletal Radiol* 22:417, 1993.

Matteson S et al: Advanced imaging methods, *Crit Rev Oral Biol Med* 7:346, 1996.

Thakker NS et al: Florid oral manifestations in an atypical familial adenomatous polyposis family with late presentation of colorectal polyps, *J Oral Pathol Med* 25:459, 1996.

Williams SC et al: Gardner's syndrome: case report and discussion of the manifestations of the disorder, *Clin Nucl Med* 19:668, 1994.

NEUROFIBROMATOSIS

D'Ambrosia JA et al: Jaw and skull changes in neurofibromatosis, *Oral Surg Oral Med Oral Pathol* 66:391, 1988.

Lee L et al: Radiographic features of the mandible in neurofibromatosis: a report of 10 cases and review of the literature, *Oral Surg Oral Med Oral Pathol Oral Radiol Endod* 81:361, 1996.

Shapiro SD et al: Neurofibromatosis: oral and radiographic manifestations, *Oral Surg* 58:493, 1984.

OSTEOBLASTOMA

Brady CL, Bronne RM: Benign osteoblastoma of the mandible, *Cancer* 30:329, 1977.

Lucas DR et al: Osteoblastoma: clinicopathologic study of 306 cases, *Hum Pathol* 25:117, 1994.

DESMOPLASTIC FIBROMA OF BONE

Gebhardt MC et al: Desmoplastic fibroma of bone: a report of eight cases and review of the literature, *J Bone Joint Surg Am* 67A:732, 1985.

Hopkins KM et al: Desmoplastic fibroma of the mandible: review and report of two cases, *J Oral Maxillofac Surg* 54:1249, 1996.

Zachariades N, Papanicolaou S: Juvenile fibromatosis, *J Craniomaxillofac Surg* 16:130, 1987.

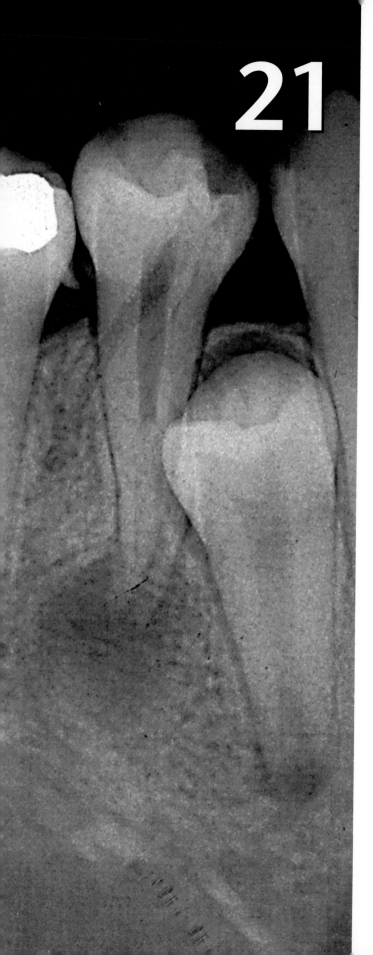

21 Malignant Diseases of the Jaws

ROBERT E. WOOD

Definition

Malignant tumors represent an uncontrolled growth of tissue. Unlike benign neoplasms, they are more locally invasive, have a greater degree of anaplasia, and have the ability to metastasize regionally to lymph nodes or distantly to other sites. Cancers may be caused by viruses, significant radiation exposure, genetic defects, and exposure to carcinogenic chemicals. For instance, using tobacco is strongly associated with oral carcinoma. Malignant tumors that arise de novo are termed *primary tumors,* and those that originate from distant primary tumors are termed *secondary* or *metastatic malignancy.*

The most convenient method of classification of cancers is based on histopathology. In the following text the malignancies that commonly affect the jaws have been divided into one of four categories: carcinomas (lesions of epithelial origin), metastatic lesions from distant sites, sarcomas (lesions of mesenchymal origin), and malignancies of the hematopoietic system. Unusual malignant tumors have been omitted to concentrate on more common lesions that a general practitioner may encounter.

Clinical Features

The following are clinical signs and symptoms that suggest that a lesion may be malignant: swelling, displaced teeth, loosened teeth over a short duration, foul smell, ulceration, presence of an indurated or rolled border, exposure of underlying bone, sensory or motor neural deficits, lymphadenopathy, weight loss, dysgeusia, dysphagia, dysphonia, hemorrhage, lack of normal healing, or pain with no demonstrable dental cause. Most oral cancers occur in men aged 50 years and older; however, malignant tumors may occur at any age in either gender.

Dentists must vigilantly watch for the possibility of malignancy in their patients. Because the prevalence of oral malignancy is low, many general practitioners practice for years without encountering a patient who has a malignant tumor. This rarity may make a dentist less likely to recognize a malignant condition when it does exist. The risks of lack of attention to this possibility are delayed diagnosis, delayed treatment, increased need for aggressive treatment with added morbidity, and, in the worst case, premature death.

Radiographic Examination

Radiology has a number of important roles in the management of the patient with cancer. First, diagnostic images may aid in the establishment of an initial diagnosis of a tumor. Diagnostic imaging also aids in the appropriate staging of disease from early small cancers to large cancers that have spread. Appropriate radiologic investigations assist the surgeon or radiation oncologist to determine the appropriate dimensions of the tumor so that it can be excised or irradiated adequately. Radiologic investigation has the potential to determine the presence of osseous involvement from soft tissue tumors and allow the practitioner to assess the presence of nodal disease and the outcome of treatment. Finally, a thorough radiographic dental examination plays a part in the management of the cancer survivor, who often is rendered xerostomic and susceptible to both dental caries and periodontal disease.

RADIOGRAPHIC FEATURES

The following features may suggest the presence of a malignant tumor. The absence of visible radiologic signs as described does not preclude malignancy. It only implies that no visible radiographic signs exist.

Location

Primary and metastatic malignant tumors may occur anywhere in the oral and maxillofacial region. Primary carcinomas are more commonly seen in the tongue, floor of the mouth, tonsillar area, lip, soft palate, or gingiva and may invade the jaws from any of these sites. Sar-

comas are more common in the mandible and in posterior regions of both jaws. Metastatic tumors are most common in the posterior mandible and maxilla. Some metastatic lesions grow at the apex of teeth or in the follicles of developing teeth (Fig. 21-1, *D*).

Periphery and Shape

The typical appearance of the periphery of a malignant lesion is an ill-defined border with lack of cortication and absence of encapsulation (a soft tissue or radiolucent periphery). This infiltrative border has uneven extensions of bone destruction. Fingerlike extension of the tumor occurs in many directions; this extension is followed by osseous destruction producing a region of radiolucency (see Fig. 21-1, *A*). Evidence of osseous destruction with adjacent soft tissue mass is highly suggestive of malignancy (see Fig. 21-1, *B*). Such a mass may exhibit a smooth or ulcerated peripheral border if cast against a radiolucent background. The shape of a malignant tumor of the jaw is irregular.

Internal Structure

Because most malignancies do not produce bone nor do they stimulate the formation of reactive bone, the internal aspect is typically radiolucent in most instances. Occasionally residual islands of bone are present, resulting in a pattern of patchy destruction with some scattered residual internal osseous structure. Some tumors, such as prostate and breast metastatic lesions, can induce bone formation, resulting in an abnormal-appearing internal osseous architecture, whereas others, such as osteogenic sarcomas, can be productive in nature, causing frank sclerosis.

Effects on Surrounding Structures

Malignancy is destructive, often rapidly so. The effect on surrounding structures mirrors this behavior. Slower-growing benign tumors or cysts may resorb or displace teeth in a bodily fashion without causing loose teeth. In contrast, rapidly growing malignant lesions generally destroy supporting alveolar bone so that teeth may appear to be floating in space (see Fig. 21-1, *F*).

Occasionally root resorption is present, this being more common in sarcomas. Internal trabecular bone is destroyed, as are cortical boundaries such as the sinus floor, inferior border of the mandible, follicular cortices, and the cortex of the inferior alveolar neurovascular canal. Because malignant tumors tend to grow rapidly, they invade by means of the easiest routes such as through the maxillary antrum or through the periodontal ligament space around teeth, resulting in irregular widening with destruction of the lamina dura (see

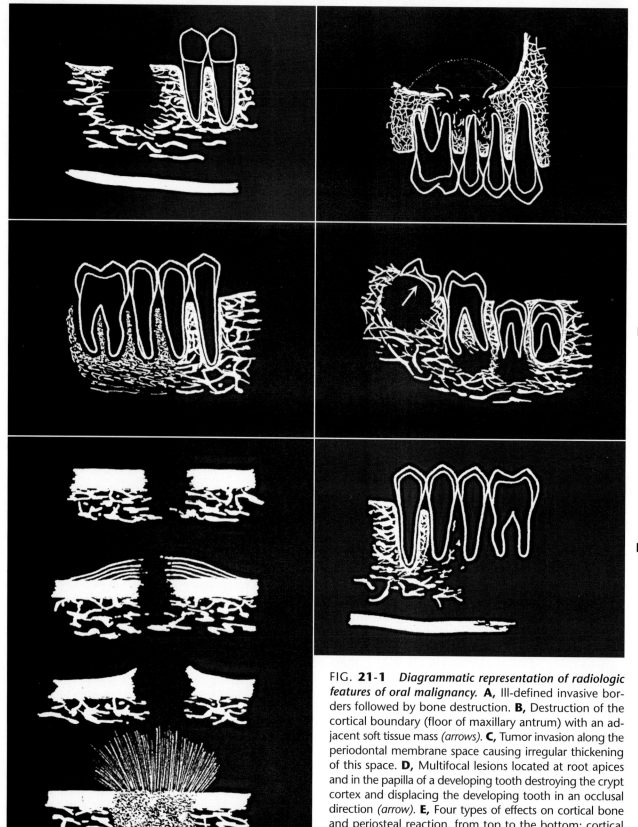

FIG. **21-1** *Diagrammatic representation of radiologic features of oral malignancy.* **A,** Ill-defined invasive borders followed by bone destruction. **B,** Destruction of the cortical boundary (floor of maxillary antrum) with an adjacent soft tissue mass *(arrows).* **C,** Tumor invasion along the periodontal membrane space causing irregular thickening of this space. **D,** Multifocal lesions located at root apices and in the papilla of a developing tooth destroying the crypt cortex and displacing the developing tooth in an occlusal direction *(arrow).* **E,** Four types of effects on cortical bone and periosteal reaction, from top to the bottom: cortical bone destruction without periosteal reaction, laminated periosteal reaction with destruction of the cortical bone and the new periosteal bone, destruction of cortical bone with periosteal reaction at the periphery forming Codman's triangles, and a spiculated or sunray type of periosteal reaction. **F,** Bone destruction around existing teeth, producing an appearance of teeth floating in space.

Fig. 21-1, *C*); they also may spread through the inferior alveolar neurovascular canal, causing similar widening. Where the tumor has destroyed the outer cortex of bone, usually no periosteal reaction occurs; however, some tumors stimulate unusual periosteal new bone formation (see Fig. 21-1, *E*). Lesions such as osteosarcoma and prostate metastatic lesions as well as other tumors can stimulate the formation of thin straight spicules of bone, giving a hair-on-end or sunburst appearance.

Carcinomas

SQUAMOUS CELL CARCINOMA ARISING IN SOFT TISSUE

Identifying Characteristics
Synonym. *Epidermoid carcinoma*

Definition. Squamous cell carcinoma, the most common oral malignancy, may be defined as a malignant tumor originating within the surface epithelium. It is characterized initially by invasion of malignant epithelial cells into the underlying connective tissue with subsequent spread into deeper soft tissues and occasionally into adjacent bone, local-regional lymph nodes, and ultimately to distant sites such as the lung, liver, and skeleton.

Clinical features. Squamous cell carcinoma appears initially as white or red (sometimes mixed) irregular patchy lesions of the affected epithelium. With time these lesions exhibit central ulceration; a rolled or indurated border, which represents invasion of malignant cells; and palpable infiltration into adjacent muscle or bone. Pain may be variable, and regional lymphadenopathy with hard lymph nodes that may or may not be tethered to underlying structures may be present. Other clinical features include a soft tissue mass, paresthesia, anesthesia, dysesthesia, pain, foul smell, trismus, grossly loosened teeth, or hemorrhage. Large lesions can obstruct the airway, the opening of the eustachian tube (leading to diminished hearing), or the nasopharynx. Patients often report a significant weight loss and feel unwell. Males are more commonly affected than females. The condition is often fatal, if untreated. Most squamous cell carcinomas occur in persons older than 50 years.

Radiographic features
Location. Squamous cell carcinoma commonly involves the lateral border of the tongue. Therefore a common site to observe bone invasion is the posterior mandible. Lesions of the lip and floor of the mouth may invade the anterior mandible. Lesions involving attached gingiva and underlying alveolar bone may mimic inflammatory disease such as periodontal disease. This condition is also seen on the tonsils, soft palate, and buccal vestibule. It is uncommon on the hard palate.

Periphery and shape. Squamous cell carcinoma may erode into underlying bone from any direction, producing a radiolucency that is polymorphous and irregular in outline. Invasion occurs in one half of cases and is characterized most commonly by an ill-defined, noncorticated border (Fig. 21-2). Rarely the border may appear smooth without a cortex, indicating underlying erosion rather than invasion. If bone involvement is extensive, the periphery appears to have fingerlike extensions preceding a zone of impressive osseous destruction. If pathologic fracture occurs, the borders show sharpened thinned bone ends with displacement of segments and an adjacent soft tissue mass. Surface carcinomas are capable of producing sclerosis in underlying osseous structures without frank invasion.

Internal structure. The internal structure of squamous cell carcinoma in jaw lesions is totally radiolucent; the original osseous structure can be completely lost. Occasionally small islands of residual normal trabecular bone are visible within this central radiolucency.

Effects on surrounding structures. Evidence of invasion of bone around teeth may first appear as widening of the periodontal ligament space with loss of adjacent lamina dura. Teeth may appear to float in a mass of radiolucent soft tissue bereft of any bony support. In extensive tumors this soft tissue mass may grow with the teeth in it as "passengers," so teeth appear to be grossly displaced from their normal position. Tumors may grow along the inferior neurovascular canal and through the mental foramen, resulting in an increase in the width and eventually the loss of the cortical boundary. Destruction of adjacent normal cortical boundaries such as the floor of the nose, maxillary sinus, or buccal or lingual mandibular plate may occur. The posterior aspect of the maxilla may also be effaced. The inferior border of the mandible may be thinned or destroyed. If the tumor is extensive, pathologic fracture may occur.

Differential diagnosis. Squamous cell carcinoma is discernible from other malignancies by its clinical and histologic features. Occasionally it is difficult to differentiate inflammatory lesions such as osteomyelitis from squamous cell carcinoma, especially when oral bacteria secondarily infect the tumor. Both osteomyelitis and squamous cell carcinoma are destructive, leaving islands of osseous structure that may appear to be consistent with sequestra. Evidence of profound bone destruction or invasive characteristics helps to identify the presence of a malignancy when a mixture of inflammatory changes and carcinoma exists. Osteomyelitis usually produces some periosteal reaction, whereas squamous cell carcinoma does not. In cases of osteoradionecrosis,

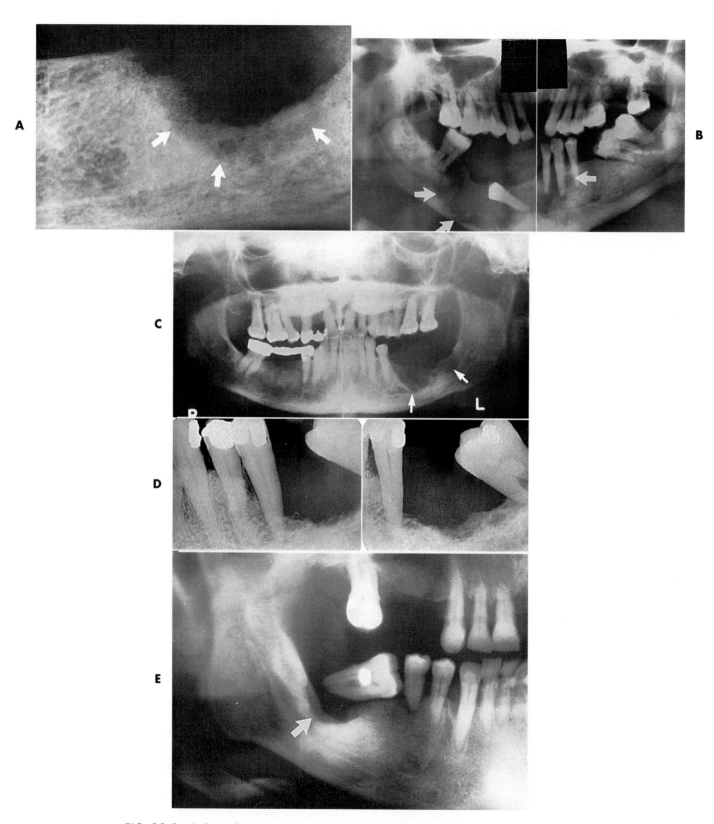

FIG. **21-2**   **A** through **E,** Squamous cell carcinoma *(arrows)* resulting in irregular resorption of bone. Note the soft tissue border of the lesion in **D. (B,** courtesy S.R. Matteson, DDS, Chapel Hill, N.C.)

where the patient has had prior malignancy, periosteal new bone is absent. If osseous destruction is present, the differentiation of this condition from squamous cell carcinoma requires advanced imaging or surgical exploration.

Management. Oral squamous cell carcinoma is usually managed using a combination of surgery and radiation therapy. The choice of which modality to use depends on the protocol of the treating center and the location and severity of the tumor. Generally, if an adequate margin of normal tissue can be obtained, surgery is the usual treatment, followed by radiation treatment. Alternately, radiation may be used as the primary treatment followed by surgical salvage. Currently, the trend is to add concomitant chemotherapy as an adjunct to either radiation or surgical treatment.

SQUAMOUS CELL CARCINOMA ORIGINATING IN BONE

Identifying Characteristics

Synonyms. *Primary intraosseous carcinoma, intra-alveolar carcinoma, primary intra-alveolar epidermoid carcinoma, primary epithelial tumor of the jaw, central squamous cell carcinoma, primary odontogenic carcinoma, intramandibular carcinoma,* and *central mandibular carcinoma*

Definition. Primary intraosseous carcinoma is a squamous cell carcinoma arising within the jaw that has no original connection with the surface epithelium of the oral mucosa. Primary intraosseous carcinomas are presumed to arise from intraosseous remnants of odontogenic epithelium. In addition, carcinoma from surface epithelium, odontogenic cysts, or distant sites (metastases) must be excluded.

Clinical features. These neoplasms are rare and may remain silent until they have reached a fairly large size. Pain, pathologic fracture, and sensory nerve abnormalities such as lip paresthesia and lymphadenopathy may occur with this tumor. It is more common in men and in patients in their fourth to eighth decade of life. The surface epithelium is invariably normal in appearance.

Radiographic features
Location. The mandible is far more commonly involved than the maxilla, with most cases being present in the molar region (Fig. 21-3) and less frequently in the anterior aspect of the jaws. Because the lesion is by definition associated with remnants of the dental lamina, it originates only in tooth-bearing parts of the jaw.

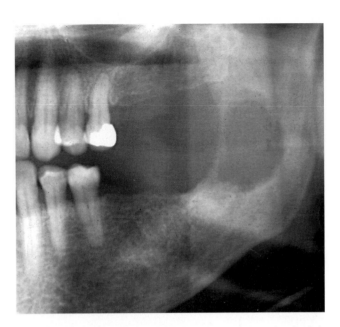

FIG. **21-3** This primary intraosseous carcinoma in the left mandible exhibits no internal structure, a poorly defined periphery, and thinning of the overlying mandibular bone.

Periphery and shape. The periphery of the majority of lesions is ill-defined, although some have been described as well-defined. They are most often rounded or irregular in shape and have a border that demonstrates osseous destruction and varying degrees of extension at the periphery. The degree of raggedness of the border may reflect the aggressiveness of the lesion. If sufficient in size, pathologic fracture occurs, with its associated step defects, thinned cortical borders, and subsequent soft tissue mass.

Internal structure. The internal structure is wholly radiolucent with no evidence of bone production and very little residual bone left within the center of the lesion. If the lesion is small, overlying buccal or lingual plates may cast a shadow that may mimic the appearance of internal trabecular bone.

Effects on surrounding structures. These lesions are capable of causing destruction of the antral or nasal floors, loss of the cortical outline of the mandibular neurovascular canal, and effacement of the lamina dura. Root resorption is unusual. Teeth that lose both lamina dura and supporting bone appear to be floating in space.

Differential diagnosis. If the lesions are not aggressive and have a smooth border and radiolucent area, they may be mistaken for periapical cysts or granulomas. Alternately, if lesions are not centered about the apex of a tooth, occasionally it is difficult to differentiate this condition from odontogenic cysts or tumors. If the border is obviously infiltrative with extensive bone destruction, a metastatic lesion must be excluded, as well as multiple myeloma, fibrosarcoma, and carcinoma arising in a dental cyst. Examination of the oral cavity and especially the surface epithelium assists in differentiating this condition from invasive squamous cell carcinoma.

Management. Generally these tumors are excised with their surrounding osseous structure in an en bloc resection. Radiation and chemotherapy may be used as adjunctive therapies.

SQUAMOUS CELL CARCINOMA ORIGINATING IN A CYST

Identifying Characteristics
Synonyms. *Epidermoid cell carcinoma* and *carcinoma ex odontogenic cyst*

Definition. Squamous cell carcinoma arising in a preexisting dental cyst is uncommon and excludes invasion from surface epithelial carcinomas, metastatic tumors and primary intraosseous carcinoma. They may arise from inflammatory periapical, residual, dentigerous, and odontogenic keratocysts. Histologically the lining squamous epithelium of the cyst gives rise to the malignant neoplasm.

Clinical features. The most common presenting sign or symptom associated with this condition is pain. The pain may be characterized as dull and of several months' duration. Swelling is occasionally reported. Pathologic fracture may occur, as may fistula formation and regional lymphadenopathy. If the upper jaw is involved, sinus pain or swelling may be present.

Radiographic features
Location. This tumor may occur anywhere an odontogenic cyst is found, namely the tooth-bearing portions of the jaws. Most cases occur in the mandible (Fig. 21-4), with a few cases reported in the anterior maxilla.

Periphery and shape. The radiologic picture of squamous cell carcinoma originating in a cyst mirrors the histologic findings. Because the lesion arises from a cyst, the shape is often round or ovoid. If it is a small lesion in a cyst wall, the periphery may be well defined and corticated. In this case the radiographic differentiation from a normal cyst is impossible. As the malignant tissue progressively replaces cyst lining, the smooth border is lost or becomes ill-defined. The advanced lesion has an ill-defined, infiltrative periphery that lacks any cortication. Its shape becomes less "hydraulic" looking and more diffuse.

Internal structure. This lesion lacks any ability to pro-

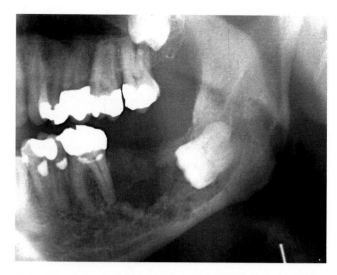

FIG. **21-4** Carcinoma arising in a preexisting dentigerous cyst related to the mandibular left third molar shows absence of a cyst cortex, invasion into adjacent bone, and ill-defined borders.

duce bone. It is wholly radiolucent, perhaps more so than invasive surface carcinoma, owing to the prior osteolysis from the cyst.

Effects on surrounding structures. Carcinoma arising in dental cysts is capable of thinning and destroying the lamina dura of adjacent teeth or adjacent cortical boundaries such as the inferior border of the jaw or floor of the nose. It can produce complete destruction of the alveolar process.

Differential diagnosis. If a dental cyst is infected, it may lose its normal cortical boundary and appear ragged and identical to a malignant lesion arising in a preexisting cyst. However, inflamed cysts usually show a reactive peripheral sclerosis because of inflammatory products present in the cyst lumen. This is not normally present in a cyst, which has undergone malignant transformation. Nevertheless, the two may be difficult to differentiate radiologically, and therefore cysts should always be submitted for histologic examination. Multiple myeloma may appear as a solitary lesion and may be difficult to distinguish, especially if it has a cystic well-defined shape. Metastatic disease may be similar, although it is commonly multifocal. Primary intraosseous carcinoma cannot be radiographically differentiated from bony involvement of an overlying invasive carcinoma but may be clinically differentiated by the presence of abnormalities of the overlying epithelium.

Management. The treatment of squamous cell carcinoma originating in a cyst is identical to that described with primary intraosseous carcinoma.

CENTRAL MUCOEPIDERMOID CARCINOMA

Identifying Characteristics

Synonym. *Mucoepidermoid carcinoma*

Definition. Central mucoepidermoid carcinoma is an epithelial tumor arising in bone; it is believed to derive from the salivary duct system. It is histologically indistinguishable from its soft tissue counterpart. The criteria for diagnosis of a central mucoepidermoid tumor is the presence of intact cortical plates, radiographic evidence of bone destruction, and typical histologic findings consistent with mucoepidermoid tumor. Additionally, the practitioner must exclude the possibility of an invasive overlying mucoepidermoid tumor or odontogenic tumor. This carcinoma has been reported to arise from the lining of a dentigerous cyst.

Clinical features. Unlike other malignant tumors of the jaws, the central mucoepidermoid tumor is more likely to manifest as a benign tumor or cyst. The most common complaint is of a painless swelling. The swelling may have been present for months or even years and has been reported to cause facial asymmetry. Occasionally it may feel as if teeth have been moved or a denture may no longer fit. Tenderness rather than severe pain may also be present. Paresthesia of the inferior alveolar nerve as well as spreading of the lesion to regional lymph nodes has been reported. Central mucoepidermoid tumor, unlike other oral malignancies, is more common in females than males.

Radiographic features

Location. The lesion is twice as common in the mandible as the maxilla, usually in the premolar and molar region with a few cases reported in the anterior mandible. The lesion most commonly occurs above the mandibular canal, similar to odontogenic tumors.

Periphery and shape. Mucoepidermoid tumor presents as a unilocular or multilocular expansile mass (Fig. 21-5). The border is most often well defined and well corticated and often crenated or undulating in nature, which is similar to odontogenic tumors. The peripheral cortication may be impressively thick, which belies its malignant nature. Rarely the periphery is not corticated and has a more malignant appearance.

Internal structure. The internal structure has features like those of a benign odontogenic tumor such as an ameloblastoma. Lesions are often described as being multilocular or having either a soap bubble or honeycomb internal structure, implying the presence of compartments separated by thin or thick cortical septa. This bone is not produced by the tumor but is merely remodeled residual bone taking the form of septa.

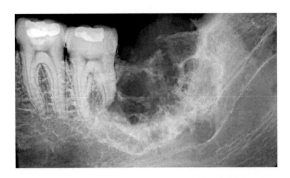

FIG. **21-5** The multilocular radiolucency in this radiograph has displaced the mandibular canal and destroyed the superior crest of the alveolar process and the distal supporting bone of the second molar.

Effects on surrounding structures. Mucoepidermoid tumor is capable of causing expansion of adjacent normal bony walls. The buccal and lingual cortical plates, inferior border of the mandible, and alveolar crest are usually intact; however, they may be thinned and grossly displaced. The mandibular canal may be depressed or pushed laterally or medially. These characteristics are more similar to benign tumors than malignant tumors. Teeth remain largely unaffected by this disease, although adjacent lamina dura may be lost in a fashion seen in inflammatory periapical disease.

Differential diagnosis. The differential diagnosis of this lesion reflects its lack of features commonly associated with oral malignancy. The chief differential is ameloblastoma, with which it shares similarities in its peripheral and internal features. It may not be possible to differentiate the two. Odontogenic myxoma and central giant cell granuloma also may be confused with mucoepidermoid tumor, as may other odontogenic cysts or tumors.

Management. Mucoepidermoid carcinoma is treated surgically with en bloc resection encompassing a margin of adjacent normal bone. Neck dissection and postoperative radiation therapy may be required for control of nodal disease.

MALIGNANT AMELOBLASTOMA AND AMELOBLASTIC CARCINOMA

Identifying Characteristics

Definition. Malignant ameloblastoma is defined as an ameloblastoma exhibiting the histologic criteria of a malignant neoplasm such as increased and abnormal mitosis and hyperchromatic, large, pleomorphic nuclei. The histologic features may not correlate with the clinical behavior. On the other hand, ameloblastic carcinoma is an ameloblastoma with typical benign histologic features that is deemed malignant because of its biologic behavior, namely, metastasis.

Clinical features. Clinically these lesions may behave as benign ameloblastomas, exhibiting a hard expansile mass of the jaw with displaced and perhaps loosened teeth and normal overlying mucosa. Tenderness of the overlying soft tissue has been reported as has the presence of bony swelling. Metastatic spread may be to the cervical lymph nodes, lung or other viscera, and the skeleton, especially the spine. Local extension may occur into adjacent bones, connective tissue, or salivary glands. These tumors occur most commonly between the first and sixth decades of life and are more common in males than females.

Radiographic features

Location. These lesions are more common in the mandible than in the maxilla, with most occurring in the premolar and molar region, where ameloblastoma is typically found.

Periphery and shape. Similar to ameloblastoma, a well-defined border occurs with cortication, presence of crenations, or scalloping in the perimeter. Malignant ameloblastoma may show some of the signs more commonly seen in malignant neoplasms, namely, loss of the cortical boundary and breaching of the cortical boundary with soft tissue spread.

Internal structure. The lesions are either unilocular or, more commonly, multilocular, giving the appearance of a honeycomb or soap-bubble pattern as seen in benign ameloblastomas. Most of the septa are robust and thick.

Effects on surrounding structures. Teeth may be moved bodily by the tumor and may exhibit root resorption similar to a benign tumor. Bony borders may be effaced or breached, and as in benign ameloblastoma, the lesions may erode lamina dura and displace normal anatomic boundaries such as the floor of the nose and maxillary sinus. The mandibular neurovascular canal may be displaced or eroded.

Differential diagnosis. The differential diagnosis of this lesion should include benign ameloblastoma, odontogenic keratocyst, odontogenic myxoma, and central mucoepidermoid tumor, from which it may not be distinguishable radiologically. If the lesion is locally invasive and this is apparent radiologically, a diagnosis of carcinoma arising in a dental cyst should be entertained. If the patient is young and the location of the lesion is anterior to the second permanent molar, central giant cell granuloma may mimic some of its radiologic features. Often the final diagnosis is the result of histologic evaluation or the detection of metastatic lesions.

Management. These lesions are most often treated with en bloc surgical resection. However, many may not be discovered to be malignant until the time of the first surgery or even later. Because the histologic appearance of these lesions may mimic benign ameloblastoma, the initial treatment often is inadequate. In addition, the metastatic lesions may not appear for many months or years after treatment of the primary tumor, adding another reason for treatment failure.

Metastatic Tumors

GENERAL METASTATIC TUMORS
Identifying Characteristics
Synonym. *Secondary malignancy*

Definition. Metastatic tumors represent the establishment of new foci of malignant disease from a distant malignant tumor. An interesting feature of these lesions is that metastatic lesions in the jaws usually arise from sites that are anatomically inferior to the clavicle. Metastatic lesions of the jaws usually occur when the distant primary lesion is already known, although on occasion a jaw metastatic tumor may reveal the presence of a silent primary lesion. Jaw involvement accounts for less than 1% of metastatic malignancies found elsewhere, with most affecting the spine, pelvis, skull, ribs, and humerus. Most frequently the tumor is a type of carcinoma, the most common primary sites being the breast, kidney, lung, colon and rectum, prostate, thyroid, stomach, melanoma, testes, bladder, ovary, and cervix. In children the tumors include neuroblastoma, retinoblastoma, and Wilms' tumor. Metastatic carcinoma must be differentiated from the more common locally invading squamous carcinoma.

Clinical features. Metastatic disease is more common in patients in their fifth to seventh decade of life. Patients may complain of dental pain, numbness or paresthesia of the third branch of the trigeminal nerve, pathologic fracture of the jaw, or hemorrhage from the tumor site.

Radiographic features
Location. The posterior areas of the jaws are more commonly affected, the mandible being favored over the maxilla. The maxillary sinus may be the next most common site, followed by the anterior hard palate and mandibular condyle. Frequently metastatic lesions of the mandible are bilateral. Also, lesions may be located in the periodontal ligament space (sometimes at the root apex), mimicking periapical inflammatory disease, or in the papilla of a developing tooth.

Periphery and shape. Metastatic lesions may be moderately well demarcated but have no cortication or encapsulation at their tumor margins; they may also have ill-defined invasive margins (Fig. 21-6). The lesions are not round but polymorphous in shape. Both prostate and breast lesions may stimulate bone formation of the adjacent bone, which will be sclerotic. The tumor may begin as a few zones of osseous destruction separated by normal bone. After a time these small areas coalesce into a larger, ill-defined mass and the jaw may become enlarged.

Internal structure. Lesions are generally radiolucent, in which case the internal structure is a combination of residual normal trabecular bone in association with areas of bone lysis. If sclerotic metastases are present (i.e., prostate and breast), the normally ragged radiolucent area may appear as an area of patchy sclerosis, the result of new bone formation. The origin of this new bone is not the tumor but stimulation of surrounding normal bone. If the tumor is seeded in multiple regions of the jaw, the result is a multifocal appearance (multiple small radiolucent lesions) with normal bone between the foci.

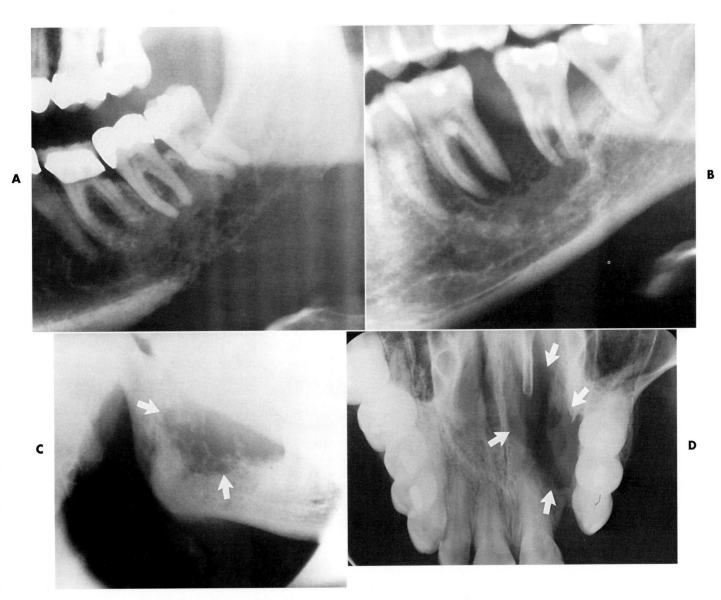

FIG. **21-6** *Metastatic carcinomas.* **A,** Metastatic breast carcinoma surrounding the apical half of the second and third molar roots and extending inferiorly. It has destroyed the inferior border of the mandible. **B,** Metastatic renal cell carcinoma that has destroyed the alveolar bone supporting the first and second molars. **C** and **D,** Lesions from gastric carcinoma. (**C** and **D,** courtesy L. Hollender, DDS, Seattle, Wash.)

Significant dissemination of metastatic tumor may give the jaws a general radiolucent appearance or even that of osteopenia.

Effects on surrounding structures. Metastatic carcinomas may stimulate a periosteal reaction that usually takes the form of a spiculated pattern (prostate and neuroblastoma). Typical of malignancy, the lesion effaces the lamina dura and can enlarge the periodontal ligament space. If the tumor has seeded in the papilla of a developing tooth, the cortices of the crypt may be totally or partially destroyed. Teeth may seem to be floating in a soft tissue mass and may be in an altered position because of loss of bony support. Extraction sockets may fail to heal and may increase in size. Resorption of teeth is rare (sometimes associated with multiple myeloma and chondrosarcoma); this is more common in benign lesions. The cortical bone of adjacent structures such as the neurovascular canal, sinus, and nasal fossa is destroyed. On occasion the tumor breaches the outer cortical plate of the jaws and extends into surrounding soft tissues or presents as an intraoral mass.

Differential diagnosis. In most cases a known primary malignancy is present, and the diagnosis of metastasis is straightforward. Multiple myeloma may be confused with metastatic tumors; however, the border of multiple myeloma is usually better circumscribed than in metastatic disease. When a lesion starts within the periodontal ligament space of a tooth, the appearance may be identical to that of a periapical inflammatory lesion. A point of differentiation is that the periodontal ligament space widening from inflammation is at its greatest width and centered about the apex of the root. In contrast, the malignant tumor usually causes irregular widening, which may extend up the side of the root. Odontogenic cysts, if secondarily infected, may have an ill-defined border giving a similar appearance to a metastatic lesion. Invasion of the jaws by primary tumors of the overlying epithelium such as squamous cell carcinoma may be indistinguishable from metastatic disease but can be differentiated by clinical examination.

Management. The presence of a metastatic tumor in the jaw indicates a poor prognosis. If metastatic disease is present, the patient will usually die within 1 to 2 years. If the radiographic appearance is suspicious, an opinion from a dental radiologist should be sought and tissue submitted for histologic analysis. Nuclear medicine may be employed to detect other metastatic lesions. Isolated malignant deposits, if symptomatic, may be treated with localized high-dose radiation treatment. In the rare occasion that the jaw is the first diagnosed site of malignant spread, it is imperative that the patient be referred quickly to an oncologist so that anticancer treatment

can be delivered promptly. This treatment may take the form of chemotherapy, radiation therapy, surgery, immunotherapy, and hormone treatment.

Sarcomas

OSTEOSARCOMA
Identifying Characteristics
Synonym. Osteogenic sarcoma

Definition. Osteosarcoma is a malignant neoplasm of bone in which osteoid is produced directly by malignant stroma as opposed to adjacent reactive bone formation. The three major histologic types are chondroblastic, osteoblastic, and fibroblastic osteosarcoma. The cause of osteosarcoma is unknown, but genetic mutation and viral causes have been suggested. It is also known to occur in association with Paget's disease and fibrous dysplasia after therapeutic irradiation.

Clinical features. Osteosarcoma of the jaws is quite rare and accounts for approximately 7% of all osteosarcomas. Despite its rarity, the dentist may be the first health professional who observes tumors involving the jaws. The lesion occurs in all racial groups worldwide and in males twice as frequently as females. Jaw lesions typically occur with a peak in the fourth decade, about 10 years later on average than long bone lesions. The most commonly reported symptom or sign is swelling, which may be present as long as 6 months before diagnosis; the swelling is usually rapid. Other indicators are pain, tenderness, erythema of overlying mucosa, ulceration, loose teeth, epistaxis, hemorrhage, nasal obstruction, exophthalmos, trismus, and blindness. Hypoesthesia has also been reported in cases involving neurovascular canals.

Radiographic features
Location. The mandible is more commonly affected than the maxilla. Although the lesion can occur in any part of either jaw, the posterior mandible, including the tooth-bearing region, angle, and vertical ramus, is most commonly affected. The posterior areas are also more commonly affected in the maxilla, with the most frequent sites being the alveolar ridge, antrum, and palate. The lesion may cross the midline.

Periphery and shape. Osteosarcoma has an ill-defined border in most instances. When viewed against normal bone, the lesion is usually radiolucent with no peripheral sclerosis or encapsulation. If the lesion involves the periosteum directly or by extension, one may see the typical sunray spicules or "hair-on-end" trabeculae (Fig. 21-7). This occurs when the periosteum is displaced,

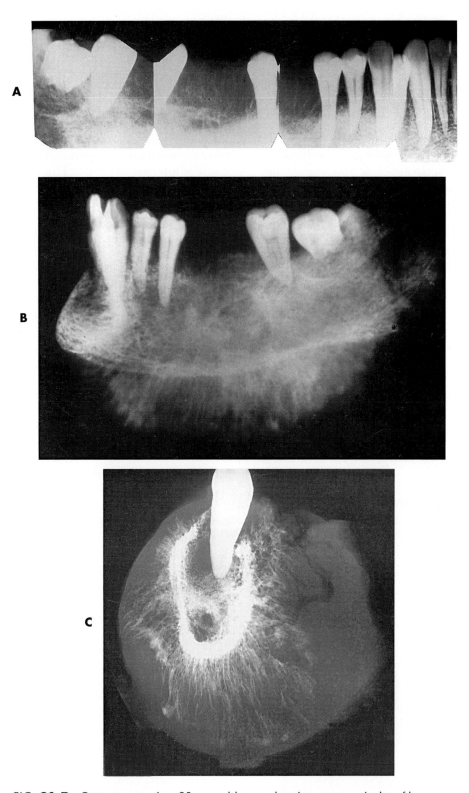

FIG. 21-7 Osteosarcoma in a 25-year-old man, showing sunray spicules of bone on periapical radiographs, **A,** and on resected jaw, **B** and **C.**

partially destroyed, and disorganized. If the periosteum is elevated and maintains its osteogenic potential but is breached in the center, a Codman's triangle at the edges is formed. Even more rarely, laminar periosteal new bone may be present. In many cases, extension is even more prominent, and a soft tissue mass is visible radiographically.

Internal structure. Osteosarcoma may be entirely radiolucent, mixed radiolucent-radiopaque, or quite radiopaque. The internal osseous structure may take the appearance of granular- or sclerotic-appearing bone, cotton bolls, wisps, or honeycombed internal structures in areas with adjacent destruction of the preexisting osseous architecture. Whatever the resultant internal structure, the normal trabecular structure of the jaws is lost.

Effects on surrounding structures. Widening of the periodontal membrane suggests osteosarcoma but is also seen in other malignancies (Fig. 21-8). The antral or nasal wall cortices may be lost in maxillary lesions. Mandibular lesions may destroy the cortex of the neurovascular canal and adjacent lamina dura. Alternatively, the neurovascular canal may be symmetrically widened and enlarged. Effects on the periosteum are discussed under the discussion on periphery.

Differential diagnosis. If internal structure is minimal or absent, fibrosarcoma or metastatic carcinoma may appear similar to osteosarcoma. If osseous structure is visible, the practitioner should also consider chondrosarcoma. If spiculated periosteal new bone is present, prostate and breast metastases should be considered. Comprehensive physical examination and laboratory tests assist in determining if the lesion is primary or metastatic. Benign tumors such as ossifying fibroma and benign conditions such as fibrous dysplasia may mimic osteosarcoma. The former conditions, however, are usually better demarcated and have a more uniform internal structure. The histopathology of osteosarcoma may be interpreted as a benign fibroosseous lesion, and in these cases, the correct diagnosis may rely on the radiographic characteristics alone. Ewing's sarcoma, solitary plasmacytoma, and even osteomyelitis share some of the radiographic characteristics of osteosarcoma. Osteosarcoma is generally not associated with signs of infection.

Management. The management of osteosarcoma is resection with a large border of adjacent normal bone. This may be possible in orthopedic cases but may be complicated by the presence of important adjacent anatomic structures in the head and neck. Generally radiation therapy and chemotherapy are used only for controlling metastatic spread or for palliation.

CHONDROSARCOMA

Identifying Characteristics
Synonym. *Chondrogenic sarcoma*

Definition. Chondrosarcoma is a malignant tumor of cartilaginous origin. The four histologic subtypes, which develop most commonly in the craniofacial region, are the clear cell, de-differentiated, myxoid, and mesenchymal forms. They may occur centrally within bone, on the periphery of bone, or less commonly in soft tissue. They can arise directly from cartilage or may occur within benign cartilaginous tumors. In the case of the latter, they are termed *secondary chondrosarcomas.*

Clinical features. Generally these tumors occur at any age, although they are more common in adults (mean age 47 years). They affect males and females equally. A patient with chondrosarcoma may have a firm or hard mass of relatively long duration. Enlargement of these lesions may cause pain, headache, and deformity. Less frequent signs and symptoms include hemorrhage from tumor or from the necks of the teeth, sensory nerve deficits, proptosis, and visual disturbances. Invariably the tumors are covered with normal overlying skin or mucosa unless secondarily ulcerated. If chondrosarcoma occurs in or near the temporomandibular joint region, trismus or abnormal joint function may result.

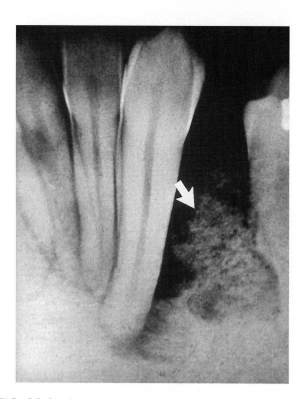

FIG. **21-8** Osteosarcoma with widening of the periodontal ligament space and production of new bone *(arrow).*

Radiographic features

Location. Chondrosarcomas are unusual in the facial bones, accounting for about 10% of all cases. They occur in the mandible and maxilla with equal frequency. Maxillary lesions typically occur in the anterior region in areas where cartilaginous tissues may be present in the maxilla. Mandibular lesions occur in the coronoid process, condylar head and neck, and occasionally the symphyseal region.

Periphery and shape. Chondrosarcomas are slow-growing tumors, and their radiologic signs may be misleading and benign in nature. The lesions are generally round, ovoid, or lobulated. Generally their borders are well defined and at times corticated, whereas at other times melding with adjacent normal bone occurs. Occasionally peripheral periosteal new bone may be present perpendicular to the original cortex, giving the so-called sunray or hair-on-end appearance. Uncommonly these lesions are ill defined and invasive. Aggressive lesions such as these have infiltrative, ill-defined, and noncorticated borders.

Internal structure. Chondrosarcomas usually exhibit some form of calcification within their center, giving them a mixed radiolucent-radiopaque appearance. At times this mixture takes the form of moth-eaten bone alternating with islands of residual bone unaffected by tumor. Lesions are rarely completely radiolucent. The central radiopaque structure has been described as "flocculent," implying snowlike features. This diffuse calcification may be superimposed on a bony background that resembles granular or ground-glass–appearing abnormal bone (Fig. 21-9). Careful examination of these areas of flocculence may reveal a central radiolucent nidus, which is probably cartilage surrounded by calcification. The result is rounded or speckled areas of calcification.

Effects on surrounding structures. Chondrosarcoma, being relatively slow growing, often expands normal cortical boundaries rather than rapidly destroying them. In mandibular cases the inferior border or alveolar process may be grossly expanded while still maintaining its cortical covering. Maxillary lesions may push the walls of the maxillary sinus or nasal fossa and impinge on the infratemporal fossa. Lesions of the condyle cause its expansion and perhaps remodeling of the corresponding articular fossa and eminence. If lesions occur in the articular disk region, a widened joint space may be present with corresponding remodeling of the condylar neck. Erosion of the articular fossa may also occur. If lesions occur near teeth, root resorption and tooth displacement may occur, as may widening of the periodontal membrane space.

Differential diagnosis. Osteosarcoma is often indistinguishable radiographically from chondrosarcoma. Although the typical calcifications of chondrosarcoma may be absent from osteosarcoma, the two share many other radiologic features. Fibrous dysplasia may also be difficult to differentiate from chondrosarcoma because of the variations in the pattern of calcifications. Generally the periphery of fibrous dysplasia is better defined and its margin with adjacent teeth differs from that of chondrosarcoma. For instance, fibrous dysplasia alters the bone pattern up to and including the lamina dura, leaving a normal or thin periodontal ligament space. The greatest danger results from the misleading benign characteristics, which may delay an accurate diagnosis.

Management. The management of chondrosarcoma is surgical. Radiation therapy and chemotherapy generally have no role to play. Patients with chondrosarcomas have a relatively good 5-year survival rate but poor 10-year survival rate.

EWING'S SARCOMA

Identifying Characteristics

Synonyms. *Endothelial myeloma* and *round cell sarcoma*

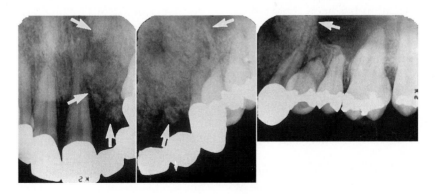

FIG. **21-9** Chondrosarcoma of the anterior maxilla, with irregular calcification in the internal structure of the tumor *(arrows)*. (Courtesy L. Hollender, DDS, Seattle, Wash.)

Definition. Ewing's sarcoma is of indeterminate histogenesis. It is a tumor of long bones and is relatively rare in the jaws. Lesions arise in the medullary portion of the bone and spread to the endosteal and later periosteal surfaces.

Clinical features. Ewing's sarcoma is most common in the second decade of life with most patients being between the ages of 5 and 30 years. Males are twice as likely to manifest the disease as females. In addition, multicentric lesions have been reported. Other reported findings at the time of presentation include, in descending frequency, swelling, pain, loose teeth, paresthesia, exophthalmos, ptosis, epistaxis, ulceration, shifted teeth, trismus, and sinusitis. Cervical lymphadenopathy has also been reported.

Radiographic features

Location. Mandibular cases outnumber maxillary cases by about two to one, with the highest frequency found in posterior areas in both jaws. Generally the lesions develop within the marrow space first and then extend to involve overlying cortical plates. This neoplasm rarely occurs in the jaws.

Periphery and shape. Ewing's sarcoma is a radiolucency that is poorly demarcated and never corticated. Its advancing edge destroys bone in an uneven fashion, resulting in a ragged border. The lesions are usually solitary and may cause pathologic fracture with adjacent radiographically visible soft tissue masses. They may be round or ovoid but generally have no typical shape.

Internal structure. Ewing's sarcoma is a destructive process with little induction of bone formation. Because it commences on the internal aspect of the bone and involves the endosteal and periosteal surfaces later in its course, it is usually entirely radiolucent.

Effects on surrounding structures. Ewing's sarcoma may stimulate the periosteum to produce new bone. This is usually the result of gross disturbances to the overlying periosteum and takes the form of Codman's triangle or sunray or hair-on-end spiculation. Laminar periosteal new bone formation has been reported to occur but is not a common feature of active Ewing's sarcoma lesions. Adjacent normal structures such as the mandibular neurovascular canal, inferior border of the mandible, and alveolar cortical plates may be effaced. If the lesion abuts teeth or tooth follicles, the cortices of these structures are destroyed. This tumor does not characteristically cause root resorption, although it does destroy the supporting bone of adjacent teeth.

Differential diagnosis. Inflammatory or infectious lesions such as osteomyelitis of the jaw may share some of the radiographic features of Ewing's sarcoma. Although both are radiolucent, osteomyelitis is likely to have demonstrable sequestra present within the confines of the lesion, whereas Ewing's sarcoma does not. Also, inflammatory lesions contain some sign of reactive bone formation, resulting in some sclerosis internally or at the periphery.

The two also differ with respect to their periosteal bone formation. Eosinophilic granuloma of the jaw is also a destructive process, which occurs in the same part of the bone. It is associated with laminar periosteal bone reaction, whereas, in the jaws, Ewing's sarcoma is not. The other central primary malignancies of bone such as osteosarcoma, chondrosarcoma, and fibrosarcoma are difficult to differentiate from this condition.

Management. Too few cases of maxillofacial Ewing's sarcoma are available at any one treatment center for any specific treatment policy to have been adopted. Surgery, radiation therapy, and chemotherapy may be used alone or in combination.

FIBROSARCOMA

Identifying Characteristics

Definition. Fibrosarcoma is a neoplasm composed of malignant fibroblasts that produce collagen and elastin. The etiology is unknown, although it may arise secondarily in tissues that have received therapeutic levels of radiation.

Clinical features. These lesions occur equally in males and females with a mean age in the fourth decade. A slowly to rapidly enlarging mass is the usual presenting symptom. The mass may be within bone, in which case it usually is accompanied by pain. Peripheral lesions or those exiting from bone may invade local soft tissues, causing a bulky, clinically obvious lesion. If central or peripheral lesions reach a large size, pathologic fracture may occur. If fibrosarcomas involve the course of peripheral nerves, sensorineural abnormalities may occur. Overlying mucosa, although initially normal, may become erythematous or ulcerated. Involvement of the temporomandibular joint or paramandibular musculature is often accompanied by trismus.

Radiographic features

Location. Most cases of fibrosarcoma of the jaws occur in the mandible, with the greatest number of these occurring in the premolar/molar region.

Periphery and shape. Fibrosarcomas have ill-defined borders that are best described as ragged (Fig. 21-10). They are poorly demarcated, noncorticated, and lack any semblance of a capsule. These tumors are generally shaped in a fashion that suggests that they have grown

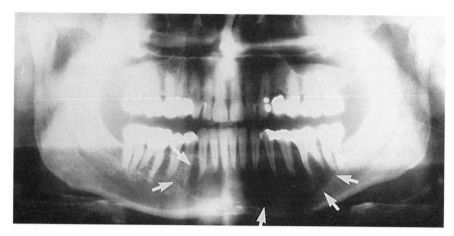

FIG. **21-10** Fibrosarcoma in the mandible, with large areas of ill-defined bone destruction (arrows).

along a bone, and so they tend to be elongated through the marrow space. The radiographic border may underestimate the extent of the tumor because these lesions typically are infiltrative. If soft tissue lesions occur adjacent to bone, they may cause a saucerlike depression in the underlying bone or invade it as would a squamous cell carcinoma. Finally, sclerosis may occur in the adjacent normal bone whether the fibrosarcoma is peripheral to bone or central.

Internal structure. Fibrosarcomas have little internal structure. In most cases the lesions are entirely radiolucent. If the lesions have been present for some time and are not overly aggressive, either residual jawbone or reactive osseous bone formation occurs.

Effects on surrounding structures. The most common effect on adjacent structures is destruction. In the mandible, the alveolar process, inferior border of the jaw, and cortices of the neurovascular canal are lost. In the maxilla, the inferior floor of the maxillary sinus, posterior wall of the maxilla, and nasal floor can be destroyed. In either jaw, lamina dura and follicular cortices are obliterated. Root resorption is uncommon. Teeth are more likely to be grossly displaced and lose their support bone so that they appear to be floating in space. In addition, widening of the periodontal membrane space occurs with this tumor, as in other malignancies. Periosteal reaction is uncommon; however, if the lesion disrupts the periosteum, a Codman's triangle or sunray spiculation may be evident.

Differential diagnosis. This solitary, ragged radiolucency with little internal structure is difficult to differentiate from other central malignancies. If the lesion does not cause enlargement of the jaw, the practitioner must rule out metastatic carcinoma, multiple myeloma, and pri-

mary or secondary intraosseous carcinoma. Another possibility is a grossly infected dental cyst, although these usually show some degree of induced peripheral sclerosis in adjacent bone. If a fibrosarcoma exhibits enlargement of the affected jaw, the practitioner must rule out chondrosarcoma and osteosarcoma, both of which have more internal structure. Ewing's sarcoma and radiolucent osteosarcomas may not be distinguishable from this tumor. Finally, peripheral invasive squamous cell carcinoma shares some of these radiologic features, but its ulcerative surface features differentiate it from fibrosarcoma, which usually lacks these.

Management. The management of fibrosarcoma is chiefly surgical. A wide margin of adjacent normal bone is taken if anatomically possible. Radiation therapy and chemotherapy are usually reserved for palliation.

Malignancies of the Hematopoietic System

MULTIPLE MYELOMA

Identifying Characteristics

Synonyms. *Myeloma, plasma cell myeloma,* and *plasmacytoma*

Definition. Multiple myeloma is a malignant neoplasm of plasma cells. It is the most common malignancy of bone in adults. Single lesions are called *plasmacytoma,* and multiple lesions are termed *multiple myeloma.*

Clinical features. Multiple myeloma is a fatal systemic malignancy. A patient with multiple myeloma is usually between the ages of 35 and 70 years (mean age 60 years). The patient may complain of fatigue, weight loss, fever, bone pain, and anemia, although the typical presenting feature is low back pain. Secondary signs include amyloidosis and hypercalcemia; in half of all patients, characteristic Bence Jones protein is present in the urine, which causes the urine to be foamy. The disease is more common in men. When this clonal proliferation occurs, these cells occupy first cancellous and later cortical bone, replacing the normally radiopaque bone with areas of radiolucency.

Orally, patients may complain of dental pain, swelling, hemorrhage, paresthesia, and dysesthesia, or they may have no complaints. The number of patients with demonstrable radiologic findings in the jaws at the time of diagnosis is relatively small.

Radiographic features

Location. Multiple myeloma is seen more frequently in the mandible (Fig. 21-11) than the maxilla but is uncommon in either. The incidence of jaw involvement has been reported to vary from 2% to 78%. In the mandible the posterior body and ramus is favored. Maxillary lesions usually appear in posterior sites.

Periphery and shape. The periphery of multiple myeloma lesions is well defined but not corticated; it

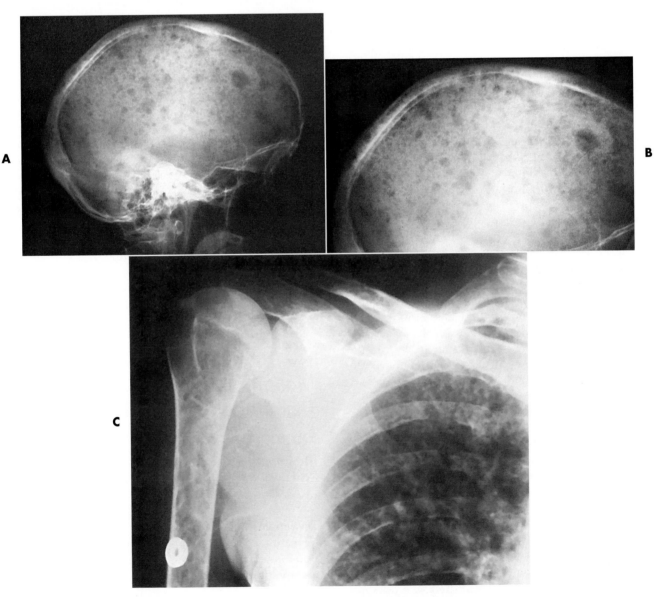

FIG. **21-11** Multiple myeloma, seen as multiple radiolucent lesions in the skull, **A** and **B**; and in the ribs and humerus, **C**. (**B** and **C,** courtesy L. Hollender, DDS, Seattle, Wash.)

lacks any sign of bone reaction (Fig. 21-12). The lesions have been described as appearing "punched out." However, many appear ragged and even infiltrative. Some lesions have an oval or cystic shape. Untreated or aggressive areas of destruction may become confluent, giving the appearance of multilocularity. If the lesion is located in the periapical periodontal ligament space, it may have a border similar to that seen in inflammatory or infectious periapical disease. Soft tissue lesions have been reported in the jaws and nasopharynx. When visible on radiographs, they appear as smooth-bordered soft tissue masses, possibly with underlying bone destruction.

Internal structure. No internal structure is radiographically visible. Occasionally islands of residual bone, yet unaffected by tumor, give the appearance of the presence of new trabecular bone within the mass. Very rarely the lesions appear radiopaque internally.

Effects on surrounding structures. If a good deal of bone mineral is lost, teeth may appear to be "too opaque" and may stand out conspicuously from their osteopenic background. Lamina dura and follicles of impacted teeth may lose their typical corticated surrounding bone in a manner analogous to that seen in hyperparathyroidism. The same may be said of the mandibular neurovascular canal, which, although usually visible, loses its cortical boundary in whole or in part. These changes are profound when there is associated renal disease. Mandibular lesions may cause thinning of the lower border of the mandible or endosteal scalloping.

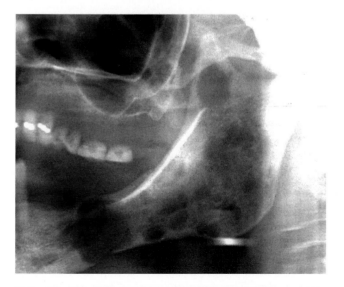

FIG. **21-12** Panoramic radiograph depicting multiple areas of well-defined bone destruction lacking any cortical boundary. The lesions are multiple, separate, and appear to be "punched out," typical of changes seen in multiple myeloma. (Courtesy G. Petrikowski, DDS, Toronto, Ontario, Canada.)

Any cortical boundary may be effaced if lesions involve them. Periosteal reaction is uncommon, but if present, takes the form of a single radiopaque line or more rarely a sunray appearance.

Differential diagnosis. The most likely disease to be mistaken for multiple myeloma is the radiolucent form of metastatic carcinoma. Knowledge of a prior malignancy in a patient may help differentiate multiple myeloma from metastatic carcinoma. Osteomyelitis, if severe, may yield a radiologic picture similar to that of multiple myeloma; however, a visible cause for it usually exists. In addition, inflammatory lesions and infections in general cause sclerosis in adjacent bone, which multiple myeloma does not. Simple bone cysts may be bilateral in the mandible and therefore may be mistaken for multiple myeloma. They are usually corticated in part and characteristically interdigitate between the roots of the teeth in a much younger population. Generalized radiolucency of the jaws may be caused by hyperparathyroidism but is differentiated based on abnormal blood chemistry. However, brown tumors of hyperparathyroidism, if present with generalized radiolucency of the jaws and similar symptomology, can readily be confused with multiple myeloma radiographically. Other metabolic diseases such as Gaucher's disease or oxalosis may cause many of the changes associated with multiple myeloma that are observed on dental radiographs.

Management. The management of multiple myeloma is usually chemotherapeutic with or without autologous or allogeneic bone marrow transplantation. Radiation therapy may be used for treatment of symptomatic osseous lesions when palliation is required.

NON-HODGKIN'S LYMPHOMA
Identfiying Characteristics
Synonyms. *Malignant lymphoma* and *lymphosarcoma*

Definition. Non-Hodgkin's lymphoma is a malignant tumor of cells normally resident in the lymphatic system. In general, lymphomas occur within lymph nodes; however, extranodal sites such as bone, skin, gastrointestinal mucosa, tonsils, and Waldeyer's ring can be involved. The term *non-Hodgkin's lymphoma* describes a family of heterogeneous tumors of varying type and severity. The classification of these diseases is difficult, and numerous means exist of subdividing these tumors. Currently the working formulation for clinical usage classifies tumors based on their histologic appearance into low-grade, intermediate-grade, or high-grade tumors, with the last being the most aggressive.

Clinical features. Non-Hodgkin's lymphoma occurs in all age groups but is rare in patients in the first decade. The maxillary sinus, palate, tonsillar area, and bone may be sites of primary or secondary lymphoma spread. Lesions occurring outside lymph nodes in the head and neck are present in as much as one out of five cases. Patients may feel unwell, experiencing night sweats, pruritus, and weight loss. Isolated lesions of the jaws may be accompanied by palpable painless swelling, lymphadenopathy, and sensorineural deficits. Lesions present for some time may cause pain and ulceration. Teeth resident in a lymphoma may become mobile as the supporting bone is lost.

Radiographic features

Location. Most non-Hodgkin's lymphomas of the head and neck occur in the lymph nodes. Those that are extranodal are likely to affect the maxillary sinus, posterior mandible, and maxillary regions.

Periphery and shape. Most non-Hodgkin's lymphomas initially take the shape and form of the host bone. If untreated, however, they are capable of causing destruction of the overlying cortex (Fig. 21-13). They may appear rounded or multiloculated and lack a defining outer cortex. Generally the borders are ill defined and invasive. Occasionally, lymphoma appears as multiple areas of destruction, which likely appear as finger-like extensions of malignant tumor cells in a buccal or lingual direction. Visible lesions occurring in the maxillary sinus or nasopharynx have a smooth periphery.

Internal structure. The internal structure of lymphoma is almost always entirely radiolucent. It is rare to see reactive osseous formation. Occasionally patchy radiopacity may be present, but this is rare.

Effects on surrounding structures. In maxillary sinus lesions the antral walls may be effaced and a soft tissue mass may be visible radiographically, either internally within the sinus or external to the maxillary sinus. Lesions involving the mandible destroy the cortex of the neurovascular canal. This tumor may grow in the periodontal ligament space of mature teeth. The cortex of the crypts of developing teeth may be lost when the lymphoma is located in the developing papilla, and the involved teeth may be displaced in an occlusal direction and exfoliated. Periosteal reaction is not common but may take the form of laminated or spiculated bone formation. Finally, resorption of the apices of teeth, although more commonly seen in odontogenic tumors and cysts, is fairly common in lymphomas affecting the alveolar processes.

Differential diagnosis. Multiple myeloma and metastatic carcinoma are easily confused with non-Hodgkin's lymphoma of the jaws. However, Ewing's sarcoma and Langerhans' histiocytosis, although also capable of producing the same effects, occur in a slightly younger age group. Osteolytic osteosarcoma and any of the central squamous cell carcinomas are not distinguishable radiographically from non-Hodgkin's lymphoma. Squamous cell carcinoma arising in the maxillary sinus may be difficult to differentiate from lymphoma of the maxillary sinus. Other lesions that can displace developing teeth in an occlusal direction include leukemia and Langerhans' histiocytosis. Differentiation from apical rarefying osteitis may be difficult; however, careful inspection of the radiographic film may reveal the presence of an infiltrative border and adjacent bone destruction.

Management. The management of extranodal or isolated nodal disease is radiation therapy with or without concomitant chemotherapy. Treatment depends on histologic variants and the location and extent of disease.

BURKITT'S LYMPHOMA

Identifying Characteristics
Synonym. *African jaw lymphoma*

Definition. Burkitt's lymphoma is a high-grade B-cell lymphoma that differs from other B-cell lymphomas with respect to its histologic appearance and clinical behavior. It was first described by Denis Burkitt in East Africa as an African jaw lymphoma.

Two separate forms of the disease have been described: the endemic African Burkitt's lymphoma and the American form. The latter is not characterized by jaw involvement (although it occurs), but by involvement of abdominal viscera. African Burkitt's lymphoma affects young children, whereas American Burkitt's lymphoma affects adolescents and young adults. Cases of endemic and nonendemic Burkitt's tumor have been described throughout the world.

Clinical features. The disease affects more males than females. Clinically the hallmark of this tumor is rapidity of growth with a tumor doubling time of less than 24 hours. It may involve children as young as 2 years and adults in their seventh decade, although it is primarily a disease of youth. Jaw tumors are rapidly growing and cause facial deformity very early in their course. They are capable of blocking nasal passages, displacing orbital contents, causing gross facial swelling, and eroding through skin. These rapidly growing tumors are more characteristic of Burkitt's lymphoma than the American form and cause pain and paresthesia. Teeth may become loosened rapidly and alveolar bone grossly distended. Paresthesia of the inferior alveolar nerve or other sensory facial nerves is common.

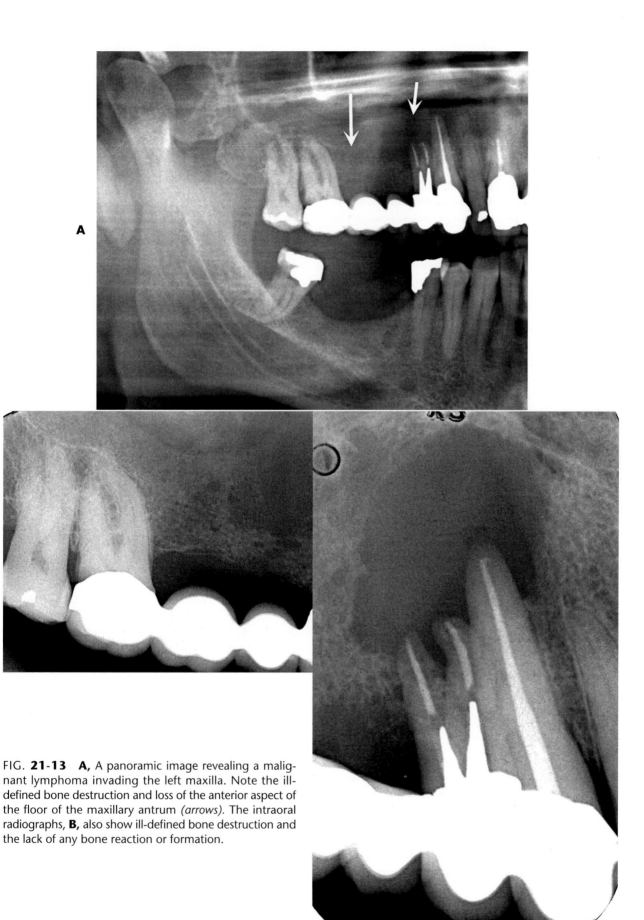

FIG. **21-13** **A,** A panoramic image revealing a malignant lymphoma invading the left maxilla. Note the ill-defined bone destruction and loss of the anterior aspect of the floor of the maxillary antrum *(arrows)*. The intraoral radiographs, **B,** also show ill-defined bone destruction and the lack of any bone reaction or formation.

Radiographic features

Location. Extranodal disease is the norm in Burkitt's tumor. African cases may involve one jaw or both the maxilla and mandible and affect the posterior parts of the jaws. By contrast, American cases may not involve the facial bones but are more likely to affect the abdominal viscera and testes.

Periphery and shape. The lesions may begin as multiple, ill-defined, noncorticated radiolucencies, which later coalesce into larger, ill-defined radiolucencies with an expansile periphery. They are of no specific shape, although they expand rapidly and have been likened to a balloon. This expansion breaches its outer cortical limits, causing gross balloonlike expansion with thinning of adjacent structures and production of a soft tissue tumor mass adjacent to the osseous lesion. Lesions that abut the orbital contents or the maxillary sinus may show a smooth surface soft tissue mass radiologically.

Internal structure. Burkitt's lymphoma does not produce bone and rarely induces production of reactive bone within its center. For this reason, the lesions are radiolucent in almost all cases. It is particularly radiolucent in the jaw of a child.

Effects on surrounding structures. Erupted teeth in the area of Burkitt's tumor are grossly displaced, as are developing tooth crypts. Tumor cells within the crypt may displace the developing tooth bud to one side of its crypt. A tumor that is located apical to a developing tooth may cause it to be displaced such that it appears to erupt with little if any root formation. After tumor involvement of the developing dental structures occurs, root development ceases. Lamina dura of teeth in the area is destroyed, and cortical boundaries such as the maxillary sinus, nasal floor, orbital walls, and inferior border of the mandible are thinned and later destroyed. The cortex of the inferior alveolar canal is lost, although it is difficult to see in the normal pediatric patient in any case. If periosteum is involved, the border may show sunray spiculation, although this is rare. Cases that involve the orbit displace the orbital contents, which is seen both clinically and radiologically.

Differential diagnosis

Differential diagnosis. Metastatic neuroblastoma may give similar changes clinically and radiologically, as may Ewing's tumor. Osteolytic osteosarcoma can grow rapidly and may be indistinguishable from Burkitt's tumor on clinical and radiologic grounds. Cherubism has more internal structure, does not breach bony borders, and grows much more slowly. Finally, non-Hodgkin's lymphoma must be considered, although it occurs in a much older age group in most cases.

Management

Management. The management of Burkitt's tumor is chemotherapeutic. Chemotherapy regimens vary from geographic locales, but the tumor is exquisitely sensitive to combinations of chemotherapeutic agents.

LEUKEMIA

Identifying Characteristics

Synonyms. *Acute myelogenous leukemia, acute lymphoblastic leukemia, chronic myelogenous leukemia,* and *chronic lymphocytic leukemia*

Definition. Leukemia is a malignant tumor of hematopoietic stem cells. These malignant cells displace normal bone marrow constituents and spill out into the peripheral blood. They are subdivided into acute leukemias and chronic leukemias and further subdivided by the cell of origin. The acute leukemias occur with a bimodal age distribution, with very young patients and very old patients being the most commonly affected. Most leukemias are associated with nonrandom chromosomal abnormalities.

Clinical features. The patient with chronic leukemia may have no presenting signs or complaints. Acute leukemia patients generally feel unwell with weakness and bone pain. They may exhibit pallor, spontaneous hemorrhage, hepatomegaly, splenomegaly, lymphadenopathy, and fever. Oral symptoms are generally absent but if present include loose teeth, petechiae, ulceration, and boggy enlarged gingiva.

Radiographic features. Radiologic signs associated with the chronic leukemias are comparatively rare.

Location. Leukemia affects the entire body because it is a malignancy of bone marrow, which discharges malignant cells into circulating blood. Its manifestations in the jaws may be seen more often in areas of developing teeth. Frequently, leukemia may be localized around the periapical region of a tooth, giving the appearance of a rarefying osteitis.

Periphery and shape. Leukemia must be considered a systemic malignancy, and as such its oral radiologic features may be present bilaterally as ill-defined patchy radiolucent areas. With time and lack of treatment, these patchy areas may coalesce to form larger areas of ill-defined radiolucent regions of bone (Fig. 21-14). The teeth may appear to stand out conspicuously from their surrounding, osteopenic bone.

Internal structure. The internal structure of leukemia is characterized by patchy areas of radiolucency and generalized radiolucency of the bone. Rarely, granular bone may be seen within these lesions. Occasionally, foci of leukemic cells may be present as a mass that may behave like a localized malignant tumor. These lesions are called *chloromas* and are rare in the jaws.

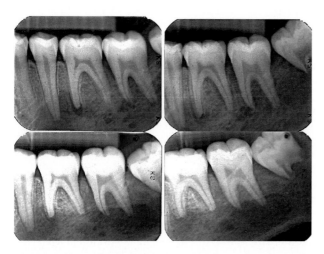

FIG. **21-14** Four periapical radiographs of the right mandible illustrating multifocal areas of bone destruction and widening of portions of the periodontal ligament space (note the mesial surface of the distal root of the first molar) characteristic of infiltration of the mandible with leukemia.

Effects on surrounding structures. Leukemia does not cause expansion of bone, although occasionally a single layer of periosteal new bone may be seen in association with this disease, this being uncommon in chronic leukemia. Developing teeth in their crypts and teeth undergoing eruption may be displaced within their crypts or into the oral cavity before root development. Less commonly, developing teeth may be displaced from their normal position. The result of this is premature loss of teeth. The lamina dura and cortical outlines of follicles may be effaced. If lesions affect the periodontal structures, the crestal bone may be lost.

Differential diagnosis. Generally, by the time oral radiologic signs of leukemia are present, a medical diagnosis has been reached. However, the development of radiologic changes may be the first indication of the relapse of treatment. Occasionally lymphoma or neuroblastoma may mimic some of the features of destruction seen in leukemia. Metabolic disorder may be considered in those cases in which generalized rarefaction of bone is seen. These conditions are all excluded based on blood testing. With apical lesions, careful examination of the involved tooth clinically and radiologically typically shows no apparent cause for rarefying osteitis.

Management. The management of leukemia is primarily through a combination of chemotherapy with or without allogeneic or autologous bone marrow transplantation. Some chronic leukemias are managed with low-dose chemotherapy.

Dental Radiology for the Cancer Survivor

The cancer survivor requires dental treatment just as any other patient. For the cancer survivor, dental radiologic examination may be more important than for a healthy patient receiving a routine examination. Some patients who have received a full course of radiation therapy are concerned about the additional exposure from a dental radiographic examination. However, this is not a valid concern because the small dose associated with dental radiographic examinations is negligible compared with the radiation dose received from cancer therapy.

The patient treated for head and neck malignancy with radiation therapy is prone to develop postradiation dental caries and osteoradionecrosis. Careful clinical examination and a thorough dental radiologic examination may be required periodically to ensure that the remaining dentition and periodontal apparatus is in good shape. Radiation caries occur in many patients and may appear clinically different from typical dental caries. If untreated, these carious teeth become nonvital and may cause infection in the underlying jaw. If they require extraction, healing can be expected to be slow and occasionally osteordionecrosis may result.

The role of radiology in these patients, however, is not restricted to examination of the teeth and supporting structures. Equally important is the monitoring of the outcome of treatment and specifically the examination of dental radiographs for evidence of tumor recurrence, development of metastases, and osteoradionecrosis.

SUGGESTED READINGS

SQUAMOUS CELL CARCINOMA

Carter RL: Patterns and mechanisms of spread of squamous carcinomas of the oral cavity, *Clin Otolaryngol* 15:185, 1990.

Marchetta FC, Sako K, Murphy JB: The periosteum of the mandible and intraoral carcinoma, *Am J Surg* 122:711, 1971.

McGregor AD, MacDonald D: Routes of entry of squamous cell carcinoma to the mandible, *Head Neck Surg* 10:284, 1988.

Noyek AM et al: The radiologic diagnosis of malignant tumors of the paranasal sinuses and related structures, *J Otolaryngol* 6:399, 1977.

O'Brien CJ et al: Invasions of the mandible by squamous carcinomas of the oral cavity and oropharynx, *Head Neck Surg* 8:247, 1986.

Worth HM: *Principles and practice of oral radiologic interpretation,* Chicago, 1963, Year Book Medical Publishers.

SQUAMOUS CELL CARCINOMA ORIGINATING IN BONE

Elzay RP: Primary intra-osseous carcinoma of the jaws, *Oral Surg Oral Med Oral Pathol* 54:299, 1982.

Yoshikazu S et al: Primary intra-osseous carcinoma: review of the literature and diagnostic criteria, *J Oral Maxillofac Surg* 52:580, 1994.

SQUAMOUS CELL CARCINOMA ORGINATING IN A CYST

Dabbs DJ et al: Squamous cell carcinoma arising in recurrent odontogenic keratocyst, *Head and Neck* 16:375, 1994.

Eversole LR, Sabre WR, Lovin S: Aggressive growth and neoplastic potential of odontogenic cysts, *Cancer* 35:270, 1975.

van der Wal, KGH, de Visscher JGAM, Eggink HF: Squamous cell carcinoma arising in a residual cyst, *Int J Oral Maxillofac Surg* 23:350, 1993.

Waldron CA, Mustoie TA: Primary intra-osseous carcinoma of the mandible with probable origin in an odontogenic cyst, *Oral Surg Oral Med Oral Pathol* 67:716, 1989.

MUCOEPIDERMOID CARCINOMA

Bilge OM, Dayi E: Central mucoepidermoid carcinoma of the jaws. Review of the literature and case report, *Ann Dentistry* 51:36, 1992.

Browand BC, Waldron CA: Central mucoepidermoid tumors of the jaws. Report of nine cases and review of the literature, *Oral Surg Oral Med Oral Pathol* 40:631, 1975.

Freije JE et al: Central mucoepidermoid carcinoma of the mandible, *Otolaryngol Head Neck Surg* 112:453, 1995.

Gingell JC et al: Central mucoepidermoid carcinoma, *Oral Surg Oral Med Oral Pathol* 57:436, 1984.

Sidoni A et al: Central mucoepidermoid carcinoma of the mandible, *J Oral Maxillofac Surg* 54:1242, 1996.

Waldron CA, Koh ML: Central mucoepidermoid carcinoma of the jaws, *J Oral Maxillofac Surg* 48:871, 1990.

MALIGNANT AMELOBLASTOMA AND AMELOBLASTIC CARCINOMA

Ameerally P, McGurk M, Shaheen O: Atypical ameloblastoma: report of 3 cases and review of the literature, *Br J Oral Maxillofac Surg* 34:235, 1996.

Buff SJ et al: Pulmonary metastasis from ameloblastoma of the mandible: report of a case and review of the literature, *J Oral Surg* 38:374, 1980.

Slootweg PJ, Muller H: Malignant ameloblastoma or ameloblastic carcinoma, *Oral Surg Oral Med Oral Pathol* 57:168, 1984.

METASTATIC TUMORS

Ciola B: Oral radiographic manifestations of a metastatic prostatic carcinoma, *Oral Surg* 52:105, 1981.

Mast HL, Nissenblatt MJ: Metastatic colon carcinoma to the jaw: a case report and review of the literature, *J Surg Oncol* 34:202, 1987.

Mucitelli DR, Zuna RE, Archard HO: Hepatocellular carcinoma presenting as an oral cavity lesion, *Oral Surg Oral Med Oral Pathol* 66:701, 1988.

Nevins A et al: Metastatic carcinoma of the mandible mimicking periapical lesion of endodontic origin, *Endod Dent Traumatol* 4:238, 1988.

Redman RS, Behrens AS, Calhoun NR: Carcinoma of the lung presenting as a mandibular metastasis, *J Oral Maxillofac Surg* 40:745, 1982.

Vigneul JC et al: Metastatic hepatocellular carcinoma of the mandible, *J Oral Maxillofac Surg* 40:745, 1982.

OSTEOGENIC SARCOMA

Batsakis JG: Osteogenic and chondrogenic sarcomas of the jaws, *Ann Otol Rhinol Laryngol* 96:474, 1987.

Bras JM et al: Juxta-cortical osteogenic sarcoma of the jaws, *Oral Surg* 50:535, 1980.

Clark JL et al: Osteosarcoma of the jaw, *Cancer* 51:2311, 1983.

Gardner DG, Mills DM: The widened periodontal ligament of osteosarcoma of the jaws, *Oral Surg* 41:652, 1976.

Seeger LL, Gold RH, Chandnani VP: Diagnostic imaging of osteosarcoma, *Clin Orthop Rel Res* 270:254, 1991.

Vener J, Rice DH, Newman AN: Osteosarcoma and chondrosarcoma of the head and neck, *Laryngoscope* 94:240, 1984.

Worth HM: *Principles and practice of oral radiologic interpretation,* Chicago, 1963, Year Book Medical Publishers.

CHONDROSARCOMA

Garrington GE, Collett WK: Chondrosarcoma. I. A selected literature review, *J Oral Pathol* 17:1, 1988.

Garrington GE, Collett WK: Chondrosarcoma. II. Chondrosarcoma of the jaws: analysis of 37 cases, *J Oral Pathol* 17:12, 1988.

Hertzanu Y et al: Chondrosarcoma of the head and neck—the value of computed tomography, *J Surg Oncol* 28:97, 1985.

Richter KJ, Freeman NS, Quick CA: Chondrosarcoma of the temporomandibular joint, *J Oral Surg* 32:777, 1974.

Vener J, Rice D, Newman AN: Osteosarcoma and chondrosarcoma of the head and neck, *Laryngoscope* 94:240, 1984.

Worth HM: *Principles and practice of oral radiologic interpretation,* Chicago, 1963, Year Book Medical Publishers.

EWING'S SARCOMA

Dahlin DC, Coventry MB, Scanlon PW: Ewing's sarcoma, *J Bone Joint Surg* 2:185, 1961.

Greer RO, Mierau GW, Favara BE: *Tumors of the head and neck in children,* New York, 1983, Praeger.

Wood RE et al: Ewing's sarcoma, *Oral Surg Oral Med Oral Pathol* 69:120, 1990.

Worth HM: *Principles and practice of oral radiologic interpretation,* Chicago, 1963, Year Book Medical Publishers.

FIBROSARCOMA

Dahlin DC: *Bone tumors,* Springfield, Ill, 1981, Charles C Thomas.

Eversole LR, Schwartz WD, Sabes WR: Central and peripheral fibrogenic and neurogenic sarcoma of the oral regions, *Oral Surg* 36:49, 1973.

Huvos AG: *Bone tumors,* Philadelphia, 1979, WB Saunders.

O'Day RA, Soule EH, Goresg RJ: Soft tissue sarcomas of the oral cavity, *Mayo Clin Proc* 39:169, 1964.

Slootweg PJ, Miller H: Fibrosarcoma of the jaws, *J Maxillofac Surg* 12:157, 1984.

Taconis WK, van Rijssel TG: Fibrosarcoma of the jaws, *Skeletal Radiol* 15:10, 1986.

van Blarcom CW, Masson JMK, Dahlin DC: Fibrosarcoma of the mandible, *Oral Surg* 32:428, 1971.

RHABDOMYOSARCOMA

Bras J, Batsakis JG, Luna MA: Rhabdomyosarcoma of the oral soft tissues, *Oral Surg* 64:585, 1987.

Dito WR, Batsakis JG: Rhabdomyosarcoma of the head and neck: an appraisal of the biologic behaviour in 170 cases, *Arch Surg* 84:582, 1962.

Grieman RB, Katsikeris NK, Symington JM: Rhabdomyosarcoma of the maxillary sinus. Review of the literature and report of a case, *J Oral Maxillofac Surg* 46:1090, 1988.

Masson JK, Soule EH: Embryonal rhabdomyosarcoma of the head and neck. Report of 88 cases, *Am J Surg* 110:585, 1965.

O'Day RA, Soule EH, Goresg RJ: Soft tissue sarcomas of the oral cavity, *Mayo Clin Proc* 39:169, 1964.

Stobbe GD, Dargeon HW: Embryonal rhabdomyosarcoma of the head and neck in children and adolescents, *Cancer* 3:826, 1950.

MULTIPLE MYELOMA

Bruce KW, Royer Q: Multiple myeloma occurring in the jaws, *Oral Surg* 6:729, 1953.

Epstein JB, Voss NJS, Stevenson-Moore P: Maxillofacial manifestations of multiple myeloma, *Oral Surg* 57:267, 1984.

Furutani M, Ohnishi M, Tanaka Y: Mandibular involvement in patients with multiple myeloma, *J Oral Maxillofac Surg* 52:23, 1994.

Huvos AG: *Bone tumors,* Philadelphia, 1979, WB Saunders.

Kaffe I, Ramon Y, Hertz M: Radiographic manifestations of multiple myeloma in the mandible, *Dentomaxillofac Radiol* 15:31, 1986.

Worth HM: *Principles and practice of oral radiologic interpretation,* Chicago, 1963, Year Book Medical Publishers.

NON-HODGKIN'S LYMPHOMA

Baker CG, Tichler JM: Malignant disease in the jaws, *J Can Assoc Radiol* 28:129, 1977.

Dahlin DC: *Bone tumors,* ed 3, Springfield, Ill, 1981, Charles C Thomas.

Daramola JO, Ajagbe HA: Presentation and behaviour of primary malignant lymphoma of the oral cavity in adult Africans.

Maxymiw WG: *Primary extra-nodal non-Hodgkin's lymphoma of the head and neck: a review of 199 cases,* (diploma essay), University of Toronto, 1995.

Wong DS et al : Extranodal Non-Hodgkin's lymphoma of the head and neck, *Am J Roentgenol* 123:471, 1975.

Worth HM: *Principles and practice of oral radiologic interpretation,* Chicago, 1963, Year Book Medical Publishers.

BURKITT'S LYMPHOMA

Adatia AK: Radiology of Burkitt's tumour in the jaws, *East Afr Med J* 43:290, 1966.

Adatia AK: Significance of jaw lesions in Burkitt's lymphoma, *Br Dent J* 145:263, 1978.

Burkitt DA: Sarcoma involving the jaws in African children, *Br J Surg* 46:218, 1958.

Levine PH et al: The American Burkitt's lymphoma registry: eight years' experience, *Cancer* 49:1016, 1982.

Sariban E, Donahue A, Magrath IT: Jaw involvement in American Burkitt's lymphoma, *Cancer* 53:1777, 1984.

LEUKEMIA

Curtis AB: Childhood leukemias: initial oral manifestations, *JADA* 83:159, 1971.

Ficarra G et al: Granulocytic sarcoma (chloroma) of the oral cavity: a case with a leukemic presentation, *Oral Surg* 53:709, 1987.

Greer RO, Mierau GW, Favara BE: *Tumors of the head and neck in children,* New York, 1983, Praeger Scientific.

Worth HM: *Principles and practice of oral radiologic interpretation,* Chicago, 1963, Year Book Medical Publishers.

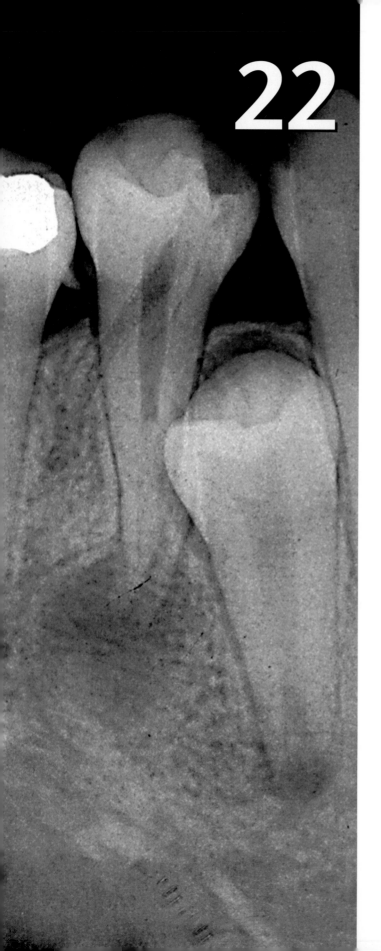

22 Diseases of Bone Manifested in the Jaws

This chapter discusses disorders of bone that do not easily fit into well-defined categories of disease.

Bone Dysplasias

Bone dysplasias constitute a group of conditions in which normal bone is replaced with fibrous tissue containing abnormal bone or cementum. These lesions must be differentiated from tumors. *Fibroosseous lesion* is a commonly used term that includes the following bone dysplasias as well as neoplasms and other lesions of bone.

FIBROUS DYSPLASIA

Definition

Fibrous dysplasia results from a localized change in normal bone metabolism that results in the replacement of all the components of cancellous bone by fibrous tissue containing varying amounts of abnormal-appearing bone. Histologically, this results in the appearance of numerous short, irregularly shaped trabeculae of woven bone. These trabeculae are not aligned in response to stress but rather have a random orientation. This histologic appearance is responsible for the internal pattern seen in radiographs. Fibrous dysplasias may be solitary or multiple (Jaffe type) or may occur in another multiple form associated with McCune-Albright syndrome, which usually comprises polyostotic fibrous dysplasia, cutaneous pigmentation (café au lait spots), and hyperfunction of one or more of the endocrine glands.

Clinical Features

The solitary (monostotic) form of fibrous dysplasia, which accounts for 70% of all cases, is the type that most often involves the jaws. The most common sites (in order) are the ribs, femur, tibia, maxilla, and mandible. The multiple (polyostotic) form usually is found in children under 10 years, whereas monostotic disease typically is discovered in a slightly older age group. The lesions usually become static when skeletal growth stops, but proliferation may continue, particularly in the polyostotic form. The lesions may become active in pregnant females or with the use of oral contraceptives; this condition has been reported to occur after surgical intervention in young patients. Studies of the sex distribution of fibrous dysplasia show no sexual predilection except for McCune-Albright syndrome, which affects females almost exclusively. Symptoms of the disease may be mild or absent. Monostotic fibrous dysplasia often is discovered as an incidental radiographic finding. Patients with jaw involvement first may complain of unilateral facial swelling or an enlarging deformity of the alveolar process. Pain and pathologic fractures are rare. If extensive craniofacial lesions have impinged on nerve foramina, neurologic symptoms such as anosmia (loss of the sense of smell), deafness, or blindness may develop.

Radiographic Features

Location. Fibrous dysplasia involves the maxilla almost twice as often as the mandible and occurs more frequently in the posterior aspect. Lesions more commonly are unilateral (Fig. 22-1) except for very rare extensive lesions of the maxillofacial region that are bilateral.

Periphery. The periphery of fibrous dysplasia lesions most commonly is ill defined, with a gradual blending of normal trabecular bone into an abnormal trabecular pattern. Occasionally the boundary between normal bone and the lesion can appear sharp and even corticated, especially in young lesions (Fig. 22-2).

Internal structure. The density and trabecular pattern of fibrous dysplasia lesions vary considerably. The variation is more pronounced in the mandible and more homogeneous in the maxilla. The internal aspect of bone may be more radiolucent, more radiopaque, or a mixture of these two variations compared with normal bone (see Fig. 22-1). The internal density is more radiopaque in the maxilla and the base of the skull. Early lesions may be more radiolucent (Fig. 22-3) than mature lesions and

in rare cases may appear to have granular internal septa, giving the internal aspect a multilocular appearance.

The abnormal trabeculae usually are shorter, thinner, irregularly shaped, and more numerous than normal trabeculae. This creates a radiopaque pattern that can vary; it may have a granular appearance (or "ground-glass" appearance, resembling the small fragments of a shattered windshield), a pattern resembling the surface of an orange (peau d'orange), a wispy arrangement (cotton wool), or an amorphous, dense pattern (Fig. 22-4). A distinctive characteristic is the organization of the abnormal trabeculae into a swirling pattern similar to a fingerprint (Fig. 22-5). Occasionally radiolucent regions resembling cysts may occur in mature lesions of fibrous dysplasia. These are bone cavities that are analogous to simple bone cysts.

Effects on surrounding structures. If the fibrous dysplasia lesion is small, it may have no effect on surrounding structures (subclinical variety). The effects on the involved bone may include expansion with maintenance of a thinned outer cortex (Fig. 22-6). Fibrous dysplasia may expand into the antrum by displacing its cortical boundary and subsequently occupying part or most of the maxillary sinus. Extension into the maxillary antrum usually occurs from the lateral wall, and the last section of the sinus to be involved usually is the most postero-superior portion. Cortical boundaries such as the floor of the antrum may be changed into the abnormal bone pattern. Often the bone surrounding the teeth is altered without affecting the dentition, and a distinct lamina dura disappears because this bone also is changed into the abnormal bone pattern (see Fig. 22-5). If the fibrous dysplasia increases the bone density, the periodontal ligament space may appear to be very narrow. Fibrous dysplasia can displace teeth or interfere with normal eruption, complicating orthodontic therapy. In rare cases, some root resorption may occur. Fibrous dysplasia appears to be unique in its ability to displace the inferior alveolar nerve canal in a superior direction (Fig. 22-7).

Differential Diagnosis

Other diseases can alter the bone pattern in a similar fashion. Metabolic bone diseases such as hyperparathyroidism may produce a similar pattern. However, these diseases are polyostotic, bilateral, and, unlike fibrous dysplasia, do not cause bone expansion. Paget's disease may produce a similar pattern and may cause expansion, but it occurs in an older age group, and when it involves the mandible, the whole mandible is involved, unlike

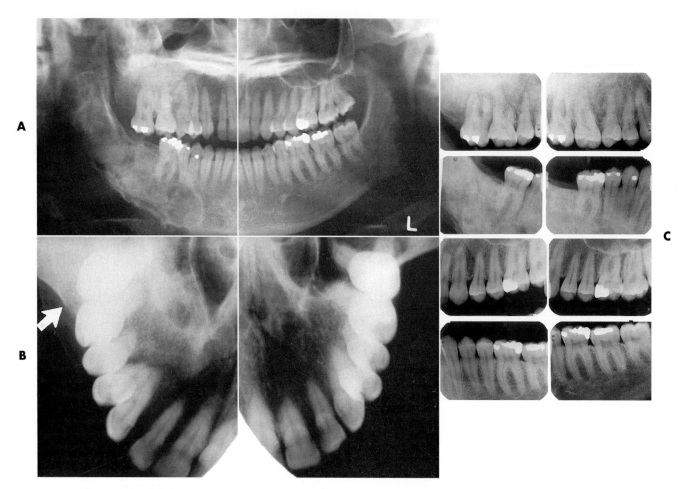

FIG. **22-1**   **A,** Unilateral fibrous dysplasia in the right maxilla and right mandible. **B,** Note the expansion of the lateral aspect of the maxilla *(arrow)* and the increased bone density caused by an increase in the number of internal trabeculae. **C,** Periapical films show a mixed radiolucent-radiopaque internal structure; however, the overall radiopacity is greater than on the left side of the jaws.

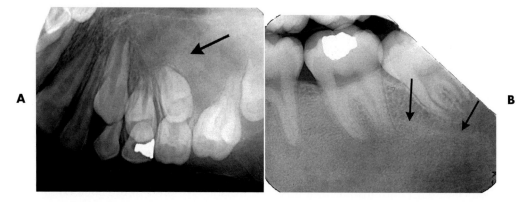

FIG. **22-2**   **A,** Fibrous dysplasia in the posterior maxilla, with an ill-defined anterior margin that blends into the normal bone pattern in the region of the unerupted cuspid. The internal pattern is granular *(arrow)*. **B,** In contrast, the margin of this case of mandibular fibrous dysplasia has a well-defined, almost corticated margin *(arrows)*.

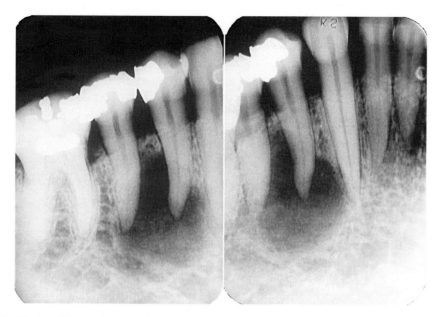

FIG. **22-3** *Fibrous dysplasia in the mandible.* At this early stage the internal structure has very little bone and therefore is radiolucent. Note that the lamina dura is less apparent. (Courtesy Dr. L. Hollender, Seattle, Wash.)

the unilateral tendency of fibrous dysplasia. Occasionally periapical cemental dysplasia may show a similar bone pattern, but the distribution is different in that it often is bilateral, with an epicenter in the periapical region. Furthermore, periapical cemental dysplasia also occurs in an older age group. With spontaneous healing of a simple bone cyst, the radiographic and histologic appearance of the new bone may be very similar to that of fibrous dysplasia.

Of paramount importance is the differentiation of osteomyelitis and osteogenic sarcoma because of both radiologic and histologic similarities. Osteomyelitis may result in enlargement of the jaws, but the additional bone is generated by the periosteum; therefore the new bone is laid down on the surface of the outer cortex, and close examination may reveal evidence of the original cortex within the expanded portion of the jaw. Fibrous dysplasia, in contrast, expands the internal aspect of bone, displacing and thinning the outer cortex so that the remaining cortex maintains its position at the outer surface of the bone. The identification of sequestra aids in the identification of osteomyelitis. Osteogenic sarcoma may produce a similar pattern but should show malignant radiologic features (see Chapter 21).

Some difficulty may arise in differentiating cemento-ossifying fibroma of the maxilla, especially the juvenile ossifying fibroma type. If the bone pattern is altered around the teeth without displacement of the teeth from one specific epicenter, the lesion probably is fibrous dysplasia. The shape of the bone expansion of fibrous dysplasia into the antrum reflects the original outer contour of the antral wall, which is different from the more convex extension of a neoplasm.

Management

In most cases the radiographic characteristics of fibrous dysplasia and the clinical information are sufficient to allow the practitioner to make a diagnosis without a biopsy. There are reports of exaggerated growth from stimulation of a lesion during surgical intervention in young patients. A consultation with a dental radiologist is advisable. The radiologist may supplement the examination with computed tomography (CT), which can give a more accurate, three-dimensional representation of the extent of the lesion and can serve as a precise baseline study for future comparisons. It is reasonable to continue occasional monitoring of the lesion or ask the patient to report any changes. With most lesions, growth is complete at skeletal maturation, therefore orthodontic treatment and cosmetic surgery may be delayed until this time. Sarcomatous changes are unusual but have been reported, especially if therapeutic radiation has been given. In the case of female patients, hormonal changes from pregnancy or the use of oral contraceptives may stimulate growth or result in the development of lesions within the area of fibrous dysplasia, such as aneurysmal bone cysts or giant cell granulomas.

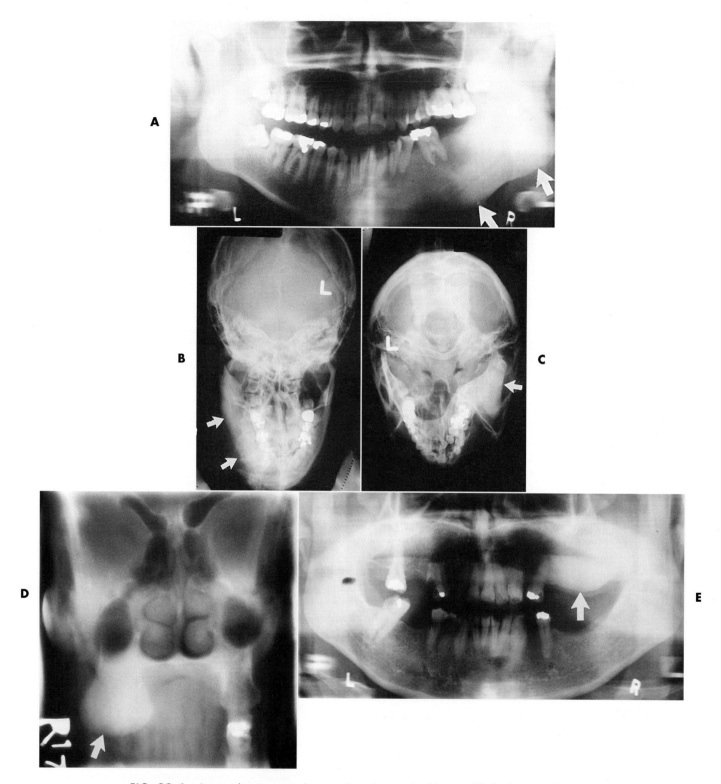

FIG. **22-4**   A very dense, amorphous pattern is seen in this mandibular lesion of fibrous dysplasia. Panoramic **(A)**, Towne's **(B)**, and submentovertex **(C)** projections also show the expansion of the mandible *(arrows)*. In another patient **(D** and **E)** a tomograph and a panoramic radiograph show a sclerotic lesion of the right maxilla.

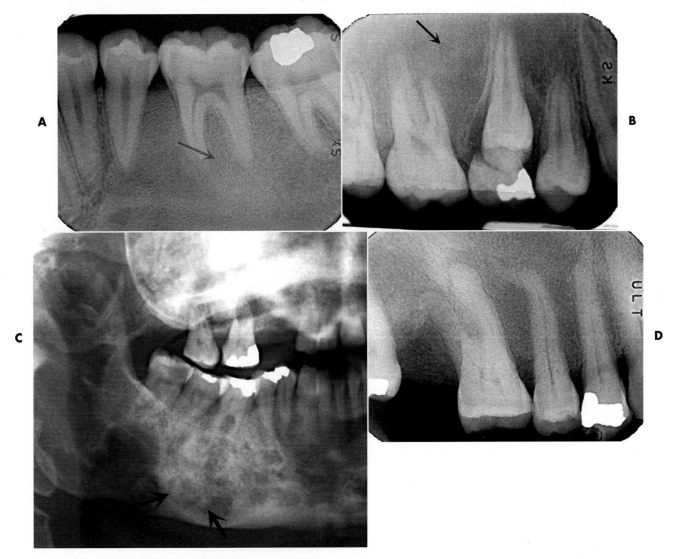

FIG. **22-5** *A series of films showing a variety of internal patterns of fibrous dysplasia.* **A,** A fingerprint pattern around the roots of the first molar *(arrow)*. Note the change in the lamina dura around the molars into the abnormal bone pattern. **B,** A granular or ground-glass pattern *(arrow)*. **C,** A cotton wool pattern. Note the almost circular radiopaque regions *(arrows)*. **D,** An orange-peel pattern.

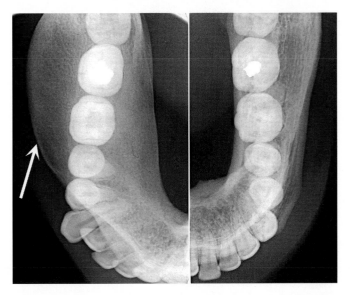

FIG. **22-6** Occlusal views of both sides of the mandible of the same patient. Note the expansion of the right side of the mandible caused by fibrous dysplasia. The outer cortical plates have been displaced and thinned but are still intact *(arrow)*.

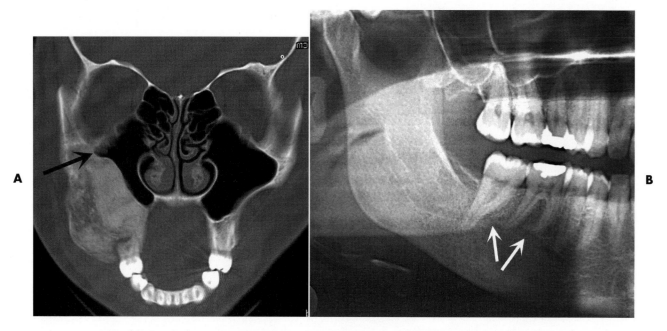

FIG. **22-7**   **A,** A coronal CT scan using bone algorithm of a maxillary lesion of fibrous dysplasia. The lesion has caused the lateral wall of the maxilla to expand into the maxillary antrum. The shape of the lateral wall of the sinus has maintained the zygomatic recess *(arrow)*. **B,** Mandibular fibrous dysplasia that has displaced the inferior alveolar nerve canal in a superior direction *(arrows)*.

CEMENTOOSSEOUS DYSPLASIAS

Periapical cemental dysplasia and florid osseous dysplasia are essentially the same process but are separated on the basis of the extent of involvement of the jaws.

Periapical Cemental Dysplasia

Synonyms. *Cementoma, fibrocementoma, sclerosing cementoma, periapical osteofibrosis, periapical fibrous dysplasia,* and *periapical fibroosteoma*

Definition. Periapical cemental dysplasia (PCD) is a localized change in normal bone metabolism that results in the replacement of the components of normal cancellous bone with fibrous tissue and cementum-like material, abnormal bone (similar to that seen in fibrous dysplasia), or a mixture of the two. By definition the lesion is located near the apex of a tooth.

Clinical features. PCD is a common bone dysplasia that typically occurs in middle age, the mean age being 39 years. It occurs nine times more often in females than in males and almost three times more often in blacks than in whites. It also frequently is seen in Asians. The involved teeth are vital, and the patient usually has no history of pain or sensitivity. The lesions usually come to light as an incidental finding during a periapical or panoramic radiographic examination made for other purposes. The lesions can become quite large, causing a

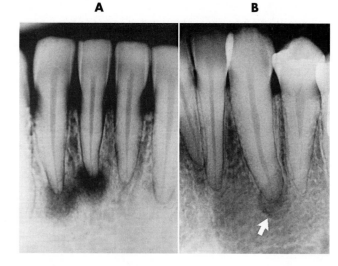

FIG. **22-8**   *PCD: radiolucent stage.* **A,** The lamina dura around the central incisor has been lost. **B,** Part of the lamina dura is present *(arrow)*.

notable expansion of the alveolar process, and may continue to enlarge slowly.

Radiographic features

Location. The epicenter of a PCD lesion usually lies at the apex of a tooth (Fig. 22-8). In rare cases the epicenter is slightly higher and over the apical third of the root. The condition has a predilection for the periapical bone

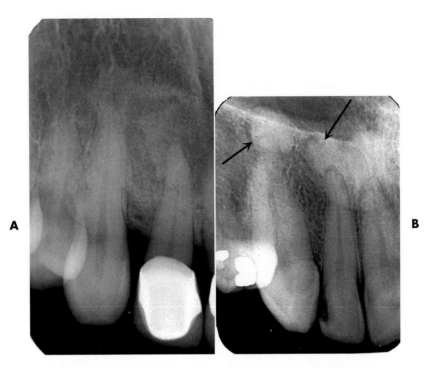

FIG. **22-9** *Examples of PCD in the maxilla.* **A,** A mixed lesion. **B,** Mature lesions *(arrows).*

of the mandibular anterior teeth, although any tooth can be involved, and in rare cases the maxillary teeth may be involved (Fig. 22-9). In most cases the lesion is multiple and bilateral, but occasionally a solitary lesion arises. If the involved teeth have been extracted, the periapical location is less evident (Fig. 22-10). In these cases the term *cemental dysplasia* may be more appropriate.

Periphery and shape. In most cases the periphery of a PCD lesion is well defined. Often a radiolucent border of varying width is present, surrounded by a band of sclerotic bone that also can vary in width (Fig. 22-11). The sclerotic bone represents a reaction of the immediate surrounding bone. The lesion may be irregularly shaped or may have an overall round or oval shape centered over the apex of the tooth.

Internal structure. The internal structure varies, depending on the maturity of the lesion. In the *early stage,* normal bone is resorbed and replaced with fibrous tissue that usually is continuous with the periodontal ligament (causing loss of the lamina dura). Radiographically, this appears as a radiolucency at the apex of the involved tooth (see Fig. 22-8).

In the *mixed stage,* radiopaque tissue appears in the radiolucent structure. This material usually is amorphous; has a round, oval, or irregular shape; and is composed of cementum or abnormal bone (see Fig. 22-11). These structures sometimes are called cementicles; however, this is a radiographic term that does not necessarily represent the histologic appearance. In rare cases the radiopaque material resembles the

abnormal trabecular patterns seen in fibrous dysplasia (Fig. 22-12).

In the *mature stage,* the internal aspect may be totally radiopaque without any obvious pattern. Usually a thin, radiolucent margin can be seen at the periphery because this lesion matures from the center outward (Fig. 22-13). Occasionally this radiolucent margin is not apparent, which makes the differential diagnosis more difficult. The internal structure may appear dramatically radiolucent if cavities resembling simple bone cysts form within the cemental lesions (Fig. 22-14). In some cases the simple bone cyst extends beyond the margin of the cemental lesion.

Effects on surrounding structures. The normal lamina dura of the teeth involved with the lesion is lost, making the periodontal ligament space either less apparent or giving it a wider appearance (see Fig. 22-8). The tooth structure usually is not affected, although in rare cases some root resorption may occur. Also, occasionally hypercementosis occurs on the root of a tooth positioned within the lesion. Some lesions stimulate a sclerotic bone reaction from the surrounding bone. Small lesions do not cause expansion of the involved jaw. However, larger lesions may cause expansion of the jaw, an area that is always bordered by a thin, intact outer cortex similar to that seen in fibrous dysplasia. This lesion may elevate the floor of the maxillary antrum.

Differential diagnosis. In early (radiolucent) PCD lesions, the most important differential diagnosis is periapical rarefying osteitis. Occasionally PCD cannot be

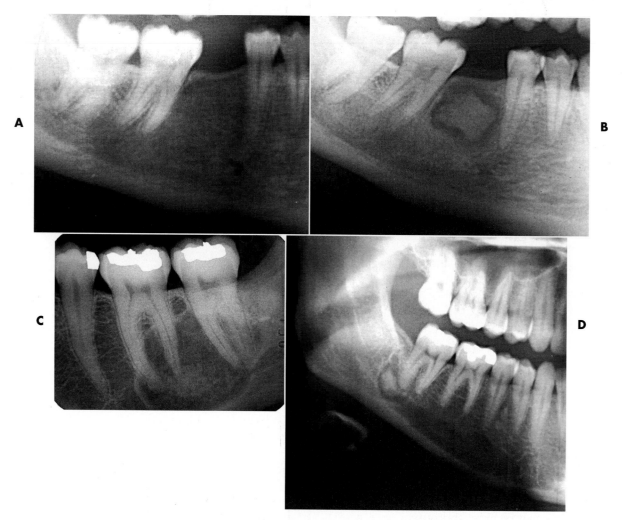

FIG. **22-10**   **A** and **B** are portions of panoramic views of the same patient taken 3 years apart. Note the development of a solitary lesion of PCD in the apical region of the first molar extraction site. **C** and **D** show solitary lesions in the posterior mandible.

distinguished from this inflammatory lesion by radiographic characteristics alone. In these cases the final diagnosis must rely on clinical information such as testing of the vitality of the involved tooth.

In the mixed and late forms of PCD the differential diagnosis may include a benign cementoblastoma. This tumor is solitary and usually is attached to the surface of the root, which may be partly resorbed. The presence or absence of clinical symptoms may help distinguish PCD from benign cementoblastoma. Another lesion to consider is an odontoma. Odontomas often start occlusal to a tooth and prevent its eruption, but some odontomas may have a periapical position. The organization of the internal aspect into toothlike structures and the identification of enamel (very radiopaque) can help in the differential diagnosis. Also, the peripheral cortex and soft tissue capsule of an odontoma are more

uniform in width and better defined than is the periphery of PCD. In mature PCD lesions, the appearance may resemble that of a dense bone island. The finding of a radiolucent periphery, even if very slight, indicates a diagnosis of PCD.

Management. The diagnosis of PCD can be made on the basis of the appropriate radiologic and clinical characteristics. In fact, a possible complication of biopsy is secondary infection, which may occur in lesions that have abundant cementum formation and poor vascularity. Normally treatment is not required. However, if the teeth have been removed and if considerable atrophy of the alveolar ridge has occurred, these segments of cementum may reach the mucosal surface, much in the same way as stones become exposed in old, worn concrete. These pieces of cementum can perforate the

A

B

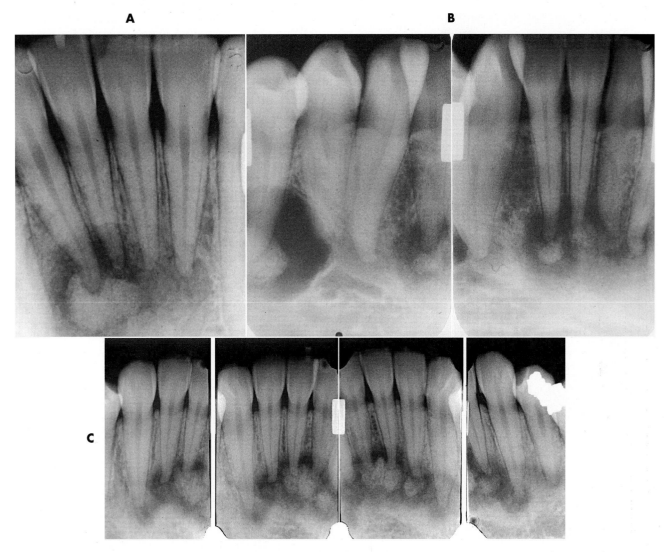

C

FIG. **22-11** *PCD: mixed stage.* **A** and **B,** Radiopacity in the center of a radiolucent area. **C,** Multiple lesions. Note the band of sclerotic bone reaction at the periphery of the lesion.

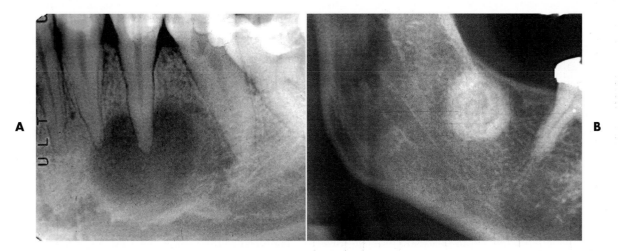

A

B

FIG. **22-12 A,** PCD with a fibrous dysplasia type of internal bone pattern. **B,** A swirling internal pattern of cemental dysplasia.

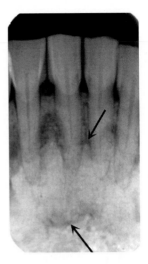

FIG. **22-13** *The mature stage of PCD.* Note the thin, radiolucent periphery *(arrows).*

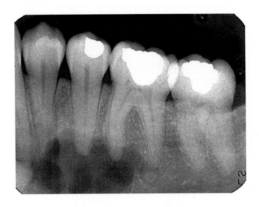

FIG. **22-14** A simple bone cyst within an area of PCD.

mucosa when positioned under a denture, and the result is secondary infection. If this occurs, the pieces of cementum may have to be removed surgically because they can act as sequestra in osteomyelitis.

Florid Osseous Dysplasia

Synonyms. *Florid cementoosseous dysplasia, gigantiform cementoma,* and *familial multiple cementomas*

Definition. Florid osseous dysplasia (FOD) appears be a widespread form of PCD. Normal cancellous bone is replaced with dense, acellular cementoosseous tissue in a background of fibrous connective tissue. The lesion has a poor vascular supply, a condition that likely contributes to its susceptibility to infection. In some cases a familial trend can be seen. No clear definition indicates when multiple regions of PCD should be termed FOD. However, if PCD is identified in three or four quadrants or is extensive throughout one jaw, it usually is considered to be FOD.

Clinical features. Several key similarities exist between FOD and PCD, including the age, sex, and racial profiles of patients and comparable radiographic and histologic appearances. Most patients with FOD are female and middle-aged (the mean age being 42 years), although the age range is broad. The condition shows a marked predilection for blacks and Asians. Often FOD produces no symptoms and is found incidentally during a radiographic examination. Occasionally patients complain of intermittent, poorly localized pain in the affected bone, especially when a simple bone cyst has developed within the lesion. Extensive lesions often have an associated bony swelling. If the lesions become secondarily infected, features of osteomyelitis may develop, including mucosal ulceration, fistulous tracts with suppuration, and pain. Teeth in the involved bone are vital unless other dental disease coincidentally affects them.

Radiographic features

Location. FOD lesions usually are bilateral and present in both jaws (Fig. 22-15). However, when they are present in only one jaw, the mandible is the more common location. The epicenter is apical to the teeth, within the alveolar process and usually posterior to the cuspid. In the mandible, lesions occur above the inferior alveolar canal.

Periphery. The periphery usually is well defined and has a sclerotic border that can vary in width, very similar to PCD. The soft tissue capsule may not be apparent in mature lesions.

Internal structure. The density of the internal structure can vary from an equal mixture of radiolucent and radiopaque regions to almost complete radiopacity. Some prominent radiolucent regions may be present, which usually represent the development of a simple bone cyst (Fig. 22-16). These cysts may enlarge with time or may fill in with abnormal dysplastic cementoosseous tissue. The radiopaque regions can vary from small oval and circular regions (cotton-wool appearance) to large, irregular, amorphous areas of calcification. These calcified masses are similar in appearance to those seen in mature PCD lesions.

Effects on surrounding structures. Large FOD lesions can displace the inferior alveolar nerve canal in an inferior direction. FOD also can displace the floor of the antrum in a superior direction and can cause enlargement of the alveolar bone by displacement of the buccal and lingual cortical plates. The roots of associated teeth may have a considerable amount of hypercementosis, which may fuse with the abnormal surrounding cemental tissue of the lesion. Extraction of these teeth may be difficult.

Differential diagnosis. The fact that FOD is bilateral and centered in the alveolar process helps in the differentiation from other lesions. Paget's disease of bone may

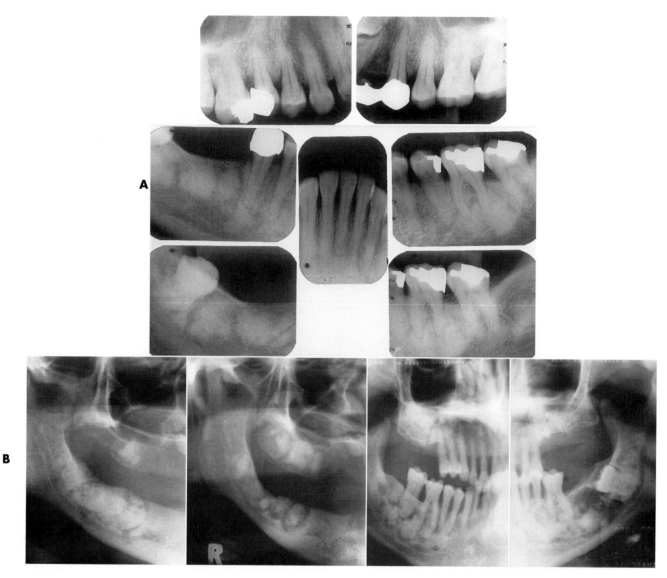

FIG. 22-15 *FOD.* **A,** Multiple radiopaque lesions in the periapical regions throughout the jaws. **B** and **C,** Lesions involving all four quadrants. Note the radiolucent periphery and the fact that the epicenter of the mandibular lesions is above the inferior alveolar canal. (Courtesy Dr. H. Abrams, Los Angeles, Calif.)

also show cotton-wool–type radiopaque regions with associated hypercementosis. However, Paget's disease affects the bone of the entire mandible, whereas FOD is centered above the inferior alveolar canal. Furthermore, Paget's disease often is polyostotic, involving other bones as well as the jaws. The well-defined nature of FOD, with its radiolucent periphery and surrounding sclerotic border, also is useful in making the differential diagnosis.

Another disease that may resemble FOD is chronic sclerosing osteomyelitis. Regions of cementum may appear that are similar to the sequestrum seen in osteomyelitis. CT imaging can aid in the differential diagnosis. Another

confusing factor may be the development of a secondary osteomyelitis that may mask the underlying FOD.

Management. Under normal circumstances, FOD does not require treatment, although there is value in obtaining a panoramic film to establish the extent of the disease. Unlike with fibrous dysplasia, no age limit is apparent for the cessation of growth of FOD. Because of the propensity to develop secondary infections in FOD, the patient should be encouraged to maintain an effective oral hygiene program to avoid odontogenic infections. Also, if the teeth are extracted and severe atrophy of the alveolar process occurs, as in PCD, the cementum

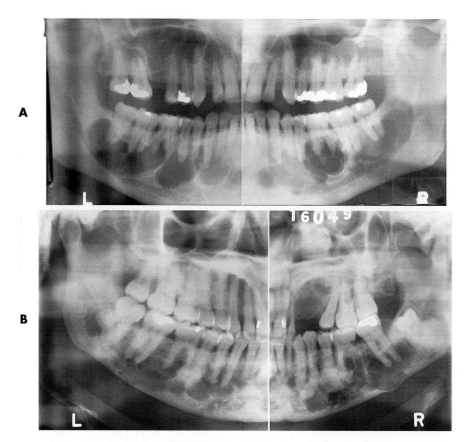

FIG. **22-16**   *FOD associated with multiple simple bone cysts.* **A,** Large cysts occupy most of the bone involved with the FOD lesions. **B,** Another example of multiple simple bone cysts in lesions of FOD.

masses emerge and the pressure of the overlying denture may cause dehiscence in the mucosa, resulting in osteomyelitis. If this occurs, the avascular cemental masses become large sequestra. The osteomyelitis may spread slowly throughout the jaw from one region of FOD to another. It may be necessary to remove large areas of cemental tissue, leaving very little residual bone for prosthetic treatment.

Other Lesions of Bone

CEMENTOOSSIFYING FIBROMA

Synonyms

Ossifying fibroma and *cementifying fibroma*

Definition

Cementoossifying fibroma (COF) is classified as and behaves like a benign bone neoplasm. However, it appears in this chapter because it often is considered to be a type of fibroosseous lesion. This bone tumor consists of highly cellular, fibrous tissue that contains varying amounts of abnormal bone or cementum-like tissue. In the past this lesion was classified as two different entities depending

on whether bone or cementum was the predominant calcified product. When the histologic appearance of most of the calcified tissue was of irregular trabeculae of woven bone, the term *ossifying fibroma* was used. The resulting internal pattern may be very similar to or indistinguishable from fibrous dysplasia. One distinguishing feature that may be present is a soft tissue capsule at the periphery not seen in fibrous dysplasia. When the predominant calcified component was cementum, the term *cementifying fibroma* was used. However, the microscopic appearance of an ossifying fibroma and a cementifying fibroma can be very similar, and the two are now thought to represent a spectrum of one disease and are combined under the name *cementoossifying fibroma*.

Juvenile ossifying fibroma is a very aggressive form of COF that occurs in the first two decades of life. Although the histopathologic definition of this entity is controversial, the radiologic appearance has similarities to that of COF.

Clinical Features

The clinical features of COF can vary from indolent to aggressive behavior. The characteristics are more like those of a tumor than a bone dysplasia. COF can occur at

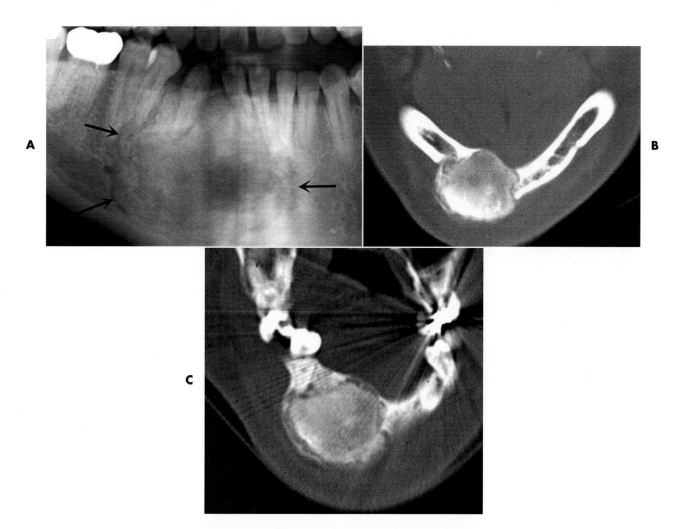

FIG. **22-17** A cementifying fibroma depicted in a panoramic film *(arrows)* **(A)**, an axial CT scan **(B)**, and a coronal CT scan **(C)**. Note the homogeneous, radiopaque internal structure and the radiolucent band at the periphery.

any age but usually is found in young adults. Females are affected more often than males. The disease usually is asymptomatic at the time of discovery. Occasionally facial asymmetry develops. Displacement of the teeth may be an early clinical feature, although most lesions are discovered during routine dental examinations. In cases of juvenile ossifying fibroma, rapid growth may occur in a young patient, resulting in deformity of the involved jaw.

Radiographic Features
Location. COF appears almost exclusively in the facial bones and most commonly in the mandible, typically inferior to the premolars and molars and superior to the inferior alveolar canal. In the maxilla it occurs most often in the canine fossa and zygomatic arch area.

Periphery. The borders of COF lesions usually are well defined. A thin, radiolucent line, representing a fibrous capsule, may separate it from surrounding bone (Fig.

22-17). Sometimes the bone next to the lesion develops a sclerotic border.

Internal structure. The internal structure of a COF lesion is a mixed radiolucent-radiopaque density with a pattern that depends on the amount and form of the manufactured calcified material. In some instances the internal structure may appear almost totally radiolucent with just a hint of calcified material (Fig. 22-18). In the type that contains mainly abnormal bone, the pattern may be similar to that seen in fibrous dysplasia, or a wispy (similar to stretched tufts of cotton) or flocculent pattern (similar to large, heavy snowflakes) may be seen (Fig. 22-19). Lesions that produce more cementum-like material may contain solid, amorphous radiopacities (cementicles) similar to those seen in cemental dysplasia (see Fig. 22-17).

Effects on surrounding structures. COF can be distinguished from the previously mentioned bone dysplasias by its tumorlike behavior. This is reflected in the growth of the lesion, which tends to be concentric within the medullary part of the bone with outward expansion approximately equal in all directions. This can result in displacement of teeth or of the inferior alveolar canal and expansion of the outer cortical plates of bone. A significant point is that the outer cortical plate, although dis-

placed and thinned, remains intact. The COF lesion can grow into and occupy the entire maxillary sinus (Fig. 22-20), expanding its walls outward; however, a bony partition always exists between the internal aspect of the remaining sinus and the tumor. The lamina dura of involved teeth usually is missing, and resorption of teeth may occur.

Differential Diagnosis

The differential diagnosis of COF includes lesions with a mixed radiolucent-radiopaque internal structure. The differentiation from fibrous dysplasia can be very difficult. The boundaries of a COF lesion usually are better defined, and these lesions occasionally have a soft tissue capsule and cortex, whereas fibrous dysplasia usually blends in with surrounding bone. The internal structure of fibrous dysplasia lesions may be more homogeneous and show less variation. Both types of lesions can displace teeth, but COF displaces from a specific point or epicenter. Fibrous dysplasia rarely resorbs teeth.

Great difficulty may arise in differentiating juvenile ossifying fibroma from fibrous dysplasia when the lesion involves the maxillary antrum. Fibrous dysplasia usually displaces the lateral wall of the maxilla into the maxillary antrum, maintaining the outer shape of the wall,

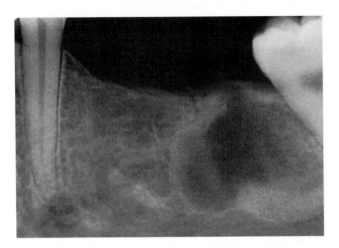

FIG. **22-18** An early radiolucent stage of a COF in an edentulous region of the alveolar process.

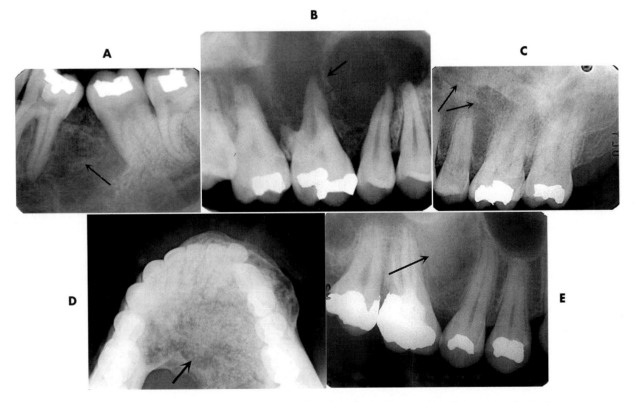

FIG. **22-19** *Various bone patterns seen in COFs.* **A,** A wispy trabecular pattern *(arrow).* **B,** Most of this pattern is radiolucent with a few wispy trabeculae *(arrow).* **C,** A fibrous dysplasia granular-like pattern *(arrows).* **D,** A flocculent pattern with larger tufts of bone formation *(arrow).* **E,** A solid, radiopaque, cementum-like pattern *(arrow).*

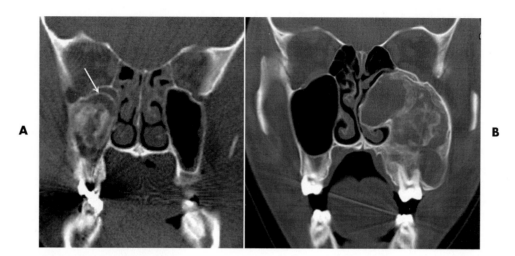

FIG. **22-20** *Large COFs involving the maxilla.* **A,** A coronal CT scan of a lesion invaginating the maxillary antrum. Note that unlike in fibrous dysplasia, the peripheral border of the lesion *(arrow)* does not parallel the original shape of the antrum. **B,** A coronal CT scan of a larger lesion expanding the maxilla, occupying all of the maxillary antrum, and extending into the nasal fossa.

whereas an ossifying fibroma has a more convex shape as it extends into the maxillary antrum (see Figs. 22-7 and 22-20). Also, fibrous dysplasia may change the bone around the teeth without moving them, which differs from the concentric growth of a tumor. The importance of this differentiation lies in the treatment, which is resection for an ossifying fibroma and observation for fibrous dysplasia.

The differential diagnosis of the type of COF that produces mainly cementum-like material from PCD may be difficult, especially with large single lesions of PCD. However, cemental dysplasia usually is multifocal whereas COF is not. Also, the presence of a simple bone cyst is a characteristic of cemental dysplasia. COF behaves in a more tumorlike fashion, with the displacement of teeth. A wide sclerotic border is more characteristic of the slow-growing cemental dysplasia.

Other lesions to be considered include those that may have internal calcifications similar to the pattern seen in COF. These include calcifying odontogenic cysts, calcifying epithelial odontogenic (Pindborg) tumors, and adenomatoid odontogenic tumors.

Occasionally the diagnosis of osteogenic sarcoma is considered. However, characteristics suggesting a malignant lesion should be seen, such as cortical bone destruction and invasion into the surrounding soft tissues and along the periodontal ligament space.

Management

The prognosis of COF is favorable with surgical enucleation or resection. Large lesions require a detailed determination of the extent of the lesion, which can be obtained with CT imaging. Even if the lesion has reached appreciable size, it usually can be separated from the surrounding tissue and completely removed. Recurrence after removal is unlikely.

CENTRAL GIANT CELL GRANULOMA

Synonyms

Giant cell reparative granuloma, giant cell lesion, and *giant cell tumor*

Definition

Central giant cell granuloma (CGCG) is thought to be a reactive lesion to an as yet unknown stimulus and not a neoplastic lesion. However, radiographically the characteristics of the lesion are similar to those of a benign tumor. The histologic appearance consists primarily of fibroblasts, numerous vascular channels, multinucleated giant cells, and macrophages. The relationship of the benign giant cell tumor to the giant cell granuloma is controversial and unclear.

Clinical Features

CGCG is a common lesion in the jaws that affects mostly adolescents and young adults; at least 60% of cases occur in individuals under 20 years of age. The most common presenting sign of CGCG is painless swelling. Palpation of the suspect bone area may elicit tenderness, although in a minority of cases the patient may complain of pain. The overlying mucosa may have a purple color. Some of these lesions cause no symptoms and are found only on routine examination. The lesion usually grows slowly, although it may grow rapidly, creating the suspicion of a malignancy.

Radiographic Features

Location. Lesions develop in the mandible twice as often as in the maxilla. The epicenter of the lesion usually is anterior to the first molar, and most maxillary lesions arise anterior to the cuspid. Lesions can cross the midline of the mandible.

Periphery. Because this neoplasm grows relatively slowly, it usually produces a well-defined radiographic margin in the mandible. In most cases the periphery shows no evidence of cortication. Lesions in the maxilla may have ill-defined, almost malignant-appearing, borders.

Internal structure. Some CGCG lesions show no evidence of internal structure (Fig. 22-21), especially small lesions. Other cases have a subtle granular pattern of calcification that may require a bright light source behind the film to enable visualization. Occasionally this granular bone is organized into ill-defined, wispy septa (Fig. 22-22). If present, these granular septa are characteristic of this lesion, especially if they emanate at right angles from the periphery of the lesion. This characteristic is even stronger if a small indentation of the expanded cortical margin is seen at the point where this right-angle septum originates (Fig. 22-23). In some instances the septa are better defined and divide the internal aspect into compartments, creating a multilocular appearance.

Effects on surrounding structures. Giant cell granulomas often displace and resorb teeth. The resorption of tooth roots is not a constant feature, but when it occurs, it may be profound and irregular in outline. The lamina dura of teeth within the lesion usually is missing. The inferior alveolar canal may be displaced in an inferior direction. This lesion has a strong propensity to expand the cortical boundaries of the mandible and maxilla. The expansion usually is uneven or undulating in nature, which may give the appearance of a double boundary when the expansion is viewed using occlusal film. In some instances the outer cortical plate of bone is destroyed instead of expanded; this occurs more often in the maxilla, where the cortical bone destruction may give the lesion a malignant appearance.

Differential Diagnosis

If the internal structure of the CGCG contains septa, the differential diagnosis may include ameloblastoma, odontogenic myxoma, and aneurysmal bone cyst. If a granular internal structure is present, COF may be considered. Useful characteristics for differentiating an ameloblastoma include the following: ameloblastomas tend to occur in an older age group and more often in the posterior mandible, and ameloblastomas have coarse, curved, well-defined trabeculae, whereas giant cell granulomas have wispy, ill-defined trabeculae, some

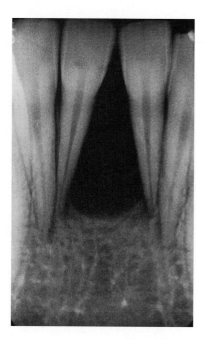

FIG. **22-21** A giant cell granuloma in the anterior mandible with no evidence of internal structure.

of which are at right angles to the periphery. Odontogenic myxomas occur in an older age group, may have sharper and straighter septa, and do not have the same propensity to expand as giant cell granulomas. Interestingly, aneurysmal bone cysts can appear identical radiographically to giant cell granulomas, especially in the appearance of the internal septa. However, aneurysmal bone cysts are comparatively rare lesions that occur more often in the posterior aspect of the jaws and usually cause profound expansion.

A small CGCG lesion with a totally radiolucent internal structure may be similar in appearance to a cyst, especially a simple bone cyst. Evidence of displacement or resorption of the adjacent teeth or expansion of the outer cortical bone is more characteristic of a giant cell granuloma. The radiographic image and histologic appearance of brown tumors of hyperparathyroidism may be identical to those of CGCG.

Management

If the lesion is in the maxilla, CT scans can be used to establish the exact extent and the involvement of surrounding structures, such as the maxillary antrum or nasal cavity. Also, CT imaging is required for large lesions, which pose the possibility of destruction of the outer cortical bone, to determine whether the adjacent soft tissue has been invaded. Occasionally this lesion behaves very aggressively. If it occurs after the second decade of life, hyperparathyroidism should be considered and serum testing for elevated calcium or parathormone or full-body technetium bone scans can be ordered.

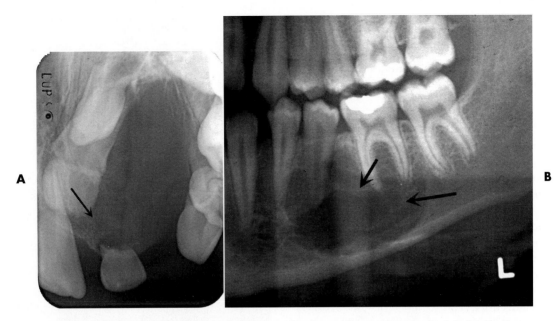

FIG. **22-22** *Various internal patterns seen in giant cell granulomas.* **A,** A lesion in the anterior maxilla with a very fine granular pattern *(arrow).* **B** and **C,** A portion of a panoramic film showing wispy, ill-defined internal septa *(arrows).*

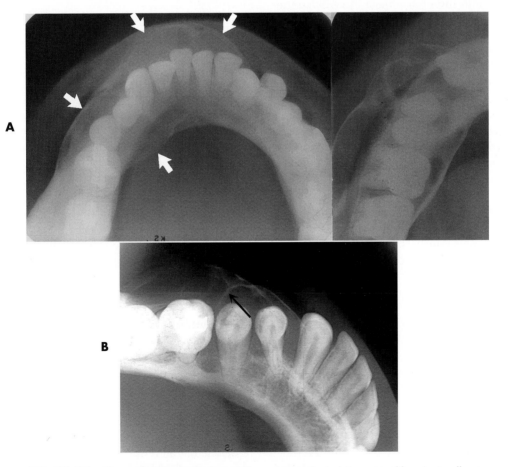

FIG. **22-23** Characteristic expansion of the outer cortical plates caused by giant cell granulomas. Note the uneven expansion in **A** *(arrows)* and the indentation of the expansion with a right-angled septum in **B** *(arrow).*

Treatment may include enucleation and curettage and in some instances resection of the jaw. The patient should be followed carefully to rule out recurrence, especially if conservative treatment is used. Recurrences are rare and are more common in the maxilla.

ANEURYSMAL BONE CYST

Definition
An aneurysmal bone cyst (ABC) usually is considered to be a reactive lesion of bone rather than a cyst or true neoplasm. Some believe that it represents an exaggerated, localized, proliferative response of vascular tissue in bone. This lesion may be related to the CGCG, which it resembles because of the histologic presence of giant cells. ABCs occasionally develop in association with other primary lesions such as fibrous dysplasia, central hemangioma, giant cell granuloma, and osteosarcoma. Its etiology remains unclear.

Clinical Features
More than 90% of reported jaw lesions have occurred in individuals under 30 years of age. The condition appears to have a predilection for females. An ABC in the jaw usually manifests as a fairly rapid bony swelling (usually buccal or labial). Pain is an occasional complaint, and the involved area may be tender on palpation.

Radiographic Features
Location. The mandible is involved more often than the maxilla (ratio of 3:2), and the molar and ramus regions are more involved than the anterior region (Fig. 22-24).

Periphery and shape. The periphery usually is well defined, and the shape is circular or "hydraulic."

Internal structure. Small initial lesions may show no evidence of an internal structure. Often the internal aspect has a multilocular appearance. The septa bear a striking resemblance to the wispy, ill-defined septa seen in giant cell granulomas (Fig. 22-25). Another similar finding is septa positioned at right angles to the outer expanded border.

Effects on surrounding structures. After an ABC becomes large, there is a strong propensity for extreme expansion of the outer cortical plates (see Fig. 22-25). This characteristic is more dramatic with these cysts than with most other lesions. ABCs can displace and resorb teeth.

Differential Diagnosis
The multilocular appearance of ABCs most resembles that of giant cell granulomas; in fact, the radiographic appearance of the two lesions may be identical. However, ABCs may expand to a greater degree, and they are more common in the posterior parts of the mandible, whereas giant

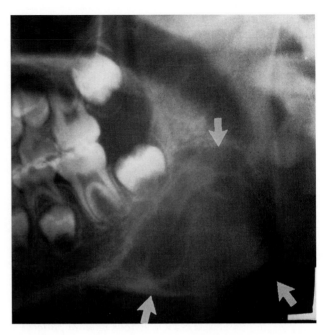

FIG. **22-24** *ABC in the angle of the mandible.* Note the ill-defined septa in the internal structure. (Courtesy Dr. H. Abrams, Los Angeles, Calif.)

cell granulomas are found more often anterior to the first molar. Ameloblastoma may be considered, but this lesion usually occurs in an older age group. ABCs may show a similarity to cherubism, which interestingly has giant cell–like features, but cherubism is a bilateral disease.

The diagnosis is based on biopsy results. A hemorrhagic aspirate favors the diagnosis of ABC. A CT scan also is recommended to better determine the extent of the lesion.

Management
Surgical curettage and partial resection are the primary means of treatment. The recurrence rate is fairly high, ranging from 19% to about 50% after curettage, and approximately 11% after resection. This indicates a need for careful follow-up.

CHERUBISM

Synonym
Familial fibrous dysplasia

Definition
Cherubism is a rare, inherited developmental abnormality that causes bilateral enlargement of the jaws, giving the child a cherubic facial appearance. Rare unilateral lesions have been reported. The term *familial fibrous dysplasia* was an unfortunate choice of early terminology because this lesion is not a bone dysplasia. It is composed of giant cell granuloma–like tissue and does not form a bone matrix. These lesions regress with age.

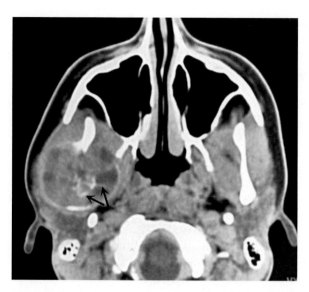

FIG. **22-25** An axial CT scan using a soft tissue algorithm demonstrating the presence of an ABC of the left mandibular condyle. Note the severe expansion and the wispy ill-defined septa *(arrows)*.

Clinical Features

Cherubism develops in early childhood between 2 and 6 years of age. The most common presenting sign is a painless, firm, bilateral enlargement of the lower face. Enlargement of the submandibular lymph nodes may occur, but no systemic abnormalities are involved. Because children's faces are rather chubby, mild cases may go undetected until the second decade. Profound swelling of the maxilla may result in stretching of the skin of the cheeks, which depresses the lower eyelids, exposing a thin line of sclera and causing an "eyes raised to heaven" appearance.

Radiographic Features

Location. This lesion is bilateral and often affects both jaws. When present in only one jaw, the mandible is the most common location. The epicenter is always in the posterior aspect of the jaws, in the ramus of the mandible or the tuberosity of the maxilla (Fig. 22-26). The lesion grows in an anterior direction and in severe cases can extend almost to the midline.

Periphery. The periphery usually is well defined and in some instances corticated.

Internal structure. The internal structure resembles that of CGCG, with fine, granular bone and wispy trabeculae forming a prominent multilocular pattern.

Effects on surrounding structures. Expansion of the cortical boundaries of the maxilla and mandible by cherubism can result in severe enlargement of the jaws. Maxillary lesions enlarge into the maxillary sinuses. Because

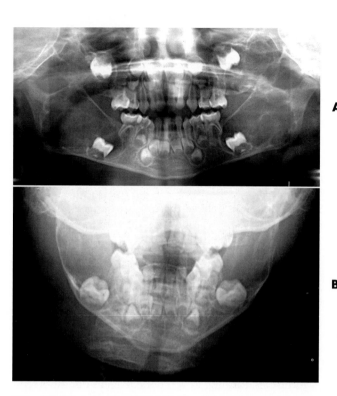

FIG. **22-26** *A case of cherubism.* **A,** A panoramic image showing four lesions in the maxilla and mandible. Note that the epicenters of the lesions are in the maxillary tuberosity and mandibular ramus; also note the anterior displacement of the unerupted maxillary first molars. The internal structure contains ill-defined septa. **B,** A portion of the posteroanterior skull view showing expansion of the mandible.

the epicenter is in the posterior aspect of the jaws, the teeth are displaced in an anterior direction. The degree of displacement can be severe, and with some lesions the tooth buds are destroyed.

Differential Diagnosis

Although the radiographic appearance of cherubism may be similar to that of giant cell granuloma, the fact that cherubism is bilateral with an epicenter in the ramus should provide a clear differentiation. The differentiation of cherubism from fibrous dysplasia should not present any difficulties because fibrous dysplasia is more commonly a unilateral disease; also, the multilocular appearance and anterior displacement of teeth are more characteristic of cherubism. Cherubism may bear some similarity to multiple odontogenic keratocysts in basal cell nevus syndrome. The bilateral symmetry of cherubism, along with the anterior displacement of teeth and pronounced multilocular appearance, help with the differential diagnosis.

Management

The distinctive radiographic features of cherubism may be more diagnostic than the histopathologic findings; therefore the diagnosis can rely on the radiologic findings alone. Treatment can be delayed because the cystlike lesions usually become static and fill in with granular bone during adolescence and at the end of skeletal growth. After skeletal growth has stopped, conservative surgical procedures, if required, may be done for cosmetic problems. Surgery also may be required to uncover displaced teeth, and orthodontic treatment may be needed.

PAGET'S DISEASE

Synonym
Osteitis deformans

Definition
Paget's disease is a condition of abnormal resorption and apposition of osseous tissue in one or more bones. The disease may involve many bones simultaneously, but it is not a generalized skeletal disease. It is initiated by an intense wave of osteoclastic activity, with resorption of normal bone resulting in irregularly shaped resorption cavities. After a period of time, vigorous osteoblastic activity ensues, forming woven bone. Paget's disease is seen most frequently in Great Britain and Australia and somewhat less often in North America.

Clinical Features
Paget's disease is primarily a disease of later middle and old age, having an incidence of about 3.5% of individuals over 40 years of age. The incidence of involvement in males is approximately twice that of females at age 65 years.

Affected bone is enlarged and commonly deformed, resulting in bowing of the legs, curvature of the spine, and enlargement of the skull. The jaws also enlarge when affected. Separation and movement of teeth may occur, causing malocclusion. Dentures may be tight or may fit poorly in edentulous patients.

Bone pain is an inconsistent symptom, most often directed toward the weight-bearing bones; facial or jaw pain is uncommon. Patients with Paget's disease may also have ill-defined neurologic pain as the result of bone impingement on foramina and nerve canals. Patients with Paget's disease often have severely elevated levels of serum alkaline phosphatase (greater than with any other disorder) during osteoblastic phases of the disease. These patients also often have high levels of hydroxyproline in the urine.

Radiographic Features
Location. Paget's disease occurs most often in the pelvis, femur, skull, and vertebrae and infrequently in the jaws (Fig. 22-27). It affects the maxilla about twice as often as the mandible. Whenever the jaws are involved, it is im-

portant to note whether all of the mandible or maxilla is affected. Although this disease is bilateral, occasionally only one maxilla is involved or the involvement may be significantly greater on one side.

Internal structure. Generally the appearance of the internal structure depends on the developmental stage of the disease. Paget's disease has three radiographic stages, although these often overlap in the clinical setting: an early radiolucent resorptive stage; a granular or ground-glass appearing second stage; and a denser, more radiopaque appositional late stage. These stages are less apparent in the jaws.

The trabeculae are altered in number and shape. Most often they increase in number, but in the early stage they may decrease. The trabeculae may be long and may align themselves in a horizontal linear pattern (Fig. 22-28), which is more common in the mandible. They also may be short, with random orientation, and may have a granular pattern similar to that of fibrous dysplasia. As a third possibility, the trabeculae may be organized into rounded, radiopaque patches of abnormal bone, creating a cotton-wool appearance (Fig. 22-29).

The overall density of the jaws may decrease (Fig. 22-30) or increase, depending on the number of trabeculae. Often the disease produces areas of bone that appear radiolucent (commonly the alveolar process) and regions of increased density in one bone.

Effects on surrounding structures. Paget's disease always enlarges an affected bone to some extent, even in the early stage. Often the bone enlargement is impressive. Prominent pagetoid skull bones may swell to three or four times their normal thickness. In enlarged jaws the outer cortex may be thinned but remains intact. The outer cortex may appear to be laminated in occlusal projections. When the maxilla is involved, the disease invariably involves the sinus floor. However, the air space usually is not diminished to a great extent. Cortical boundaries such as the sinus floor may be more granular and less apparent as sharp boundaries. The lamina dura may become less evident and may be altered into the abnormal bone pattern. Often hypercementosis develops on a few or most of the teeth in the involved jaw. This hypercementosis may be exuberant and irregular, which is characteristic of Paget's disease (Fig. 22-31). As previously mentioned, the teeth may become spaced or displaced in the enlarging jaw.

Differential Diagnosis
Paget's disease may appear similar to fibrous dysplasia. However, Paget's disease occurs in an older age group and is almost always bilateral. In the maxilla, fibrous dys-

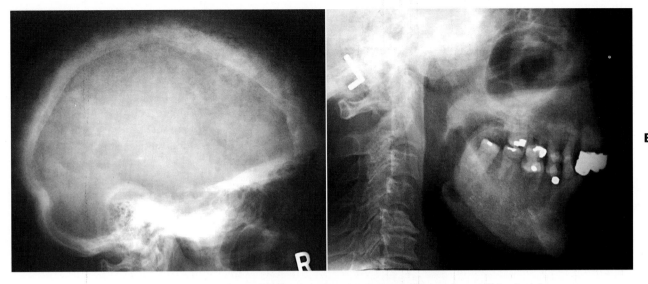

FIG. **22-27**   *A case of Paget's disease involving the skull, maxilla, and mandible.* **A,** A lateral view of the skull showing an increase in density and dimension between the internal and outer cortex of the skull. A cotton wool pattern can be seen. **B,** A lateral view of the jaws of the same patient showing the increase in jaw size and density. There is a subtle linear orientation of the trabeculae of the mandible.

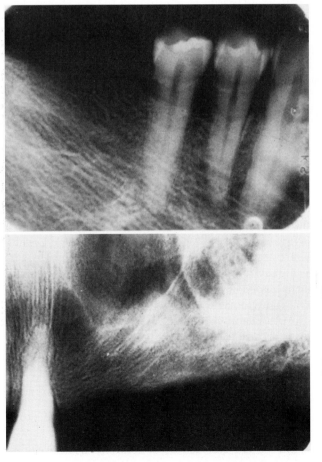

FIG. **22-28**   *Paget's disease with an altered trabecular pattern.* The trabeculae are aligned in linear striations, which follow an approximately horizontal direction in the mandible but are randomly oriented in the maxilla. (Courtesy Dr. H.G. Poyton, Toronto, Canada.)

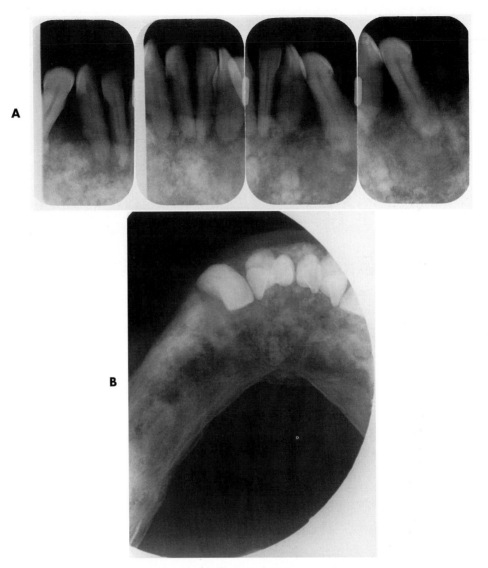

FIG. **22-29** *Paget's disease.* **A,** Multiple radiopaque masses in the mandible that have a cotton-wool appearance. **B,** Note the expansion of the mandible and the maintenance of a thin outer cortical plate.

plasia has a tendency to encroach upon the antral air space, whereas Paget's disease does not. The linear trabeculae and cotton-wool appearance of Paget's disease are distinctive. FOD may have a cotton-wool pattern, but these lesions are centered above the inferior alveolar nerve canal and most commonly have a radiolucent capsule. The changes seen in FOD do not affect all of the jaw, unlike with Paget's disease. The bone pattern in Paget's disease may show some similarities to the bone pattern in metabolic bone diseases, and both conditions may be bilateral. However, Paget's disease enlarges bone, and metabolic diseases do not.

The specific bone pattern changes, the late age of onset, the enlargement of the involved bone, and the extreme elevation of serum alkaline phosphatase aid in the differential diagnosis.

Management

Currently Paget's disease usually is managed medically, using either calcitonin or sodium etidronate. Calcitonin relieves pain and reduces the serum alkaline phosphatase levels and osteoclastic activity. Sodium etidronate covers bone surfaces and retards bone resorption and formation. Surgery may be required to correct deformities of the long bones and treat fractures.

There are complications of this disease that are of concern. Extraction sites heal slowly. The incidence of jaw osteomyelitis is higher than for nonaffected individuals. About 10% of cases with polyostotic disease develop osteogenic sarcoma. Characteristics such as invasion and bone destruction, as described in Chapter 21, indicate the presence of a malignant neoplasm.

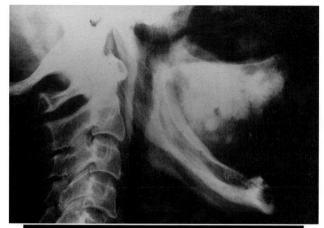

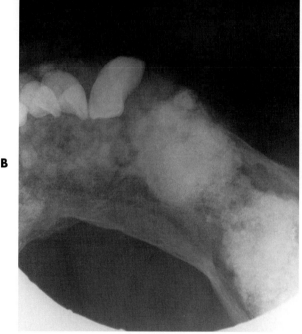

FIG. **22-30** Paget's disease with very radiopaque lesions in the maxilla **(A)** and mandible **(B)**. (Courtesy Dr. H.G. Poyton, Toronto, Canada.)

LANGERHANS' CELL HISTIOCYTOSIS

Synonyms

Histiocytosis X, idiopathic histiocytosis, and *Langerhans' cell disease*

Definition

The disorders included in the category of Langerhans' cell histiocytosis (LCH) are abnormalities that result from the abnormal proliferation of Langerhans' cells or their precursors. Langerhans' cells are specialized cells of the histiocytic cell line that normally are found in the skin. The abnormal proliferation of Langerhans' cells and eosinophils results in a spectrum of clinical diseases. Historically, histiocytosis X was classified into three distinct clinical

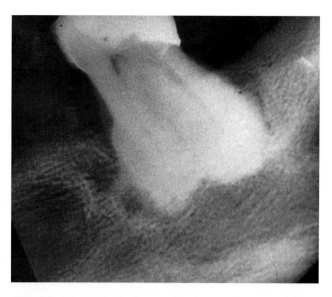

FIG. **22-31** Paget's disease showing exuberant hypercementosis of the roots of a mandibular molar.

forms: eosinophilic granuloma (solitary), Hand-Schüller-Christian disease (chronic disseminated), and Letterer-Siwe disease (acute disseminated).

A newly proposed LCH classification creates two categories: nonmalignant disorders, such as unifocal or multifocal eosinophilic granuloma, and malignant disorders, including Letterer-Siwe disease and variants of histiocytic lymphoma. Recent research has shown that all forms of LCH are clonal and thus may represent a form of malignancy.

Clinical Features

Head and neck lesions are common at initial presentation, and approximately 10% of all patients with LCH have oral lesions. Often the oral changes are the first clinical signs of the disease.

Eosinophilic granuloma (EG) usually appears in the skeleton (ribs, pelvis, long bones, skull, and jaws) and in rare cases in soft tissue. This condition occurs most often in older children and young adults but may develop later in life. The lesions often form quickly and may cause a dull, steady pain. In the jaws the disease may cause bony swelling, a soft tissue mass, gingivitis, bleeding gingiva, pain, and ulceration. Loosening or sloughing of the teeth often occurs after destruction of alveolar bone by one or more foci of EG. The sockets of teeth lost to the disease generally do not heal normally. EG may have a single focus or may develop into a multifocal, aggressive disease. The disseminated form may involve multiple bone lesions, diabetes insipidus, and exophthalmos, a condition previously defined as Hand-Schüller-Christian disease.

Letterer-Siwe disease is a malignant form of LCH that most often occurs in infants under 3 years of age. Soft

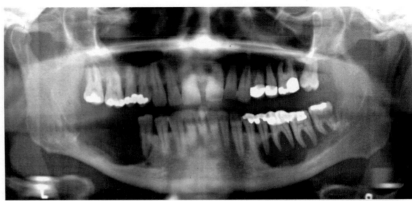

FIG. **22-32** *A panoramic film of multiple lesions of Langerhans' cell histiocytosis.* Note the scooped-out shape of the bone destruction in the mandible. The floor of the right maxillary antrum has been destroyed.

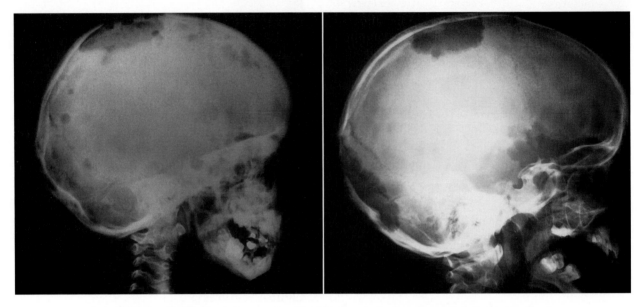

FIG. **22-33** Skull lesions of Langerhans' cell histiocytosis showing well-defined, punched-out lesions. (Courtesy Dr. H.G. Poyton, Toronto, Ontario.)

tissue and bony granulomatous reactions disseminate throughout the body, and the condition is marked by intermittent fever, hepatosplenomegaly, anemia, lymphadenopathy, hemorrhage, and failure to thrive. Lesions in bone are rare. Death usually occurs within several weeks of the onset of the disease.

Radiographic Features

For ease of discussion, the author divides LCH jaw lesions into two groups: those that occur in the alveolar process and intraosseous lesions that occur elsewhere in the jaws. The radiographic features of this condition generally are similar to those of malignant neoplasms.

Location. The alveolar type of LCH lesions are commonly multiple, whereas the intraosseous type usually is solitary. The mandible is a more common site than the maxilla, and the posterior regions are more involved than the an-

terior regions (Fig. 22-32). The mandibular ramus is a common site of intraosseous lesions. Solitary lesions of the jaws may be accompanied by lesions in other bones.

Periphery and shape. The periphery of EG lesions varies from moderately to well defined but without cortication; the periphery sometimes appears punched out (Fig. 22-33). The margins may be smooth or somewhat irregular. The alveolar lesions commonly start in the midroot region of the teeth. The bone destruction progresses in a circular shape, and after it includes a portion of the superior border of the alveolar process, it may give the impression that a section of the alveolar process has been scooped out (see Figs. 22-32 and 22-34). The shape of intraosseous lesions may be irregular, oval, or round.

Internal structure. The internal structure usually is totally radiolucent.

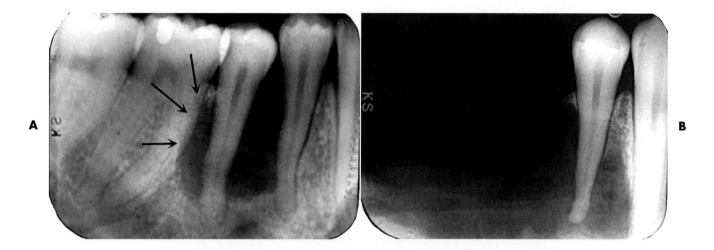

FIG. **22-34** *Two periapical films of the same area of the mandible taken approximately 1 year apart in a patient with Langerhans' cell histiocytosis.* **A,** The earlier phase of the disease produces a scooped-out shape *(arrows)*, which shows that the epicenter of the lesion is in the midroot area of the involved teeth, unlike in periodontal disease. **B,** One year later, bone destruction is extensive, resulting in loss of teeth. (Courtesy Dr. D. Stoneman, Toronto, Ontario, Canada.)

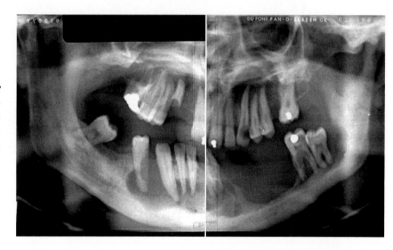

FIG. **22-35** *A panoramic film showing the bone destruction that can occur with Langerhans' cell histiocytosis.* Note that the bone around many of the remaining mandibular teeth has been destroyed, leaving the teeth apparently unsupported. (Courtesy Dr. D. Stoneman.)

Effects on surrounding structures. LCH destroys bone. In alveolar lesions the bone around teeth, including the lamina dura, is destroyed, and as a result the teeth appear to be standing in space. The lesion does not displace teeth, although teeth may move because they are bereft of bone support (Fig. 22-35). Only minor root resorption has been reported. Of note is the ability of these lesions to stimulate periosteal new bone formation; this occurs more commonly with the intraosseous type of lesion (Fig. 22-36). The periosteal new bone formation is indistinguishable from the appearance seen in inflammatory lesions of the jaws. This lesion can destroy the outer cortical plate and in rare cases extends into the surrounding soft tissues in the CT examination.

Differential Diagnosis

The major differential diagnosis of alveolar type lesions is periodontal disease and squamous cell carcinoma. An important characteristic in differentiation of periodontal disease is the fact that the epicenter of the bone destruction in LCH is approximately in the midroot region, resulting in a scooped-out appearance. In contrast, the bone destruction in periodontal disease starts at the alveolar crest and extends apically down the root surface. Differentiation of a squamous cell carcinoma may not be possible by radiographic characteristics alone, although the borders of an LCH lesion typically are better defined. Multiple lesions in a younger age group (usually the first three decades) are more likely to be LCH than squamous cell carcinoma, which typically appears as a single lesion in middle or old age. LCH may bear a superficial resemblance to simple bone cysts, but the alveolar crest is maintained in simple bone cysts, and a partial cortex may be present.

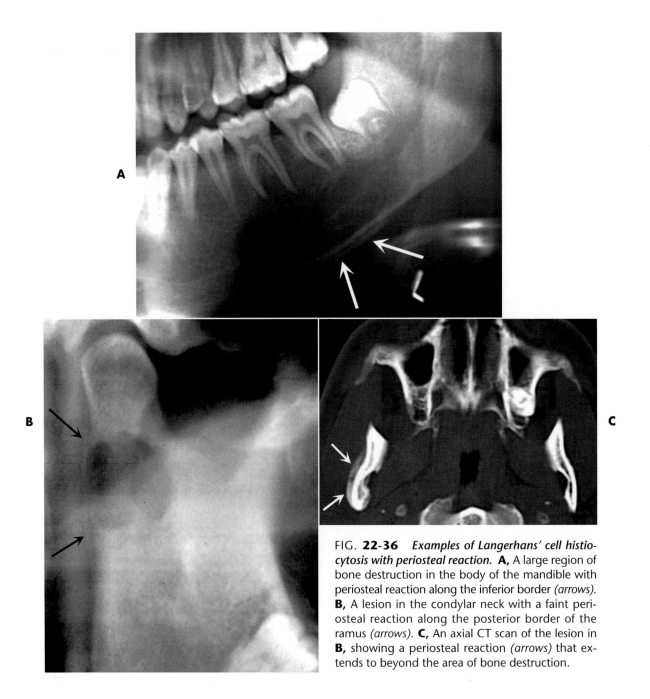

FIG. **22-36** *Examples of Langerhans' cell histiocytosis with periosteal reaction.* **A,** A large region of bone destruction in the body of the mandible with periosteal reaction along the inferior border *(arrows).* **B,** A lesion in the condylar neck with a faint periosteal reaction along the posterior border of the ramus *(arrows).* **C,** An axial CT scan of the lesion in **B,** showing a periosteal reaction *(arrows)* that extends to beyond the area of bone destruction.

The differential diagnosis of solitary intraosseous lesions includes metastatic malignant neoplasia and malignant tumors from adjacent soft tissues. However, the well-defined borders and the periosteal reaction seen in histiocytosis helps in the differential diagnosis.

Patients suspected of having LCH should be referred to an oral and maxillofacial radiologist for a complete workup; this may include nuclear imaging to detect other possible bone lesions. The radiologic workup should be followed by a biopsy. The histologic appearance of histiocytosis may be hidden by changes caused by secondary infection from the oral cavity in alveolar lesions. Therefore it is important to correlate the radiographic findings with the histologic appearance of the biopsy.

Management

Treatment of localized lesions usually consists of surgical curettage or limited radiation therapy. Surgical management of jaw lesions usually is preferable because it has a low recurrence rate. The earlier EG of the mandible is diagnosed and controlled, the fewer teeth are lost to bone destruction. Disseminated disease is treated with chemotherapy.

SUGGESTED READINGS

FIBROUS DYSPLASIA

Ebata K et al: Chondrosarcoma and osteosarcoma arising in polyostotic fibrous dysplasia, *J Oral Maxillofac Surg* 50:761, 1992.

Eversole L et al: Fibrous dysplasia: a nosologic problem in the diagnosis of fibroosseous lesions of the jaws, *J Oral Pathol* 1:189, 1972.

Mendelshon D et al: Computed tomography of craniofacial fibrous dysplasia, *J Comput Assist Tomogr* 8:1062, 1984.

Obisean A et al: The radiologic features of fibrous dysplasia of the craniofacial bones, *Oral Surg* 44:949, 1977.

Present D et al: Osteosarcoma of the mandible arising in fibrous dysplasia: a case report, *Clin Orthop* 204:238, 1986.

Waldron C, Giansanti J: Benign fibroosseous lesions of the jaws: a clinical-radiologic-histologic review of sixty-five cases. I. Fibrous dysplasia of the jaws, *Oral Surg* 35:190, 1973.

PERIAPICAL CEMENTAL DYSPLASIA

Waldron C, Giansanti J: Benign fibroosseous lesions of the jaws: a clinical-radiologic-histologic review of sixty-five cases. II. Benign fibroosseous lesions of periodontal ligament origin, *Oral Surg* 35:340, 1973.

FLORID OSSEOUS DYSPLASIA

Fun-Chee L, Jinn-Fei Y: Florid osseous dysplasia in Orientals, *Oral Surg Oral Med Oral Pathol* 68:748, 1989.

MacDonald-Jankowski DS: Gigantiform cementoma occurring in two populations, London and Hong Kong, *Clin Radiol* 45:316, 1992.

Melrose RJ et al: Florid osseous dysplasia: a clinical-pathologic study of 34 cases, *Oral Surg* 41:62, 1976.

Thompson SH, Altini M: Gigantiform cementoma of the jaws, *Head Neck* 11:538, 1989.

CEMENTOOSSIFYING FIBROMA

Eversole L et al: Radiographic characteristics of central ossifying fibroma, *Oral Surg* 59:522, 1985.

Hamner J et al: Benign fibroosseous jaw lesions of periodontal membrane origin: an analysis of 249 cases, *Cancer* 22:861, 1968.

Sciubba JJ, Younai F: Ossifying fibroma of the mandible and maxilla: review of 18 cases, *J Oral Pathol Med* 18:315, 1989.

GIANT CELL GRANULOMA

Cohen MA, Hertzanu Y: Radiologic features, including those seen with computed tomography, of central giant cell granuloma of the jaws, *Oral Surg Oral Med Oral Pathol* 65:255, 1988.

Horner K: Central giant cell granuloma of the jaws: a clinico-radiological study, *Clin Radiol* 40:622, 1989.

Waldron CA, Shafer WG: The central giant cell granuloma of the jaws: an analysis of 38 cases, *Am J Clin Pathol* 45:437, 1966.

ANEURYSMAL BONE CYST

Buraczewski J, Dabska P: Pathogenesis of aneurysmal bone cyst: relationship between the aneurysmal bone cyst and fibrous dysplasia of bone, *Cancer* 28:597, 1971.

Dahlin D, McLeod R: Aneurysmal bone cyst and other non-neoplastic conditions, *Skeletal Radiol* 8:243, 1982.

Giddings NA et al: Aneurysmal bone cyst of the mandible, *Arch Otolaryngol Head Neck Surg* 115:865, 1989.

Struthers P et al: Aneurysmal bone cyst of the jaws. I. Clinico-pathological features, *Int J Oral Surg* 13:85, 1984.

Struthers P et al: Aneurysmal bone cyst of the jaws. II. Pathogenesis, *Int J Oral Surg* 13:92, 1984.

Tillman BP: Aneurysmal bone cyst: an analysis of 95 cases, *Mayo Clin Proc* 43:478, 1968.

CHERUBISM

Bianchi SD et al: The computed tomographic appearances of cherubism, *Skeletal Radiol* 16:6, 1987.

Faircloth WJ Jr et al: Cherubism involving a mother and daughter: case reports and review of the literature, *J Oral Maxillofac Surg* 49:535, 1991.

Katz JO et al: Cherubism: report of a case showing regression without treatment, *J Oral Maxillofac Surg* 50:301, 1992.

Reade P et al: Unilateral mandibular cherubism: brief review and case report, *Br J Oral Maxillofac Surg* 22:189, 1984.

PAGET'S DISEASE

Barker D: The epidemiology of Paget's disease, *Metab Bone Dis Rel Res* 3:231, 1981.

Kanis J et al: Paget's disease of bone: diagnosis and management, *Metab Bone Dis Rel Res* 3:219, 1981.

Rao V, Karasick D: Hypercementosis: an important clue to Paget's disease of the maxilla, *Skeletal Radiol* 9:126, 1982.

Singer F, Millo B: Evidence for a viral etiology of Paget's disease of bone, *Clin Orthop* 178:245, 1983.

Smith B, Eveson J: Paget's disease of bone with particular reference to dentistry, *J Oral Pathol* 10:233, 1981.

Sofaer J: Dental extractions in Paget's disease of bone, *Int J Oral Surg* 13:79, 1984.

LANGERHANS' CELL HISTIOCYTOSIS

Bottomley WK et al: Histiocytosis X: report of an oral soft tissue lesion without bony involvement, *Oral Surg Oral Med Oral Pathol* 63:228, 1987.

Cline MJ: Histiocytes and histiocytosis, *Blood* 84:2840, 1996.

Domboski M: Eosinophilic granuloma of bone manifesting mandibular involvement, *Oral Surg Oral Med Oral Pathol* 50:116, 1980.

Gorsky M et al: Histiocytosis X: occurrence and oral involvement in six adolescent and adult patients, *Oral Surg Oral Med Oral Pathol* 55:24, 1983.

Hartman KS: Histiocytosis X: a review of 114 cases with oral involvement, *Oral Surg Oral Med Oral Pathol* 49:38, 1980.

Wong GB et al: Eosinophilic granuloma of the mandibular condyle: report of three cases and review of the literature, *J Oral Maxillofac Surg* 55:870, 1997.

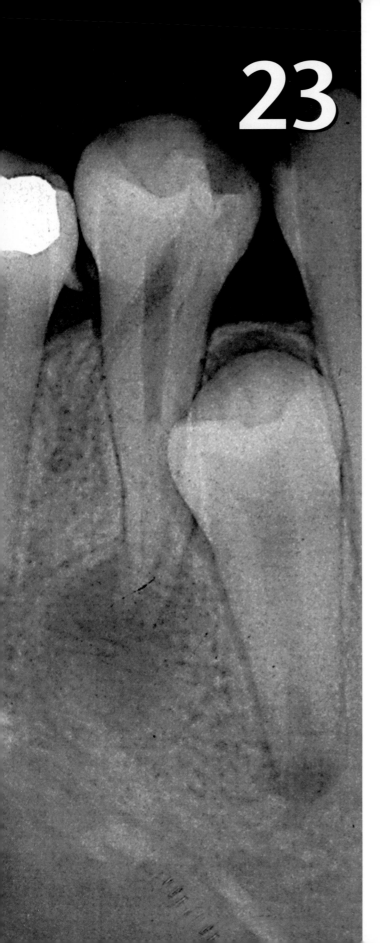

23 Systemic Diseases Manifested in the Jaws

Definition

Disorders of the endocrine system, bone metabolism, and other systemic diseases may have an effect on the form and function of bone and teeth. The function of bone not only includes support, protection, and an environment for hemopoiesis but also serves as a major reserve of calcium for the body. More than 99% of the total body calcium is contained within the skeletal structure. When considering the influence of systemic conditions on the jaws, it is important to consider that bone is constantly remodeling. Approximately 5% to 10% of the total bone mass is replaced each year. The turnover rate of trabecular bone is higher than for cortical bone; 20% of its mass is replaced per year, compared with 5% for cortical bone. The effects of systemic diseases of bone are brought about by changes in the number and activity of osteoclasts, osteoblasts, and osteocytes.

Radiographic Features

Because systemic disorders affect the entire body, the radiographic changes manifested in the jaws are generalized (Table 23-1). In most cases it is not possible to identify diseases based on radiographic characteristics. The general changes include the following:

1. A change in size and shape of the bone
2. A change in the number, size, and orientation of trabeculae
3. Altered thickness and density of cortical structures
4. An increase or decrease in overall bone density

Changes in these elements can result in a decrease or increase in bone density.

Because many parameters in the production of a radiograph influence the density of the image, it is difficult to detect genuine changes in the density of bone. Systemic conditions that result in a *decrease* in bone density do not affect the teeth; therefore the image of the teeth may stand out with normal density against a generally radiolucent jaw. In severe cases the teeth may appear to be bereft of any bony support. Also, cortical structures appear thin, less defined, and occasionally disappear. On the other hand, a true *increase* in bone density may be detected by a loss of contrast of the inferior cortex of the mandible as the radiopacity of the cancellous bone approaches that of cortical bone. Often the inferior alveolar nerve canal appears more distinct in contrast to the surrounding dense bone.

Some systemic diseases that occur during tooth formation may result in dental alterations. Lamina dura is part of the bone structure of the alveolar process, but because it is usually examined in conjunction with the periodontal membrane space and roots of teeth, it is included with the description of the dental structures (Table 23-2). Changes to teeth and associated structures include the following:

TABLE 23-1
Radiographic Changes in Bone Observed in Systemic Disease*

| | BONE | | | | |
| | | | | TRABECULAE | |
SYSTEMIC DISEASE	DENSITY	SIZE OF JAWS	INCREASE	DECREASE	GRANULAR
Hyperparathyroidism	decrease	no	yes	yes	yes
Hypoparathyroidism	rare increase	no	no	no	no
Hyperpituitarism	no	large	no	no	no
Hypopituitarism	no	small	no	no	no
Hypothyroidism	decrease	no	no	no	no
Hyperthyroidism	no	small	no	no	no
Cushing's syndrome	decrease	no	no	yes	yes
Osteoporosis	decrease	no	no	yes	no
Rickets	decrease	no	no	yes	no
Osteomalacia	rare decrease	no	no	rare decrease	no
Hypophosphatasia	decrease	no	no	yes	no
Renal osteodystrophy	decrease; rare increase	no	rare	yes	yes
Hypophosphatemia	decrease	no	no	yes	yes

*This table summarizes the major radiographic changes to bone with endocrine and metabolic bone diseases. It does not include all the possible variable appearances.

TABLE 23-2
Effects of Systemic Disease on Dental Structures*

| | EFFECTS ON TEETH AND ASSOCIATED STRUCTURES | | | | | |
SYSTEMIC DISEASE	HYPOCALCIFICATION	HYPOPLASIA	LARGE PULP CHAMBER	LOSS OF LAMINA DURA	LOSS OF TEETH	ERUPTION
Hyperparathyroidism	no	no	no	yes	rare	no
Hypoparathyroidism	no	yes	no	no	no	delayed
Hyperpituitarism	no	no	no	no	no	super eruption
Hypopituitarism	no	no	no	no	no	delayed
Hypothyroidism	no	no	no	no	yes	early

*This table summarizes the major radiographic changes that can occur to teeth and associated structures with endocrine and metabolic bone diseases. It does not include all the possible variable appearances.

Continued.

TABLE **23-2**
Effects of Systemic Disease on Dental Structures—cont'd

	EFFECTS ON TEETH AND ASSOCIATED STRUCTURES					
SYSTEMIC DISEASE	HYPOCALCIFICATION	HYPOPLASIA	LARGE PULP CHAMBER	LOSS OF LAMINA DURA	LOSS OF TEETH	ERUPTION
Hyperthyroidism	no	no	no	thin	yes	delayed
Cushing's syndrome	no	no	no	partial	no	permature
Osteoporosis	no	no	no	thin	no	no
Rickets	yes—enamel	yes—enamel	no	thin	no	delayed
Osteomalacia	no	no	no	no	no	no
Hypophosphatasia	yes	yes	yes	yes	yes	no
Renal osteodystrophy	yes	yes	no	yes	yes	no
Hypophosphatemia	yes	yes	yes	yes	yes	no
Osteopetrosis	no	rare	no	no	no	delayed

1. Accelerated or delayed eruption
2. Hypoplasia
3. Hypocalcification
4. Loss of a distinct lamina dura

Often bone and teeth exhibit no detectable radiographic changes associated with systemic diseases. However, on occasion the first symptoms of a disease may present as a dental problem.

Endocrine Disorders

HYPERPARATHYROIDISM

Identifying Characteristics

Definition. Hyperparathyroidism is an endocrine abnormality in which there is an excess of circulating parathyroid hormone (PTH). An excess of serum PTH increases bone remodeling in preference of osteoclastic resorption, which mobilizes calcium from the skeleton. In addition, PTH increases renal tubular reabsorption of calcium and renal production of the active vitamin D metabolite $1,25(OH)_2D$. The net result of these functions is in an increase in serum calcium.

Primary hyperparathyroidism usually results from a benign tumor (adenoma) of one of the four parathyroid glands, which produces excess PTH. Less frequently, individuals may have hyperplastic parathyroid glands that secrete excess PTH. The combination of hypercalcemia and an elevated serum level of PTH is diagnostic of primary hyperparathyroidism. The incidence of primary hyperparathyroidism is about 0.1%.

Secondary hyperparathyroidism results from a compensatory increase in the output of PTH in response to hypocalcemia. The underlying hypocalcemia may result from an inadequate dietary intake or poor absorption of vitamin D or from deficient metabolism of vitamin D in the liver or kidney. This condition produces clinical and radiographic effects similar to those of primary hyperparathyroidism.

Clinical features. Women are two to three times more commonly affected than men by primary hyperparathyroidism. The condition occurs mainly in those 30 to 60 years of age. Clinical manifestations of the disease cover a broad range, but most patients have renal calculi, peptic ulcers, psychiatric problems, or bone and joint pain. These clinical symptoms are mainly related to hypercalcemia. Gradual loosening, drifting, and loss of teeth may occur. Definite consistent hypercalcemia is virtually pathognomonic of primary hyperparathyroidism. (Rarely, multiple myeloma and metastatic tumors may produce the same serum alterations.) Because of daily fluctuations, the serum calcium level should be tested at different intervals. The serum alkaline phosphatase level, a reliable indicator of bone turnover, may also be elevated in hyperparathyroidism.

Radiographic features. Only about one in five patients with hyperparathyroidism has radiographically observable bone changes.

General radiographic features. The following are the major manifestations of hyperparathyroidism:

1. The earliest and most reliable changes of hyperparathyroidism are subtle erosions of bone from the subperiosteal surfaces of the phalanges of the hands.
2. Demineralization of the skeleton results in an unusual radiolucent appearance.

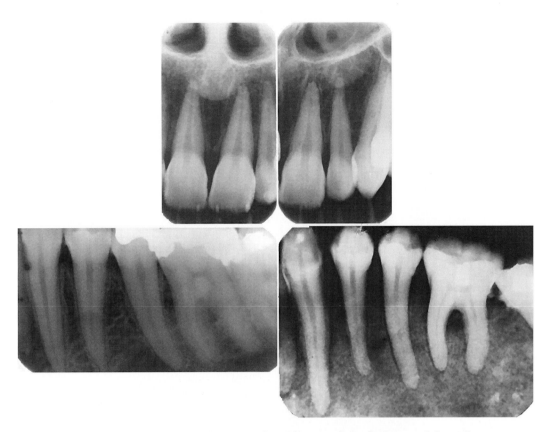

FIG. **23-1** The loss of bone in hyperparathyroidism results in the image of the radiopaque teeth standing out in contrast to the radiolucent jaws. Note the loss of a distinct lamina dura and the granular texture of the bone pattern. (*Bottom right radiograph* courtesy H.G. Poyton, DDS, Toronto, Ontario.)

3. Osteitis fibrosa cystica are localized regions of bone loss produced by osteoclastic activity resulting in a loss of all apparent bone structure.
4. Brown tumors occur late in the disease and in about 10% of cases. These peripheral or central tumors of bone are radiolucent. The gross specimen has a brown or reddish-brown color.
5. Pathologic calcifications in soft tissues have a punctate or nodular appearance and occur in the kidneys and joints.
6. In prominent hyperparathyroidism, the entire calvarium has a granular appearance caused by the loss of central (diploic) trabeculae and thinning of the cortical tables.

Radiographic features of the jaws. Demineralization and thinning of cortical boundaries often occur in the jaws in cortical boundaries such as the inferior border, mandibular canal, and the cortical outlines of the maxillary sinuses. The density of the jaws is decreased, resulting in a radiolucent appearance that contrasts with the density of the teeth. The teeth stand out in contrast to the radiolucent jaws (Fig. 23-1). A change in the normal trabecular pattern may occur, resulting in a ground-glass appearance of numerous, small, randomly oriented trabeculae.

Brown tumors of hyperparathyroidism may appear in any bone but are frequently found in the facial bones and jaws, particularly in long-standing cases of the disease. These lesions may be multiple within a single bone. They have variably defined margins and may produce cortical expansion (Fig. 23-2). If solitary, the tumor may resemble a central giant cell granuloma or an aneurysmal bone cyst. It is interesting to note that the histologic appearance of the brown tumor is identical to that of the giant cell granuloma. Therefore, if a giant cell granuloma occurs later than the second decade, the patient should be screened for an increase in serum calcium, PTH, and alkaline phosphatase.

Radiographic features of the teeth and associated structures. Occasionally periapical radiographs reveal loss of the lamina dura in patients (only about 10%) with hyperparathyroidism (see Fig. 23-1). Depending on the duration and severity of the disease, loss of the lamina dura may occur around one tooth or all the remaining

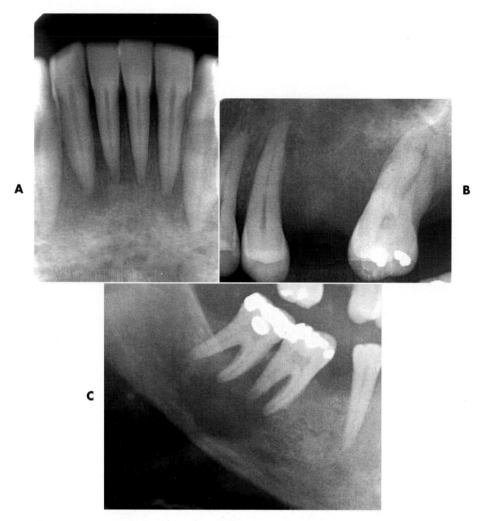

FIG. 23-2 *Hyperparathyroidism.* **A** and **B** reveal a granular bone pattern that was characteristic in all intraoral films. Note the loss of a distinct lamina dura and floor of the maxillary antrum. **C,** This panoramic view of the same case reveals a brown tumor related to the apical region of the second and third molars.

teeth. The loss may be either complete or partial around a particular tooth. The result of lamina dura loss may give the root a tapered appearance because of loss of image contrast. Although PTH mobilizes minerals from the skeleton, mature teeth are immune to this systemic demineralizing process.

Management. After successful surgical removal of the causative parathyroid adenoma, almost all radiographic changes revert to normal. The only exception may be the site of a brown tumor, which often heals with bone that is radiographically more sclerotic than normal. Many people with this disease are being diagnosed earlier, resulting in fewer severe cases.

HYPOPARATHYROIDISM AND PSEUDOHYPOPARATHYROIDISM

Identifying Characteristics

Definition. Hypoparathyroidism is an uncommon condition in which insufficient secretion of PTH occurs. Several causes exist, but the most common is damage or removal of the parathyroid glands during thyroid surgery. In pseudohypoparathyroidism there is a defect in the response of the tissue target cells to normal levels of PTH.

Clinical features. Both hypoparathyroidism and pseudohypoparathyroidism produce hypocalcemia, which has a variety of clinical manifestations. Most often this includes sharp flexion (tetany) of the wrist and ankle joints

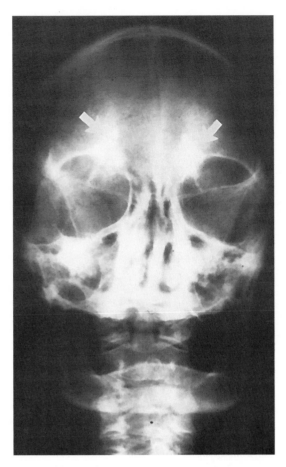

FIG. **23-3** Hypoparathyroidism-induced calcification of the basal ganglia, seen in this posteroanterior skull view. (Courtesy H.G. Poyton, DDS, Toronto, Ontario.)

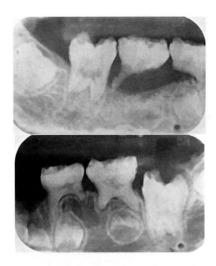

FIG. **23-4** Pseudohypoparathyroidism-induced dental anomalies. (Courtesy Dr. S. Bricker, San Antonio, Tex.)

(carpopedal spasm). Some patients have sensory abnormalities consisting of paresthesia of the hands, feet, or area around the mouth. Neurologic changes may include anxiety and depression, epilepsy, parkinsonism, and chorea. Chronic forms may produce a reduction in intellectual capacity. Some patients show no changes at all. Patients with pseudohypoparathyroidism often have early closure of certain bony epiphyses and thus manifest short stature or extremity disproportions.

Radiographic features. The principal radiographic change is calcification of the basal ganglia (Fig. 23-3). On skull radiographs this calcification appears flocculent and paired within the cerebral hemispheres on the posteroanterior view. Radiographic examination of the jaws may reveal dental enamel hypoplasia, external root resorption, delayed eruption, or root dilaceration (Fig. 23-4).

Treatment. These conditions are managed with orally administered supplemental calcium and vitamin D.

HYPERPITUITARISM

Identifying Characteristics
Synonyms. *Acromegaly* and *giantism*

Definition. Hyperpituitarism results from hyperfunction of the anterior lobe of the pituitary gland, which increases the production of growth hormone. An excess of growth hormone causes overgrowth of all tissues in the body still capable of growth. The usual cause of this problem is a benign, functioning tumor of the acidophilic cells in the anterior lobe of the pituitary gland.

Clinical features. Hyperpituitarism in children involves generalized overgrowth of most hard and soft tissues, a condition termed *giantism*. Active growth occurs in those bones in which the epiphyses have not united with the bone shafts. Throughout adolescence, generalized skeletal growth is excessive and may be prolonged. Those affected may ultimately attain heights of 7 to 8 feet or more yet exhibit remarkably normal proportions. The eyes and other parts of the central nervous system do not enlarge, except in rare cases in which the condition is manifested in infancy.

Adult hyperpituitarism, called *acromegaly*, has an insidious clinical course, quite different from the clinical profile seen in the childhood disease. In adults the clinical effects of a pituitary adenoma develop quite slowly because many types of tissues have lost the capacity for growth. This is true of much of the skeleton; however, an excess of growth hormone can stimulate the mandible and the phalanges of the hand. Mandibular condylar

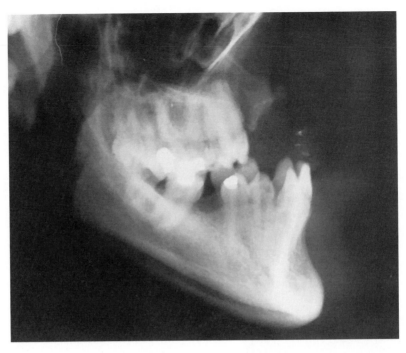

FIG. 23-5 Acromegaly manifested as excessive growth of the mandible, resulting in a class III skeletal relationship of the jaws.

growth may be very prominent. Also, the supraorbital ridges and the underlying frontal sinus may be enlarged. Excess growth hormone in adults may also produce hypertrophy of some soft tissues. The lips, tongue, nose, and soft tissues of the hands and feet typically overgrow in adults with acromegaly, sometimes to a striking degree.

Radiographic features
General radiographic features. The pituitary tumor responsible for hyperpituitarism often produces enlargement ("ballooning") of the sella turcica. It is important to note that in some examples the sella may not expand at all. Skull radiographs characteristically reveal enlargement of the paranasal sinuses (especially the frontal sinus). These air sinuses are more prominent in acromegaly than in pituitary giantism because sinus growth in giantism tends to be more in step with the generalized enlargement of the facial bones. Hyperpituitarism in adults also produces diffuse thickening of the outer table of the skull.

Radiographic features of the jaws. Hyperpituitarism causes enlargement of the jaws, most notably the mandible. The increase in the length of the dental arches results in spacing of the teeth. In acromegaly the angle between the ramus and body of the mandible may increase. This, in combination with enlargement of the tongue (macroglossia), may result in anterior flaring of the teeth and the development of an anterior open bite. The sign of incisor flaring is a helpful point of differentiation between acromegalic prognathism and inherited prognathism. In acromegaly the most profound growth occurs in the condyle and ramus, often resulting in a class III skeletal relationship between the jaws (Fig. 23-5). The thickness and height of the alveolar processes may also increase.

Radiographic changes associated with the teeth. The tooth crowns are usually normal in size, although the roots of posterior teeth often enlarge as a result of hypercementosis. This hypercementosis may be the result of functional and structural demands on teeth instead of a secondary hormonal effect. Supereruption of the posterior teeth may occur in an attempt to compensate for the growth of the mandible.

HYPOPITUITARISM

Identifying Characteristics
Definition. Hypopituitarism results from reduced secretion of pituitary hormones.

Clinical features. Individuals with this condition show dwarfism but have relatively well-proportioned bodies. One study reported a marked failure of development of the maxilla and the mandible. The dimensions of these bones in these adults were approximately those of normal children 5 to 7 years of age.

Radiographic features. Eruption of the primary dentition occurs at the normal time, but exfoliation is delayed by several years. The crowns of the permanent teeth form normally, but their eruption is delayed several years. The third molar buds may be completely absent. In hypopituitarism the jaws, especially the mandible, are small, which results in crowding and malocclusion.

Treatment. Treatment is usually directed toward removal of the cause or replacement of the pituitary hormones or those of its target gland. The response of the dentition to treatment with growth hormone is variable but seems to parallel skeletal response.

HYPERTHYROIDISM

Identifying Characteristics
Synonyms. *Thyrotoxicosis* and *Graves' disease*

Definition. Hyperthyroidism is a syndrome that involves excessive production of thyroxin in the thyroid gland. This condition occurs most commonly with diffuse toxic goiter (Graves' disease) and less frequently with toxic nodular goiter or toxic adenoma, a benign tumor of the thyroid gland. Each of these conditions results in increased levels of circulating thyroxin. Excessive thyroxin causes a generalized increase in the metabolic rate of all body tissues, resulting in tachycardia, increased blood pressure, sensitivity to heat, and irritability. Hyperthyroidism is more common in females.

Radiographic features. Hyperthyroidism results in an advanced rate of dental development and early eruption, with premature loss of the primary teeth. Adults may show a generalized decrease in bone density or loss of some areas of edentulous alveolar bone.

HYPOTHYROIDISM

Identifying Characteristics
Synonyms. *Myxedema* and *cretinism*

Definition. Hypothyroidism usually results from insufficient secretion of thyroxin by the thyroid glands, despite the presence of thyroid-stimulating hormone.

Clinical features. In children, hypothyroidism may result in retarded mental and physical development. The base of the skull shows delayed ossification, and the paranasal sinuses only partially pneumatize. Dental development is delayed, and the primary teeth are slow to exfoliate.

Hypothyroidism in the adult results in myxedematous swelling but not the dental or skeletal changes seen in children. Adult symptoms may range from lethargy, poor memory, inability to concentrate, constipation, and cold intolerance to the more florid clinical picture of dull and expressionless face, periorbital edema, large tongue, sparse hair, and skin that feels "doughy" to the touch.

Radiographic features. Radiographic features in children include delayed closing of the epiphyses and skull sutures with the production of numerous wormian bones (accessory bones in the sutures). Effects on the teeth include delayed eruption, short roots, and thinning of the lamina dura. The maxilla and mandible are relatively small. Patients with adult hypothyroidism may show periodontal disease, loss of teeth, separation of teeth as a result of enlargement of the tongue, and external root resorption.

DIABETES MELLITUS

Identifying Characteristics
Definition. Diabetes mellitus is a metabolic disorder that has two primary forms. Type I, insulin-dependent diabetes mellitus (previously known as *juvenile-onset diabetes*), results from an absence or insufficiency of insulin, a hormone normally produced by the beta cells of the islets of Langerhans in the pancreas. Type II, non-insulin-dependent diabetes mellitus, results from insulin resistance. Patients with type I diabetes have virtually no beta cells (in the islets), whereas patients with type II diabetes have approximately half the normal number. A shortage of insulin adversely affects carbohydrate metabolism. The principal clinical laboratory signs of the disease are hyperglycemia and glycosuria, both reflecting a complex biochemical imbalance between tissue demand for glucose and the release of this nutrient by the liver.

Clinical features. Untreated diabetes may manifest classic symptoms and signs such as polydipsia (excessive intake of fluids), polyuria (excessive urination), and, in more severe cases, acetone present in the urine and on the breath. This metabolic disorder, if not adequately treated, lowers the resistance of the body to infection. Diabetes may demonstrate a number of adverse effects in the oral cavity. Most prominently, uncontrolled diabetes acts as a continuing factor that predisposes to, aggravates, and accelerates periodontal disease. Patients with controlled diabetes do not appear to have more periodontal problems than do persons without diabetes. Some children with uncontrolled diabetes have an increased likelihood of caries activity because of a high-carbohydrate diet. Another occasional oral complication of diabetes mellitus is xerostomia resulting from a reduced salivary flow (about one third of normal).

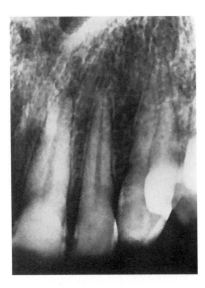

FIG. **23-6** Cushing's syndrome manifested in the jaws as thinning of the lamina dura. (Courtesy H.G. Poyton, DDS, Toronto, Ontario.)

Radiographic features. Diabetes mellitus exhibits no characteristic radiographic features of the jaws or teeth. Periodontal disease associated with diabetes is indistinguishable radiographically from periodontal disease in patients without diabetes.

CUSHING'S SYNDROME

Identifying Characteristics
Definition. Cushing's syndrome arises from an excess of secretion of glucocorticoids by the adrenal glands. This may result from any of the following:

1. An adrenal adenoma
2. An adrenal carcinoma
3. Adrenal hyperplasia (usually bilateral)
4. A basophilic adenoma of the anterior lobe of the pituitary gland (Cushing's disease), producing excess adrenocorticotropic hormone (ACTH)
5. Medical therapy with exogenous corticosteroids

The increased level of glucocorticoid results in a loss of bone mass from reduced osteoblastic function and either directly or indirectly increased osteoclastic function.

Clinical features. Patients with Cushing's syndrome often show obesity (which spares the extremities), kyphosis of the thoracic spine ("buffalo hump"), weakness, hypertension, striae, or concurrent diabetes. This condition affects females three to five times as frequently as males. Onset may occur at any age but is usually seen in the third or fourth decade.

Radiographic features. The primary radiographic feature of Cushing's syndrome is generalized osteoporosis, which may have a granular bone pattern. This demineralization may result in pathologic fractures. The skull can show diffuse thinning accompanied by a mottled appearance. The teeth may erupt prematurely, and partial loss of the lamina dura may occur (Fig. 23-6).

Metabolic Bone Diseases

OSTEOPOROSIS
Identifying Characteristics
Definition. Osteoporosis is a generalized decrease in bone mass in which the histologic appearance of bone is normal. An imbalance occurs in bone resorption and formation. Decrease in bone formation results in a lower trabecular bone volume and thinning of cortical bone and trabeculae.

Osteoporosis occurs with the aging process of bone and can be considered a variation of normal (primary osteoporosis). Bone mass normally increases from infancy to about 35 to 40 years of age. At this time there begins a gradual and progressive decline, occurring at the rate of about 8% per decade in women and 3% per decade in men. The loss of bone mass with age is so gradual that it is virtually imperceptible until it reaches significant proportions.

Secondary osteoporosis may result from nutritional deficiencies, hormonal imbalance, inactivity, or corticosteroid or heparin therapy.

Clinical features. The most important clinical manifestation of osteoporosis is fracture. The most common locations are the distal radius, proximal femur, ribs, and vertebrae. Patients may suffer from bone pain. The population most at risk is postmenopausal women.

Radiographic features. Osteoporosis results in an overall reduction in the density of bone. This reduction may be observed in the jaws by using the unaltered density of teeth as a comparison. There may be evidence of a reduced density and thinning of cortical boundaries such as the inferior mandibular cortex (Fig. 23-7). Reduction in the volume of cancellous bone is more difficult to assess. Reduction in the number of trabeculae is least evident in the alveolar process, possibly because of the constant stress applied to this region of bone by the teeth. On occasion the lamina dura may appear thinner than normal. In other regions of the mandible a reduction in the number of trabeculae may be evident. Accurate assessment of bone mass loss is difficult but may be done with sophisticated techniques such as dual energy photon absorption (DEXA) or quantitative computed tomography (QCT) programs.

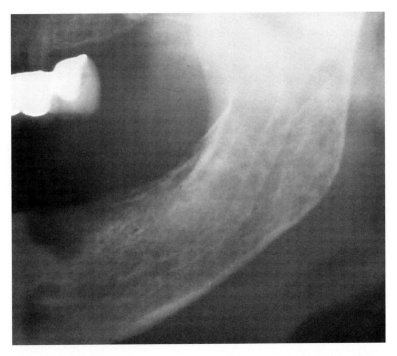

FIG. **23-7** Osteoporosis evident as a loss of the normal thickness and density of the inferior cortex of the mandible.

Treatment. The administration of estrogens and calcium supplements after menopause helps in preventing further cortical and trabecular bone loss. Exercise programs are also effective.

RICKETS AND OSTEOMALACIA

Identifying Characteristics

Definition. Rickets and osteomalacia result from inadequate serum and extracellular levels of calcium and phosphate, minerals required for the normal calcification of bone and teeth. Both abnormalities result from a defect in the normal activity of the metabolites of vitamin D, especially $1,25(OH)_2D$, required for resorption of calcium in the intestine. Failure of normal mineralization is seen histologically as wide uncalcified osteoid (new bone matrix) seams. The term *rickets* is usually applied when the disease affects the growing skeleton in infants and children. The term *osteomalacia* is used when this disease affects the mature skeleton in adults.

Failure of normal activity of vitamin D may occur as a result of the following:

1. Lack of vitamin D in the diet
2. Lack of absorption of vitamin D resulting from various gastrointestinal malabsorption problems
3. Lack of metabolism of the active metabolite $1,25(OH)_2D$ that is required for intestinal absorption of calcium

Interference may occur anywhere along the metabolic pathway for $1,25(OH)_2D$:

1. Lack of exposure to ultraviolet light required for conversion of provitamin D_3
2. Lack of conversion of vitamin D_3 to $25(OH)D$ in the liver because of liver disease
3. Lack of metabolism of $25(OH)D_2$ to $1,25(OH)_2D$ by the kidney because of kidney diseases
4. A defect in the intestinal target cell response to $1,25(OH)_2D$ or inadequate calcium supply

Clinical features

Rickets. In the first 6 months of life, tetany or convulsions are the most common clinical problems resulting from the hypocalcemia of rickets. Later in infancy the skeletal effects of the disease may be more clinically prominent. Craniotabes, a softening of the posterior of the parietal bones, may be the initial sign of the disease. The wrists and ankles typically swell. Children with rickets usually have short stature and deformity of the extremities. Development of the dentition is delayed, and the eruption rate of the teeth is retarded.

Osteomalacia. Most patients with osteomalacia have some degree of bone pain. The majority of patients with osteomalacia have muscle weakness of varying severity. Other clinical features include a peculiar waddling or "penguin" gait, tetany, and greenstick bone fractures.

Radiographic features

General radiographic features. In *rickets* the earliest and most prominent radiographic manifestation is a widening and fraying of the epiphyses of the long bones. The soft weight-bearing bones such as the femur and tibia undergo a characteristic bowing. Greenstick fractures (an incomplete fracture) occur in many patients with rickets.

In *osteomalacia* the cortex of bone may be thin. Pseudofractures, which are poorly calcified, ribbonlike zones extending into bone at approximate right angles to the margin of the bone, may also be present. Pseudofractures occur most commonly in the ribs, pelvis, and weight-bearing bones and rarely in the mandible.

Radiographic features of the jaws. In *rickets*, jaw cortical structures, such as the inferior mandibular border or the walls of the mandibular canal, may thin. Changes in the jaws generally occur after changes in the ribs and long bones. Within the cancellous portion of the jaws, the trabeculae become reduced in density, number, and thickness. In severe cases, the jaws appear so radiolucent that the teeth appear to be bereft of bony support.

Most cases of *osteomalacia* produce no radiographic manifestations in the jaws. However, when present there may be an overall radiolucent appearance and sparse trabeculae.

Radiographic changes associated with the teeth. Rickets in infancy or early childhood may result in hypoplasia of developing dental enamel (Fig. 23-8). If the disease occurs before 3 years, such enamel hypoplasia is fairly common. Radiographs may reveal this early manifestation of rickets in unerupted and erupted teeth. Radiographs may also document retarded tooth eruption in early rickets. The lamina dura and the cortical boundary of tooth follicles may be thin or missing.

Osteomalacia does not alter the teeth because they are fully developed before the onset of the disease. The lamina dura may be especially thin in individuals with long-standing or severe osteomalacia (Fig. 23-9).

HYPOPHOSPHATASIA

Identifying Characteristics

Definition. Hypophosphatasia is a rare inherited disorder that is caused by either a reduced production or a defective function of alkaline phosphatase. This enzyme is required for normal mineralization of osteoid. Patients have a low level of serum alkaline phosphatase activity and elevated urinary excretion of phosphoethanolamine. The usual pattern of inheritance is an autosomal dominant mode of disease transmission.

Clinical features. The disease in individuals with homozygous involvement usually begins in utero, and affected patients often die within the first year. These in-

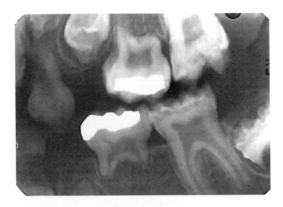

FIG. **23-8** Rickets may cause thinning (hypoplasia) or decreased mineralization (hypocalcification) of the enamel as is seen in this bitewing view. (Courtesy H.G. Poyton, DDS, Toronto, Ontario.)

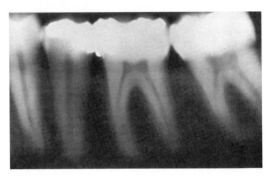

FIG. **23-9** Osteomalacia may cause a loss of bone, resulting in an increased radiolucency of the alveolar bone and lamina dura.

fants demonstrate bowed limb bones and a marked deficiency of skull ossification. Individuals with heterozygous disease show the biochemical defects but a milder disease clinically. These children show poor growth, fractures, and deformities similar to rickets. A history may exist of fractures, delayed walking, or ricketslike deformities that heal spontaneously. About 85% of these children show premature loss of the primary teeth, particularly the incisors, and delayed eruption of the permanent dentition. This is often the first clinical sign of hypophosphatasia.

Radiographic features

General radiographic features. In young children with hypophosphatasia the long bones show irregular defects in the epiphysis, and the skull is poorly calcified. In older children with premature closure of the skull sutures, multiple lucent areas of the calvarium may exist, called *gyral* or *convolutional* markings. These markings resemble hammered copper. The skull may assume a brachycephalic shape. A generalized reduction in bone density may occur in adults.

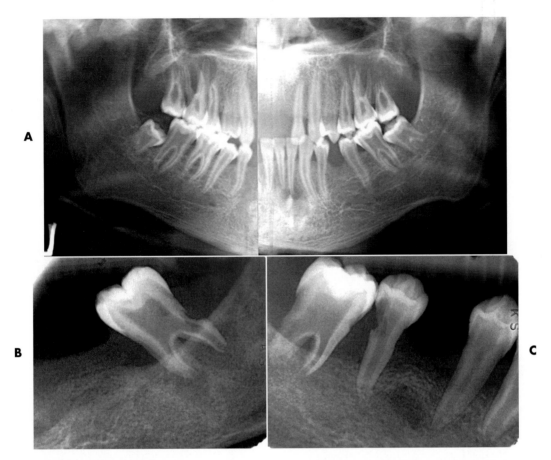

FIG. **23-10** **A,** A panoramic image of hypophosphatemic rickets. Note the radiolucent appearance of the jaws and hence the lack of bone density and the large pulp chambers. **B** and **C,** These periapical films of a case of hypophosphatemic rickets demonstrate apparent bone loss around the teeth, a granular bone pattern, large pulp chambers, and external root resorption.

Radiographic features of the jaws. A generalized radiolucency of the mandible and maxilla is evident. The cortical bone and lamina dura are thin, and the alveolar bone is poorly calcified and may appear deficient.

Radiographic changes associated with the teeth. Both primary and permanent teeth have a thin enamel layer and large pulp chambers and root canals (Fig. 23-10). The teeth may also be hypoplastic.

RENAL OSTEODYSTROPHY

Identifying Characteristics
Synonym. *Renal rickets*

Definition. In renal osteodystrophy, bone changes result from chronic renal failure. The kidney disease interferes with the hydroxylation of 25(OH)D into 1,25(OH)₂D, which normally occurs in the kidney. The vitamin D metabolite 1,25(OH)₂D is responsible for the active

transport of calcium in the duodenum and upper jejunum. Affected patients often have hypocalcemia as a result of impaired calcium absorption and hyperphosphatemia resulting from reduction in renal phosphorus excretion. A prolonged low serum level of calcium stimulates the parathyroid glands to produce PTH. The result is a secondary hyperparathyroidism.

Clinical features. The clinical features of renal osteodystrophy are those of chronic renal failure. In children, growth retardation and frequent bone fractures may occur. Adults may experience a gradual softening and bowing of the bones.

Radiographic features
General radiographic features. The radiographic features of renal osteodystrophy are quite variable. Some changes of the skeleton resemble those seen in rickets, and other changes are consistent with hyperparathyroidism, including generalized loss of bone density and thinning of

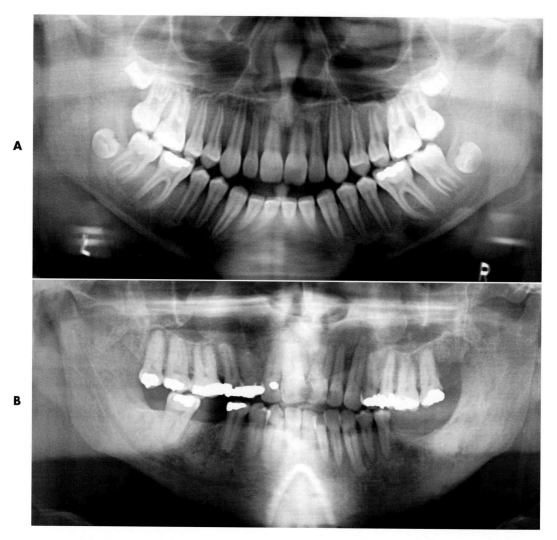

FIG. **23-11**   Two cases of renal osteodystrophy. **A,** This panoramic image reveals areas of radiolucency corresponding to loss of bone mass, loss of distinct lamina dura, and a sclerotic bone pattern around the roots of the teeth. **B,** This panoramic image reveals a diffuse sclerotic (radiopaque) bone pattern throughout the jaws. Note the loss of a distinct inferior cortex of the mandible resulting from an increase in the radiopacity of the internal aspect of the bone.

bony cortices. Of interest is the occasional finding of an increase in bone density (Fig. 23-11). There may be brown tumors, similar to those seen in primary hyperthyroidism, but these are less frequent.

Radiographic features of the jaws. In renal osteodystrophy the density of the mandible and maxilla may be less than normal and occasionally may be greater than normal. Manifestations include a decrease or an increase in the number of internal trabeculae, and the trabecular bone pattern may be granular. The cortical boundaries may be thinner or less apparent. It is important to note that these bone changes may persist after a successful renal transplant because of hyperplasia of the parathyroid glands, resulting in a continued elevation of PTH.

Radiographic changes associated with the teeth. Hypoplasia and hypocalcification of the teeth are possible, sometimes resulting in loss of any radiographic evidence of enamel. The lamina dura may be absent or less apparent in instances of bone sclerosis.

HYPOPHOSPHATEMIA

Identifying Characteristics
Synonym. *Vitamin D–resistant rickets*

Definition. Hypophosphatemia represents a group of inherited conditions that produce renal tubular disorders resulting in excessive loss of phosphorus. There is a failure to reabsorb phosphorus in the distal renal tubules, resulting in a decrease in serum phosphorus (hypophosphatemia). Normal calcification of the osseous structures requires the correct amount and ratio of serum calcium and phosphorus. Multiple myeloma may induce hypophosphatemia as a result of secondary damage to the kidneys.

Clinical features. Children with hypophosphatemia show reduced growth and ricketslike bony changes. These include bowing of the legs, enlarged epiphyses, and skull changes. Adults have bone pain, muscle weakness, and vertebral fractures.

Radiographic features

General radiographic features. In children with hypophosphatemia, radiographic findings are indistinguishable from those of rickets. In adults the long bones may show persistent deformity, fractures, or pseudofractures.

Radiographic features of the jaws. The jaws are usually osteoporotic and in extreme cases are remarkably radiolucent. Cortical boundaries may be unusually radiolucent or not apparent. Other possibilities include fewer visible trabeculae and a granular trabecular pattern.

Radiographic features associated with the teeth. The teeth may be poorly formed, with thin enamel caps and large pulp chambers and root canals. In addition, periapical and periodontal abscesses occur frequently. The occurrence of periapical rarefying osteitis without an etiology may be a result of large pulp chambers and defects in the formation of dentin. This may allow for the ingress of oral microorganisms and subsequent pulp necrosis. If the disease is severe, the patient experiences premature loss of the teeth. The lamina dura may become sparse, and cortical boundaries around tooth crypts may be thin or entirely absent.

OSTEOPETROSIS

Identifying Characteristics

Synonyms. *Albers-Schönberg* and *marble bone disease*

Definition. Osteopetrosis is a disorder of bone that results from a defect in the differentiation and function of osteoclasts. The lack of normally functioning osteoclasts results in abnormal formation of the primary skeleton and a generalized increase in bone mass. The failure of normal bone remodeling results in dense, fragile bones that are susceptible to fracture and infection. Obliteration of the marrow compromises hematopoiesis and compresses cranial nerves. This disorder is inherited as an autosomal recessive type (osteopetrosis congenita) and autosomal dominant type (osteopetrosis tarda).

Clinical features. The more severe, recessive form of osteopetrosis is seen in infants and young children, and the more benign, dominant form appears later. The severe form is invariably fatal early in life. The patient experiences progressive loss of the bone marrow and its cellular products and a severe increase in bone density. The narrowing of bony canals results in hydrocephalus, blindness, deafness, vestibular nerve dysfunction, and facial nerve paralysis. The benign, dominant form is milder and may be entirely asymptomatic. It may be discovered any time from childhood into adulthood. The disease may be found as an incidental finding or appear as a pathologic fracture of a bone. In some of the more chronic cases, bone pain and cranial nerve palsies caused by neural compression may be clinical problems. Osteomyelitis may complicate this disease because of the relative lack of vascularity of the dense bone. This problem is more common in the mandible, whereas osteomyelitis is usually secondary to dental or periodontal disease.

Radiographic features

General radiographic features. In the classic radiographic presentation of osteopetrosis, all bones show greatly increased density, which is bilaterally symmetric. The increased density throughout the skeleton is homogeneous and diffuse (Fig. 23-12). The internal aspect of the involved bone may be so dense or radiopaque that the trabecular patterns of the medullary cavity may not be visible. The internal radiopacity also reduces the contrast between the outer cortical border and the cancellous portion of the bone. The entire bone may be mildly enlarged.

Radiographic features of the jaws. The increased radiopacity of the jaws may be so great that the radiographic image may fail to reveal any internal structure and even the roots of the teeth may not be apparent. The increased bone density and relatively poor vascularity results in a susceptibility of the mandible to osteomyelitis, usually from odontogenic inflammatory lesions.

Radiographic features associated with the teeth. Effects on teeth may include delayed eruption, early tooth loss, missing teeth, malformed roots and crowns, and teeth that are poorly calcified and prone to caries (Fig. 23-13). The normal eruption pattern of the primary and secondary dentition may be delayed as a result of bone density or ankylosis. The lamina dura and cortical borders may appear thicker than normal.

Differential diagnosis. The differential diagnosis includes other sclerosing bone dysplasias such as sclerosteosis, infantile cortical hyperostosis, pyknodysostosis, craniometaphyseal dysplasia, diaphyseal dysplasia,

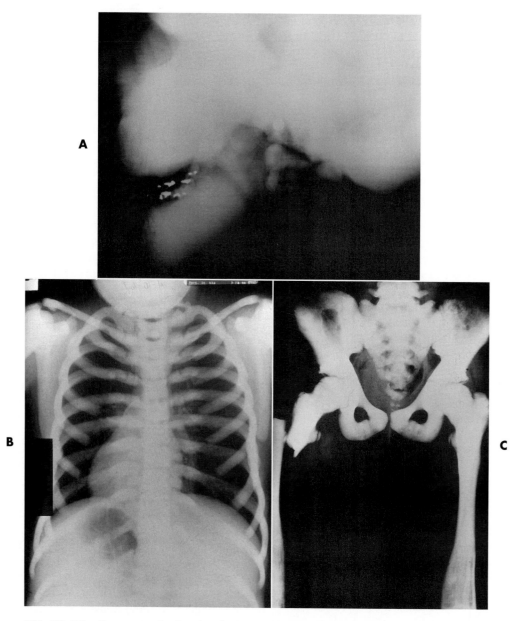

FIG. 23-12 *Osteopetrosis, showing dense calcification of all the bones.* **A,** Skull and facial bones. **B,** Chest. **C,** Pelvis and femurs (note the fracture of the proximal right femur).

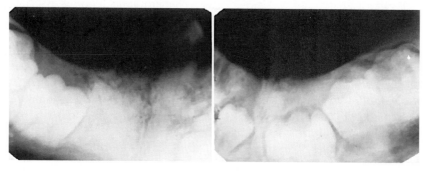

FIG. 23-13 Osteopetrosis, showing dense alveolar bone and embedded, poorly formed teeth. (Courtesy H.G. Poyton, DDS, Toronto, Ontario.)

melorheostosis, and osteopathia striata. Osteosclerosis from fluoride poisoning and secondary hyperparathyroidism from renal disease also may have a general sclerotic appearance.

Treatment. Treatment of osteopetrosis consists of bone marrow transplants to attempt to stimulate the formation of functional osteoclasts and systemic steroids for the hematologic component. The osteomyelitis is difficult to treat, and a combination of antibiotics and hyperbaric oxygen therapy is used. It is imperative that affected patients avoid odontogenic inflammatory disease.

Other Systemic Diseases

PROGRESSIVE SYSTEMIC SCLEROSIS
Identifying Characteristics
Synonym. *Scleroderma*

Definition. Progressive systemic sclerosis (PSS) is a generalized connective tissue disease that causes hardening (sclerosis) of the skin and other tissues. The involvement of the gastrointestinal tract, heart, lungs, and kidneys usually results in more serious complications. The cause of the disease is unknown.

Clinical features. PSS is a disease of middle age with the greatest incidence between the ages of 30 and 50 years. It is seen rarely in adolescence or the elderly. Women are affected about three times as often as men.

In most patients with moderate to severe PSS, the involved skin has a thickened, leathery quality. The skin is not mobile over the underlying soft tissues, and involvement of the facial region may inhibit normal mandibular opening. Patients with diffuse disease are also likely to have xerostomia; increased numbers of decayed, missing, or filled teeth; and carious lesions. Further, patients with systemic disease are more likely to have deeper periodontal pockets and higher gingivitis scores. Patients with cardiac and pulmonary problems may have varying degrees of heart failure and respiratory insufficiencies. Renal involvement usually leads to some degree of uremia, with or without hypertension.

Radiographic features
Radiographic features of the jaws. A radiographic feature in some cases of PSS is an unusual pattern of mandibular erosions at regions of muscle attachment such as the angles, coronoid process, digastric region, or condyles (Fig. 23-14). This type of resorption is typically bilateral and fairly symmetric. Most of these erosive borders are smooth and sharply defined. This resorption may be progressive with the disease.

Radiographic changes associated with the teeth. The most common oral radiographic manifestation of PSS is an increase in the width of the periodontal ligament (PDL) spaces around the teeth (Fig. 23-15). Approximately two thirds of patients with PSS show this change. The PDL spaces affected by PSS usually are at least twice as thick as normal and both anterior and posterior teeth are affected, although it is more pronounced around the posterior teeth. The lamina dura remains normal. Despite the widening of the PDL spaces, the clinician finds that involved teeth are often not mobile and their gingival attachments are usually intact. Almost half of the patients with PDL space thickening also had some mandibular erosive bone changes.

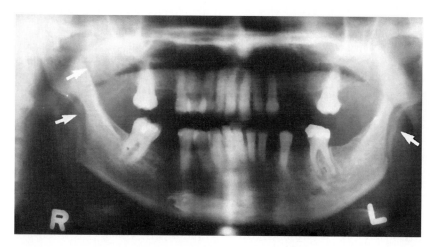

FIG. **23-14** PSS, demonstrating a loss of bone in the region of the angle of the mandible *(right arrow)* and at the right coronoid process *(left arrows)*, which are locations of muscle attachments.

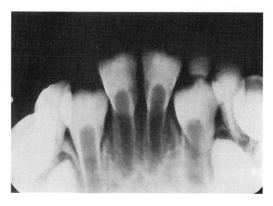

FIG. 23-15 PSS may be manifested as a marked thickening of the PDL space.

Differential diagnosis. Other causes of widening of the periodontal membrane space include tooth mobility, orthodontic tooth movement, intermaxillary fixation with arch bars, and invasion of the PDL by malignant neoplasms. Widening of the PDL space with malignant neoplasia differs in destruction of the lamina dura and irregular widening.

Management. The aforementioned thickening of PDL spaces does not seem to present any clinical difficulties. The progressive loss of bone in the region of the mandibular angle, however, is more serious because of potential fracture. It is reasonable to obtain initial and periodic panoramic radiographs in all patients with PSS to assess mandibular integrity.

SICKLE CELL ANEMIA

Identifying Characteristics

Definition. Sickle cell anemia is an autosomal recessive, chronic, hemolytic blood disorder. Patients with this disorder have abnormal hemoglobin (deoxygenated hemoglobins), which under low oxygen tension results in sickling of the red blood cells. These blood cells have a reduced capacity to carry oxygen to the tissues and, because of damage to their membrane lipids and proteins, adhere to vascular endothelium and obstruct capillaries. The spleen traps and readily destroys these abnormal red cells. The hematopoietic system responds to the resultant anemia by increasing the production of red blood cells, which requires compensatory hyperplasia of the bone marrow.

Clinical features. The homozygous form of sickle cell anemia occurs in approximately 1 in every 400 African-Americans. Although the gene is present in the heterozygous state in about 6% to 8% of African-Americans, those who manifest this form of the sickle cell trait do not show related clinical findings.

Although symptoms and signs vary considerably, most patients with the disease normally manifest mild, chronic features. Long, quiet spells of hemolytic latency occur, occasionally punctuated by exacerbations known as *sickle cell crises*. During the crisis state, patients often experience severe abdominal, muscle, and joint pain, have a high temperature, and may even undergo circulatory collapse. During milder periods the patient may complain of fatigability, weakness, shortness of breath, and muscle and joint pain. As in the other chronic anemias, the heart is usually enlarged and a murmur may be present. The disease occurs mostly in children and adolescents. It is compatible with a normal life span, although many patients die of complications of the disease before the age of 40 years.

Radiographic features. The hyperplasia of the bone marrow at the expense of cancellous bone is the primary reason for the radiographic manifestations of sickle cell anemia. The extent of bone changes in sickle cell anemia relates to the degree of this hyperplasia.

General radiographic features. The thinning of individual cancellous trabeculae and cortices is most common in the vertebral bodies, long bones, skull, and jaws. The skull may have widening of the diploic space and thinning of the inner and outer tables (Fig. 23-16). Loss of the outer table and a hair-on-end appearance may occur in about 5% of cases. Small areas of infarction may be present within bones after blockage of the microvasculature; these are seen radiographically as areas of localized bone sclerosis. Osteomyelitis may complicate sickle cell anemia if infection begins in an area of pronounced hypovascularity. There may also be retardation of generalized bone growth.

Radiographic features of the jaws. The radiographic manifestations of sickle cell anemia in the jaws include general osteoporosis (Fig. 23-17). This occurs because of a decrease in the volume of trabecular bone and, to a lesser extent, thinning of the cortical plates. In most cases the change is mild or moderate, with extreme radiographic manifestations being unusual. The bone pattern may be altered to one with fewer but coarser trabeculae. Radiographs of the jaws of children with sickle cell anemia have been reported to show a high frequency of sometimes severe osteoporosis. Rarely, bone marrow hyperplasia may cause enlargement and protrusion of the maxillary alveolar ridge.

THALASSEMIA

Identifying Characteristics

Synonyms. *Cooley's anemia, Mediterranean anemia* and *erythroblastic anemia*

Definition. Thalassemia is a hereditary disorder that results in a defect in hemoglobin synthesis. This defect

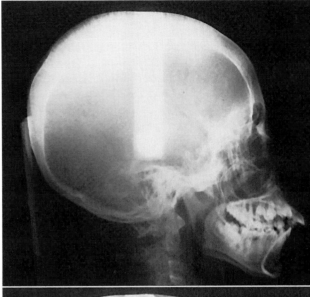

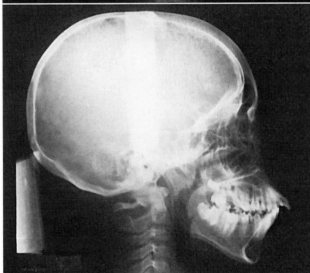

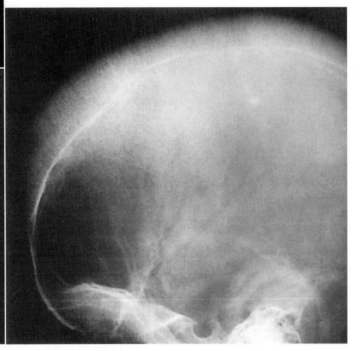

FIG. **23-16**   **A,** Radiograph of a patient with sickle cell anemia, showing a thickened diploic space and thinning of the skull cortex. **B,** Normal skull for comparison. **C,** Skull showing the hair-on-end bone pattern. (**B** courtesy Dr. B. Sarnat, Los Angeles, Calif; **C** courtesy H.G. Poyton, DDS, Toronto, Ontario.)

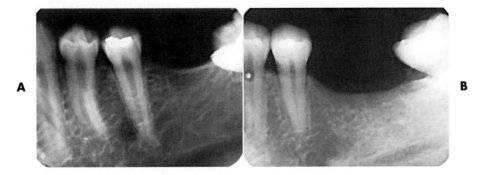

FIG. **23-17**   **A,** Radiograph of a patient with sickle cell anemia with enlarged bone marrow spaces in the mandible. **B,** Normal mandible for comparison. (**A** and **B** courtesy Dr. B. Sarnat, Los Angeles, Calif.)

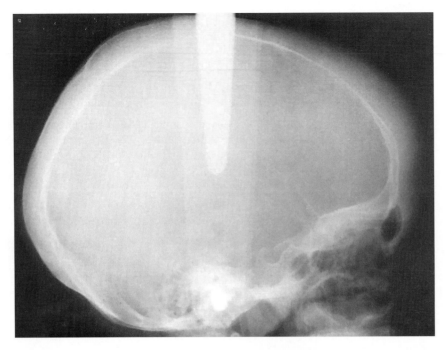

FIG. **23-18**   Radiograph of a patient with thalassemia showing a granular appearance of the skull and thickening of the diploic space. (Courtesy H.G. Poyton, DDS, Toronto, Ontario.)

may involve either the alpha or beta globulin genes. The resultant red blood cells have reduced hemoglobin content, are thin, and have a shortened life span. The heterozygous form of the disease (thalassemia minor) is mild. The homozygous form (thalassemia major) may be severe. A less severe form, thalassemia intermedia, also occurs.

Clinical features. In the severe form of the disease, the onset is in infancy and the survival time may be short. The face develops prominent cheekbones and a protrusive premaxilla resulting in a "rodent-like" face. The milder form of the disease occurs in adults.

Radiographic features
General radiographic features. Similar to sickle cell anemia, the radiographic features of thalassemia generally result from hyperplasia of the ineffective bone marrow and its subsequent failure to produce normal red cells. However, these changes are usually more severe than with other anemias. There is a generalized radiolucency of the long bones with cortical thinning. In the skull the diploic space exhibits marked thickening, especially in the frontal region. The skull shows a generalized granular appearance (Fig. 23-18), and occasionally a hair-on-end effect may develop.

Radiographic appearance of the jaws. Severe bone marrow hyperplasia prevents pneumatization of the paranasal

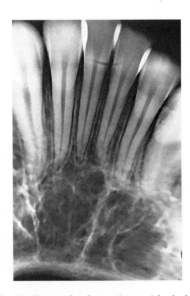

FIG. **23-19**   Radiograph of a patient with thalassemia with thick trabeculae and large bone marrow spaces. (Courtesy H.G. Poyton, DDS, Toronto, Ontario.)

sinuses, especially the maxillary sinus, and causes an expansion of the maxilla that results in malocclusion. The jaws appear radiolucent, with thinning of the cortical borders and enlargement of the marrow spaces. The trabeculae are large and coarse (Fig. 23-19). The lamina dura is thin, and the roots of the teeth may be short.

SUGGESTED READINGS

Aegerter E, Kirkpatrick JA: *Orthopedic diseases,* ed 4, Philadelphia, 1975, WB Saunders.

Keller EE, Stafne EC, Gibilisco JA: Oral radiographic manifestations of systemic disease. In Gibilisco JA, Turlington EG, editors: *Stafne's oral roentgenographic diagnosis,* ed 5, Philadelphia, 1985, WB Saunders.

Paterson CR: *Metabolic disorders of bone,* Oxford, 1974, Blackwell Scientific.

Trapnell DH, Boweman JE: *Dental manifestation of systemic disease,* London, 1973, Butterworth.

DIABETES MELLITUS

Lamey PJ, Darwazeh AM, Frier BM: Oral disorders associated with diabetes mellitus, *Diabet Med* 9:410, 1992.

Mackenzie RS, Millard HD: Interrelated effects of diabetes, arteriosclerosis and calculus on alveolar bone loss, *J Am Dent Assoc* 54:191, 1963.

Murrah VA: Diabetes mellitus and associated oral manifestations: a review, *J Oral Pathol* 14:271, 1985.

Stahl SS: Roentgenographic and bacteriologic aspects of periodontal changes in diabetics, *J Periodontol* 19:130, 1948.

HYPERPARATHYROIDISM

Bilezikian JP: Hyper- and hypoparathyroidism. In Rakel R, editor: *Conn's current therapy,* Philadelphia, 1985, WB Saunders.

Boonstra CE, Jackson CE: Serum calcium survey for hyperparathyroidism: results in 50,000 clinic patients, *Am J Clin Pathol* 55:523, 1971.

Cooper D, Wood L: Hyperthyroidism. In Rakel R, editor: *Conn's current therapy,* Philadelphia, 1985, WB Saunders.

Rosenberg E, Guralnick W: Hyperparathyroidism: a review of 220 proved cases with special emphasis on findings in the jaws, *Oral Surg Oral Med Oral Pathol* 15(suppl 2):84, 1962.

Steinbach HL et al: Primary hyperparathyroidism: a correlation of roentgen, clinical and pathologic features, *Am J Roentgenol* 86:329, 1961.

HYPOPARATHYROIDISM

Frensilli J, Stoner R, Hinrichs E: Dental changes of idiopathic hypoparathyroidism, *J Oral Surg* 29:727, 1971.

Glynne A, Hunter I, Thomson J: Pseudohypoparathyroidism with paradoxical increase in hypocalcemic seizures due to long-term anticonvulsant therapy, *Postgrad Med J* 48:632, 1972.

Silverman S, Ware W, Gillody C: Dental aspects of hyperparathyroidism, *Oral Surg Oral Med Oral Pathol* 26:184, 1968.

HYPOPHOSPHATASIA

Eastman JR, Bixler D: Clinical, laboratory, and genetic investigations of hypophosphatasia: support for autosomal dominant inheritance with homozygous lethality, *J Craniofac Genet Dev Biol* 3:213, 1983.

Jedrychowski JR, Duperon D: Childhood hypophosphatasia with oral manifestations, *J Oral Med* 34:18, 1979.

Macfarland JD, Swart JGN: Developmental aspects of hypophosphatasia: a case report, family study, and literature review, *Oral Surg Oral Med Oral Pathol* 67:521, 1989.

HYPOPITUITARISM

Conley H et al: Clinical and histologic findings of the dentition in a hypopituitary patient: report of case, *ASDC J Dent Child* 57:376, 1990.

Edler RJ: Dental and skeletal ages in hypopituitary patients, *J Dent Res* 56:1145, 1977.

Kosowicz J, Rzymski K: Abnormalities of tooth development in pituitary dwarfism, *Oral Surg Oral Med Oral Pathol* 44:853, 1977.

Myllarniemi S, Lenko HL, Perheentupa J: Dental maturity in hypopituitarism, and dental response to substitution treatment, *Scand J Dent Res* 86:307, 1978.

OSTEOPOROSIS

Gallagher C: Osteoporosis. In Rakel R, editor: *Conn's current therapy,* Philadelphia, 1985, WB Saunders.

Garn S, Rohmann C, Wagner B: Bone loss as a general phenomenon in man, *Fed Proc* 26:1729, 1967.

Law AN, Bollen AM, Chen SK: Detecting osteoporosis using dental radiographs: a comparison of four methods, *J Am Dent Assoc* 127:1734, 1996.

Mohammad AR, Alder M, McNally MA: A pilot study of panoramic film density at selected sites in the mandible to predict osteoporosis, *Int J Prosthodont* 9:290, 1996.

Taguchi A et al: Oral signs as indicators of possible osteoporosis in elderly women, *Oral Surg Oral Med Oral Pathol Oral Radiol Endod* 80:612, 1995.

Taguchi A et al: Usefulness of panoramic radiography in the diagnosis of postmenopausal osteoporosis in women. Width and morphology of inferior cortex of the mandible, *Dentomaxillofac Radiol* 25:263, 1996.

OSTEOPETROSIS

Dick H, Simpson W: Dental changes in osteopetrosis, *Oral Surg* 34:408, 1972.

Ruprecht A, Wagner H, Engel H: Osteopetrosis: report of a case and discussion of the differential diagnosis, *Oral Surg Oral Med Oral Pathol* 66:674, 1988.

Steiner M, Gould A, Means W: Osteomyelitis of the mandible associated with osteopetrosis, *J Oral Maxillofac Surg* 41:395, 1983.

Younai F, Eisenbud L, Sciubba JJ: Osteopetrosis: a case report including gross and microscopic findings in the mandible at autopsy, *Oral Surg Oral Med Oral Pathol* 65:214, 1988.

PROGRESSIVE SYSTEMIC SCLEROSIS

Alexandridis C, White SC: Periodontal ligament changes in patients with progressive systemic sclerosis, *Oral Med Oral Pathol* 58:113, 1984.

Rout PG, Hamburger J, Potts AJ: Orofacial radiological manifestations of systemic sclerosis. *Dentomaxillofac Radiol* 25:193, 1996.

Ruprecht A, Dolan K, Lilly GE: Osteolysis of the mandible associated with progressive systemic sclerosis, *Dentomaxillofac Radiol* 19:31, 1990.

White SC, Frey NW, Blaschke DD, et al: Oral radiographic changes in patients with progressive systemic sclerosis (scleroderma), *J Am Dent Assoc* 94:1178, 1977.

Wood RE, Lee P: Analysis of the oral manifestations of systemic sclerosis (scleroderma), *Oral Med Oral Pathol* 65:172, 1988.

RENAL OSTEODYSTROPHY

Bras J et al: Radiographic interpretation of the mandibular angular cortex: a diagnostic tool in metabolic bone loss. II, Renal osteodystrophy, *Oral Surg* 53:647, 1982.

Scutellari PN et al: Radiographic manifestations in teeth and jaws in chronic kidney insufficiency, *Radiol Med (Torino)* 92:415, 1996.

Syrjanen S, Lampainen E: Mandibular changes in panoramic radiographs of patients with end stage renal disease, *Dentomaxillofac Radiol* 12:51, 1983.

RICKETS

Harris R, Sullivan H: Dental sequelae in deciduous dentition in vitamin-D resistant rickets, *Aust Dent J* 5:200, 1960.

Marks SC, Lindahl RL, Bawden JW: Dental and cephalometric findings in vitamin D resistant rickets, *J Dent Child* 32:259, 1965.

SICKLE CELL ANEMIA

Brown DL, Sebes JI: Sickle cell gnathopathy: radiologic assessment, *Oral Surg Oral Med Oral Pathol* 61:653, 1986.

Halstead CL: Oral manifestations of hemoglobinopathies. A case of homozygous hemoglobin C disease diagnosed as a result of dental radiographic changes, *Oral Surg Oral Med Oral Pathol* 30:615, 1970.

Mourshed F, Tuckson C: A study of radiographic features of the jaws in sickle-cell anemia, *Oral Surg Oral Med Oral Pathol* 37:812, 1974.

Sanger RG, Bystrom EB: Radiographic bone changes in sickle cell anemia, *J Oral Med* 32:32, 1977.

Sanger RG, Greer R, Averbach R: Differential diagnosis of some simple osseous lesions associated with sickle-cell anemia, *Oral Surg Oral Med Oral Pathol* 43:538, 1977.

Sears RS, Nazif MM, Zullo T: The effects of sickle-cell disease on dental and skeletal maturation. *ASDC J Dent Child* 48:275, 1981.

THALASSEMIA

Caffey J: Cooley's anemia: a review of the roentgenographic findings in the skeleton, *AJR Am J Roentgenol* 78:381, 1957.

Poyton HG, Davey KW: Thalassemia: changes visible in radiographs used in dentistry, *Oral Surg Oral Med Oral Pathol* 25:564, 1968.

Sommermater JI, Bacon W: Dentomaxillary and maxillofacial manifestations of thalassemia major apropos of a case, *Actual Odontostomatol* 35:489, 1981.

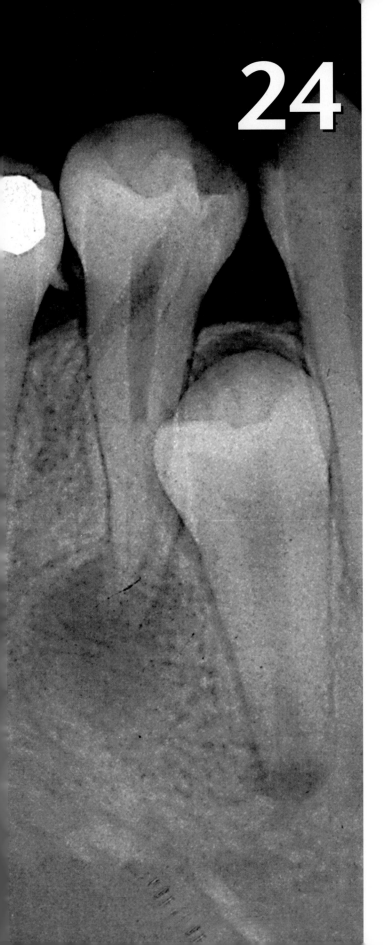

24

Disorders of the Temporomandibular Joint

C. GRACE PETRIKOWSKI

Disorders of the temporomandibular joint are abnormalities that interfere with the normal form or function of the joint. The most common of these disorders are dysfunction of the articular disk and associated ligaments and muscles, joint arthritides, inflammatory lesions, neoplasms, and growth or developmental abnormalities.

Clinical Features

Temporomandibular joint (TMJ) dysfunction is the most common jaw disorder, with 28% to 86% of adults and adolescents showing one or more clinical signs or symptoms. A higher incidence of the disorder has been reported in females, although the reason for this preponderance is not clear. Signs and symptoms of dysfunction include pain in the TMJ or ear or both, headache, muscle tenderness, joint stiffness, clicking or other joint noises, reduced range of motion, locking, and subluxation. In most cases the clinical signs and symptoms are transitory, and treatment is not indicated. A small group of patients (5%) suffers severe dysfunction (e.g., severe pain, marked functional impairment, or both), which requires a thorough diagnostic workup, including diagnostic imaging, before treatment is begun.

The clinical signs and symptoms of other disorders of the TMJ may include swelling in and around the joint, an elevated temperature, and redness of the overlying skin.

Application of Diagnostic Imaging

TMJ imaging may be necessary to supplement information obtained from the clinical examination, particularly when an osseous abnormality or infection is suspected, conservative treatment has failed, or symptoms are worsening. Diagnostic imaging also should be considered for patients with a history of trauma, significant dysfunction, alteration in range of motion, sensory or motor abnormalities, or significant changes in occlusion. TMJ imaging is not indicated for joint sounds if other signs or symptoms are absent or for asymptomatic children and adolescents before orthodontic treatment. The purposes of TMJ imaging are to evaluate the integrity and relationships of the hard and soft tissues, confirm the extent or stage of progression of known disease, and evaluate the effects of treatment. The clinician must correlate the radiographic information with the patient's history and clinical findings to arrive at a final diagnosis and plan the management of the underlying disease process.

Radiographic Anatomy of the TMJ

A thorough understanding of the radiographic anatomy of the TMJ is essential so that a normal variant is not mistaken for an abnormality. The TMJs are unique in that although they constitute two separate joints anatomically, they function together as a single unit. Each condyle articulates with the mandibular fossa of the temporal bone. A disk composed of fibrocartilage is interposed between the condyle and mandibular fossa. A fibrous capsule lined with synovial membrane surrounds and encloses the joint. Ligaments and muscles restrict or allow movement of the condyle.

CONDYLE

The condyle is a bony, ellipsoid structure connected to the mandibular ramus by a narrow neck (Fig. 24-1). The condyle is approximately 20 mm long mediolaterally and 8 to 10 mm thick anteroposteriorly. The shape of the condyle varies considerably; the superior aspect may be flattened, rounded, or markedly convex, whereas the mediolateral contour usually is slightly convex. These variations in shape may cause difficulty with radiographic interpretation; this underlines the importance of understanding the range of normal appearance. The extreme aspects of the condyle are called the *medial pole* and *lateral poles*. The long axis of the condyle is slightly rotated on the condylar neck such that the medial pole is angled posteriorly, forming an angle of 15 to 33 degrees with the sagittal plane. The two condylar axes typically intersect near the anterior border of the foramen magnum in the submentovertex projection.

Most condyles have a pronounced ridge oriented mediolaterally on the anterior surface, marking the anteroinferior limit of the articulating area. This ridge is the upper limit of the pterygoid fovea, a small depression on the anterior surface at the junction of the condyle and neck. It is the attachment site of the superior head of the lateral pterygoid muscle and should not be mistaken for an osteophyte (spur), which indicates degenerative joint disease.

Although the mandibular and temporal components of the TMJ are calcified by 6 months of age, complete calcification of cortical borders may not be completed until 20 years of age. As a result, radiographs of condyles in children may show little or no evidence of a cortical border. In the absence of disease, the cortical borders in adults are visible radiographically. A layer of fibrocartilage covers the condyle but is not visible radiographically.

MANDIBULAR FOSSA

The mandibular (glenoid) fossa is located at the inferior aspect of the squamous part of the temporal bone and is composed of the articular fossa and articular eminence of the temporal bone (Fig. 24-2, *A*). It is sometimes described as the *temporal component* of the TMJ. The articular eminence forms the anterior limit of the mandibular fossa and is convex in shape. Its most inferior aspect is called the *summit* or *apex* of the eminence. In a normal TMJ, the roof of the fossa, the posterior slope of the articular eminence, and the eminence itself form an S shape when viewed in the sagittal plane. The most lateral aspect of the eminence consists of a protuberance, called the *articular tubercle*, that is a ligamentous attachment. The squamotympanic fissure and its medial extension, the petrotympanic fissure, form the posterior limit of the fossa. The middle portion of the roof of the fossa forms a small portion of the floor of the middle cranial fossa, and only a thin layer of cortical bone separates the joint cavity from the intracranial subdural space. The spine of the sphenoid forms the medial limit of the fossa. Fossa depth varies, and the development of the articular eminence relies on functional stimulus from the condyle. For example, the mandibular fossa is very flat and underdeveloped in patients with micrognathia or condylar agenesis. The fossa and articular eminence develop during the first 3 years and reach mature shape by the age of 4 years; young infants lack a definite fossa and articular eminence.

All aspects of the temporal component may be pneumatized with small air cells derived from the mastoid air cell complex (Fig. 24-2, *B*). Pneumatization of the articular eminence is seen radiographically in approximately 2% of patients. Like the condyle, the mandibular fossa is covered with a thin layer of fibrocartilage.

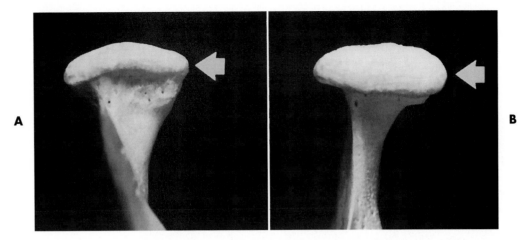

FIG. **24-1** *Mandibular condyle.* The medial pole *(arrow)* is on the right in each case. **A,** Anterior aspect. **B,** Superior aspect.

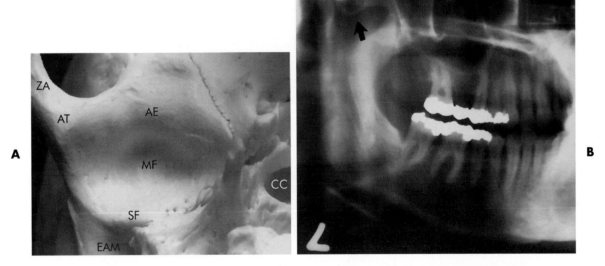

FIG. **24-2** **A,** Basal view of the skull showing the mandibular fossa. *AE,* Articular eminence; *AT,* articular tubercle; *CC,* carotid canal; *EAM,* external auditory meatus; *MF,* mandibular fossa; *SF,* squamotympanic fissure; *ZA,* zygomatic arch. **B,** Pneumatization of the articular eminence with a mastoid air cell (panoramic view) *(arrow).* (**B** courtesy Dr. D. Tyndall and Dr. S.R. Matteson, Chapel Hill, N.C.)

INTERARTICULAR DISK

The interarticular disk (meniscus), composed of fibrous connective tissue, is located between the condylar head and mandibular fossa. The disk divides the joint cavity into two compartments, called the *inferior* (lower) and *superior* (upper) *joint spaces,* which are located below and above the disk, respectively (Fig. 24-3). A normal disk has a biconcave shape with a thick anterior band, thicker posterior band, and a thin middle part. The disk also is thicker medially than laterally. The medial and lateral margins of the disk blend with the capsule. The thin central portion normally serves as an articulating cush-

ion between the condyle and articular eminence. The anterior band is thought to be attached to the superior head of the lateral pterygoid muscle, and the posterior band attaches to the posterior retrodiskal tissues (also called the *posterior attachment*). The junction between the posterior band and posterior attachment lies within 10 degrees of vertical above the condylar head in normal individuals. The disk and posterior attachment are collectively called the *soft tissue component* of the TMJ.

During mandibular opening, as the condyle translates downward and forward, the disk also moves forward so that its thin central portion remains between the

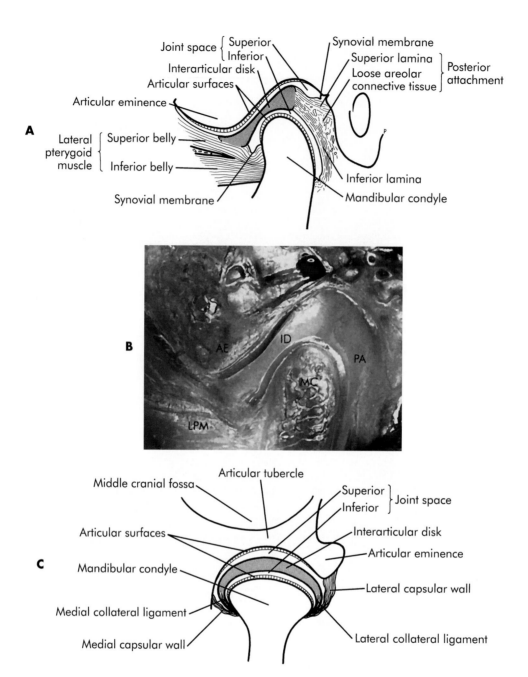

FIG. **24-3** *TMJ anatomy.* **A,** Lateral view. **B,** Sectioned cadaver specimen in the same orientation. *AE,* Articular eminence; *ID,* interarticular disk; *LPM,* lateral pterygoid muscle; *MC,* mandibular condyle; *PA,* posterior attachment. **C,** Coronal view. (Courtesy Dr. W.K. Solberg, Los Angeles, Calif.)

articulating convexities of the condylar head and articular eminence. Laterally and medially the disk attaches to the condylar poles, helping to ensure passive movement of the disk with the condyle so that the condyle and disk translate forward together to the summit of the articular eminence. As the mandible opens, the condyle also rotates against the lower surface of the disk in the inferior joint space. On mandibular closing, this process reverses, with the disk moving back with the condyle into the mandibular fossa.

POSTERIOR ATTACHMENT (RETRODISKAL TISSUES)

The posterior attachment consists of a bilaminar zone of vascularized and innervated loose fibroelastic tissue. The superior lamina, which is rich in elastin, inserts into the posterior wall of the mandibular fossa. The superior lamina stretches and allows the disk to move forward with condylar translation. The inferior lamina attaches to the posterior surface of the condyle. The posterior attachment is covered with a synovial membrane that secretes synovial fluid, which lubricates the joint. As the condyle moves forward, tissues of the posterior attach-

ment expand in volume, primarily as a result of venous distention, and as the disk moves forward, tension is produced in the elastic posterior attachment. This tension is thought to be responsible for the smooth recoil of the disk posteriorly as the mandible closes.

TMJ BONY RELATIONSHIPS

Radiographic joint space is a general term used to describe the radiolucent area between the condyle and temporal component (see Fig. 24-3). This general term should not be confused with the terms *superior joint space* and *inferior joint space* described earlier, which refer to soft tissue spaces above and below the disk. The radiographic joint space contains the soft tissue components of the joint. Clinicians sometimes use comparison of radiographic joint space dimensions with corrected tomograms to determine the condylar position in the fossa, with the opposite joint used for comparison. A condyle is positioned concentrically when the anterior and posterior aspects of the radiolucent joint space are uniform in width. The condyle is retruded when the posterior joint space width is less than the anterior (Fig. 24-4) and protruded when the posterior joint space is wider than the anterior.

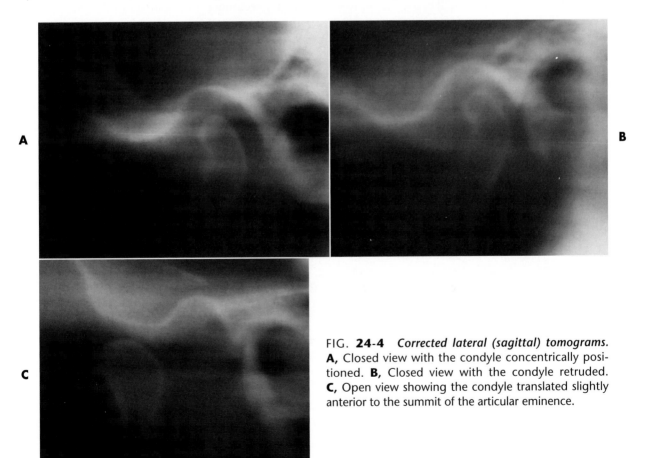

FIG. **24-4** *Corrected lateral (sagittal) tomograms.* **A,** Closed view with the condyle concentrically positioned. **B,** Closed view with the condyle retruded. **C,** Open view showing the condyle translated slightly anterior to the summit of the articular eminence.

The diagnostic significance of mild or moderate condylar eccentricity is not clear; condylar eccentricity is seen in one third to one half of asymptomatic individuals and is not a reliable indicator of the soft tissue status of the joint, particularly because the shape of the condylar head is not concentric to the shape of the fossa. Markedly eccentric condylar positioning usually represents an abnormality. For example, inferior condylar positioning (widened joint space) may be seen in cases involving fluid or blood within the joint, and superior condylar positioning (decreased joint space or no joint space, with osseous contact of joint components) may indicate loss, displacement, or perforation of intracapsular soft tissue components. Marked posterior condylar positioning is seen in some cases of disk displacement, and marked anterior condylar positioning may be seen in juvenile rheumatoid arthritis.

CONDYLAR MOVEMENT

The condyle undergoes complex movement during mandibular opening. Downward and forward translation (sliding) of the condyle occurs whereby the superior surface of the disk slides against the articular eminence; at the same time a hingelike, rotatory movement occurs with the superior surface of the condyle against the inferior surface of the disk. The extent of normal condylar translation varies considerably. In most individuals, at maximal opening the condyle moves down and forward to the summit of the articular eminence or slightly anterior to it (see Fig. 24-4). The condyle typically is found within a range of 2 to 5 mm posterior and 5 to 8 mm anterior to the crest of the eminence. Reduced condylar translation, in which the condyle has little or no downward and forward movement and does not leave the mandibular fossa, is seen

in patients who clinically have a reduced degree of mouth opening. Hypermobility of the joint may be suspected if the condyle translates more than 5 mm anterior to the eminence. This may permit anterior locking or dislocation of the condyle if a superior movement also occurs above and anterior to the summit of the articular eminence.

Diagnostic Imaging of the TMJ

The type of imaging technique selected depends on the specific clinical problem, whether imaging of hard or soft tissues is desired, the amount of diagnostic information available from a particular imaging modality, the cost of the examination, and the radiation dose. In most cases the imaging protocol begins with hard tissue imaging to evaluate the osseous contours, the positional relationship of the condyle and fossa, and the range of motion, although a combination of imaging techniques may be indicated. Soft tissue imaging is indicated when information about disk position, morphology, or integrity is needed or to image abnormalities in the muscles or surrounding tissues. A summary of the diagnostic information provided by each imaging technique is presented in Table 24-1.

HARD TISSUE IMAGING

Panoramic Projection

Because the panoramic projection provides an overall view of the teeth and jaws, it serves as a screening projection to identify odontogenic diseases and other disorders that may be the source of TMJ symptoms. Some panoramic machines have specific TMJ programs, but these are of limited usefulness because of thick image layers and the oblique, distorted view of the joint they

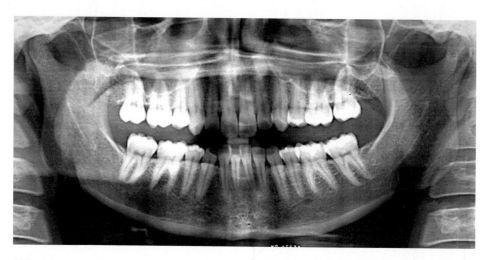

FIG. **24-5** *Panoramic view.* The right condyle is smaller than the left and is not smoothly corticated. Tomograms later showed marked erosive changes of the right condylar head.

TABLE **24-1**
Diagnostic Information Provided by Various TMJ Imaging Techniques

ABNORMALITY	IMAGING TECHNIQUE*									
	PANORAMIC	TRANS-CRANIAL	TRANS-PHARYNGEAL	TRANS-ORBITAL	SUBMENTO-VERTEX	SKULL VIEWS	CONVENTIONAL TOMOGRAPHY	COMPUTED TOMOGRAPHY	ARTHROG-RAPHY	MAGNETIC RESONANCE IMAGING
Hard Tissue										
Bony ankylosis	−	−	−	−	−	−	++	+++	−	+
Arthridites	+	++	+	+	−	−	++	+++	−	+++
Remodeling	+	++	+	+	−	−	++	++	−	−
Developmental abnormalities	++	+	+	+	+	+	++	+++	−	+
Neoplasm	+	+	+	+	+	+	++	+++	−	+++
Trauma (fracture)	++	+	+	+++	++	++	++	+++	−	++
Range of motion	−	+++	+	−	−	−	+++	−	+++	++
Asymmetry	++	+	+	+	++	++	++	+	−	−
Soft Tissue										
Disk position	−	−	−	−	−	−	−	+	+++	+++
Disk perforation	−	−	−	−	−	−	−	−	+++	−
Fibrous ankylosis	−	−	−	−	−	−	−	−	+++	+++
Joint effusion	−	−	−	−	−	−	−	−	+++	+++
Inflammatory conditions	−	−	−	−	−	−	−	−	++†	+++
Joint space calcifications	−	+	+	−	−	−	++	+++	−	+

Modified from Brooks SL et al: Imaging of the temporomandibular joint, position paper of the American Academy of Oral and Maxillofacial Radiology, *Oral Surg Oral Med Oral Pathol Oral Radiol Endod* 83:609, 1997.
*−, Does not provide diagnostic information for the abnormality; +, only occasionally useful; ++, often useful; +++, almost always useful.
†When including arthrocentesis.

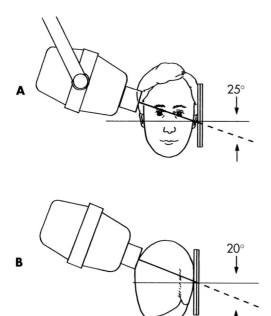

FIG. **24-6** *Transcranial projection.* **A,** The central ray is oriented at a 25-degree positive angle from the opposite side **(B)** and anteriorly 20 degrees, centered over the TMJ of interest.

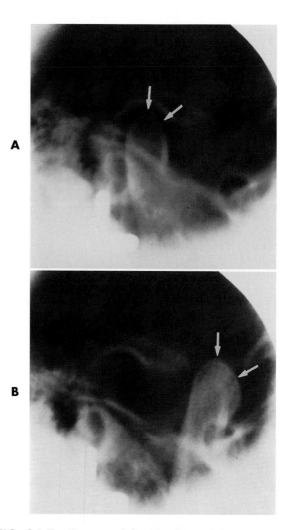

FIG. **24-7** *Transcranial projections of the right TMJ.* In each case, the condyle is indicated by arrows. **A,** Closed view. **B,** Open view.

provide, which severely limits image quality. Gross osseous changes in the condyles may be identified, such as asymmetries, extensive erosions, large osteophytes, or fractures (Fig. 24-5). However, no information about condylar position or function is provided because the mandible is partly opened and protruded when this radiograph is exposed. Also, mild osseous changes may be obscured, and only marked changes in articular eminence morphology can be seen because of superimposition by the skull base and zygomatic arch. For these reasons, the panoramic view does not provide an adequate examination of the hard tissues of the joints.

Transcranial Projection

The transcranial projection provides a sagittal view of the lateral aspects of the condyle and temporal component. The patient is positioned in a cephalostat; the x-ray beam is directed downward from the opposite side, through the cranium and above the petrous ridge of the temporal bone, at a 25-degree positive angle centered through the joint. The horizontal beam may be individually corrected for the condylar long axis (see Conventional Tomography, p. 502), or an average 20-degree anterior angle may be used. The film cassette is placed on the side to be imaged (Fig. 24-6). A routine transcranial series includes projections of both TMJs in the closed and maximally open positions (Fig. 24-7).

Because of the positive beam angulation, the central and medial aspects of the joint are projected inferiorly,

and only lateral joint contours are visible in this projection. The ipsilateral petrous ridge often is superimposed over the condylar neck, which may obscure osseous changes in the condyle or temporal component. The image of the condyle, temporal component, and joint space is distorted, and condylar position cannot be reliably determined, particularly if the horizontal beam angle is not individualized for each patient. The transcranial projection is useful for identifying gross osseous changes on the lateral aspect of the joint only, displaced condylar fractures, and range of motion (open views).

Transpharyngeal (Parma) Projection

The transpharyngeal (Parma) projection provides a sagittal view of the medial pole of the condyle. The x-ray beam is directed superiorly at −5 degrees through the sigmoid notch of the opposite side and 7 to 8 degrees from the anterior (Fig. 24-8); the film cassette is placed on the side being imaged. The patient opens the mouth

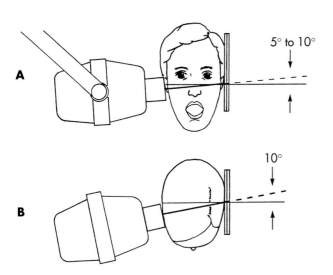

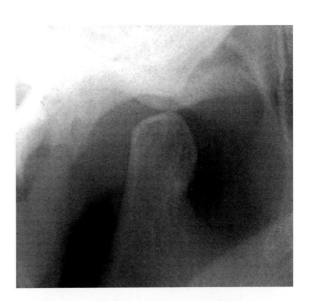

FIG. **24-8** *Transpharyngeal projection.* **A,** The central ray is oriented superiorly 5 to 10 degrees and **(B)** posteriorly approximately 10 degrees, centered over the TMJ of interest. Note that the mandible is positioned at maximal opening.

FIG. **24-9** Transpharyngeal projection showing the condyle at the articular eminence. The zygomatic arch is superimposed over the glenoid fossa.

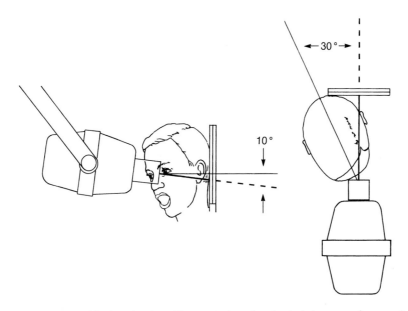

FIG. **24-10** *Transorbital projection.* The central ray is oriented downward approximately 10 degrees and laterally approximately 30 degrees through the ipsilateral orbit, centered over the TMJ of interest.

maximally to avoid superimposition of the condyle on the temporal component. Because of the negative beam angulation, this view depicts the medial aspect of the condyle. The transpharyngeal view provides limited diagnostic information because the temporal component is not imaged well (Fig 24-9). The transpharyngeal projection is effective for visualizing erosive changes of the condyle rather than more subtle changes.

Transorbital Projection

The transorbital projection is similar to the transmaxillary projection in that both provide an anterior view of the TMJ, perpendicular to transcranial and transpharyngeal projections. In the transorbital view, the patient's head is tilted downward 10 degrees so that the canthomeatal line is horizontal (Fig. 24-10). The x-ray beam is directed from the front of the patient through

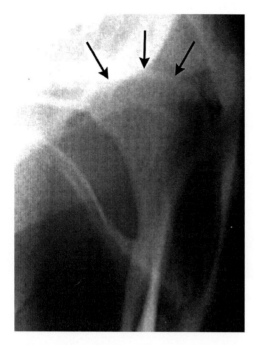

FIG. **24-11** Transorbital view showing the condyle *(arrows)* below the articular eminence. The mastoid process partly obscures the articulating surface on the mediosuperior aspect.

the ipsilateral orbit and TMJ of interest. The film cassette is placed behind the patient's head, perpendicular to the x-ray beam. The patient opens maximally or, as an alternative, protrudes the mandible, thereby positioning the condyle at the summit of the articular eminence and avoiding superimposition of the articular eminence or skull base on the condyle.

The entire mediolateral dimension of the articular eminence, condylar head, and condylar neck is visible, which makes this view particularly useful for visualizing condylar neck fractures. The morphology of the convex surface of the condylar head can be evaluated, making this projection a useful adjunct to transcranial and transpharyngeal projections in the diagnosis of gross degenerative changes or other anomalies (Fig. 24-11). The usefulness of this projection is limited by the ability of the condyle to move to the summit of the articular eminence. If condylar motion is limited, only the condylar neck is visible because areas of the joint articulating surfaces are obscured by superimposition of the temporal component on the condylar head. A similar projection is the reverse Towne's projection, which sometimes is used to image condylar neck fractures, particularly if medial displacement has occurred, because the condylar head and neck is visualized in the frontal plane.

Submentovertex (Basal) Projection

The submentovertex (SMV) projection provides a view of the skull base and condyles superimposed on the condylar necks and mandibular rami. For this reason the SMV projection often is used to determine the angulations of the long axis of the condylar head for corrected tomography (see Chapter 10 for technique). This view may be used as an adjunct to views depicting the TMJs in the lateral plane and is particularly useful for evaluating facial asymmetries, condylar displacement, or rotation of the mandible in the horizontal plane associated with trauma or orthognathic surgery.

Conventional Tomography

Tomography is a radiographic technique that produces multiple thin image slices, permitting visualization of an anatomic structure essentially free of superimpositions of overlapping structures (see Chapter 12). Because this technique can provide multiple image slices at right angles through the joint, it is superior to the transcranial view in depicting true condylar position and revealing osseous changes. For these reasons, tomography is a valuable adjunct to plain film radiography and can provide information that may not be available with plain films alone.

Tomographs typically are exposed in the sagittal (lateral) plane with several image slices in the closed (maximal intercuspation) position and usually only one image in the maximal open position. In "corrected" sagittal tomography, the condylar long axis with respect to the midsagittal plane is determined using an SMV projection (Fig. 24-12). The patient's head is then rotated to this angle, permitting alignment of image slices perpendicular to the condylar long axis. This minimizes geometric distortion of the joint and allows accurate assessment of condylar position. Although a corrected tomographic technique is preferred, when not available, a 20-degree head rotation toward the side of interest is superior to image slices parallel to the midsagittal plane. To minimize patient movement in open views, a bite-block may be inserted between the patient's anterior teeth because it takes several seconds to complete each tomographic exposure.

It may be desirable to supplement this examination with coronal (frontal) tomographs, particularly when morphologic abnormalities or erosive changes of the condylar head are suspected. For coronal tomographs, the patient is in a maximal open or protruded position, which brings the condyle to the summit of the articular eminence, free of superimposition of the posterior slope of the eminence. The entire condylar head is visible in the mediolateral plane (Fig. 24-13).

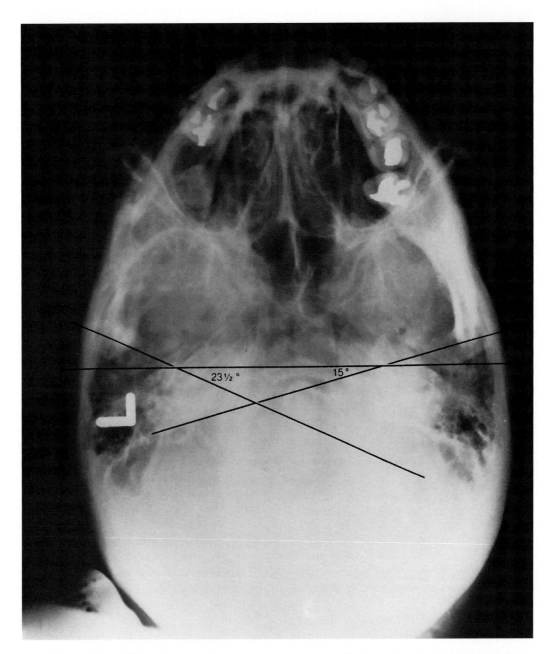

FIG. **24-12** *SMV projection.* Tracing of angles between the long axis of each condyle and the midsagittal plane. For tomographic views the patient is rotated according to the measured angles to produce an undistorted radiographic view of each TMJ.

Computed Tomography

Computed tomography (CT) is indicated when more information is needed about the three-dimensional shape and internal structure of the osseous components of the joint. CT produces digital image slices (see Chapter 12). Multiple image slices are made in both the axial and coronal planes, although the coronal images are the more useful. Data from axial and coronal scans can be manipulated to produce (reformat) images in the sagit-

tal plane. Three-dimensional reformatted images also can be produced. These are useful for assessing osseous deformities of the jaws or surrounding structures. CT cannot produce accurate images of the articular disk.

CT may be considered for determining the presence and extent of ankylosis and neoplasms and the extent of bone involvement in some arthritides, imaging complex fractures, and evaluating complications from the use of polytetrafluoroethylene or silicon sheet implants

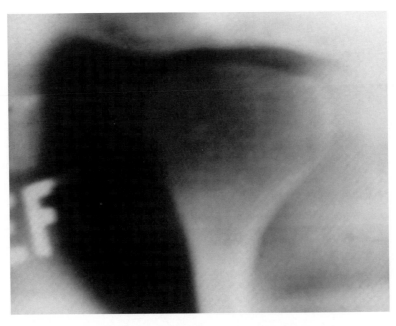

FIG. **24-13** Frontal tomographic section of the mandibular condyle.

such as erosions into the middle cranial fossa and ectopic bone growth.

SOFT TISSUE IMAGING

The soft tissues of the joint can be imaged with magnetic resonance imaging (MRI) or arthrography. Conventional imaging techniques do not demonstrate disk position, morphology, or function. Soft tissue imaging is indicated when TMJ pain and dysfunction are present or when the clinical findings suggest disk displacement along with symptoms that are unresponsive to conservative therapy.

MRI and arthrography should be used only when information about the condition of the soft tissue components of the joint is required to formulate a treatment plan. The choice of technique depends on patient factors, such as allergy to contrast agents and claustrophobia, as well as on the cost, availability, and objectives of the imaging technique. Arthrography is superior for diagnosis of small disk perforations and joint adhesions. MRI can indicate a pathologic condition of the soft tissue through altered tissue signal, allowing evaluation of the disk and surrounding muscles, and can image joint effusion. The technique is noninvasive and does not use ionizing radiation. Arthrography with videofluoroscopy provides a superior motion study of the joint, although some MRI techniques can provide limited dynamic information.

Arthrography

Imaging of the hard tissues should be completed before arthrographic imaging is performed.

Arthrography is a technique in which an indirect image of the disk is obtained by injecting a radiopaque contrast agent into one or both joint spaces under fluoroscopic guidance (Fig. 24-14). A perforation is detected by the flow of contrast agent into the superior joint space from the lower space, and adhesions are detected by the manner in which contrast agent fills the joint space. After both spaces are filled, disk function is studied using fluoroscopy during open and closing movements. The fluoroscopic study usually is supplemented with tomographs of the joint.

Arthrography is indicated when information about disk position, function, morphology, and the integrity of diskal attachments is required for treatment planning. The risks of this procedure include allergic reaction to the nonionic iodine contrast agent and infection.

Magnetic Resonance Imaging

MRI uses a magnetic field and radiofrequency pulses rather than ionizing radiation to produce multiple digital image slices (see Chapter 12). Because MRI can provide superb images of soft tissues, this technique can be used for imaging the articular disk. MRI allows construction of images in the sagittal and coronal planes without repositioning the patient (Fig 24-15). These images usually are acquired in open and closed mandibular positions using surface coils to improve image reso-

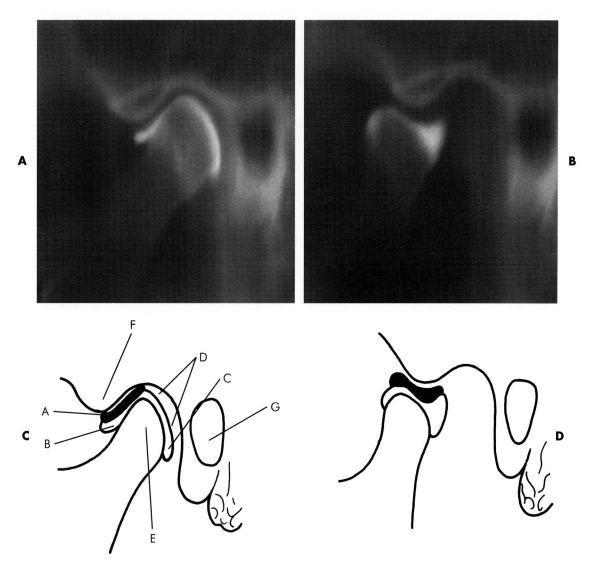

FIG. **24-14** *Lower joint space arthrograms of a normal TMJ.* **A,** Closed view. **B,** Open view. The disk is visualized by observing the superior margin of the contrast agent, which defines the inferior border of the disk and its attachments. **C** and **D** show the structures in the arthrograms. *A,* Disk; *B,* anterior, and *C,* posterior, recesses of the lower compartment, filled with contrast agent; *D,* bilaminar zone; *E,* condylar head; *F,* articular eminence; *G* auditory canal. (Courtesy Dr. Alan G. Lurie, Farmington, Conn.)

lution. Sagittal slices can be directed perpendicular to the condylar long axis. The examinations usually are performed using T1-weighted, proton-weighted, or T2-weighted pulse sequences. T1-weighted images best demonstrate osseous and diskal tissues, whereas T2-weighted images demonstrate inflammation and joint effusion. Motion MRI studies during opening and closing can be obtained by having the patient open in a series of stepped distances and using rapid image acquisition ("fast scan") techniques. Medial disk displacements can be detected by MRI. The change in tis-

sue signal that results from changes in the disk and retrodiskal tissue may make accurate identification of the disk difficult.

MRI does not have the morbidity associated with the introduction of needles into the joint (as occurs in arthrography), but MRI is a more expensive examination and is contraindicated in patients who are pregnant or who have pacemakers, intracranial vascular clips, or metal particles in vital structures. Some patients may not be able to tolerate the procedure because of claustrophobia or an inability to remain motionless.

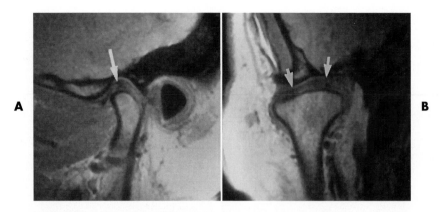

FIG. **24-15**   *MRI of a normal TMJ.* **A,** Closed view showing the condyle and temporal component. The biconcave disk is located with its posterior band *(arrow)* over the condyle. **B,** Coronal image showing the osseous components and disk *(arrows)* superior to the condyle. (Courtesy Dr. Per-Lennart Westesson, Rochester, N.Y.).

Radiographic Abnormalities of the TMJ

DEVELOPMENTAL ABNORMALITIES

Developmental abnormalities may be broadly categorized as anomalies in the form and size of joint components. The most striking radiographic changes usually are seen in the condyle, although the temporal component also may be deformed, often remodeling to accommodate the abnormal condyle. Condylar articular cartilage is a mandibular growth site, and, as a result, developmental abnormalities at this location may manifest as altered growth on the affected side of the condyle, mandibular ramus, mandibular body, and alveolar process.

Condylar Hyperplasia

Definition. Condylar hyperplasia is a developmental abnormality that results in enlargement and occasionally deformity of the condylar head; this may have a secondary effect on the mandibular fossa as it remodels to accommodate the abnormal condyle. The etiology may be overactive cartilage or persistent cartilaginous rests, which increases the thickness of the entire cartilaginous and precartilaginous layers. This condition usually is unilateral and may be accompanied by varying degrees of hyperplasia of the ipsilateral mandible.

Clinical features. Condylar hyperplasia is more common in males, and it usually is discovered before the age of 20 years. The condition is self-limiting and tends to arrest with termination of skeletal growth, although in a small number of cases continued growth and adult onset have been reported. The condition may progress slowly or

rapidly. Patients have a mandibular asymmetry that varies in severity, depending on the degree of condylar enlargement. The chin may be deviated to the unaffected side, or it may remain unchanged but with an increase in the vertical dimension of the ramus, mandibular body, or alveolar process of the affected side. As a result of this growth pattern, patients may have a posterior open bite on the affected side. Patients may also have symptoms related to TMJ dysfunction and may complain of limited or deviated mandibular opening or both caused by restricted mobility of the enlarged condyle.

Radiographic features. The condyle may appear relatively normal but symmetrically enlarged, or it may be altered in shape (e.g., conical, spherical, elongated, lobulated) or irregular in outline. It may be more radiopaque because of the additional bone present. A morphologic variation manifesting as elongation of the condylar head and neck with a compensating forward bend, forming an inverted L, may be seen. Also, the condylar neck may be elongated and thickened and may bend laterally when viewed in the coronal (anteroposterior) plane (Fig. 24-16). The cortical thickness and trabecular pattern of the enlarged condyle usually are normal, which helps to distinguish this condition from a condylar neoplasm. The glenoid fossa may be enlarged, usually at the expense of the posterior slope of the articular eminence. The ramus and mandibular body on the affected side also may be enlarged, resulting in a characteristic depression of the inferior mandibular border at the midline, where the enlarged side joins the contralateral normal mandible. The affected ramus may have increased vertical depth and may be thicker in the anteroposterior dimension.

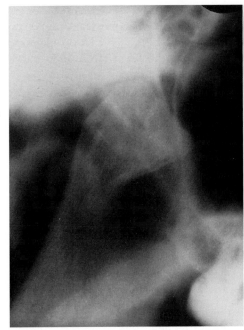
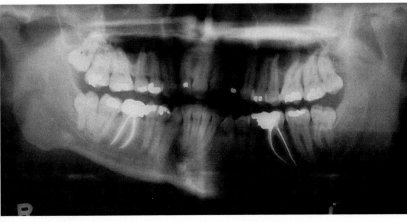

FIG. **24-16** **A,** Condylar hyperplasia (transpharyngeal projection). The condylar head is enlarged, and the neck is thick. **B,** Associated hyperplasia of the affected side of the mandible. Note the depression of the inferior mandibular border at the midline where the enlarged side joins the contralateral normal mandible.

Differential diagnosis. A condylar tumor, most notably an osteochondroma, is included in the differential diagnosis. An osteochondroma usually is more irregular in shape compared with a hyperplastic condyle. Surface irregularities and continued growth after cessation of skeletal growth should increase suspicion of this tumor. Occasionally a condylar osteoma or large osteophyte that occurs in chronic degenerative joint disease may simulate condylar hyperplasia.

Treatment. Treatment consisting of orthodontics combined with orthognathic surgery ideally should be attempted after condylar growth is complete. Determining when condylar growth has stopped may be difficult; imaging may include longitudinal radiographic studies to assess the dimensions of the condyle and mandible, nuclear imaging techniques, or both. A lack of bone activity, demonstrated in a technetium bone scan, is a useful indication of arrested condylar growth.

Condylar Hypoplasia
Definition. Condylar hypoplasia is failure of the condyle to attain normal size because of congenital and developmental abnormalities or acquired diseases that affect condylar growth. The condyle is small, but condylar morphology usually is normal. The condition may be inherited or may appear spontaneously. Some cases have been attributed to early injury or injury to the articular cartilage by birth trauma or intraarticular inflammatory lesions.

Clinical features. Condylar hypoplasia usually is a component of a mandibular growth deficiency and therefore often is associated with an underdeveloped ramus and (occasionally) mandibular body. Congenital abnormalities may be unilateral or bilateral and usually are a manifestation of a more generalized condition (e.g., micrognathia, Treacher Collins syndrome); they also may be associated with congenital defects of the ear and zygomatic arch. Developmental abnormalities that manifest during growth usually are unilateral. Acquired abnormalities are the result of damage during the growth period from sources such as therapeutic radiation or infection that diminish or prevent further condylar growth and development. Patients with condylar hypoplasia have mandibular asymmetry and may have symptoms of TMJ dysfunction. The chin commonly is deviated to the affected side, and the mandible deviates to the affected side during mandibular opening. Degenerative joint disease is a common long-term sequela.

Radiographic features. The condyle may be normal in shape and structure but is diminished in size, and the mandibular fossa also is proportionally small. The condylar neck and coronoid process usually are very slender and are shortened or elongated in some cases. The posterior border of the ramus and condylar neck may have a dorsal (posterior) inclination. The ramus and mandibular body on the affected side may also be small, resulting in a mandibular asymmetry and occasional dental crowding, depending on the severity of mandibular underdevelopment. The antegonial notch

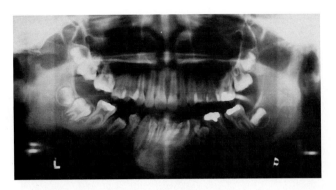

FIG. **24-17** Condylar hypoplasia on the left side, resulting in loss of vertical height of the mandibular ramus.

is deepened. The associated mandibular hypoplasia is more pronounced if the effect takes place early in life (Fig. 24-17).

Differential diagnosis. Condylar destruction from juvenile rheumatoid arthritis may appear similar to that of hypoplasia. A survey of other joints or testing for rheumatoid factor may be helpful. Changes in condylar morphology in severe degenerative joint disease may have a similar appearance, although arthritic disease does not cause hypoplasia of the affected side of the mandible.

Treatment. Orthognathic surgery, bone grafts, and orthodontic therapy may be required.

Juvenile Arthrosis
Synonyms. *Boering's arthrosis* and *arthrosis deformans juvenilis*

Definition. Juvenile arthrosis, a condylar growth disturbance first described by Boering, manifests as hypoplasia and characteristic morphologic abnormalities. This condition may be a form of condylar hypoplasia but is thought to differ in that the affected condyle at one time was normal and then became abnormal during growth. Juvenile arthrosis may be unilateral or bilateral, and it predisposes the TMJ to secondary degenerative changes.

Clinical features. Juvenile arthrosis affects children and adolescents during the period of mandibular growth. It is more common in females. It may be an incidental finding in a panoramic projection, or the patient may have mandibular asymmetry, signs and symptoms of TMJ dysfunction, or both.

Radiographic features. The condylar head develops a characteristic "toadstool" appearance, with marked flattening and apparent elongation of the articulating condylar surface and dorsal (posterior) inclination of the

condyle and neck. The condylar neck is shortened or even absent in some cases, with the condyle resting on the upper margin of the ramus (Fig. 24-18). The articulating surface of the temporal component often is flattened. Progressive shortening of the ramus occurs on the affected side, and the antegonial notch may be deepened, indicating mandibular hypoplasia. In long-standing cases, superimposed degenerative changes may be present.

Differential diagnosis. The radiographic appearance of juvenile arthrosis may be very similar to, and in some cases is indistinguishable from, developmental hypoplasia of the condyle. Destruction of the anterior aspect of the condylar head from rheumatoid arthritis and severe degenerative joint disease or severe condylar degeneration after orthognathic surgery or joint surgery also may simulate juvenile arthrosis.

Treatment. Orthognathic surgery and orthodontic therapy may be required to correct the mandibular asymmetry. Caution should be exercised in undertaking orthodontic therapy because stress on the joint may result in further degeneration and orthodontic relapse.

Coronoid Hyperplasia
Definition. Coronoid process hyperplasia may be acquired or developmental, resulting in elongation of the coronoid process. In the developmental variant, the condition usually is bilateral. Acquired types may be unilateral or bilateral and usually are a response to restricted condylar movement caused by abnormalities such as ankylosis.

Clinical features. Bilateral coronoid hyperplasia is more common in males, often commencing at the onset of puberty, although the condition was reported in a 3-year-old. Patients complain of a progressive inability to open the mouth and may have an apparent closed lock. The condition is painless.

Radiographic features. Coronoid hyperplasia is best seen in panoramic, Waters', and lateral tomographic views and on CT scans. The coronoid processes are elongated, and the tips extend at least 1 cm above the inferior rim of the zygomatic arch (Fig. 24-19). As a result, the coronoid processes may impinge on the medial surface of the zygomatic arch during opening, restricting condylar translation. The coronoid processes may have a large but normal shape or may curve anteriorly and may appear very radiopaque. The posterior surface of the zygomatic process of the maxilla may be remodeled to accommodate the enlarged coronoid process during function. The radiographic appearance of the TMJs usually is normal.

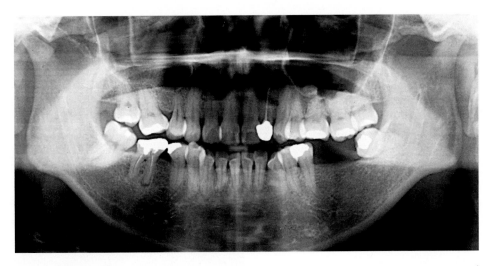

FIG. **24-18** *Juvenile arthrosis.* The condylar heads have a "toadstool" appearance and are posteriorly inclined. The condylar necks are absent.

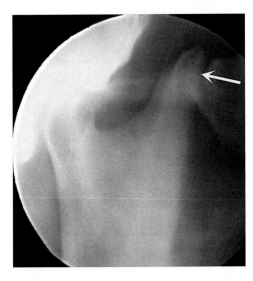

FIG. **24-19** *Coronoid hyperplasia (sagittal tomogram).* The coronoid process is elongated and extends above the inferior rim of the zygomatic arch *(arrow)* but otherwise is shaped normally.

Differential diagnosis. Unilateral cases should be differentiated from a tumor of the coronoid process such as an osteochondroma or osteoma. Unlike coronoid hyperplasia, tumors usually have an irregular shape. The differential diagnosis also includes any cause of inability to open, such as soft tissue abnormalities and ankylosis, emphasizing the importance of including the coronoid process in images of the TMJs. An axial CT image with the patient in a wide open position is useful in establishing coronoid interference to opening.

Treatment. Treatment consists of osteotomy or surgical removal of the coronoid process and postoperative physiotherapy.

Bifid Condyle

Definition. A bifid condyle has a vertical depression, notch, or deep cleft in the center of the condylar head, seen in the frontal or sagittal plane, or actual duplication of the condyle, resulting in the appearance of a "double" or "bifid" condylar head. This condition may be unilateral or bilateral. It may result from an obstructed blood supply or other embryopathy, although a traumatic cause has been postulated as a result of a longitudinal linear fracture of the condyle.

Clinical features. Bifid condyle usually is an incidental finding in panoramic views or anteroposterior projections. Some patients have signs and symptoms of temporomandibular dysfunction, including joint noises and pain.

Radiographic features. A depression or notch is present on the superior condylar surface, giving the anteroposterior silhouette a heart shape; in more severe cases a duplicate condylar head is present in the mediolateral plane (Fig. 24-20). The mandibular fossa may remodel to accommodate the altered condylar morphology.

Differential diagnosis. A slight medial depression on the superior condylar surface may be considered a normal variation; the point at which the depth of the depression signifies a bifid condyle is unclear. The differential diagnosis also includes a vertical fracture through the condylar head.

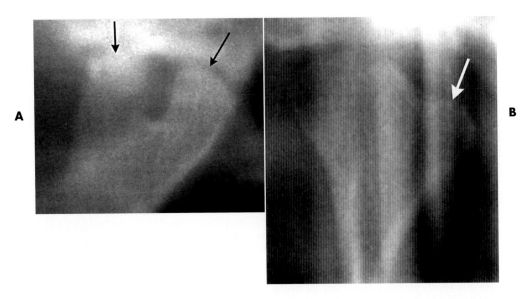

FIG. **24-20** *Bifid condyle.* **A,** Sagittal tomogram showing a deep central notch with duplication of the condylar head *(arrows).* The glenoid fossa has remodeled (enlarged) to accommodate the abnormal condyle. **B,** Coronal tomogram. Another example showing a notch in the center of the condylar head with a small medial condylar pole *(arrow).* (**A** courtesy Dr. M.J. Pharoah, Toronto, Canada.)

Treatment. Treatment is not indicated unless pain or functional impairment is present.

Soft Tissue Abnormalities

INTERNAL DERANGEMENTS

Definition

An internal derangement is an abnormality in the position and sometimes the morphology of the articular disk that may interfere with normal function. The disk most often is displaced in an anterior direction, but it may be displaced anteromedially, medially, or anterolaterally. Lateral and posterior displacements are extremely rare. Some hypothesize that disk displacements may be considered a normal variation based on the frequency of this finding in asymptomatic patients. The cause of internal derangements is unknown, although parafunction, jaw injuries (e.g., direct trauma), whiplash injury, and forced opening beyond the normal range have been implicated.

Internal derangements can be diagnosed using either arthrography or MRI. In some instances the disk may resume a normal position with respect to the condyle (called *reduction* of the disk) during mandibular opening; when the disk remains displaced throughout the entire range of mandibular movement, the term *nonreduction* is used (Fig. 24-21). A chronically displaced disk may become deformed, losing its normal biconcave shape, and it may become thickened and fibrotic. Possible complications in long-standing chronic disk displacement are degenerative joint disease and

perforation through the disk or (more commonly) the posterior attachment.

Clinical Features

Disk displacement has been found both in symptomatic patients and in healthy volunteers, suggesting that it may be a normal variant and not necessarily a predisposing factor in TMJ dysfunction. It is not known why some disks remain displaced or why symptoms of pain and dysfunction are not found in all affected patients. Symptomatic patients may have a decreased range of mandibular motion. Internal derangements can be unilateral or bilateral; unilateral cases may manifest clinically with mandibular deviation to the affected side on opening. Joint noises are common and may manifest as a click as the disk reduces to a normal position during mandibular opening and occasionally as a softer click as the disk becomes displaced again during mandibular closing. Noises may be absent in chronically displaced, nonreducing disks, or crepitus may be heard. Patients may complain of pain in the preauricular region or headaches and may have episodes of closed or open locking of the joint. Patients may have to manipulate the mandible to open it fully past an apparent closed lock by applying medially directed pressure to the affected joint or mandible with the hand.

Radiographic Features

The disk cannot be visualized with conventional radiography or tomography; arthrography or MRI are the techniques of choice. Although a retruded condylar position

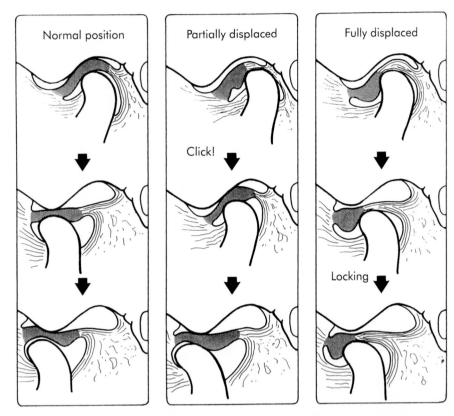

FIG. **24-21** *Position and movement of the disk during jaw opening.* Normal position *(left);* partially displaced anteriorly (with reduction, *middle*); fully displaced anteriorly (without reduction, *right*). (Courtesy Dr. W.K. Solberg, Los Angeles, Calif.)

has been associated with disk displacement, the condylar position in maximal intercuspation is not a reliable indicator of disk displacement. Likewise, diminished range of motion at maximal opening is not a reliable indication of a nonreducing disk.

Disk Displacement

Identifying the disk may be difficult in cases of gross deformation of the disk and other soft tissue components. Anterior displacement is the most common disk displacement. When the mandible is in maximal intercuspation, partial or full anterior disk displacement is indicated by anterior location of the posterior band of the disk from the normal position, which is directly superior to the condylar head. The normal articulating surface of the disk (thin intermediate zone) is somewhat anteriorly positioned, and as a result the osseous structures of the joint articulate with the posterior band of the disk or the retrodiskal tissue. Anteromedial displacement is indicated in sagittal image slices when the disk is in a normal position in the medial images of the joint but anteriorly positioned in the lateral images of the same joint. Medial displacement is indicated in MRI coronal images when the body of the disk is positioned at the medial aspect of the condyle.

Disk Reduction and Nonreduction

Arthrography allows a motion study of the condyle and disk during mandibular movement. Videofluoroscopy of mandibular movements during arthrography may show a sudden movement of the disk from an anterior displacement to a normal position during mandibular opening and back to the abnormal anterior (displaced) position during mandibular closing (Figs. 24-22 and 24-23). Often coinciding opening and closing (reciprocal) clicks are heard.

If the disk remains anteriorly displaced (nonreduction) on opening, it may bend or deform as the condyle pushes against it (Fig. 24-24). The nonreduced disk is readily seen on MRI scans, although fibrotic changes of the bilaminar zone may alter the signal to approximate the signal of the disk and thus make identification of the disk itself difficult. In such cases the disk may be erroneously interpreted as occupying a normal position at maximal opening.

Disk Perforation and Deformities

Arthrography can reveal a tear in the joint capsule or a perforation in the disk or posterior attachment by demonstrating the flow of contrast agent from the inferior to the superior joint space during the injection phase (Fig. 24-25). Disk perforations are not reliably de-

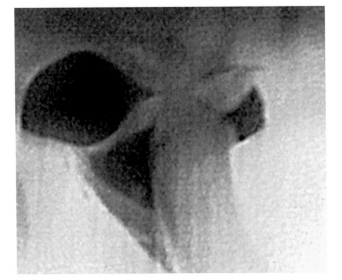

FIG. **24-22** A digital image of an arthrogram that included injection of both joint spaces. This is a reverse-density image that gives the contrast agent a radiolucent appearance; the disk is radiopaque.

A   **B**   **C**

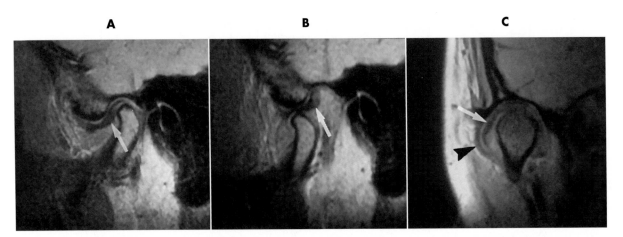

FIG. **24-23** *MRI of anterior disk displacement with reduction.* **A,** Closed sagittal view showing the disk with its posterior band *(arrow)* anterior to the condyle. **B,** Open view showing the normal relationship of the disk and condyle and the posterior band of the disk *(arrow).* **C,** Coronal view showing the disk *(white arrow)* laterally displaced. The joint capsule *(black arrowhead)* bulges laterally. (Courtesy Dr. Per-Lennart Westesson, Rochester, N.Y.)

A   **B**

FIG. **24-24** *Lower joint space arthrograms of a nonreducing, anteriorly displaced disk.* **A,** Closed position. The disk is located anterior to the condylar head. **B,** Open view. The disk is compressed, represented by a change in the shape of the contrast agent anterior to the condyle. Minimal condylar translation is apparent, and the disk remains anterior to the condyle. (Courtesy Dr. Alan G. Lurie, Farmington, Conn.)

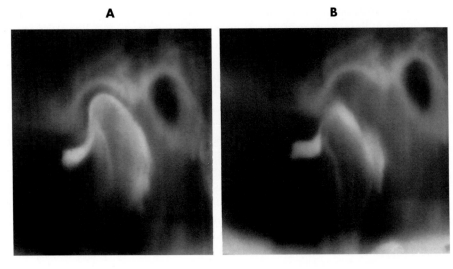

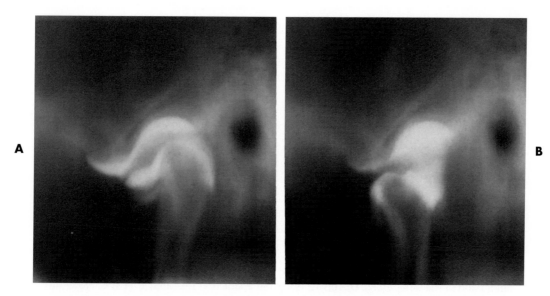

FIG. **24-25** Lower joint space arthrograms of a disk in closed position **(A)** and open position **(B)**, with loss of attachment between the posterior band and the bilaminar zone. These images were obtained after opacification of the lower joint space; both lower and upper joint spaces filled simultaneously. Contrast material can be seen redistributing between the compartments in the open and closed images. The disk is displaced anteriorly in the closed position and reduces on opening. (Courtesy Dr. Alan G. Lurie, Farmington, Conn.)

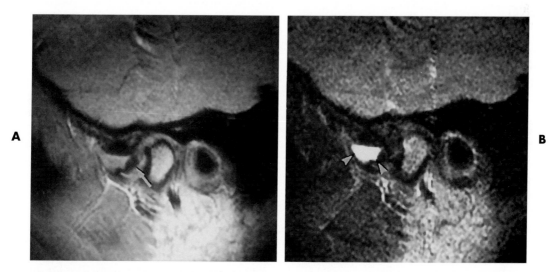

FIG. **24-26** *MRI of disk displacement without reduction in the presence of joint effusion.* **A,** The disk *(arrow)* is anteriorly displaced in this closed view. **B,** A T2-weighted image of the same section shows the collection of joint effusion *(arrowheads)* in the anterior recess of the upper joint space. *Continued.*

tected with MRI. Both MRI and arthrography can indicate alteration in the normal biconcave outline of the disk, which may vary from enlargement of the posterior band to a bilinear or biconvex disk outline.

Fibrous Adhesions and Effusion

Fibrous adhesions are masses of fibrous tissue or scar tissue that form in the joint space, particularly after TMJ

surgery. Adhesions may be detected in MRI studies as tissue with low signal intensity or during arthrography by resistance to injection of contrast agent. The pressure of injected contrast agent may tear some of these adhesions, resulting in increased joint mobility after the procedure. MRI can detect accumulation of fluid in joint spaces, which appears as a high signal in the joint spaces in T2-weighted images (Fig. 24-26).

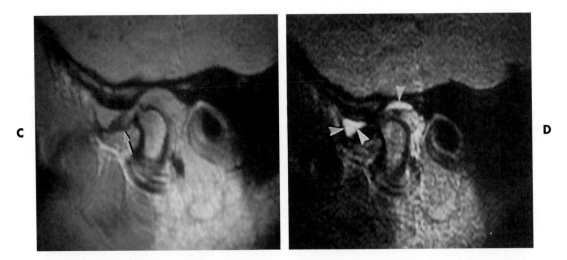

FIG. **24-26, cont'd   C,** Open view showing the disk anterior to the condyle and the posterior band of the disk *(arrow).* **D,** This T2-weighted image is at the same level as **C.** Note the joint effusion *(arrowheads)* in the anterior and posterior recesses of the upper joint space. (Courtesy Dr. Per-Lennart Westesson, Rochester, N.Y.)

Remodeling and Arthritic Conditions

REMODELING

Definition

Remodeling is an adaptive response of cartilage and osseous tissue to forces applied to the joint that may be excessive, resulting in alteration of the shape of the condyle and articular eminence. This adaptive response may result in flattening of curved joint surfaces, which effectively distributes forces over a greater surface area. The number of trabeculae also increases, increasing the density of subchondral cancellous bone (sclerosis) to better resist applied forces. No destruction or degeneration of articular soft tissues occurs. TMJ remodeling occurs throughout adult life and is considered abnormal only if accompanied by clinical signs and symptoms of pain or dysfunction or if the degree of remodeling seen radiographically is judged to be severe. Remodeling may be unilateral and does not invariably serve as a precursor to degenerative joint disease.

Clinical Features

Remodeling may be asymptomatic, or patients may have signs and symptoms of temporomandibular dysfunction that may be related to the soft tissue components, associated muscles, or ligaments. Accompanying internal derangement of the disk may be a factor.

Radiographic Features

Radiographic changes may affect the condyle, temporal component, or both; they first occur on the anterosuperior surface of the condyle and posterior slope of the articular eminence. The lateral aspect of the joint is affected in early stages, and the central and medial aspects become involved as remodeling progresses. The radiographic appearance may include one or a combination of the following: flattening, cortical thickening of articulating surfaces, and subchondral sclerosis (Fig. 24-27).

Differential Diagnosis

Severe joint flattening and subchondral sclerosis may be difficult to differentiate from early degenerative joint disease. It is known that the microscopic changes of degeneration occur before they can be detected radiographically. The radiographic appearance of bone erosions, osteophytes, and loss of joint space are signs signifying degenerative joint disease.

Treatment

When no clinical signs or symptoms are present, treatment is not indicated. Otherwise, treatment directed to relieve stress on the joint, such as splint therapy, may be considered. This should be preceded by an attempt to discover the cause of the joint stress.

DEGENERATIVE JOINT DISEASE

Synonym

Osteoarthritis

Definition

Degenerative joint disease (DJD) is a noninflammatory disorder of joints characterized by joint deterioration and proliferation. Joint deterioration is characterized by abrasion, loss of articular cartilage, and bone ero-

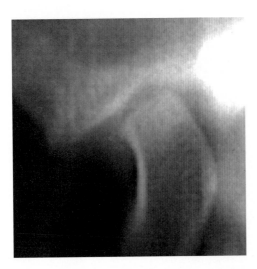

FIG. **24-27** *Remodeling.* Flattening of the articulating surface of the condyle with flattening and subchondral sclerosis of the temporal component.

sion. The proliferative component is characterized by new bone formation at the articular surface and in the subchondral region. Usually a variable combination of deterioration and proliferation occurs, but occasionally one aspect predominates; deterioration is more common in acute disease, and proliferation predominates in chronic disease. DJD is thought to occur when the ability of the joint to adapt to excessive forces (remodel) is exceeded. The etiology of DJD is unknown, although a number of factors may be important, including acute trauma, hypermobility, and loading of the joint such as occurs in parafunction. Internal derangements may be contributing etiologic factors, but this theory is controversial.

Clinical Features

DJD can occur at any age, although the incidence increases with age. DJD has a female preponderance. The disease may be asymptomatic, or patients may complain of signs and symptoms of TMJ dysfunction, including pain on palpation and movement, joint noises (crepitus), limited range of motion, and muscle spasm. The onset of symptoms may be sudden or gradual, and symptoms may disappear spontaneously, only to return in recurring cycles. Some studies report that the disease eventually "burns out" and that symptoms disappear or markedly decrease in severity in long-standing cases.

Radiographic features. When the patient is in maximal intercuspation, the joint space may be narrow or absent, which often correlates with an internal derangement and frequently with a perforation of the disk or posterior attachment, resulting in bone-to-bone contact of the joint components. Signs of previous remodeling, such as flattening and subchondral sclerosis, may be evident,

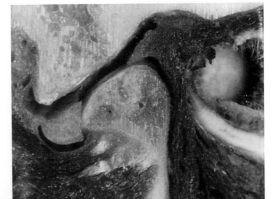

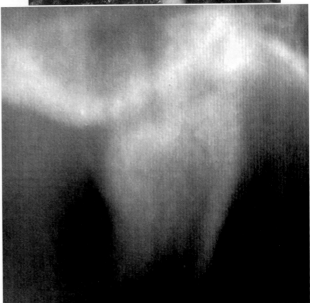

FIG. **24-28** *DJD.* **A,** A cadaver specimen. Note the flattened temporal component and anterosuperior condylar surface, with destruction of the disk between the condyle and temporal component. **B,** Sagittal tomogram showing sclerosis, flattening, and erosions of the condyle and temporal component. (**A** courtesy Dr. Carol Bibb, Los Angeles, Calif.)

although degenerative changes may obscure these findings. Loss of cortex or erosions of the articulating surfaces of the condyle or temporal component (or both) are characteristic of this disease (Fig. 24-28). In some cases small, round, radiolucent areas with irregular margins surrounded by a varying area of increased density are visible deep to the articulating surfaces. These lesions are called Ely cysts but are not true cysts; they are areas of degeneration that contain fibrous tissue, granulation tissue, and osteoid (Fig. 24-29).

Later in the course of the disease, bony proliferation occurs at the periphery of the articulating surface, increasing the articulating surface area. This new bone is called an *osteophyte*, which typically appears on the anterosuperior surface of the condyle, lateral aspect of the temporal component, or both (Fig. 24-30). Osteophytes

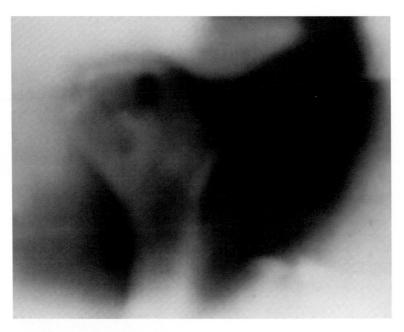

FIG. **24-29** *Pseudocyst (Ely cyst).* Coronal view. The "cyst" is seen as a radiolucency on the mediosuperior aspect of the condylar head. Note also the erosion of the lateral condylar pole.

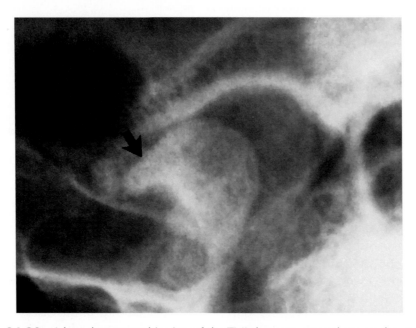

FIG. **24-30** A lateral tomographic view of the TMJ shows an osteophyte on the anterior surface of the condyle *(arrow)*.

also may form on the lateral, medial, and posterosuperior aspect of the condyle. In severe cases, osteophyte formation originating in the glenoid fossa extends from the articular eminence to almost encase the condylar head. Osteophytes may break off and lie free within the joint space (these fragments are known as "joint mice"), and these must be differentiated from other conditions that cause joint space radiopacities (Fig. 24-31).

In severe DJD, the glenoid fossa may appear grossly enlarged because of erosion of the posterior slope of the articular eminence, and the condyle may be markedly diminished in size and altered in shape because of destruction and erosion of the condylar head. This in turn may allow the condylar head to move forward and superiorly into an abnormal anterior position that may result in an anterior open bite.

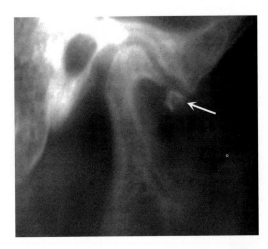

FIG. **24-31** A "joint mouse" (separated osteophyte) *(arrow)* positioned anterior to the condyle in the joint space.

Differential Diagnosis

DJD can have a spectrum of appearances ranging from substantial subchondral sclerosis and osteophyte formation (proliferative component) to extensive erosions (degenerative component). A more erosive appearance may simulate inflammatory arthritides such as rheumatoid arthritis, whereas a more proliferative appearance with extensive osteophyte formation may simulate a benign tumor such as osteoma or osteochondroma.

Treatment

Treatment is directed toward relieving joint stress (e.g., splint therapy), relieving secondary inflammation with antiinflammatory drugs, and increasing joint mobility and function (e.g., physiotherapy).

RHEUMATOID ARTHRITIS

Definition

Rheumatoid arthritis (RA) is a heterogeneous group of systemic disorders that manifests mainly as synovial membrane inflammation in several joints. The TMJ becomes involved in approximately half of affected patients. The characteristic radiographic findings are a result of villous synovitis, which leads to formation of synovial granulomatous tissue (pannus) that grows into fibrocartilage and bone, releasing enzymes that destroy articular surfaces and underlying bone.

Clinical Features

RA is more common in females and can occur at any age but increases in incidence with increasing age. A juvenile variant is discussed separately. Usually the small joints of the hands, wrists, knees, and feet are affected in a bilateral, symmetric fashion, whereas TMJ involve-

ment varies. Patients with TMJ involvement complain of swelling, pain, tenderness, stiffness on opening, limited range of motion, and crepitus. The chin appears receded, and an anterior open bite is a common finding because of the bilateral destruction and anterosuperior positioning of the condyles. TMJ involvement usually is bilateral and symmetric.

Radiographic Features

The initial changes may be generalized osteopenia (decreased density) of the condyle and temporal component. The pannus may destroy the disk, resulting in diminished width of the joint space. Bone erosions by the pannus most often involve the articular eminence and the anterior aspect of the condylar head, which permits anterosuperior positioning of the condyle when the teeth are in maximal intercuspation and results in an anterior open bite (Fig. 24-32). Erosion of the anterior and posterior condylar surfaces at the attachment of the synovial lining may result in a "sharpened pencil" appearance of the condyle. Erosive changes may be so severe that the entire condylar head is destroyed, with only the neck remaining as the articulating surface. Similarly, the articular eminence may be destroyed to the extent that a concavity replaces the normally convex eminence. Joint destruction eventually leads to secondary DJD. Subchondral sclerosis and flattening of articulating surfaces may occur, as well as subchondral "cyst" and osteophyte formation. Fibrous ankylosis or, in rare cases, osseous ankylosis, may occur; reduced mobility is related to the duration and severity of the disease.

Differential Diagnosis

The differential diagnosis includes severe DJD and psoriatic arthritis. Osteopenia and severe erosions, particularly of the articular eminence, are more characteristic of RA. Psoriatic arthritis may be ruled out by the patient's history.

Treatment

Treatment is directed toward pain relief (analgesics), reduction or suppression of inflammation (nonsteroidal antiinflammatory drugs, gold salts, corticosteroids), and preservation of muscle and joint function (physiotherapy). Joint replacement surgery may be necessary in patients with severe joint destruction.

JUVENILE CHRONIC ARTHRITIS

Synonyms

Juvenile rheumatoid arthritis and *Still's disease*

Definition

Juvenile chronic arthritis (JCA), formerly called *juvenile rheumatoid arthritis*, is a chronic inflammatory disease

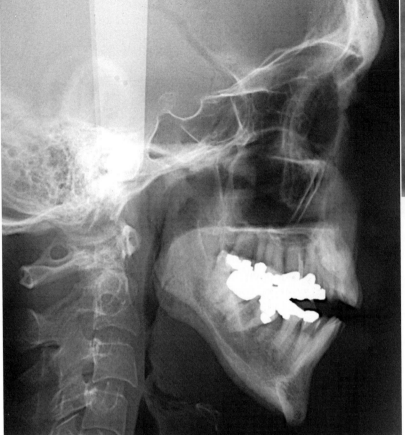

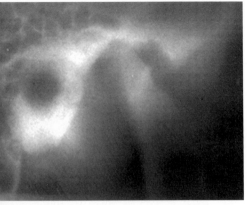

FIG. **24-32** *RA.* **A,** Lateral cephalometric view illustrating a steep mandibular plane and anterior open bite. **B,** Lateral tomogram illustrating a large erosion of the anterosuperior condylar head accompanied by severe erosions of the temporal component, including the articular eminence.

that appears before the age of 16 years (the mean age is 5 years). It is characterized by chronic, intermittent synovial inflammation that results in synovial hypertrophy, joint effusion, and swollen, painful joints. As the disease progresses, cartilage and bone are destroyed. Rheumatoid factor may be absent, hence the preferred terminology of *JCA* rather than *juvenile rheumatoid arthritis.* JCA differs from adult RA in that it has an earlier onset, and systemic involvement usually is more severe. TMJ involvement occurs in approximately 40% of patients and may be unilateral or bilateral.

Clinical Features

The patient usually has pain and tenderness in the affected joint or joints, although the disease can be asymptomatic. Unilateral onset is common, but contralateral involvement may occur as the disease progresses. Severe TMJ involvement results in inhibition of mandibular growth. Affected patients may have micrognathia and posteroinferior chin rotation, resulting in a facial appearance known as "bird face," which may also be accompanied by an anterior open bite. The degree of micrognathia is proportional to the severity of joint involvement and the early onset of disease. Additionally, when only one TMJ is involved or if one side is more

severely affected, the patient may have a mandibular asymmetry with the chin deviated to the affected side.

Radiographic Features

Osteopenia (decreased density) of the affected TMJ components may be the only initial radiographic finding. Radiographic findings are similar to those for the adult form except for the addition of impaired mandibular growth. Erosions may extend to the mandibular fossa, and the articular eminence may be destroyed. Similarly, erosion of the anterior or superior aspect of the condyle may occur, and in more severe cases only a pencil-shaped small condyle remains; the condyle may be destroyed (Fig. 24-33). Because the inflammation is intermittent, during quiescent periods the cortex of the joint surfaces may reappear, and the surfaces will appear flattened. As a result of bone destruction, the condylar head typically is positioned anterosuperiorly in the mandibular fossa. Hypomobility at maximal opening is common, and fibrous ankylosis may occur in some cases. Secondary degenerative changes manifesting as sclerosis and osteophyte formation may be superimposed on the rheumatoid changes, and ankylosis may occur. Manifestations of inhibited mandibular growth, such as deepening of the antegonial notch, diminished height of the ramus, and dorsal bending of the ramus and condylar neck, also may occur unilaterally or bilaterally, resulting in an obtuse angle between the mandibular body and ascending ramus.

PSORIATIC ARTHRITIS AND ANKYLOSING SPONDYLITIS

Psoriatic arthritis and ankylosing spondylitis are seronegative, systemic arthritides that may affect the TMJs. The radiographic changes seen in these disorders may be indistinguishable from those caused by RA, although occasionally a profound sclerotic change is seen in psoriatic arthritis.

SEPTIC ARTHRITIS

Synonym

Infectious arthritis

Definition

Septic arthritis is infection and inflammation of a joint that can result in joint destruction. It is rare in comparison to the incidence of degenerative disease and RA in the TMJ. Septic arthritis may be caused by direct spread of organisms from an adjacent cellulitis or from parotid, otic, or mastoid infections. It also may occur by direct extension of osteomyelitis of the mandibular body and ramus, although hematogenous spread from a distant nidus is more common. Most cases are caused by hematogenous spread of gonococci or by direct extension of a middle ear infection.

Clinical Features

Individuals can be affected at any age, and the condition shows no gender predilection. It usually occurs unilaterally. The patient may have redness and swelling over the joint; trismus; severe pain on opening; inability to occlude the teeth; large, tender cervical lymph nodes; fever; and malaise. The mandible may be deviated to the unaffected side as a result of joint effusion.

Radiographic Features

No radiographic signs may be present in early stages of the disease, although the space between the condyle and the roof of the mandibular fossa may be widened because of inflammatory exudate in the joint spaces. Osteopenic (radiolucent) changes of the joint components and mandibular ramus may be evident. More obvious bony changes are seen approximately 7 to 10 days after the onset of clinical symptoms. As a result of the osteolytic effects of inflammation, the condylar articular cortex may become slightly radiolucent, and discontinuity or subtle irregularity of the anterior cortical surface may

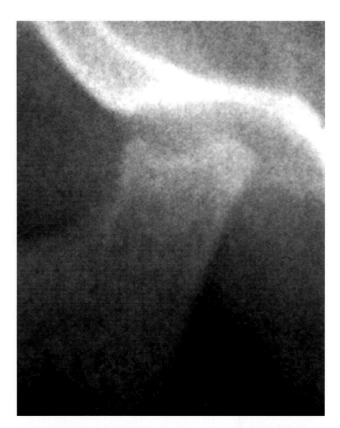

FIG. **24-33** *JCA.* Sagittal tomogram (closed position) showing osteopenia and characteristic erosion of the anterosuperior condylar surface. Note the anterior position of the condyle.

be evident. As the disease progresses, the condyle and articular eminence, including the disk, may be destroyed. Osseous ankylosis may occur after the infection subsides. If the disease occurs during the period of mandibular growth, radiographic manifestations of inhibited mandibular growth may be evident.

Differential Diagnosis

The radiographic changes caused by septic arthritis may mimic those of severe DJD or RA, although septic arthritis usually occurs unilaterally, and the patient often has clinical signs and symptoms of infection. Inflammatory changes that may accompany septic arthritis may be seen in CT images, such as involvement of mastoid air cells, osteomyelitis of the mandible, and inflammation of surrounding soft tissue.

Treatment

Treatment includes antimicrobial therapy, drainage of effusion, and joint rest. Physiotherapy to reestablish joint mobility is initiated after the acute phase of infection has passed.

Articular Loose Bodies

Articular loose bodies are radiopacities of varying origin located in the synovium, within the capsule in the joint spaces or outside the capsule in soft tissue. They appear radiographically as soft tissue calcifications positioned around the condylar head. The loose bodies may represent bone that has separated from joint components, as in DJD (joint mice), hyaline cartilage metaplasia (calcification) that occurs in synovial chondromatosis, crystals deposited in the joint space in crystal-associated arthropathy (pseudogout), or tumoral calcinosis associated with renal disease. In rare cases chondrosarcoma also may mimic the appearance of articular loose bodies.

SYNOVIAL CHONDROMATOSIS

Synonyms
Synovial chondrometaplasia and *osteochondromatosis*

Definition
Synovial chondromatosis is an uncommon disorder characterized by metaplastic formation of multiple cartilaginous and osteocartilaginous nodules within connective tissue of the synovial membrane of joints. Some of these nodules may detach and form loose bodies in the joint space, where they persist and may increase in size, being nourished by synovial fluid. This condition is more common in the axial skeleton than in the TMJ. When the cartilaginous nodules ossify, the term *synovial osteochondrometaplasia* may be used.

Clinical Features
Patients may be asymptomatic or may complain of preauricular swelling, pain, and decreased range of motion. Some patients have crepitus or other joint noises. The condition usually occurs unilaterally.

Radiographic Features
The osseous components may appear normal or may exhibit osseous changes similar to those in DJD. The joint space may be widened, and if ossification of the cartilaginous nodules has occurred, a mass of radiopacity or several radiopaque loose bodies may be seen surrounding the condylar head (Fig. 24-34). CT imaging can identify the location of the calcifications. Occasionally erosion through the glenoid fossa into the middle cranial fossa may occur, which is best detected with CT imaging.

Differential Diagnosis
The appearance of synovial chondromatosis cannot be differentiated from chondrocalcinosis. Conditions that appear similar include DJD with joint mice or chondrosarcoma. Chondrosarcoma may be accompanied by

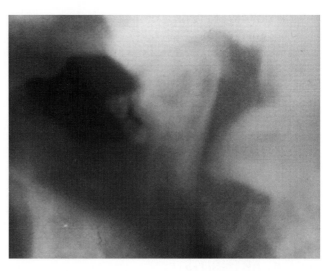

FIG. **24-34** Synovial chondromatosis, seen as radiopaque bodies anterior to the condyle.

severe bone destruction, which may help in differentiating the condition from osteochondromatosis.

Treatment
Treatment consists of removal of the loose bodies and resection of abnormal synovial tissue in the joint by arthroscopic or open joint surgery.

CHONDROCALCINOSIS

Synonyms
Pseudogout and *calcium pyrophosphate dihydrate deposition disease*

Definition
Chondrocalcinosis is characterized by acute or chronic synovitis and precipitation of calcium pyrophosphate dihydrate crystals in the joint space. It differs from gout, in which urate crystals are precipitated; hence the term *pseudogout*.

Clinical Features
The joints more commonly affected are the knee, wrist, hip, shoulder, and elbow; TMJ involvement is uncommon. The condition occurs unilaterally and is more common in males. Patients may be asymptomatic or may complain of pain and joint swelling.

Radiographic Features
The radiographic appearance of chondrocalcinosis may simulate synovial chondromatosis, described above. Bone erosions as well as a severe increase in condylar bone density also have been described. Erosions of the glenoid fossa may be present, which require CT for detection.

Differential Diagnosis

The differential diagnosis is the same as for synovial chondromatosis.

Treatment

Treatment consists of surgical removal of the crystalline deposits. Steroids, aspirin, and nonsteroidal antiinflammatory agents may provide relief. Colchicine may be used to alleviate attacks and for prophylaxis.

Trauma

EFFUSION

Definition

Effusion is an influx of fluid into the joint, usually as a result of trauma (hemorrhage) or inflammation (exudate).

Clinical Features

The patient may have swelling over the affected joint; pain in the TMJ, preauricular region, or ear; and limited range of motion. Patients may also complain of the sensation of fluid in the ear, tinnitus, and hearing difficulties, as well as difficulty occluding the posterior teeth.

Radiographic Features

Joint effusion is more commonly seen in conjunction with internal derangements, although it has been described in normal joints. The joint space is widened, and T2-weighted MRI studies may show a bright signal (white), indicating fluid adjacent to the disk or posterior to the condyle (see Fig. 24-26).

Differential Diagnosis

Effusion must be differentiated from septic arthritis; in the latter case the accompanying signs and symptoms of infection are present.

Treatment

Treatment may include antiinflammatory drugs, although surgical drainage of the effusion occasionally is necessary.

DISLOCATION

Definition

Dislocation is abnormal positioning of the condyle out of the mandibular fossa but within the joint capsule. It usually occurs bilaterally and most commonly in an anterior direction. Dislocation may be caused by a failure of muscular coordination, subluxation, or external trauma and may be associated with a condylar fracture.

Clinical Features

Patients are unable to close the mandible to maximal intercuspation; some patients cannot reduce the disloca-tion, whereas others may be able to reduce the mandible by manipulation. In the former case associated pain and muscle spasm often are present.

Radiographic Features

In bilateral cases both condyles are located anterior and superior to the summits of the articular eminentia. Clinical information is important because the normal range of motion may extend anterior to the summit of the articular eminence.

Differential Diagnosis

The diagnosis is confirmed by the radiographic findings, although some fracture dislocations may be difficult to visualize, particularly if the dislocation is very slight.

Treatment

Treatment consists of manual manipulation of the mandible to reduce the dislocation. Surgery occasionally is necessary to reduce the condyle in the case of a fracture dislocation, although treatment may not be indicated for this type of dislocation if mandibular function is adequate.

FRACTURE

Definition

Fractures of the TMJ usually occur at the condylar neck and often are accompanied by dislocation of the condylar head. Fractures may be divided into those involving the condylar head and those involving the condylar neck, although occasionally both may be involved. On rare occasions the fracture may involve the temporal component.

Clinical Features

Unilateral fractures, which are more common than bilateral fractures, may be accompanied by a parasymphyseal or mandibular body fracture on the contralateral side. The patient may have swelling over the TMJ, pain, limited range of motion, and an anterior open bite. Some TMJ fractures are relatively asymptomatic and may not be discovered at the time of trauma; instead, these come to light as incidental findings at a later time when radiographs are taken for other reasons. Condylar fractures should be ruled out if the patient has a history of a blow to the mandible, especially to the anterior aspect.

Radiographic Features

In relatively recent condylar neck fractures, a radiolucent line limited to the outline of the neck is visible. This line may vary in width, depending on whether the bone fragments are still aligned (narrow line) or displacement/dislocation has occurred (wider line). If the bone fragments overlap, an area of apparent increase in ra-

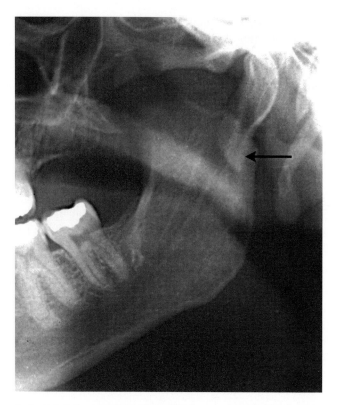

FIG. 24-35 *Condylar fracture (panoramic view).* The arrow points to overlapped fragments, as evidenced by increased radiopacity.

diopacity may be seen instead of a radiolucent line (Fig. 24-35). Also, the outer cortical boundary may have an irregular outline or a step defect. Approximately 60% of condylar fractures show evidence of fragment angulation and a variable degree of displacement (dislocation) of the fracture ends. Fractures of the condylar head are less common and may be of the vertical (responsible for the traumatic type of bifid condyle) or compressive type. Multiple right-angle radiographic projections from the lateral, frontal, and basilar aspects are required to detect a fracture and to determine fragment displacement. CT is also an excellent imaging modality for detecting condylar fractures.

The amount of remodeling seen in the TMJ after a condylar fracture with medial displacement varies considerably. In some cases the condyle remodels to a form that is essentially normal, whereas in other cases the condyle and mandibular fossa become flattened, with loss of vertical height on the affected side. The condyle eventually may show degenerative changes, including flattening, erosion, and osteophytes, and ankylosis. These changes are more severe if the condyle is displaced.

Differential Diagnosis

Occasionally old fractures that have remodeled may be difficult to differentiate from developmental abnormalities of the condyle. The most common difficulty is in determining whether a fracture is indeed present. Transorbital or open Towne's views are mandatory and aid in fracture identification, particularly if the condylar fragment has been displaced.

Treatment

Treatment may not be indicated if mandibular mobility is adequate; otherwise, the fracture is reduced surgically.

Trauma to the Developing Condyle

If a condylar fracture occurs during the period of mandibular growth, growth may be inhibited because of damage to the condylar growth center. The degree of subsequent hypoplasia is related to the stage of mandibular development at the time of injury (younger patients have more profound hypoplasia) and the severity of the injury. Injury to the joint may result in hemorrhage or effusion into the joint spaces that eventually may form bone during the healing process, which in turn may result in severe hypoplasia and limited joint function.

NEONATAL FRACTURES

The use of forceps during delivery of neonates may result in fracture and displacement of the rudimentary condyle, which later manifests as severe mandibular hypoplasia and lack of development of the glenoid fossa and articular eminence. Such cases have a characteristic radiographic appearance in the panoramic image, having the appearance of a partly opened pair of scissors in place of a normal condyle. This presentation results from the overlapping images of the medially displaced "carrot-shaped" condyle and remnants of the condylar neck.

Differential Diagnosis

This condition often is not diagnosed until later in life, at which time a diagnosis of fracture may be made without the realization that the fracture occurred at the time of birth. The condition must be differentiated from a developmental hypoplasia of the mandible, which is unrelated to birth injury.

Treatment

The fracture usually is not treated, but the mandibular asymmetry may be corrected with a combination of orthodontics and orthognathic surgery.

ANKYLOSIS

Definition

Ankylosis is a condition in which condylar movement is limited by a mechanical problem in the joint ("true" ankylosis) or by a mechanical cause not related to joint components ("false" ankylosis). True ankylosis may be bony or fibrous. In bony ankylosis the condyle or ramus is attached to the temporal bone by an osseous bridge. In fibrous ankylosis a soft tissue (fibrous) union of joint components occurs; the bone components appear normal. False ankylosis may result from conditions that inhibit condylar movement such as muscle spasm, myositis ossificans, or coronoid process hyperplasia.

Clinical Features

Most unilateral cases are caused by mandibular trauma or infection. The most common cause of bilateral TMJ ankylosis is RA, although in rare cases bilateral fractures may be the cause. Most if not all cases of TMJ ankylosis in infancy occur secondary to birth injury. Patients have a history of progressively restricted jaw opening, or they may have a long-standing history of limited opening. Some degree of mandibular opening usually is possible through flexing of the mandible, although opening may be restricted to only a few millimeters, particularly in the case of bony ankylosis.

Radiographic Features

In fibrous ankylosis the osseous components of the joint may appear normal or the articulating surfaces may be irregular because of erosions; joint space is markedly decreased. Little or no condylar movement is seen. Radiographic signs of remodeling occasionally are visible as the joint components adapt to repeated attempts at mandibular opening. In bony ankylosis the joint space may be partly or completely obliterated by the osseous bridge, which can vary from a slender segment of bone to a large, bony mass. This extensive new bone may fuse the condyle to the cranial base (Fig. 24-36). Secondary degenerative changes of the joint components are common. Often morphologic changes occur, such as compensatory progressive elongation of the coronoid processes and deepening of the antegonial notch in the mandibular ramus on the affected side as a result of muscle function during attempted mandibular opening. If ankylosis occurs before mandibular growth is complete, growth of the affected side of the mandible is inhibited (see Trauma to the Developing Condyle, p. 522).

Differential Diagnosis

The major differential diagnosis is a condylar tumor. However, a history of trauma, infection, or other joint diseases should help rule out neoplastic disease. Detection of fibrous ankylosis is difficult because fibrous tissue is not visible in the radiographic image and therefore may be difficult to differentiate from false ankylosis.

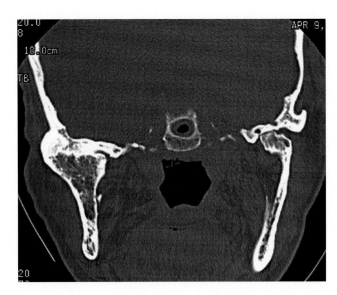

FIG. 24-36 *Bony ankylosis (CT, coronal image slice).* The right condyle and ramus are markedly enlarged. The articulating surface is irregular, and the central and lateral aspects are fused to the roof of the glenoid fossa, as evidenced by a lack of joint space. Note that the left condylar articulating surface is eroded, and the joint space is decreased on the medial aspect; these changes are consistent with DJD.

Treatment

Joint mobility is improved by surgical removal of the osseous bridge or creation of a pseudarthrosis.

Tumors

Benign and malignant tumors originating in or involving the TMJ are rare. Tumors may be intrinsic or extrinsic (adjacent) to the TMJ. Intrinsic tumors may develop in the condyle, temporal bone, or coronoid process. Extrinsic tumors may affect the morphology, structure, or function of the joint without invading the joint itself. Radiographic changes in the TMJ or ramus may be a result of indirect effects on growth, such as those seen with vascular lesions, pressure, or the effects of mandibular positioning.

BENIGN TUMORS

The most common benign intrinsic tumors affecting the TMJ are osteomas, osteochondromas, and osteoblastomas. Chondroblastomas, fibromyxomas, benign giant cell lesions, and aneurysmal bone cysts also occur. Benign tumors and cysts of the mandible (e.g., ameloblastomas, odontogenic keratocysts, simple bone cysts) may involve the entire ramus and in rare cases the condyle. In cases of false ankylosis in which the TMJs appear radiographically normal, hyperplasia or a tumor of the coronoid process must be ruled out.

Clinical Features

Condylar tumors grow slowly and may attain considerable size before becoming clinically noticeable. Patients may complain of TMJ swelling, which may be accompanied by pain and decreased range of motion. The clinical examination may reveal facial asymmetry, malocclusion, and deviation of the mandible to the unaffected side; these may be accompanied by symptoms of TMJ dysfunction. Tumors of the coronoid process typically are painless, but patients may complain of progressive limitation of motion.

Radiographic Features

Condylar tumors cause condylar enlargement that often is irregular in outline. The trabecular pattern may be altered, resulting in regions of destruction seen as radiolucencies or new abnormal bone formation, which may increase the radiopacity of the condyle with abnormal trabeculae. An osteoma or osteochondroma appears as an abnormal, pedunculated mass attached to the condyle (Fig. 24-37). Osteochondromas often extend from the anterior or superior surface of the condyle. Tumors of the coronoid process may affect TMJ function, which emphasizes the need to image and evaluate the

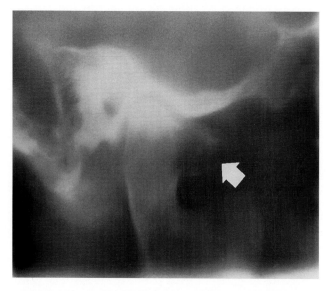

FIG. 24-37 Sagittal tomographic view of the TMJ showing a globular osteochondroma on the anterior condylar surface *(arrow)*.

coronoid process when evaluating joint abnormalities. The most common benign tumor is the osteochondroma. This tumor may interfere with joint function and erode adjacent osseous structures.

Differential Diagnosis

Condylar neoplasms may simulate unilateral condylar hyperplasia because of condylar enlargement, although osteomas and osteochondromas give an irregular appearance, such as bulbous or globular expansion of the condyle or, more commonly, a pedunculated growth. Also, the characteristic condylar shape and proportions are better preserved in condylar hyperplasia. Coronoid tumors must be differentiated from coronoid hyperplasia, which differs from a condylar tumor in that the coronoid process remains regular in shape.

Treatment

Treatment consists of surgical excision of the tumor and occasionally excision of the condylar head or coronoid process.

MALIGNANT TUMORS

Malignant tumors of the jaws may be primary or, more commonly, metastatic. Primary intrinsic malignant tumors of the condyle are extremely rare and include chondrosarcoma, osteogenic sarcoma, synovial sarcoma, and fibrosarcoma of the joint capsule. Extrinsic malignant tumors may represent direct extension of adjacent parotid salivary gland malignancies, rhabdomyosarcoma (particularly in children), or other regional carcinomas from the skin, ear, and nasopharynx. The most common metastatic lesions include neoplasms originating in the breast, kidney, lung, colon, prostate, and thyroid gland.

Clinical Features

Malignant tumors (primary or metastatic) may be asymptomatic or patients may have symptoms of TMJ dysfunction such as pain, limited mandibular opening, mandibular deviation, and swelling. Unfortunately, a patient occasionally is treated for TMJ dysfunction without recognition that the underlying condition is a malignancy.

Radiographic Features

Malignant primary and metastatic TMJ tumors appear as a variable degree of bone destruction with ill-defined, irregular margins. Most lack tumor bone formation, with the exception of osteogenic sarcoma. Chondrosarcoma may appear as an indistinct, essentially radiolucent destructive lesion of the condyle with surrounding discrete soft tissue calcifications that may simulate the appearance of the articular loose bodies seen in chondrocalcinosis or pseudogout (Fig. 24-38). In the case of metastatic tumors, the radiographic appearance usually is nonspecific condylar destruction (with a few exceptions, such as metastatic prostate carcinoma) and does not indicate the site of origin.

Differential Diagnosis

Joint destruction caused by a malignant tumor must be differentiated from the osseous destruction seen in severe DJD. Malignant tumors cause profound central bone destruction, whereas DJD causes more peripheral bone destruction. Proliferative changes such as osteophyte formation may be seen in DJD, but unlike with a malignant tumor, no soft tissue mass or swelling is evident. Chondrosarcoma may simulate joint space calcifications (discussed earlier), but in the case of malignancy, severe bone destruction also occurs.

Treatment

In the case of primary malignant tumors, treatment consists of wide surgical removal of the tumor. Tumor extension to vital anatomic structures may compromise survival. Metastatic tumors of the TMJ rarely are treated surgically; treatment mainly is palliative and may include radiotherapy and chemotherapy.

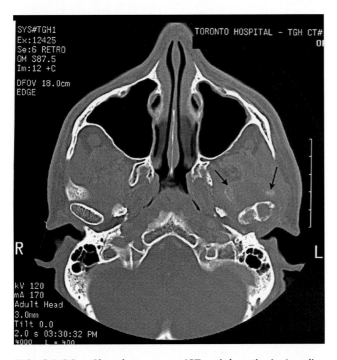

FIG. 24-38 *Chondrosarcoma (CT, axial section).* A radiolucent destructive lesion is present in the left condylar head, and faint radiopacities (soft tissue calcifications) are visible anterior to the condylar head *(arrows).* (Courtesy M.J. Pharoah, DDS, Toronto, Canada.)

SUGGESTED READINGS

DISORDERS OF THE TEMPOROMANDIBULAR JOINT

Brooks SL et al: Imaging of the temporomandibular joint, position paper of the American Academy of Oral and Maxillofacial Radiology, *Oral Surg Oral Med Oral Pathol Oral Radiol Endod* 83:609, 1997.

Helkimo M: Studies on function and dysfunction of the masticatory system. II. Index for anamnestic and clinical dysfunction and occlusal state, *Swed Dent J* 67:101, 1974.

McNeill C et al: Temporomandibular disorders: diagnosis, management, education, and research, *J Am Dent Assoc* 120:253, 1990.

Petrikowski CG, Grace MG: Temporomandibular joint radiographic findings in adolescents, *J Craniomand Pract* 14:30, 1996.

Rugh JD, Solberg WK: Oral health status in the United States: temporomandibular disorders, *J Dent Educ* 49:398, 1985.

Wänman A, Agerberg G: Mandibular dysfunction in adolescents. I. Prevalence of symptoms, *Acta Odontol Scand* 44:47, 1986.

ANATOMY OF THE TEMPOROMANDIBULAR JOINT

Blaschke DD, Blaschke TJ: A method for quantitatively determining temporomandibular joint bony relationships, *J Dent Res* 60:35, 1981.

Drace JE, Enzmann DR: Defining the normal temporomandibular joint: closed, partially open, and open mouth MR imaging of asymptomatic subjects, *Radiology* 177:67, 1990.

Hansson LG et al: A comparison between clinical and radiologic findings in 259 temporomandibular joint patients, *J Prosthet Dent* 50:89, 1983.

Ingervall B et al: Postnatal development of the human temporomandibular joint. II. A microradiographic study, *Acta Odont Scand* 34:133, 1976.

Larheim TA: Radiographic appearance of the normal temporomandibular joint in newborns and small children, *Acta Radiol Diagn* 22(5):593, 1981.

Pullinger AG et al: A tomographic study of mandibular condyle position in an asymptomatic population, *J Prosthet Dent* 53:706, 1985.

Taylor RC et al: A study of temporomandibular joint morphology and its relationship to the dentition, *Oral Surg* 33:1002, 1972.

Ten Cate AR: Gross and micro anatomy. In Zarb GA et al, editors: *Temporomandibular joint and masticatory muscle disorders,* ed 2, Copenhagen, 1994, Munksgaard.

Westesson P-L et al: Cryosectional observations of functional anatomy of the temporomandibular joint, *Oral Surg Oral Med Oral Pathol* 68:247, 1989.

Yale SH et al: An epidemiological assessment of mandibular condyle morphology, *Oral Surg* 21:169, 1966.

DIAGNOSTIC IMAGING OF THE TEMPOROMANDIBULAR JOINT

Brooks SL et al: Imaging of the temporomandibular joint, position paper of the American Academy of Oral and Maxillofacial Radiology, *Oral Surg Oral Med Oral Pathol Oral Radiol Endod* 83:609, 1997.

Helms CA, Kaplan P: Diagnostic imaging of the temporomandibular joint: recommendations for use of the various techniques, *AJR Am J Roentgenol* 154:319, 1990.

Katzberg RW: Temporomandibular joint imaging, *Radiology* 170:297, 1989.

Hard tissue imaging

Bean L et al: The transmaxillary projection in temporomandibular joint radiography, *Dentomaxillofac Radiol* 4:13, 1975.

Christiansen EL et al: Computed tomography of the normal temporomandibular joint, *Scand J Dent Res* 95:499, 1987.

Coin CG: Tomography of the temporomandibular joint, *Dent Radiol Photogr* 47:23, 1974.

Hansson L-G, Petersson A: Radiography of the temporomandibular joint using the transpharyngeal projection, *Dentomaxillofac Radiol* 7:69, 1987.

Mongini F: The importance of radiography in the diagnosis of TMJ dysfunctions: a comparative evaluation of transcranial radiographs and serial tomography, *J Prosthet Dent* 45:186, 1981.

Soft tissue imaging

Conway WF et al: Dynamic magnetic resonance imaging of the temporomandibular joint using FLASH sequences, *J Oral Maxillofac Surg* 46:930, 1988.

Hansson L-G et al: Comparison of tomography and midfield magnetic resonance imaging for osseous changes of the temporomandibular joint, *Oral Surg Oral Med Oral Pathol Oral Radiol Endod* 82:698, 1996.

Moses JJ et al: Magnetic resonance imaging or arthrographic diagnosis of internal derangement of the temporomandibular joint, *Oral Surg Oral Med Oral Pathol* 75:268, 1993.

Schellhas KP et al: The diagnosis of temporomandibular joint disease: two-compartment arthrography and MR, *AJR Am J Roentgenol* 151:341, 1988.

Westesson P-L: Double-contrast arthrography of the temporomandibular joint: introduction of an arthrographic technique for visualization of the disc and articular surfaces, *J Oral Maxillofac Surg* 41:163, 1983.

Westesson P-L, Bronstein SL: Temporomandibular joint: comparison of single- and double-contrast arthrography, *Radiology* 164:65, 1987.

RADIOGRAPHIC ABNORMALITIES OF THE TEMPOROMANDIBULAR JOINT

Condylar hyperplasia

Gray RJM et al: Histopathological and scintigraphic features of condylar hyperplasia, *Int J Oral Maxillofac Surg* 19:65, 1990.

Jonck LM: Facial asymmetry and condylar hyperplasia, *Oral Surg* 40:567, 1975.

Rubenstein LK, Campbell RL: Acquired unilateral condylar hyperplasia and facial asymmetry: report of a case, *ASDC J Dent Child* 52:114, 1985.

Condylar hypoplasia

Jerell RG et al: Acquired condylar hypoplasia: report of a case, *ASDC J Dent Child* 58:147, 1991.

Worth HM: Radiology of the temporomandibular joint. In Zarb GA, Carlsson GE, editors: *Temporomandibular joint function and dysfunction,* Copenhagen, 1979, Munksgaard.

Juvenile arthrosis

Boering G: Temporomandibular joint arthrosis and facial deformity, *Trans Int Conf Oral Surg* 258, 1967.

Worth HM: Radiology of the temporomandibular joint. In Zarb GA, Carlsson GE, editors: *Temporomandibular joint function and dysfunction,* Copenhagen, 1979, Munksgaard.

Coronoid hyperplasia

McLoughlin PM et al: Hyperplasia of the mandibular coronoid process: an analysis of 31 cases and a review of the literature, *J Oral Maxillofac Surg* 53:250, 1995.

Bifid condyle

Loh FC, Yeo JF: Bifid mandibular condyle, *Oral Surg Oral Med Oral Pathol* 69:24, 1990.

SOFT TISSUE ABNORMALITIES

Dolwick MF, Sanders B: TMJ internal derangement and arthrosis. In *Surgical atlas,* St Louis, 1985, Mosby.

Helms CA et al: Temporomandibular joint: morphology and signal intensity characteristics of the disk at MR imaging, *Radiology* 172:817, 1989.

Katzberg RW: Temporomandibular joint imaging, *Radiology* 170:297, 1989.

Katzberg RW et al: Internal derangements of the temporomandibular joint: findings in the pediatric age group, *Radiology* 154:125, 1985.

Larheim TA: Current trends in temporomandibular joint imaging, *Oral Surg Oral Med Oral Pathol Oral Radiol Endod* 80:555, 1995.

Nuelle DG et al: Arthroscopic surgery of the temporomandibular joint, *Angle Orthod* 56:118, 1986.

Rammelsberg P et al: Variability of disk position in asymptomatic volunteers and patients with internal derangements of the TMJ, *Oral Surg Oral Med Oral Pathol Oral Radiol Endod* 83:393, 1997.

Sano T, Westesson P-L: Magnetic resonance imaging of the temporomandibular joint: increased T2 signal in the retrodiskal tissue of painful joints, *Oral Surg Oral Med Oral Pathol Oral Radiol Endod* 79:511, 1995.

Wilkes CH: Internal derangements of the temporomandibular joint: pathological variations, *Arch Otolaryngol Head Neck Surg* 115:469, 1989.

REMODELING AND ARTHRITIC CONDITIONS

Remodeling

Brooks SL et al: Prevalence of osseous changes in the temporomandibular joint of asymptomatic persons without internal derangement, *Oral Surg Oral Med Oral Pathol* 73:118, 1992.

Moffett BC et al: Articular remodeling in the adult human temporomandibular joint, *Am J Anat* 115:119, 1964.

Degenerative joint disease

deLeeuw R et al: Temporomandibular joint osteoarthrosis: clinical and radiographic characteristics 30 years after non-surgical treatment—a preliminary report, *J Craniomand Pract* 11:15, 1993.

Mayne JG, Hatch GS: Arthritis of the temporomandibular joint, *J Am Dent Assoc* 79:125, 1969.

Radin EL et al: Role of mechanical factors in pathogenesis of primary osteoarthritis, *Lancet* 1(749):519, 1972.

Sato H et al: Temporomandibular joint osteoarthritis: a comparative clinical and tomographic study pre- and post-treatment, *J Oral Rehab* 21:383, 1994.

Rheumatoid arthritis

Gynther GW et al: Radiographic changes in the temporomandibular joint in patients with generalized osteoarthritis and rheumatoid arthritis, *Oral Surg Oral Med Oral Pathol Oral Radiol Endod* 81:613, 1996.

Larheim TA et al: Rheumatic disease of the temporomandibular joint: MR imaging and tomographic manifestations, *Radiology* 175:527, 1990.

Syrjänen SM: The temporomandibular joint in rheumatoid arthritis, *Acta Radiologica Diagnosis* 26(3):235, 1985.

Juvenile chronic arthritis

Ganik R, Williams FA: Diagnosis and management of juvenile rheumatoid arthritis with TMJ involvement, *J Craniomandib Pract* 4:255, 1986.

Hu Y-S, Schneiderman ED: The temporomandibular joint in juvenile rheumatoid arthritis. I. Computed tomographic findings, *Pediatr Dent* 17:46, 1995.

Hu Y-S et al: The temporomandibular joint in juvenile rheumatoid arthritis. II. Relationship between computed tomographic and clinical findings, *Pediatr Dent* 18:312, 1996.

Karhulahti T et al: Mandibular condyle lesions related to age at onset and subtypes of juvenile rheumatoid arthritis in 15-year-old children, *Scand J Dent Res* 101:332, 1993.

Psoriatic arthritis

Koorbusch GF et al: Psoriatic arthritis of the temporomandibular joints with ankylosis, *Oral Surg Oral Med Oral Pathol* 71:267, 1991.

Wilson AW et al: Psoriatic arthropathy of the temporomandibular joint, *Oral Surg Oral Med Oral Pathol* 70:555, 1990.

Ankylosing spondylitis

Locher MC et al: Involvement of the temporomandibular joints in ankylosing spondylitis (Bechterew's disease), *J Craniomaxillofac Surg* 24:205, 1996.

Ramos-Remus C et al: Temporomandibular joint osseous morphology in a consecutive sample of ankylosing spondylitis patients, *Ann Rheum Dis* 56(2):103, 1997.

Septic arthritis

Leighty SM et al: Septic arthritis of the temporomandibular joint: review of the literature and report of two cases in children, *Int J Oral Maxillofac Surg* 22:292, 1993.

ARTICULAR LOOSE BODIES

Carls FR et al: Loose bodies in the temporomandibular joint, *J Craniomaxillofac Surg* 23:215, 1995.

Chuong R, Piper MA: Bilateral pseudogout of the temporomandibular joint: report of a case and review of the literature, *J Oral Maxillofac Surg* 53:691, 1995.

Dijkgraaf LC et al: Calcium pyrophosphate dihydrate crystal deposition disease: a review of the literature and a light and electron microscopic study of a case of the temporomandibular joint with numerous intracellular crystals in the chondrocytes, *Osteoarthritis Cartilage* 3:35, 1995.

Lustmann J, Zeltser R: Synovial chondromatosis of the temporomandibular joint: review of the literature and case report, *Int J Oral Maxillofac Surg* 18:90, 1989.

Orden A et al: Chronic preauricular swelling, *J Oral Maxillofac Surg* 47:390, 1989.

Pynn BR et al: Calcium pyrophosphate dihydrate deposition disease of the temporomandibular joint: a case report and review of the literature, *Oral Surg Oral Med Oral Pathol Oral Radiol Endod* 79:278, 1995.

TRAUMA

Effusion

Schellhas KP, Wilkes CH: Temporomandibular joint inflammation: comparison of MR fast scanning with T1- and T2-weighted imaging techniques, *AJNR* 10:589, 1989.

Schellhas KP et al: Facial pain, headache, and temporomandibular joint inflammation, *Headache* 29:229, 1989.

Takaku S et al: Magnetic resonance images in patients with acute traumatic injury of the temporomandibular joint: a preliminary report, *J Craniomaxillofac Surg* 24:173, 1996.

Westesson P-L, Brooks SL: Temporomandibular joint: relationship between MR evidence of effusion and the presence of pain and disk displacement, *AJR Am J Roentgenol* 159:559, 1992.

Dislocation

Kai S et al: Clinical symptoms of open lock position of the condyle: relation to anterior dislocation of the temporomandibular joint, *Oral Surg Oral Med Oral Pathol* 74:143, 1992.

Kallal RH et al: Cranial dislocation of mandibular condyle, *Oral Surg* 43:2, 1977.

Wijmenga JP et al: Protracted dislocation of the temporomandibular joint, *Int J Oral Maxillofac Surg* 15:380, 1986.

Fracture

Dahlstrom L et al: Fifteen years follow-up on condylar fractures, *Int J Oral Maxillofac Surg* 18:18, 1989.

Horowitz I et al: Demonstration of condylar fractures of the mandible by computed tomography, *Oral Surg* 54:263, 1982.

Lindahl L, Hollender L: Condylar fractures of the mandible. II. A radiographic study of remodeling processes in the temporomandibular joint, *Int J Oral Surg* 6:153, 1977.

Raustia AM et al: Conventional radiographic and computed tomographic findings in cases of fracture of the mandibular condylar process, *J Oral Maxillofac Surg* 48:1258, 1990.

Schellhas KP: Temporomandibular joint injuries, *Radiology* 173:211, 1989.

TRAUMA TO THE DEVELOPING CONDYLE

Pharoah MJ: Radiology of the temporomandibular joint. In Zarb GA et al, editors: *Temporomandibular joint and masticatory muscle disorders,* ed 2, Copenhagen, 1994, Munksgaard.

Neonatal fractures

Pharoah MJ: Radiology of the temporomandibular joint. In Zarb GA et al, editors: *Temporomandibular joint and masticatory muscle disorders,* ed 2, Copenhagen, 1994, Munksgaard.

Worth HM: Radiology of the temporomandibular joint. In Zarb GA, Carlsson GE, editors: *Temporomandibular joint function and dysfunction,* Copenhagen, 1979, Munksgaard.

Ankylosis

Rowe NL: Ankylosis of the temporomandibular joint, *J R Coll Surg Edinb* 27:67, 1982.

Wood RE et al: The radiologic features of true ankylosis of the temporomandibular joint: an analysis of 25 cases, *Dentomaxillofac Radiol* 17:121, 1988.

TUMORS

Benign tumors

James RB et al: Osteochondroma of the mandibular coronoid process: report of a case, *Oral Surg* 37:189, 1974.

Nwoku ALN, Koch H: The temporomandibular joint: a rare localisation for bone tumors, *J Maxillofac Surg* 2:113, 1974.

Pharoah MJ: Radiology of the temporomandibular joint. In Zarb GA et al, editors: *Temporomandibular joint and masticatory muscle disorders,* ed 2, Copenhagen, 1994, Munksgaard.

Svensson B, Isacsson G: Benign osteoblastoma associated with an aneurysmal bone cyst of the mandibular ramus and condyle, *Oral Surg Oral Med Oral Pathol* 76:433, 1993.

Thoma KH: Tumors of the temporomandibular joint, *J Oral Surg* 22:157, 1964.

Worth HM: Radiology of the temporomandibular joint. In Zarb GA, Carlsson GE, editors: *Temporomandibular joint function and dysfunction,* Copenhagen, 1979, Munksgaard.

Malignant tumors

Morris MR et al: Chondrosarcoma of the temporomandibular joint: case report, *Head Neck Surg* 10:113, 1987.

Rubin MM et al: Metastatic carcinoma of the mandibular condyle presenting as temporomandibular joint syndrome, *J Oral Maxillofac Surg* 47:507, 1989.

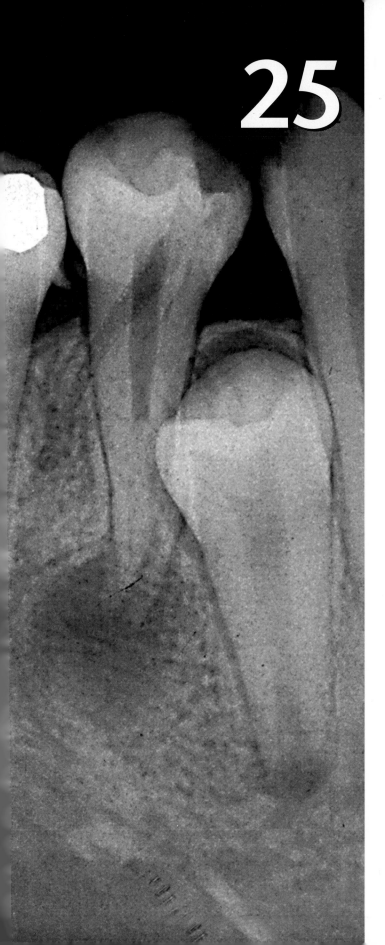

25

Paranasal Sinuses

AXEL RUPRECHT

The paranasal sinuses, especially the maxillary sinuses located near the dental structures, are important to the dentist. Diseases of the sinuses may extend to the jaws and may mimic odontogenic diseases. Conversely, odontogenic diseases may spread to the sinuses and mimic diseases of the sinuses. Part or all of the paranasal sinuses appear on many dental radiographs, for example, maxillary periapical radiographs and panoramic films made for dental treatment. All of the paranasal sinuses can appear on cephalometric skull radiographs made for orthodontic or orthognathic surgical purposes, although not necessarily in the most diagnostic fashion. Therefore the dentist should have some familiarity with the normal appearances and more common diseases of the paranasal sinuses.

Normal Development and Variations

The paranasal sinuses develop as invaginations from the nasal fossae into their respective bones (frontal, ethmoid, sphenoid, and maxillary). The first to develop are the *maxillary sinuses* (sometimes called the *maxillary antra* or *antra of Highmore)*, which become apparent by day 17 in utero. They begin just above the inferior concha and grow laterally. At birth each is quite small and slitlike; its greatest diameter, in an anteroposterior direction, is no more than 8 mm.

Initially the sinuses lie in the most medial aspect of the maxilla, but as they grow they extend laterally under the orbits. They reach laterally to the infraorbital canals during the second year and to the zygomatic bones by the ninth year. By approximately this time the inferior borders have extended to the level of the floor of the nasal fossae. Lateral growth usually ceases by the fifteenth year. The average volume of the adult maxillary sinus is about 15 ml. The sinuses may continue to enlarge throughout life. In some cases the sinuses may extend into the zygomatic bones, alveolar processes, sometimes the alveolar crests, and occasionally into the palatal processes of the maxilla.

Hypoplasia of the maxillary sinuses occurs unilaterally in about 1.7% of patients and bilaterally in 7.2%. In patients with hypoplasia of the maxillary sinus, the radiographic images of the affected sinus are more radiopaque than normal because of the relatively large amount of remaining maxillary bone. The configuration of the walls of the maxillary sinus frequently helps in distinguishing between a hypoplastic sinus and one that is pathologically radiopaque. On the occipitomental (Waters') view the walls of the hypoplastic sinus bow inward, resulting in a small air cavity, which appears to be more radiopaque than usual.

The *ethmoid sinuses* are better known as the ethmoid air cells because, unlike the other paranasal sinuses, they consist of multiple interconnected, or sometimes separate, small chambers. They start developing as outgrowths or extensions of the nasal fossae into the ethmoid bones during the fifth fetal month. These air cells continue to enlarge and extend into the ethmoid bone until the end of puberty. The number of ethmoid air cells varies considerably. Most often each ethmoid bone contains approximately 8 to 15 cells. The ethmoid air cells often extend into the neighboring maxillary, lacrimal, frontal, sphenoid, and palatine bones.

The development of the *frontal sinuses* does not usually begin until the fifth or sixth year. The frontal sinuses may develop either directly as extensions from the nasal fossae or from anterior ethmoid air cells. As with the other paranasal sinuses, a right and left frontal sinus cavity develop separately. As these cavities expand, they approach each other in the midline, where a thin bony septum separates them. This intersinus septum may be absent in some individuals. In about 4% of people the frontal sinuses fail to develop. In the adult the frontal sinuses are usually seen as two asymmetric cavities above the level of the supraorbital ridges and the nasion. The sinuses may also extend posteriorly in the roofs of the orbits. Depending on their source of extension, these sinuses drain directly into the nasal fossae via their frontonasal ducts (in about half the cases) or into the anterior ethmoid cells, then into the nasal fossae through the infundibula.

The *sphenoid sinuses* begin growth from the nasal cavities in the fourth fetal month. The invaginations for the sphenoid sinuses are from the sphenoethmoid recesses of the nasal cavities. They are present at birth as minute cavities in the body of the sphenoid bone. The main development takes place after puberty. Like the frontal sinuses, the right and left sphenoid sinuses, separated by a bony septum, are usually asymmetric in size and shape. Also, the overall size of the sinuses is quite variable. The sinuses may extend beyond the body of the sphenoid bone into the dorsum sellae, the greater or lesser wings, and the pterygoid processes. The sinuses communicate with the nasal cavities through ostia (singular, ostium), which are usually 2 to 3 mm in diameter. This may explain why, as with the maxillary sinuses, mucoceles (destructive growths resulting from blockage of the drainage from the sinuses) are uncommon in the sphenoid sinuses (see the section on mucoceles later in this chapter).

Various functions have been ascribed to these sinuses, including the following:

- Air conditioning (heating and humidification)
- Acting as an air reservoir
- Ventilation
- Aiding in olfaction
- Reduction in weight of the cranium
- Addition of resonance to the voice
- Protection
- Insulation of the cerebrum and orbits
- Participation in formation of the cranium

They may also have no function—that is, they may be evolutionary unwanted space. The maxillary and ethmoid sinuses may assist in respiration, with the growth of the maxillary sinuses also representing an adjustment to the changing size of the maxillofacial area. The frontal sinuses participate in the growth and development of the cerebral cranium, and the sphenoid sinuses allow for adjustments of the buckling in the cranial base in evolution.

The mucous membrane of the sinuses is similar to that of the nasal cavity, but with slightly fewer mucous glands. In the absence of disease the epithelial cilia move mucus toward its respective communications with the nasal fossae.

Diseases Associated with the Paranasal Sinuses

Because the maxillary sinus is of most concern to the dentist, the following text emphasizes diseases related to the maxillary sinus.

DEFINITION

Diseases associated with the maxillary sinus include both intrinsic diseases (originating within the sinus) and those that originate outside the sinus (most commonly odontogenic disease) and extend into the sinus. The types of diseases include inflammatory disease, odontogenic cysts, neoplasia, bone dysplasias, and trauma.

CLINICAL FEATURES

Clinical signs and symptoms that indicate the presence of a disease associated with the maxillary antrum range from a feeling of stuffiness, altered voice characteristics, pain on movement of the head or percussion of the teeth or cheek region, to loss of sensation in the region and swelling of the facial structures adjacent to the maxilla.

When the clinical signs indicate that the disease may be related to the odontogenic apparatus or the alveolar process of the maxilla, it is reasonable for the general practitioner to proceed with the initial radiologic investigation. If there are positive findings, the patient should be referred to an oral and maxillofacial radiologist to complete the examination. The application of specific imaging modalities is reviewed in the following section.

APPLIED DIAGNOSTIC IMAGING

The intraoral periapical film provides a detailed view of the floor of the maxillary antrum (a description of the normal appearance is in Chapter 9). If during this examination the dental practitioner suspects an abnormality, the maxillary lateral occlusal projection may be used for a more extensive view of the antrum. Also, the panoramic view provides a view of both maxillary sinuses, revealing internal structure and parts of the inferior, posterior, and anteromedial walls. It is difficult to compare the internal radiopacities of the sinus with these views.

Specialized skull views are the next step in the investigation. The Waters' projection is optimal for visualization of the maxillary sinuses, especially to compare the internal radiopacity. Other images that may be included are the submentovertex, posteroanterior, and lateral skull views. The lateral skull view allows examination of all four pairs of the paranasal sinuses, but with each member of a pair superimposed on the other. Other skull views are specifically designed for the investigation of the other sinuses.

In recent years, computed tomography (CT) and magnetic resonance imaging (MRI) have become increasingly important for evaluation of sinus disease and have virtually replaced conventional tomography. Because these modalities provide multiple sections through the sinuses at different planes, they contribute to the final diagnosis and the determination of the extent of the disease. High-resolution axial and coronal CT and MRI examinations are the most revealing, noninvasive techniques for the paranasal sinuses and adjacent structures and areas. CT examination is appropriate to determine the extent of disease in patients who have chronic or recurrent sinusitis. It provides superior imaging of the anterior ethmoid air cells and the upper two thirds of the nasal cavity. CT is also best for demonstrating any reaction in the surrounding bone in the presence of sinus diseases. MRI provides superior imaging of soft tissue, especially the extension of infiltrating neoplasms into surrounding soft tissues, or the differentiation of retained fluids from soft tissue masses in the sinuses.

Inflammatory Changes

Whether of infectious, chemical, or allergic origin, introduction of a foreign body, or facial trauma, insults to the paranasal sinuses cause changes and disorders that are detectable by radiographic examination. Such changes include thickened mucous membranes, fluid levels in the sinuses, polyps, empyema, and retention pseudocysts. However, viral infections may not cause a radiographic change in a sinus.

THICKENED MUCOUS MEMBRANE

Identifying Characteristics

Synonym. *Mucositis*

Definition. The lining mucous membrane of the paranasal sinuses is composed of respiratory epithelium. It is normally about 1 mm thick. Normal sinus mucous membrane is not usually apparent in a radiograph, and the bony walls appear well defined. However, when the mucous membrane becomes inflamed from either an infectious or allergic process, it may increase in thickness 10 to 15 times. This inflammation is called *mucositis*. Mucous membrane thickening greater than 3 mm is most likely pathologic. Dental inflammatory lesions such as periodontal disease or periapical disease may cause a localized mucositis in the adjacent floor of the maxillary antrum. This is a result of the extension of the inflammatory products (exudate) beyond the cortical floor of the antrum and into the periosteum and the mucous membrane of the sinus.

Clinical features. Most of the inflammatory or allergic episodes that result in thickening of the sinus lining are unrecognized by the patient and are discovered only incidentally on a radiograph. Also, the depth of a thickened mucous membrane in an asymptomatic individual may vary considerably over a relatively short time. Consequently, the discovery of a thickened mucous membrane in an individual who is otherwise without symptoms does not necessarily imply that further investigation or treatment is required. The localized type of mucositis related to dental inflammatory disease usually clears up in days or weeks after successful treatment of the underlying cause.

Radiographic features. The image of the thickened mucous membrane is readily detectable in the radiograph as a band noticeably more radiopaque than the air-filled sinus, paralleling the bony wall of the sinus (Fig. 25-1).

PERIOSTITIS

Identifying Characteristics
Definition. As described above, the inflammatory exudate from dental inflammatory lesions can extend into the maxillary antrum through the cortical boundary of the floor. The exudate can strip and elevate the periosteal lining of the cortical bone of the floor of the maxillary antrum. The presence of inflammatory products next to the periosteum stimulates the periosteum to produce a thin elevated layer of new bone adjacent to the root apex of the involved tooth (Fig. 25-2).

Radiographic features. Although the periosteal tissue is not visible in the radiographic image, the presence of a halolike layer of new bone indicates inflammation of the periosteum. This new bone may take the form of one thin radiopaque line or may be very thick or rarely laminated (similar to onion skin).

SINUSITIS

Identifying Characteristics
Definition. Sinusitis is a condition involving generalized inflammation of the paranasal sinus mucous membrane. This term is usually restricted to conditions that are primarily inflammatory, produce symptoms, and persist longer than 7 days, the duration of a typical viral upper respiratory tract infection. Sinusitis is usually caused by blockage of drainage from the ostiomeatal complex, the region of the ostium of the maxillary sinus and the ethmoidal ostium. The inflammation leads to ciliary dysfunction and retention of the mucous membrane secretions, followed by bacterial invasion and overgrowth. Perhaps 10% of inflammatory episodes of the maxillary sinuses are extensions of dental infections. Although not universally accepted, sinusitis has been divided into three subtypes, based on length of time the disease has been present. *Acute sinusitis* refers to those present for less than 2 weeks; *subacute sinusitis,* to conditions present from 2 weeks to 3 months; and *chronic sinusitis,* to conditions that have been present for more than 3 months. The term *pansinusitis* describes sinusitis affecting all the paranasal sinuses. Pansinusitis in children suggests the possibility of cystic fibrosis.

Clinical features. *Acute maxillary sinusitis* is often a complication of a common cold. It is often accompanied by

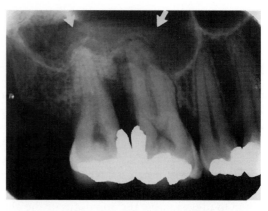

FIG. **25-1** The thickened mucous membrane is seen as a radiopaque band on the floor of the maxillary antrum. It develops in response to a localized area of periodontal disease.

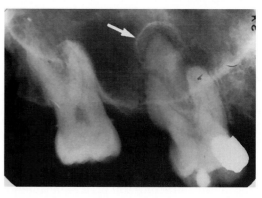

FIG. **25-2** This halolike appearance of bone *(arrow)* is the result of elevation of the periosteal lining in the floor of the maxillary antrum and the formation of new bone by the periosteum. The source of the inflammatory lesion responsible for this periosteal reaction is the first molar.

purulent nasal discharge or pharyngeal drainage. After a few days, the stuffiness and nasal discharge increase, and the patient may complain of pain and tenderness to pressure or swelling over the involved sinus. The pain, however, may be referred to the premolar and molar teeth on the affected side, and these teeth may also be sensitive to percussion. This finding requires that these teeth be ruled out as a possible source of the pain or infection. However, the key signs and symptoms are those of sepsis: fever, chills, malaise, and an elevated leukocyte count. Acute sinusitis is the most common of the sinus conditions that cause pain.

Chronic maxillary sinusitis is typically a sequela of an acute infection that fails to resolve by 3 months. In general, no external signs occur, except during periods of acute exacerbations when increased pain and discomfort

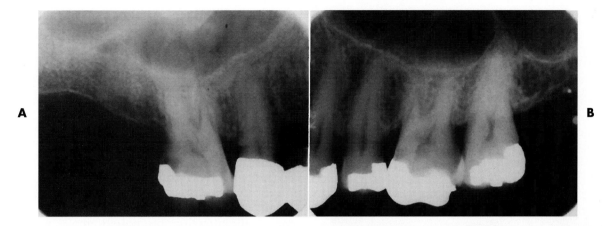

FIG. **25-3** Sinusitis results in thickening of the mucous membrane, which makes the internal structure of the antrum more radiopaque (soft tissue compared to air). Compare the internal radiopacity of the maxillary sinus, **A,** with the normal sinus, **B.**

are apparent. Chronic sinusitis is often associated with anatomic derangements that inhibit the outflow of mucus, including deviation of the nasal septum and presence of a concha bullosa (pneumatization of the middle concha). Chronic sinusitis is also often associated with allergic rhinitis, asthma, cystic fibrosis, and dental infections.

Radiographic features. The thickening of the mucous membrane and the accumulation of secretions that accompany sinusitis reduce the air content of the sinus and cause it to become increasingly radiopaque (Figs. 25-3 and 25-4). The most common radiopaque patterns that occur in the Waters' view are the following:

1. Localized mucosal thickening at the base of the sinus
2. Generalized thickening of the mucous membrane around the entire wall of the sinus
3. Complete filling of the sinus except about the ostium on the medial wall
4. Complete filling of the sinus

Such changes are best seen in the maxillary sinus, but the frontal and sphenoid sinuses may be similarly affected. Scrutinizing the area around the maxillary ostium on any of the views from Waters' projections to CT scans may reveal the presence of thickening of the mucosal tissue, which may cause blockage of the ostium. Mucosal thickening in just the base of the sinus may not represent sinusitis. Rather, it may represent the more localized thickening that can occur in association with rarefying osteitis from a tooth with a nonvital pulp. This may, however, progress to involve the entire sinus.

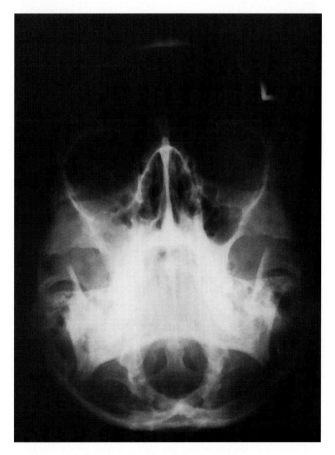

FIG. **25-4** Sinusitis of the right maxillary antrum has resulted in a more radiopaque internal density in the right sinus compared with the left sinus as seen in this Waters' view.

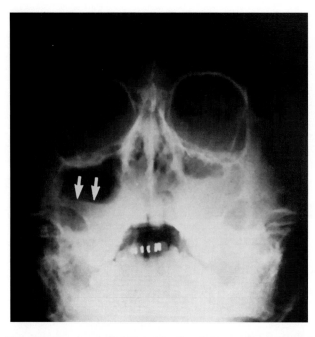

FIG. **25-5** An air-fluid level in the right maxillary antrum *(arrows)*. Note the thickening of the mucous membrane of the left sinus resulting in an increase in the density of the internal structure.

The image of the thickened mucous membrane on the radiograph may be uniform or polypoid. In the case of an allergic reaction, and if the antral cavity is apparent, the mucous membrane tends to be more lobulated. In contrast, in cases of infection, the thickened mucous membrane outline tends to be smoother, with its contour following that of the sinus wall.

An air-fluid level resulting from the accumulation of secretions may be present. Because the radiopacities of transudates, exudates, blood, and pathologically altered mucous membrane are similar, the differentiation among them relies on their shape and distribution. When present, fluid appears radiopaque and occupies the inferior aspect of the sinus. The border between the radiopaque fluid and the relatively radiolucent antrum is horizontal and straight, or with a meniscus (Fig. 25-5). It is possible to confirm that one is viewing an air-fluid interface by tilting the head and making another radiograph. This changes the orientation of the fluid level, which eliminates any doubt as to its fluid nature.

However, when attempting to verify that such a shadow is an air-fluid level, the dentist should allow sufficient time between when the head is tilted and the second radiograph is made. If the fluid in question is thick mucus, some minutes may be required before it attains its new level. To demonstrate an air-fluid level, the central ray of the x-ray beam must be horizontal and at the level of the air-fluid interface.

The resolution of acute sinusitis becomes apparent on the radiograph as a gradual increase in the radiolucency of the sinus. This can first be recognized when a small clear area appears in the interior of the sinus; the thickened mucous membrane gradually shrinks so that it begins to follow the outline of the bony wall. In time the mucous membrane again becomes radiographically invisible, and the sinus appears normal. Chronic sinusitis may result in persistent radiopacification of the sinus and sclerosis or thickening of the surrounding bone. Resorption of the bony border is unusual.

Management. The goals of treatment of sinusitis are to control the infection, promote drainage, and relieve pain. Acute sinusitis is usually treated medically with decongestants to reduce swelling of the mucous membranes and with antibiotics against bacteria. Chronic sinusitis is primarily a disease of obstruction of the ostia; thus the goal is ventilation and drainage. This is often accomplished through endoscopic surgery to enlarge obstructed ostia. When dental disease, either of pulpal or periodontal origin, is the cause of sinusitis, it should be treated promptly.

EMPYEMA

Identifying Characteristics
Definition. An empyema is a cavity filled with pus. It may result as a possible sequela of a sinus ostium blocked by a thickened, inflamed mucous membrane or some other pathologic process, especially in the maxillary sinus. Empyema is probably a variant of a mucocele or pyocele.

POLYPS

Identifying Characteristics
Definition. The thickened mucous membrane of a chronically inflamed sinus frequently forms into irregular folds called *polyps*. Polypoid hyperplasia of the mucous membrane may develop in an isolated area or a number of areas throughout the sinus.

Clinical features. Polyps may cause displacement or destruction of bone. Polyps in the maxillary sinus can displace or destroy the medial or lateral wall. In the ethmoid air cells, they may cause destruction of the medial wall of the orbit (lamina papyracea) with subsequent unilateral proptosis.

Radiographic features. A polyp may be differentiated from a retention pseudocyst on a radiograph by noting that a polyp usually occurs with a thickened mucous membrane lining (Fig. 25-6) because the polypoid mass is no more than an accentuation of the mucosal thickening. In

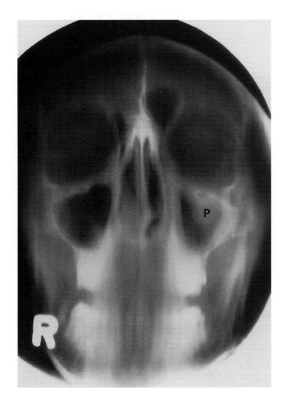

FIG. **25-6** A frontal tomograph at the level of the maxillary sinuses demonstrates thickened mucous membrane of all the borders of the left maxillary sinus and a polyp (*P*) suspended from the superior border of the sinus. (Courtesy A.G. Farman, DDS, C.J. Nortje, DDS, and R.E. Wood, DDS.)

the case of a retention pseudocyst, however, the adjacent mucous membrane lining is not usually apparent.

The radiographic image of the bone destruction associated with polyps frequently mimics that of a benign or malignant neoplasm. Because many sinus neoplasms are asymptomatic, examination of a paranasal sinus that reveals bone destruction associated with radiopacification is an indication for biopsy, not delayed by initial conservative treatment.

ANTROLITHS

Identifying Characteristics
Definition. Antroliths occur within the maxillary sinuses and are the result of calcification of masses of stagnant mucus in sites of previous inflammation, root fragments and bone chips, or foreign objects.

Clinical features. The smaller antroliths are asymptomatic and usually are discovered on routine examination. If they continue to grow, the patient may experience an associated sinusitis, bloodstained nasal discharge, nasal obstruction, or facial pain.

Radiographic features
Location. Antroliths occur within the maxillary sinus and thus are positioned above the floor of the maxillary antrum in either periapical films or panoramic images.

Periphery and shape. Antroliths are well defined and may have a smooth or irregular shape.

Internal structure. The internal aspect may vary in density from a barely perceptible radiopacity to an extremely radiopaque structure. The internal density may be homogenous or heterogenous, and some instances may see evidence of alternating layers of radiolucency and radiopacity in the form of laminations.

Differential diagnosis. Antroliths may be distinguished from root fragments in the sinus by inspection of the mass for the usual root anatomy such as the presence of a pulp canal. A displaced root fragment in the sinus may move when radiography is performed with the head in different positions, unless it is lodged between the bone and the sinus lining. Rhinoliths are similar calcifications but are found within the nasal fossa. A posteroanterior skull view helps identify the location of a rhinolith.

Management. An otolaryngologist may need to remove symptomatic antroliths.

RETENTION PSEUDOCYSTS

Identifying Characteristics
Synonyms. Benign mucous cyst, mucous retention cyst, mesothelial cyst, pseudocyst, interstitial cyst, lymphangiectatic cyst, false cyst, retention cyst of the maxillary sinus, benign cyst of the antrum, benign mucosal cyst of the sinus, serous nonsecretory retention pseudocyst, and *mucosal antral cyst*

Definition. The term *retention pseudocysts* is used to describe several related conditions. Blockage of the secretory ducts of seromucous glands in the sinus mucous membrane may result in a pathologic accumulation of secretions and result in swelling of the mucous membrane. The serous nonsecretory retention cyst arises as a cystic degeneration within an inflamed, thickened sinus lining. Both types of lesions are called *pseudocysts* because although they are fluid-filled pathologic cavities, they are often not lined with epithelium. The actual pathogenesis of these lesions is controversial. Because their clinical and radiographic features are the same, no attempt is made here to distinguish them.

Clinical features. Retention pseudocysts may be found in any of the sinuses at any time of the year but occur more often around April and November. This suggests that they might have to do with changes in season or heating or air conditioning in buildings. Most studies have found that the retention pseudocyst is more common in males.

The retention pseudocyst rarely causes any signs or symptoms, and thus the patient is usually unaware of the lesion. It often is noticed as an incidental finding on radiographs made for other purposes. However, when the pseudocyst completely fills the maxillary sinus cavity, it may prolapse (extrude) through the ostium and cause nasal obstruction and postnasal discharge. This may be the only clinical evidence of the presence of the pseudocyst.

As either type of retention pseudocyst enlarges and fills the sinus cavity, it frequently ruptures as a result of abrupt pressure changes caused by sneezing or blowing the nose. If this does not happen, the expanding pseudocyst may herniate through the ostium into the nasal cavity, where it subsequently ruptures. The pseudocyst may be present on radiographic examination of the maxillary sinus, perhaps absent only a few days later, only to reappear on subsequent examinations.

The maxillary sinus is the most common site of antral retention pseudocysts, although they are occasionally found in the frontal or sphenoid sinuses. Antral retention pseudocysts are not related to extractions or associated with periapical disease.

Radiographic features

Location. Partial images of retention pseudocysts of the maxillary antrum may appear on maxillary posterior periapical projections, but it is best demonstrated in panoramic radiographs. Although these pseudocysts may occur bilaterally, usually only a single pseudocyst develops. Occasionally more than one pseudocyst may form in a sinus. These pseudocysts usually project from the floor of the sinus, although some may form on the lateral walls. Retention pseudocysts vary in size, from that of a fingertip to completely filling the sinus and making it radiopaque.

Periphery and shape. Both varieties of pseudocysts usually appear as smooth and dome-shaped radiopaque masses. Because the lesion originates within the maxillary sinus, no osseous border surrounds it. The base of the lesions may be narrow or more commonly broad.

Internal structure. The internal aspect is homogeneous and more radiopaque than the surrounding air of the sinus cavity (Fig. 25-7). The radiopacity of the lesion is caused by the accumulation of fluid and, as such, normal osseous landmarks may often be seen through its image.

Effects on surrounding structures. Usually no effects are present on the surrounding structures, and thus it is of note that the sinus floor is intact.

Differential diagnosis. It is important to distinguish retention pseudocysts from odontogenic cysts (for example, radicular or dentigerous cysts or keratocysts), antral polyps, or any rounded neoplastic mass. This can usually be done radiographically and by the patient's history.

The retention pseudocyst is dome shaped and does not have the thin marginal radiopaque line representing the corticated border characteristic of the odontogenic cyst. The odontogenic cyst is also more rounded or tear shaped. The lamina dura of the tooth or teeth associated with a radicular cyst is not intact in the apical area; it may be continuous with the corticated outline of the odontogenic cyst. In contrast, the roots of healthy teeth projecting over an area of an antral cavity occupied by a retention pseudocyst usually have the intact lamina dura apparent. Also, commonly the floor of the antrum is missing or displaced by the odontogenic cyst.

Antral polyps of infectious or allergic origin may be distinguished radiographically from a retention pseudocyst in that they are more often multiple. They are commonly associated with a thickened mucous membrane, which is less frequently observed with retention pseudocysts.

Neoplasms may also mimic a retention pseudocyst. If benign and originating from outside the sinus, they are separated from the cavity of the sinus by a radiopaque border, similar to the odontogenic cysts. Malignant neoplasms, if originating outside the sinus, destroy the osseous border of the sinus. If the neoplasm originates within the sinus, the condition of the border varies from completely intact to displaced and disrupted. The neoplasm is less likely to be as dome shaped as the retention pseudocyst.

Management. Retention pseudocysts in the maxillary sinus usually require no treatment because they customarily resolve spontaneously without any residual effect on the antral mucous membrane. Surgical intervention should be considered only in the case of persistent pain, headache, or expansion.

MUCOCELE

Identifying Characteristics
Synonyms. *Pyocele* and *mucopyocele*

Definition. A mucocele is an expanding, destructive lesion that results from a blocked ostium of a sinus. The blockage may result from intra-antral or intranasal inflammation, polyps, or bony neoplasms. The whole sinus thus becomes the pathologic cavity or cystlike lesion. As this lesion continues to accumulate mucus and after the sinus cavity has filled, the pressure increases and the lesion becomes destructive, thinning, displacing, and, in some cases, destroying the sinus walls. If a mucocele becomes infected, it is called a *pyocele* or a *mucopyocele.*

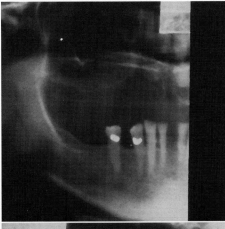

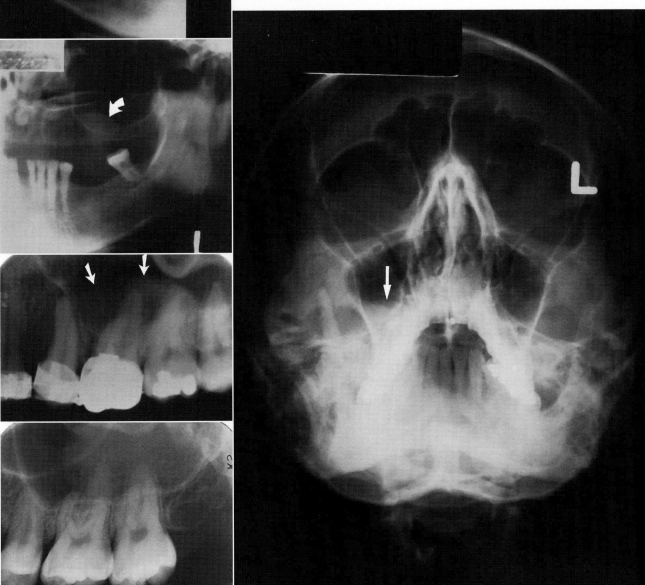

FIG. **25-7** Mucous retention cyst in the maxillary antrum *(arrows)* seen as a soft tissue opacity with a circular (hydraulic) border without a peripheral cortex. This indicates that the cyst originated within the sinus, seen in the panoramic **(A)**, periapical **(B** and **C)**, and Waters' **(D)** projections.

Clinical features. A mucocele in the maxillary sinus may exert pressure on the superior alveolar nerves when resorbing the sinus walls and thus cause radiating pain. The patient may first complain of a sensation of fullness in the cheek, and the area may swell. This swelling may first become apparent over the anteroinferior aspect of the antrum, the area where the wall is thin and may be destroyed. If the lesion expands inferiorly, it may cause loosening of the posterior teeth in the area. If it expands the medial wall of the sinus, the lateral wall of the nasal cavity is deformed and the nasal airway may be obstructed. Should it expand into the orbit, it may cause diplopia (double vision) and proptosis (protrusion of the globe of the eye).

Radiographic features
Location. About 90% of these bone-destroying lesions occur in the ethmoidal and frontal sinuses and are rare in the maxillary and sphenoid sinuses.

Periphery and shape. The normal shape of the sinus is changed into a more circular shape as the mucocele grows.

Internal structure. The internal aspect of the sinus cavity is uniformly radiopaque.

Effects on surrounding structures. The shape of the sinus changes with the bony expansion. Septa and the bony walls may be destroyed. When the mucocele is associated with the maxillary antrum, teeth may be displaced or resorbed. In the frontal sinus the usually scalloped border is smoothed by erosion, and the intersinus septum may be displaced. The supramedial border of the orbit is destroyed or displaced. In the ethmoid air cells, displacement of the lamina papyracea may occur, displacing the contents of the orbit. In the sphenoid sinus the expansion may be in a superior direction, suggesting a pituitary neoplasm.

Differential diagnosis. Although it may not be possible to distinguish between a mucocele in the maxillary antrum and a malignant neoplasm, any suggestion that the lesion is associated with an occluded ostium should strengthen the likelihood of a mucocele. Blockage of the ostium is usually the result of a previous surgical procedure, although a deviated nasal septum or polyps may be a factor. A large odontogenic cyst filling the maxillary antrum and causing expansion of the walls may mimic a mucocele. Look for any remnants of the internal aspect of the antrum between the wall of the cyst and the wall of the antrum. CT is the imaging method of choice for making these distinctions.

Management. Treatment of the mucocele is usually surgical, using a Caldwell-Luc operation to allow excision of the lesion. The prognosis is excellent.

Odontogenic Cysts

Odontogenic cysts are the most common group of extrinsic cysts that encroach on the maxillary sinuses. These cysts comprise almost half of the lesions involving the maxillary sinuses. Most are radicular cysts, followed by dentigerous cysts and odontogenic keratocysts.

GENERAL ODONTOGENIC CYSTS
Identifying Characteristics
Radiographic features
Location. These cysts are not within the maxillary sinuses but merely encroach on the space of the sinuses by displacing their borders. The cortex of the cysts and the sinus wall fuse, and thus as the cyst enlarges, the sinus decreases in size (Fig. 25-8, *A*). This results in a radiopaque line between the lumen of the cyst and the air space of the sinus, and thus the contents of the cyst are separated from the internal aspect of the sinus. This is in contrast to a retention pseudocyst, which, being inside the sinus, does not have a cortex around its periphery. In some cases the cyst may enlarge to the point that it has encroached on almost the entire sinus, so the remaining sinus sits like a thin saddle over the cyst (see Fig. 25-8, *B*).

Periphery and shape. The invaginating cyst has a curved or oval shape and a cortical boundary.

Internal structure. The internal structure is homogeneous and radiopaque. The degree of radiopacity may appear to be that of bone resulting from the extreme contrast to the radiolucent air within the sinus.

Effects on surrounding structures. The cyst may displace the floor of the maxillary antrum. If the cyst grows to a size large enough to displace the entire sinus, the cyst may expand the walls of the maxillary antrum.

Differential diagnosis. A common lesion to differentiate is the retention pseudocyst, which can have the same shape but does not have a cortex at the periphery. If the odontogenic cyst were to become infected, the cortex may be lost. At this point it may become difficult to determine whether the lesion is from outside or inside the sinus. The relationship to neighboring teeth may help to make this decision. This is true for all odontogenic cysts, including radicular cysts, dentigerous cysts, and keratocysts. Very large cysts may occupy all the internal aspect of the sinus. When this occurs, no radiographic evidence may exist of the air space left, and it may appear as if the cyst is the sinus. In this case, because of the radiopacity of the cyst, the appearance may resemble sinusitis with radiopacification of the sinus. Evaluation of such conditions is aided by noting that the wall of the cyst is often thicker and more uniform than that of a sinus. In addition, the normal vascular markings on

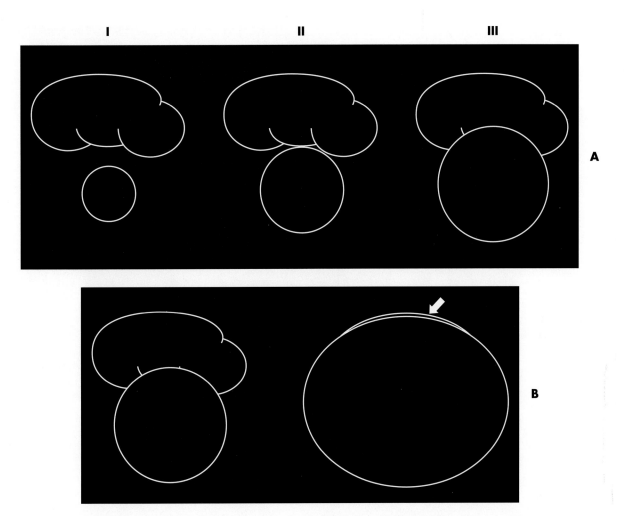

FIG. **25-8**   **A,** The odontogenic cyst starts near the sinus *(I).* As it enlarges, the cyst comes up against the border of the maxillary sinus *(II)* and then displaces the border of the sinus as it continues to enlarge *(III).* The border of the cyst and the border of the sinus are now the same line of bone. **B,** The odontogenic cyst, as it continues to enlarge, may encroach on almost all the space of the sinus, leaving a small saddlelike sinus over the cyst *(arrow).* The appearance may mimic sinusitis.

the wall of the maxillary sinus are not present on the walls of a cyst.

An antral loculation may occasionally have a round shape and sometimes appear to have a cortex. However, because the loculation contains air, which is more radiolucent than the fluid within a cyst, the loculation appears more radiolucent than the surrounding antrum.

RADICULAR CYST

The radicular cyst is described in Chapter 19. When it occurs in the maxilla, it may encroach on the maxillary sinus as it enlarges (see Figs. 25-8 and 25-9), as described previously for cysts in general. The radicular cyst may be interpreted by its relationship to the root of the tooth from which it has arisen. Commonly involved teeth in-

clude the maxillary lateral incisors and first molars. Because of the posterior inclination of the root of the lateral incisor, cysts often expand in a posterior direction and into the antrum. The maxillary first molar is often cariously involved and has a close relationship to the sinus.

DENTIGEROUS CYST

As described in Chapter 19, the dentigerous cyst forms around all or part of the crown of an unerupted tooth. Although such cysts are not nearly as common in the maxilla as in the mandible, when they do occur in the upper jaw, it is most often in association with impacted third molars. Consequently, this cyst is usually associated with a tooth missing from the arch. When the cyst en-

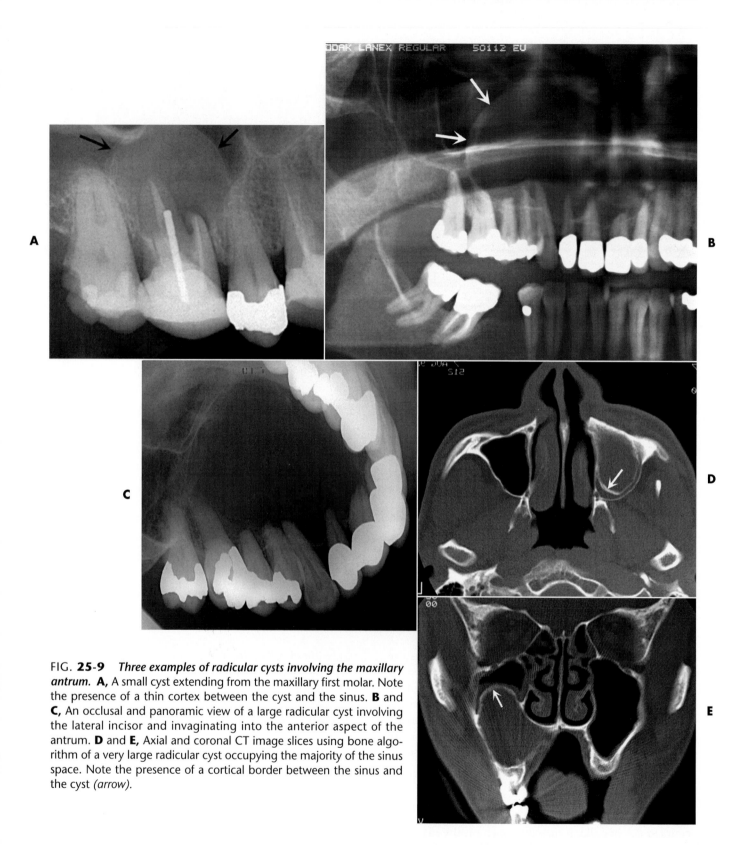

FIG. **25-9** *Three examples of radicular cysts involving the maxillary antrum.* **A,** A small cyst extending from the maxillary first molar. Note the presence of a thin cortex between the cyst and the sinus. **B** and **C,** An occlusal and panoramic view of a large radicular cyst involving the lateral incisor and invaginating into the anterior aspect of the antrum. **D** and **E,** Axial and coronal CT image slices using bone algorithm of a very large radicular cyst occupying the majority of the sinus space. Note the presence of a cortical border between the sinus and the cyst *(arrow).*

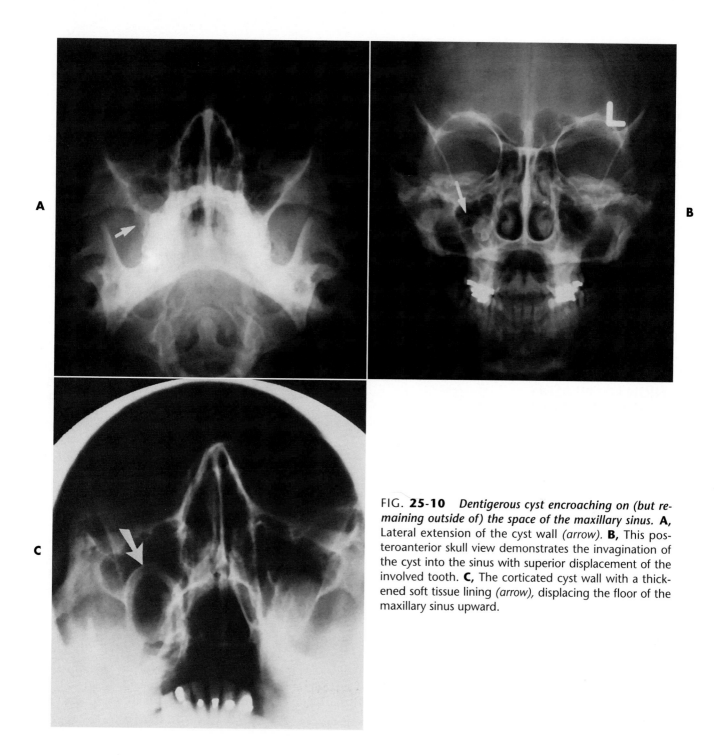

FIG. **25-10** *Dentigerous cyst encroaching on (but remaining outside of) the space of the maxillary sinus.* **A,** Lateral extension of the cyst wall *(arrow).* **B,** This posteroanterior skull view demonstrates the invagination of the cyst into the sinus with superior displacement of the involved tooth. **C,** The corticated cyst wall with a thickened soft tissue lining *(arrow),* displacing the floor of the maxillary sinus upward.

croaches on the sinus, the radiograph usually shows a radiolucent area elevating an intact wall or floor of a maxillary sinus, in a manner similar to that of the radicular cyst described previously (Fig. 25-10). Within this area is the crown of the associated tooth. The tooth is usually displaced in a superior direction and, in large cysts, may be pushed to the floor of the orbit.

ODONTOGENIC KERATOCYSTS

A description of the odontogenic keratocyst cyst can be found in Chapter 19. This cyst may also encroach on the maxillary sinus. These cysts are usually unilocular in the maxilla. They may act aggressively and replace most of the sinus, cause resorption of cortical plates, and involve adjacent soft tissue. In some cases this cyst may be associated with an impacted and displaced tooth and cannot be differentiated from a dentigerous cyst.

Neoplasms

Benign neoplasms of the paranasal sinuses other than inflammatory polyps are rare. The radiographic images of such benign neoplasms are nonspecific. Usually the involved portion of the sinus appears radiopaque because of the presence of a mass. Bone resorption may occur as a result of pressure from the mass.

The most common malignant neoplasms of the paranasal sinuses are squamous cell carcinomas and, to a lesser extent, malignant salivary gland neoplasms. Of carcinomas of the paranasal sinuses, 74% originate in the maxillary sinus. Although radiopacification is a feature of both the inflammatory conditions and neoplasms, bone destruction is more common with malignant neoplasms.

BENIGN NEOPLASMS OF THE PARANASAL SINUSES

Epithelial Papilloma

Definition. The epithelial papilloma is a rare neoplasm of respiratory epithelium that occurs in the nasal cavity and paranasal sinuses. It occurs predominantly in men.

Clinical features. Unilateral nasal obstruction, nasal discharge, pain, and epistaxis may occur. The patient may have complained of recurring sinusitis for years and a subsequent nasal obstruction on the same side as the sinusitis. The epithelial papilloma, although benign and relatively rare, has a 10% incidence of associated carcinoma.

Radiographic features. The features may not be specific, and the diagnosis can be made only by histopathologic examination of the tissue.

Location. The epithelial papilloma is usually in the ethmoidal or maxillary sinus. It may also appear as an isolated polyp in the nose or sinus.

Internal structure. This neoplasm appears as a homogeneous radiopaque mass of soft tissue density.

Effects on surrounding structures. If bone destruction is apparent, it is the result of pressure erosion.

OSTEOMA

Identifying Characteristics

Definition. The osteoma is the most common of the mesenchymal neoplasms in the paranasal sinuses. For a detailed description, see Chapter 20.

Clinical features. Most osteomas are usually slow growing and asymptomatic and thus usually detected as an incidental finding in an examination made for another purpose. When symptoms do occur, they are the result of obstruction of the sinus ostium or infundibulum or are secondary to erosion or deformity, orbital involvement, or intracranial extension. Those growing in the maxillary sinus may extend into the nose and cause nasal obstruction or a swelling of the side of the nose. They may expand the sinus and produce swelling of the cheek or hard palate. In cases extending to the orbit, the patient may have proptosis. In some cases, external fistulae have occurred. Osteomas of the maxillary sinus have been described after Caldwell-Luc operations. Osteomas are almost twice as common in males as females and are most common in the second, third, and fourth decades.

Radiographic features

Location. Although osteomas occasionally develop in the maxillary sinus, they more often occur in the frontal and ethmoidal sinuses. The incidence in the maxillary antrum varies between 3.9% and 28.5% of the incidence in all paranasal sinuses.

Periphery and shape. The osteoma is usually lobulated or rounded and has a sharply defined margin.

Internal structure. The internal aspect is homogeneous and extremely radiopaque (see Fig. 20-36 in Chapter 20).

Differential diagnosis. The differential interpretation includes the antrolith, mycolith, teeth, or odontogenic neoplasms, including odontoma, although these are all usually not as homogeneous in appearance as the osteoma.

AMELOBLASTOMA

Identifying Characteristics

Definition. Although rare and classified as benign, ameloblastoma is the most common extrinsic benign odontogenic neoplasm affecting the maxillary sinus. For a detailed description of ameloblastomas, see Chapter 20.

Clinical features. When this neoplasm occurs in the maxilla, it may cause painless facial deformity, nasal obstruction, and displacement of teeth. The lack of bony barriers and the relatively good blood supply are probably also responsible for efficient local spread. Death may occur because of direct invasion into adjacent vital structures.

Radiographic features

Location. When located in the maxilla, about 85% of ameloblastomas originate posterior to the canines. Thus

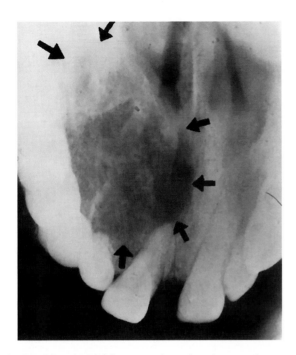

FIG. 25-11 Ameloblastoma obscuring the anterior aspect of the maxillary antrum *(arrows)*. (Courtesy L. Hollender, DDS, Seattle, Wash.)

a high probability exists that the ameloblastoma will invade the sinus, which is in close proximity.

Internal structure. When an ameloblastoma involves the maxillary sinus, the sinus has a radiopaque appearance equivalent to a soft tissue density (Fig. 25-11). Rarely the curved, coarse septa characteristic of ameloblastoma may be present.

Effects on surrounding structures. The bony walls of the sinus are thinned and eroded, and adjacent structures may be invaded. A tooth or part of a tooth may be embedded in the neoplasm.

Management. Although treatment of the ameloblastoma in the mandible is generally successful, the prognosis for this entity in the maxillary sinus is less favorable. It lies in close proximity to the nasal cavity, the other paranasal sinuses, orbit, pharyngeal tissues, and base of the skull, and invasion of any of these structures complicates its excision, the most accepted mode of treatment.

MALIGNANT NEOPLASMS OF THE PARANASAL SINUSES

Malignant neoplasms of the paranasal sinuses are rare, accounting for less than 1% of all malignancies in the body. Squamous cell carcinoma, comprising 80% to 90% of the cancers in this site, is by far the most common primary malignant neoplasm of the paranasal sinuses. Other primary neoplasms include adenocarci-

noma, carcinomas of salivary gland origin, soft and hard tissue sarcomas, melanoma, and malignant lymphoma. Factors that contribute to a poor prognosis for cancer of the paranasal sinuses include the advanced stage of the disease when it is finally diagnosed and the close anatomic proximity of vital structures. The clinical signs and symptoms may masquerade as an inflammatory sinusitis. The early primary lesions may only appear as a soft tissue mass in the sinus before they cause bone destruction. The lesion may become extensive, involving the entire sinus, with radiographic evidence of bone destruction before symptoms become apparent. Therefore any unexplained radiopacity in the maxillary sinus of an individual older than 40 years should be investigated thoroughly.

SQUAMOUS CELL CARCINOMA

Identifying Characteristics

Definition. Squamous cell carcinoma likely originates from metaplastic epithelium of the sinus mucous membrane lining.

Clinical features. The most common symptoms of cancer in the maxillary sinus are facial pain or swelling, nasal obstruction, and a lesion in the oral cavity. The mean age of the patient is 60 years (range 25 to 89 years). Twice as many men as women are affected. Lymph nodes are involved in about 10% of cases, and the symptoms are present for about 5 months before diagnosis.

The symptoms produced by neoplasms in the maxillary sinus depend on which wall(s) of the sinus is involved. The medial wall is usually the first to become eroded, leading to such nasal signs and symptoms as obstruction, discharge, bleeding, and pain. These symptoms may appear trivial, and their significance may not be appreciated. Lesions that arise on the floor of the sinus may first produce dental signs and symptoms, including expansion of the alveolar process, unexplained pain and numbness of the teeth, loose teeth, and swelling of the palate or alveolar ridge and malfitting dentures. The neoplasm may erode the floor and penetrate into the oral cavity. Such oral manifestations appear in 25% to 35% of patients with cancer in the maxillary sinus. When the lesion penetrates the lateral wall, facial and vestibular swelling becomes apparent and the patient may complain of pain and hyperesthesia of the maxillary teeth. Involvement of the sinus roof and the floor of the orbit causes symptoms related to the eye: diplopia, proptosis, pain, and hyperesthesia or anesthesia and pain over the cheek and upper teeth. Invasion and penetration of the posterior wall lead to invasion of the muscles of mastication, causing painful trismus, obstruction of the eustachian tube causing a

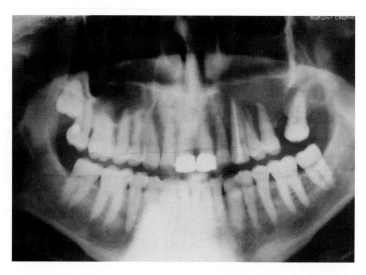

FIG. **25-12**   *Squamous cell carcinoma of the left maxillary sinus.* Note the radiopaque internal structure in the sinus and the destruction of its walls. Compare this sinus with the radiolucent internal aspect and outline of the right maxillary sinus. (Courtesy C. Bohnfolk, DDS, Dallas, Tex.)

stuffy ear, and referred pain and hyperesthesia over the distribution of the second and third divisions of the fifth nerve.

Radiographic features. Sometimes the radiographic findings, especially in early malignant disease of the paranasal sinuses, are nonspecific. It may not be possible to differentiate the early manifestations in radiographs of the maxillary sinus from the radiopacity of the sinus that develops in sinusitis and polyp formation. Evidence relies on changes seen in the surrounding bone, the sinus walls, and the maxillary alveolar process.

Location. Most carcinomas occur in the maxillary sinuses, but involvement of the frontal and sphenoid sinuses is also comparatively common.

Internal structure. The internal aspect of the maxillary sinus has a soft tissue radiopaque appearance.

Effects on surrounding structures. As the lesion expands, it is capable of destroying the sinus walls and in general causing irregular radiolucent areas in the surrounding bone. A detailed examination of the adjacent alveolar process may reveal bone destruction around the teeth or irregular widening of the periodontal ligament space. Frequently the medial wall of the maxillary sinus is thinned or destroyed, although there may also be destruction of the floor and anterior or posterior walls that may be detected in the panoramic film. The medial wall of the maxillary sinus is best seen on the Caldwell and Waters' projections. In addition to loss of the medial wall, it may extend into the nasal cavity.

Additional imaging. If a conventional radiograph of any radiopacified sinus reveals the slightest suggestion of bone destruction, advanced imaging is imperative (Fig. 25-12). On CT, the most characteristic sign of malignancy is invasion into the soft tissue facial planes beyond the sinus walls. Consequently CT is useful in revealing the extent of paranasal sinus neoplasms, especially when extension into the orbit, infratemporal fossa, or cranial cavity has occurred. MRI examinations are excellent for revealing the extent of soft tissue penetration into adjacent structures and in differentiating mucous accumulation from the soft tissue mass of the neoplasm (Fig. 25-13).

Differential diagnosis. The differential interpretation includes all the conditions that may cause radiopacity of the antrum, such as sinusitis, large retention pseudocysts, and odontogenic cysts. It is important to note that bone destruction may also occur in infectious and benign as well as malignant conditions. Neoplasms should be suspected in any older patient in whom chronic sinusitis develops for the first time without obvious cause.

Management. Treatment of squamous cell carcinoma in the paranasal sinuses generally combines surgery and radiation therapy. Malignant neoplasms in the paranasal sinuses usually have a poor prognosis because they are usually well advanced by the time of diagnosis. Other factors contributing to the poor prognosis include frequently inaccurate preoperative staging and the complex anatomy of the region.

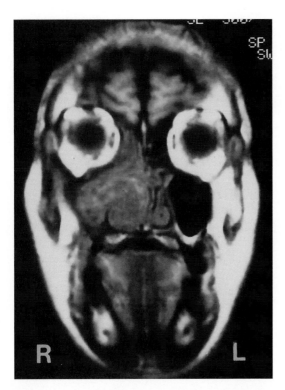

FIG. **25-13** *Frontal MRI at the level of the maxillary sinuses.* Note the squamous cell carcinoma filling the entire maxillary sinus and eroding its medial wall to fill the right half of the nasal fossa and the superior portion of the left nasal cavity as well as the right ethmoid air cells. Compare the gray image of the carcinoma on right side with the normal black air-filled maxillary and ethmoid air cells on left. (Courtesy A.G. Farman, DDS, C.J. Nortje, DDS, and R.E. Wood, DDS.)

PSEUDOTUMOR

Identifying Characteristics
Synonyms. *Invasive fungal sinusitis, inflammatory pseudotumor, fibroinflammatory pseudotumor, plasma cell granuloma, sinonasal fungal disease, mucormycosis, aspergillosis, zygomycosis of the paranasal sinuses,* and *Rhizopus sinusitis*

Definition. *Pseudotumor* is a descriptive name for a group of apparently related diseases of fungal origin that occur in the paranasal sinuses, as well as other parts of the head and neck.

Clinical features. Pseudotumor often occurs after a series of recurrent infections. The symptoms may not be very specific. There may be recurring pain and a mass simulating a neoplasm. The latter may cause erosion of the walls of the involved sinus and proptosis if the orbit is involved. Altered nerve function resulting from involvement of the nerve or occlusion of blood vessels by

the mass has also been reported. Although cases have been reported in otherwise healthy individuals, many cases appear in patients who are immunocompromised or have systemic diseases such as diabetes mellitus, von Willebrand disease, or myelodysplasia.

Radiographic features. The radiographic findings in pseudotumor include masses simulating malignant neoplasms that cause erosion of bony walls of the involved sinuses.

Differential diagnosis. The differential interpretation includes benign and malignant neoplasms.

Management. The treatment of pseudotumor, which can include debridement of the sinuses and administration of amphotericin B, a 7-week course of deoxycholate amphotericin B and rifampin, a Caldwell-Luc surgical approach, and therapy, reflects the differences in the specific lesions included under the term *pseudotumor of the sinuses,* the exact location of the disease, the organism involved, and the medical status of the patient.

Fibrous Dysplasia

Fibrous dysplasia may extend into or near one of the paranasal sinuses. Monostotic fibrous dysplasia may arise in the maxillary, sphenoid, frontal, ethmoid, and temporal bones. For a detailed description of fibrous dysplasia, see Chapter 22.

GENERAL FIBROUS DYSPLASIA

Identifying Characteristics
Clinical features. The involvement of the facial skeleton with fibrous dysplasia can result in facial asymmetry, nasal obstruction, proptosis, pituitary gland compression, impingement on cranial nerves, or sinus obliteration. The sinus obliteration results when the expanding lesion of dysplastic bone encroaches on it. The lesion may displace the roots of teeth and cause teeth to separate or migrate, but it usually does not cause root resorption. Fibrous dysplasia is more common in children and young adults and tends to stop growing when skeletal growth ceases, although cases in adults are found.

Radiographic features
Location. The posterior maxilla is the most common location for fibrous dysplasia.
  Periphery. The lesion itself is usually not well defined, tending to blend into the surrounding bone. The external cortex of the bone is, however, maintained intact, although it may be displaced.

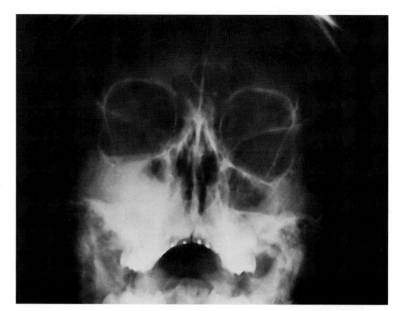

FIG. **25-14**   Fibrous dysplasia, invaginating into the right maxillary sinus and increasing the radiopacity of the sinus through an increase in bone with a ground-glass–like pattern. (Courtesy L. Hollender, DDS, Seattle, Wash.)

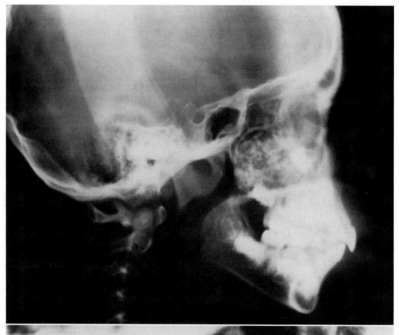

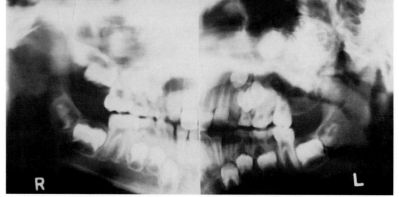

A

B

FIG. **25-15**   *Complex odontoma encroaching on the maxillary sinus.* This lesion is composed of amorphous radiopacities surrounding and partially obscuring unerupted teeth. **A,** Lateral skull view; **B,** panoramic view.

Internal structure. The normal radiolucent maxillary antrum may be partially or totally replaced by the increased radiopacity of this lesion. The degree of radiopacity depends on its stage of development and the relative amounts of bone present. Usually the radiopaque areas have the characteristic "ground-glass" appearance on extraoral radiographs or an "orange-peel" appearance on intraoral views (Fig. 25-14).

Effects on surrounding structures. Fibrous dysplasia may replace most of the sinus by encroaching on and displacing the antral walls, elevating the orbital floor or obstructing the nasal fossa.

Differential diagnosis. Such a painless, solitary enlargement in the jaw of a relatively young person is difficult to confuse with other radiopaque entities. Paget's disease of bone does not usually obliterate the sinus as does fibrous dysplasia. A complex odontoma (Fig. 25-15) is usually associated with one or more unerupted teeth and is surrounded by a radiolucent line, in turn surrounded by a radiopaque line. An ossifying fibroma similar to fibrous dysplasia may have a uniform radiopaque appearance but usually has a definite border (Fig. 25-16). However, in some cases the differential diagnosis of ossifying fibroma involving the antrum and fibrous dysplasia can be extremely difficult. The shape of the new bone encroaching on the internal aspect of the antrum often parallels the original shape of the external walls of the antrum in fibrous dysplasia.

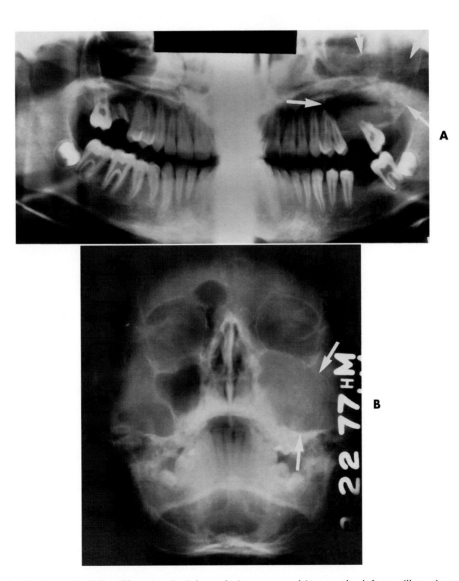

FIG. **25-16** *Ossifying fibroma.* **A,** A large lesion encroaching on the left maxillary sinus with well-defined borders and internal bone formation, causing displaced teeth and root resorption *(arrows).* **B,** A Waters' view of the radiopaque sinus and expansion of the maxilla *(arrows).*

Continued.

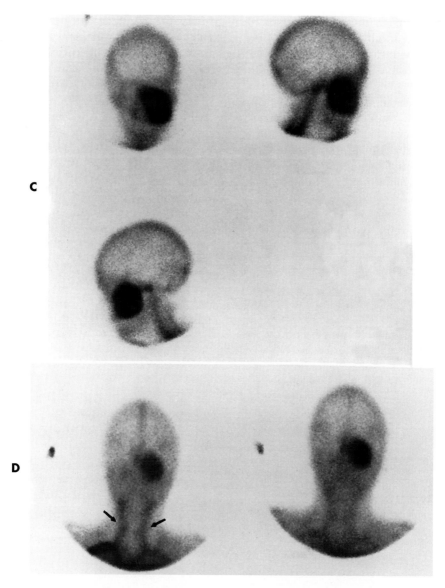

FIG. **25-16, cont'd**   **C,** A positive bone scan demonstrates an increase in bone meta-bolic activity. **D,** Early perfusion scans demonstrate that the lesion is very vascular *(arrows point to the great vessels).*

Traumatic Injuries to the Paranasal Sinuses

DENTAL STRUCTURES DISPLACED INTO THE SINUS

Identifying Characteristics
Definition. Dental roots may be fractured due to various forms of trauma, including iatrogenic causes. Fractured roots may be forced into the sinus during extraction or subsequent attempts to retrieve them.

Clinical features. No specific features may be visible if the root was forced into the sinus recently. However, the dentist may note the absence of the root fragment on examining the extracted tooth and be unable to locate it anywhere else. Sometimes asking the patient to hold his or her nose while attempting to breathe out through it, similar to a Valsalva maneuver, will cause bubbles to appear within the blood contained within the fresh extraction socket.

If the patient has had the root or tooth in the sinus for a number of days, he or she may present with sinusitis (see the previous discussion on sinusitis).

Radiographic features
Location. Roots or teeth in the sinus are associated with premolars and molars because the sinus is often in close

proximity to the roots. The dental structure may be found anywhere within the sinus but is more often on the floor of the sinus because of gravity. Sometimes it may be submucosal, between the osseous wall of the sinus and the mucoperiosteum.

Lateral maxillary occlusal views are useful for examining root tips in the maxillary sinus. Other films in a different anatomic plane, such as a Waters' projection, may help in the three-dimensional localization.

Periphery and shape. No immediate evidence may be present of any change in the sinus, even when an oroantral fistula has been created. The disruption of the sinus wall may be difficult or impossible to see on periapical or occlusal radiographs if it is not in the mesial, distal, or superior (apical) part of the alveolus. The outer shape of the radiopacity should be similar to the tooth structure. No evidence should exist of a periodontal ligament space or a lamina dura at the periphery of the structure.

Internal structure. In the early stages no internal structural changes are present, except that the dental fragment may appear as a radiopaque mass of a size corresponding to the missing dental fragment. The tooth structure may have a layer of enamel or a pulp canal.

Effects on surrounding structures. The dental fragment usually has no effect on surrounding structures; however, a sinusitis may result (see changes described under Sinusitis, p. 532). The floor of the maxillary sinus may break, caused by the displacement of the tooth or fragment into the sinus.

Differential diagnosis. Bony masses, which are exostosis of the sinus wall or floor, and septa within the sinus, may mimic dental root fragments or even whole teeth. Antroliths may also present a similar appearance. The presence of a pulp canal or a layer of enamel may help in the differential diagnosis. Also it may be possible to cause the tooth fragment to move by having the patient move the head abruptly between views. If the root tip remains in its socket, it may be superimposed radiographically over the maxillary sinus, but the presence of a lamina dura and periodontal ligament space indicate a position within the alveolar process.

The root may be subperiosteal, and thus within the osseous cavity of the sinus, but not within the antral lumen. Alternatively, the root may have been forced out of the socket, into the surrounding bone, or even through the bone to lie between the soft tissue of the oral mucosa and the bone of the alveolar process. Also, the fragment may be forced into surrounding structures such as the infratemporal space. Another possible result is that the fragment may have been displaced into a cyst that was preoperatively mistaken for a loculus of the sinus cavity. Use of radiographs at different angles should help to localize the dental structure.

Management. Management ranges from following the patient to see if a small root tip will be removed from the sinus via the ostium by ciliary action to surgically entering the sinus via a Caldwell-Luc procedure to remove the dental structure. Sinusitis may develop and should be managed with the appropriate treatment.

For other trauma involving the paranasal sinuses, see Chapter 27.

SUGGESTED READINGS

NORMAL DEVELOPMENT AND VARIATIONS

Dodd GD, Jing BS: *Radiology of the nose, paranasal sinus and nasopharynx,* Baltimore, 1977, Williams & Wilkins.

DuBrul EL: *Sicher's oral anatomy,* ed 7, St Louis, 1980, Mosby.

Grant JCB: *A method of anatomy,* Baltimore, 1958, Williams & Wilkins.

Hengerer AS: Embryonic development of the sinuses, *Ear Nose Throat J* 63:134, 1984.

Karmody CS, Carter B, Vincent ME: Developmental anomalies of the maxillary sinus, *Trans Am Acad Ophthalmol Otolaryngol* 84:723, 1977.

Lusted LB, Keats TE: *Atlas of roentgenographic measurement,* ed 3, Chicago, 1972, Year Book Medical Publishers.

Ritter FN: *The paranasal sinuses: anatomy and surgical technique,* St Louis, 1973, Mosby.

Shapiro R: *Radiology of the normal skull,* Chicago, 1981, Year Book Medical Publishers.

Som PM: The paranasal sinuses. In Bergeron RT, Osborn AG, Som PM, editors: *Head and neck imaging: excluding the brain,* St Louis, 1984, Mosby.

Takahashi R: The formation of the human paranasal sinuses, *Acta Otolaryngol Suppl (Stockh)* 408:1, 1984.

APPLIED DIAGNOSTIC IMAGING

Lloyd GA: Diagnostic imaging of the nose and paranasal sinuses, *J Laryngol Otol* 103:453, 1989.

Zinreich SJ: Imaging of chronic sinusitis in adults: x-ray, computed tomography, and magnetic resonance imaging, *J Allergy Clin Immunol* 90:445, 1992.

INFLAMMATORY CHANGES

Robinson K: Roentgenographic manifestations of benign paranasal sinus disease, *Ear Nose Throat J* 63:144, 1984.

THICKENED MUCOUS MEMBRANE
Mucositis

Dolan K, Smoker W: Paranasal sinus radiology: part 4A, maxillary sinuses, *Head Neck Surg* 5:345, 1983.

Killey HC, Kay LA: *The maxillary sinus and its dental implications,* Bristol, 1975, John Wright.

PERIOSTITIS
Sinusitis

Druce HM: Diagnosis and medical management of recurrent and chronic sinusitis in adults. In Gershwin ME, Incaudo GA, editors: *Diseases of the sinuses,* Ottawa, Canada, 1996, Humana Press.

Fireman P: Diagnosis of sinusitis in children: emphasis on the history and physical examination, *J Allergy Clin Immunol* 90:433, 1992.

Incaudo G, Gershwin ME, Nagy SM: The pathophysiology and treatment of sinusitis, *Allergol Immunopathol (Madr)* 14:423, 1986.

Kennedy DW: Surgical update, *Otolaryngol Head Neck Surg* 103:884, 1990.

Killey HC, Kay LA: *The maxillary sinus and its dental implications,* Bristol, 1975, John Wright.

Palaceos E, Valvassori G: Computed axial tomography in otorhinolaryngology, *Adv Otorhinolaryngol* 24:1, 1978.

Paparella MM: Mucosal cyst of the maxillary sinus, *Arch Otolaryngol* 77:650, 1963.

Poyton H: Maxillary sinuses and the oral radiologist, *Dent Radiol Photogr* 45:43, 1972.

Reilly JS: The sinusitis cycle, *Otolaryngol Head Neck Surg* 103:856, 1990.

Shapiro GG, Rachelefsky GS: Introduction and definition of sinusitis, *J Allergy Clin Immunol* 90:417, 1992.

Zinreich SJ: Imaging of chronic sinusitis in adults: x-ray, computed tomography, and magnetic resonance imaging, *J Allergy Clin Immunol* 90:445, 1992.

EMPYEMA

Ash JE, Raum M: *An atlas of otolaryngic pathology,* New York, 1956, American Registry of Pathology.

Groves J, Gray RF: *A synopsis of otolaryngology,* Bristol, 1985, John Wright.

POLYPS

Potter GD: Inflammatory disease of the paranasal sinuses. In Valvassori GE, Potter GD, Hanefee WN, editors: *Radiology of the ear, nose and throat,* Philadelphia, 1982, WB Saunders.

RETENTION PSEUDOCYSTS

Allard RHB, Van der Kwast WAM, Van der Wall JI: Mucosal antral cysts: review of the literature and report of a radiographic survey, *Oral Surg* 51:2, 1981.

Dolan K, Smoker W: Paranasal sinus radiology: part 4A, maxillary sinuses, *Head Neck Surg* 5:345, 1983.

Gothberg K et al: A clinical study of cysts arising from mucosa of the maxillary sinus, *Oral Surg* 41:52, 1976.

Hardy G: Benign cysts of the antrum, *Ann Otol Rhinol Laryngol* 48: 649, 1939.

Kadymova MI: Lymphangietctatic (false) cysts of the maxillary sinuses and their relation with allergy, *Vestn Otorinolaringol* 28:58, 1966.

Kaffe I, Littner MM, Moskona D: Mucosal-antral cysts: radiographic appearance and differential diagnosis, *Clin Prev Dent* 10:3, 1988.

McGregor GW: Formation and histologic structure of cysts of the maxillary sinus, *Arch Otolaryngol* 8:505, 1928.

Mills CP: Secretory cysts of the maxillary antrum and their relationship to the development of antrochoanal polypi, *J Laryngol Otol* 73:324, 1959.

Poyton HG: *Oral radiology,* Baltimore, 1982, Williams & Wilkins.

Ruprecht A, Batniji S, El-Neweihi E: Mucous retention cyst of the maxillary sinus, *Oral Surg Oral Med Oral Pathol* 62:728, 1986.

Shafer WG, Hine MK, Levy BM: *A textbook of oral pathology,* ed 4, Philadelphia, 1983, WB Saunders.

Van Norstrand AWP, Goodman WS: Pathologic aspects of mucosal lesions of the maxillary sinus, *Otolaryngol Clin North Am* 9:21, 1976.

MUCOCELE

Atherino C, Atherino T: Maxillary sinus mucopyoceles, *Arch Otolaryngol* 110:200, 1984.

Jones JL, Kaufman PW: Mucopyocele of the maxillary sinus, *J Oral Surg* 39:948, 1981.

Zizmor JK, Noyek AM: The radiologic diagnosis of maxillary sinus disease, *Otolaryngol Clin North Am* 9:93, 1976.

ODONTOGENIC CYSTS

Killey HC, Kay LA: *The maxillary sinus and its dental implications,* Bristol, 1975, John Wright.

Poyton H: Maxillary sinuses and the oral radiologist, *Dent Radiol Photogr* 45:43, 1972.

Van Alyea OE: *Nasal sinuses,* Baltimore, 1951, Williams & Wilkins.

Odontogenic keratocysts

MacDonald-Jankowski DS: The involvement of the maxillary antrum by odontogenic keratocysts, *Clin Radiol* 45:31, 1992.

NEOPLASMS

Goepfert H et al: Malignant salivary gland tumors of the paranasal sinuses and nasal cavity, *Arch Otolaryngol* 109:662, 1983.

St-Pierre S, Baker S: Squamous cell carcinoma of the maxillary sinus: analysis of 66 cases, *Head Neck Surg* 5:508, 1983.

Epithelial papilloma

Rogers JH, Fredrickson JM, Noyek AM: Management of cysts, benign tumors, and bony dysplasia of the maxillary sinus, *Otolaryngol Clin North Am* 9:233, 1976.

Osteoma

Dolan K, Smoker W: Paranasal sinus radiology: part 4B, maxillary sinuses, *Head Neck Surg* 5:428, 1983.

Goodnight J, Dulguerov P, Abemayor E: Calcified mucor fungus ball of the maxillary sinus, *Am J Otolaryngol* 14:209, 1993.

Reuben B: Odontoma of the maxillary sinus: a case report, *Quint Int* 14:287, 1983.

Samy LL, Mostofa H: Osteoma of the nose and paranasal sinuses with a report of twenty-one cases, *J Laryngol Otol* 85:449, 1971.

Ameloblastoma

Hames RS, Rakoff SJ: Diseases of the maxillary sinus, *J Oral Med* 27:90, 1972.

Reanue C et al: Ameloblastoma of the maxillary sinus, *J Oral Surg* 38:520, 1980.

Malignant neoplasms of the paranasal sinuses

Batsakis JG: *Tumors of the head and neck,* ed 2, Baltimore, 1979, Williams & Wilkins.

St-Pierre S, Baker S: Squamous cell carcinoma of the maxillary sinus: analysis of 66 cases, *Head Neck Surg* 5:508, 1983.

Zizmor J, Noyek AM: Cysts, benign tumors and malignant tumors of the paranasal sinuses, *Otolaryngol Clin North Am* 6:487, 1973.

Squamous cell carcinoma

Batsakis JG, Rice DH, Solomon AR: The pathology of head and neck tumors: squamous and mucous-gland carcinomas of the nasal cavity, paranasal sinuses and larynx: part 6, *Head Neck Surg* 2:497, 1980.

Boone MLM, Harle TS: Malignant tumors of the paranasal sinuses, *Semin Roentgenol* 3:202, 1968.

Bridger M, Beale F, Bryce D: Carcinoma of the paranasal sinuses: a review of 158 cases, *J Otolaryngol* 7:379, 1978.

Eddleston B, Johnson R: A comparison of conventional radiographic imaging and computed tomography in malignant disease of the paranasal sinuses and the post-nasal space, *Clin Radiol* 56:161, 1983.

Haso A: CT of tumors and tumor-like conditions of the paranasal sinuses, *Radiol Clin North Am* 22:119, 1984.

Larheim T, Kolbenstvdt A, Lien H: Carcinoma of maxillary sinus, palate and maxillary gingiva, occurrence of jaw destruction, *Scand J Dent Res* 92:235, 1984.

Lund V, Howard D, Lloyd G: CT evaluation of paranasal sinus tumors for cranio-facial resection, *Br J Radiol* 56:439, 1983.

Mancuso A et al: Extensions of paranasal sinus tumors and inflammatory disease: an evaluation by CT and pluridirectional tomography, *Neuroradiology* 16:449, 1978.

St-Pierre S, Baker S: Squamous cell carcinoma of the maxillary sinus: analysis of 66 cases, *Head Neck Surg* 5:508, 1983.

Thomas GK, Kasper KA: Ossifying fibroma of the frontal bone, *Arch Otolaryngol* 83:43, 1966.

Tsaknis PJ, Nelson JF: The maxillary ameloblastoma: an analysis of 24 cases, *J Oral Surg* 38:336, 1980.

Webeer A et al: Malignant tumors of the sinuses: radiologic evaluation, including CT scanning, with clinical and pathologic correlation, *Neuroradiology* 16:443, 1978.

Pseudotumor

Butugan O et al: Rhinocerebral mucormycosis: predisposing factors, diagnosis, therapy, complications and survival, *Rev Laryngol Otol Rhinol (Bord)* 117:53, 1996.

Del Valle Zapico A et al: Mucormycosis of the sphenoid sinus in an otherwise healthy patient. Case report and literature review, *J Laryngol Otol* 110:471, 1996.

Ishida M et al: Five cases of mucormycosis in paranasal sinuses, *Acta Oto-Laryngologica* 501(suppl):92, 1993.

Lee BL, Holland GN, Glasgow BJ: Chiasmal infarction and sudden blindness caused by mucormycosis in AIDS and diabetes mellitus, *Am J Ophthalmol* 122:895, 1996.

Muzaffar M, Hussain SI, Chughtai A: Plasma cell granuloma: maxillary sinuses, *J Laryngol Otol* 108:357, 1994.

Ng TT et al: Successful treatment of sinusitis caused by *Cunninghamella bertholetiae, Clin Infect Dis* 19:313, 1994.

Ozhan S et al: Pseudotumor of the maxillary sinus in a patient with von Willebrand's disease, *AJR Am J Roentgenol* 166:950, 1996.

Perolada Valmana JM et al: Mucormycosis of the paranasal sinuses, *Rev Laryngol Otol Rhinol (Bord)* 117:51, 1996.

Som PM et al: Inflammatory pseudotumor of the maxillary sinus: CT and MR findings in six cases, *AJR Am J Roentgenol* 163:689, 1994.

Tkatch LS, Kusne S, Eibling D: Successful treatment of zygomycosis of the paranasal sinuses with surgical debridement and amphotericin B colloidal dispersion, *Am J Otolaryngol* 14:249, 1993.

Utas C et al: Acute renal failure associated with rhinosinuso-orbital mucormycosis infection in a patient with diabetic nephropathy [letter], *Nephron* 71:235, 1995.

Zapater E et al: Invasive fungal sinusitis in immunosuppressed patients. Report of three cases, *Acta Oto-Rhino-Laryngologica Belgica* 50:137, 1996.

FIBROUS DYSPLASIA

Malcolmson KG: Ossifying fibroma of the sphenoid, *J Laryngol* 81:87, 1967.

Thomas GK, Kasper KA: Ossifying fibroma of the frontal bone, *Arch Otolaryngol* 83:43, 1966.

Wong A, Vaughan CW, Strong MS: Fibrous dysplasia of temporal bone, *Arch Otolaryngol* 81:131, 1965.

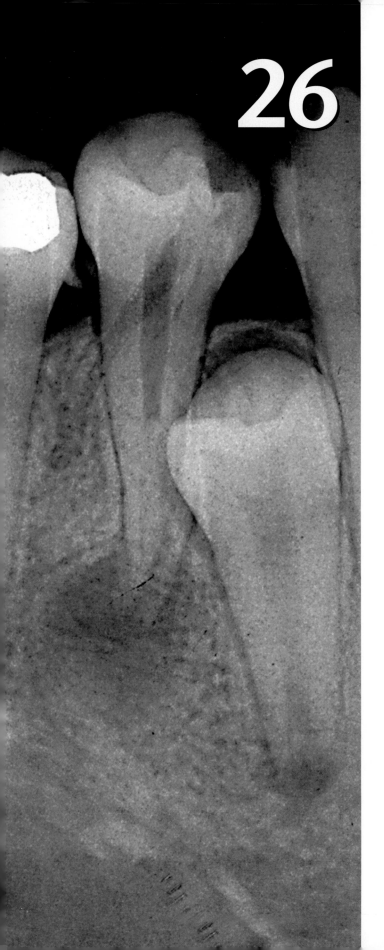

26 Soft Tissue Calcification and Ossification

The deposition of calcium salts, primarily calcium phosphate, usually occurs in the skeleton. When it occurs in an unorganized fashion in soft tissue, it is referred to as *heterotopic calcification*. This soft tissue mineralization may develop in a wide variety of unrelated disorders and degenerative processes. Soft tissue calcifications may be divided into three categories:

- Dystrophic calcification
- Idiopathic calcification
- Metastatic calcification

Pathologic calcification that forms in degenerating and dead tissue despite normal serum calcium and phosphate levels is classified as *dystrophic calcification*. The soft tissue may be damaged by blunt trauma, inflammation, injections, parasitic calcification, soft tissue changes arising from disease, and many other causes. The calcification usually is localized to the site of injury. The deposition of calcium in normal tissue despite normal serum calcium and phosphate levels is referred to as *idiopathic calcinosis* or *calcification*. Examples include chondrocalcinosis and phleboliths. When the minerals precipitate into normal tissue as a result of higher than normal serum levels of calcium (e.g., hyperparathyroidism) or phosphate (e.g., chronic renal failure), the process is called *metastatic calcification*. This calcification usually occurs bilaterally and symmetrically.

When the mineral is deposited in soft tissue as organized, well-formed bone, the process is known as *heterotopic ossification*. The term *heterotopic* indicates normal bone formed in an abnormal location. The bone may be circumscribed compact bone, or it may show some trabeculae and fatty marrow. The deposits may range from 1 mm to several centimeters in diameter, and one or more may be present. The causes range from post-traumatic ossification, bone produced by tumors, and ossification caused by diseases such as progressive myositis ossificans and ankylosing spondylitis.

Clinical Features

Sites of heterotopic calcification or ossification may not cause significant signs or symptoms; they most often are detected as incidental findings during radiographic examination.

Radiographic Features

Soft tissue opacities are fairly common, present on about 4% of panoramic radiographs. In most cases the goal is to identify the calcification correctly to determine whether treatment or further investigation is required. When the soft tissue calcification is adjacent to bone, it sometimes is difficult to determine whether the calcification is within bone or soft tissue. Another radiographic view at right angles is useful. The important criteria to consider in arriving at the correct interpretation are the anatomic location, number, distribution, and shape of the calcifications. Analysis of the location requires a knowledge of soft tissue anatomy, such as the position of lymph nodes, stylohyoid ligaments, blood vessels, and the major ducts of the salivary glands.

Dystrophic Calcification

GENERAL DYSTROPHIC CALCIFICATION OF THE ORAL REGIONS

Definition

When calcium salts precipitate into primary sites of chronic inflammation or dead and dying tissue, the process is called *dystrophic calcification*. It usually is associated with a high local concentration of phosphatase, as in normal bone calcification, and with anoxic conditions within the devitalized tissue. A long-standing, chronically inflamed cyst is a common location of dystrophic calcification.

Clinical Features

Common soft tissue sites include the gingiva, tongue, and cheek. The condition may produce no signs or symptoms, although occasionally enlargement and ulceration of overlying soft tissues may occur, and a solid mass of calcium salts sometimes can be palpated.

Radiographic Features

Such dystrophic calcification varies from barely perceptible, fine grains of radiopacities to larger, irregular radiopaque particles that rarely exceed 0.5 cm in diameter. One or more of these radiopacities may be seen, and the calcification may be homogeneous or may contain punctate areas. The outline of the calcified area usually is irregular or indistinct. Common sites are long-standing, chronically inflamed cysts (Fig. 26-1) and polyps (Fig. 26-2).

CALCIFIED LYMPH NODES

Definition

Calcified lymph nodes are a type of dystrophic calcification that occurs in lymph nodes that have been chronically inflamed because of various diseases. In the past, tuberculosis was the most common disease causing calcified lymph nodes.

Clinical Features

A calcified lymph node usually is asymptomatic, and these nodes are first discovered as an incidental finding on a panoramic radiograph. The most commonly involved nodes are the submandibular and cervical nodes and, rarely, the nodes in the parotid region. When these nodes can be palpated, they are hard round or oblong masses.

Radiographic Features

Location. The most common location is the submandibular region, often near or below the angle of the mandible, or a more inferior location when the cervical lymph nodes are involved. The image of the calcified node sometimes overlaps the inferior aspect of the ramus. In rare cases the calcified node is found posterior to the ramus. The lesion may be single or multiple, lying in a roughly linear orientation (Fig. 26-3).

Periphery. The periphery is well defined and usually irregular, occasionally having a lobulated appearance similar to the outer shape of cauliflower.

Internal structure. The internal aspect is without pattern but may vary in the degree of radiopacity, giving the impression of a collection of spherical or irregular masses. Occasionally the lesion has a laminated appearance.

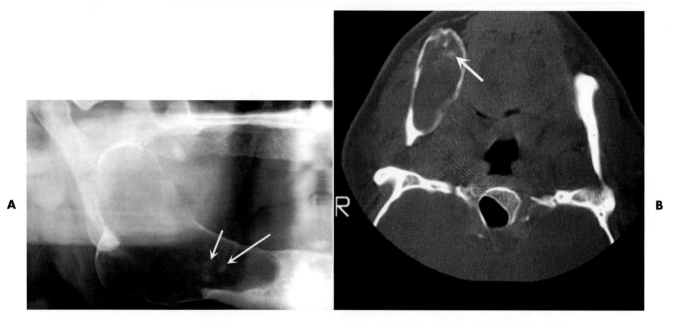

FIG. **26**-1   **A,** A large residual cyst with ill-defined calcifications seen in a panoramic image *(arrows).* **B,** A coronal computed tomography image of the same case that demonstrates the dystrophic calcification within the cyst *(arrow).*

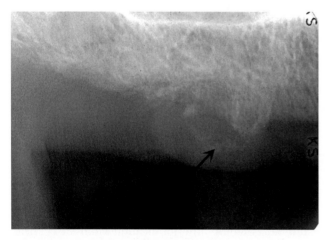

FIG. **26**-2   A periapical film showing the soft tissue mass shadow of a polyp emanating from the edentulous ridge. The soft tissue mass contains a dystrophic calcification *(arrow).*

Differential Diagnosis

Differentiation between a single calcified lymph node and a sialolith in the hilar region of the submandibular gland may be difficult. Usually a sialolith has a smooth outline, whereas a calcified lymph node is usually irregular and sometimes lobulated. The differentiation can be made if the patient has symptoms related to the submandibular salivary gland (see Chapter 29). Occasionally sialography

may be necessary to make the differentiation. Another calcification that may have a similar appearance in this region is a phlebolith; however, a phlebolith is usually smaller, it often has concentric radiopaque and radiolucent rings, and its shape may mimic a portion of a blood vessel.

Management
Calcified lymph nodes do not require treatment.

DYSTROPHIC CALCIFICATION IN THE TONSILS

Synonyms
Tonsillar calculi, tonsil concretions, and *tonsilloliths*

Definition
The mechanism for deposition of dystrophic calcification in the tonsils is similar to that for lymph nodes and is the result of chronic inflammation.

Clinical Features
Small calcifications usually produce no clinical signs or symptoms. However, pain, swelling, and dysphagia have been reported with larger calcifications. These calcifications have been reported to occur between 20 and 68 years of age; they are found more often in older age groups.

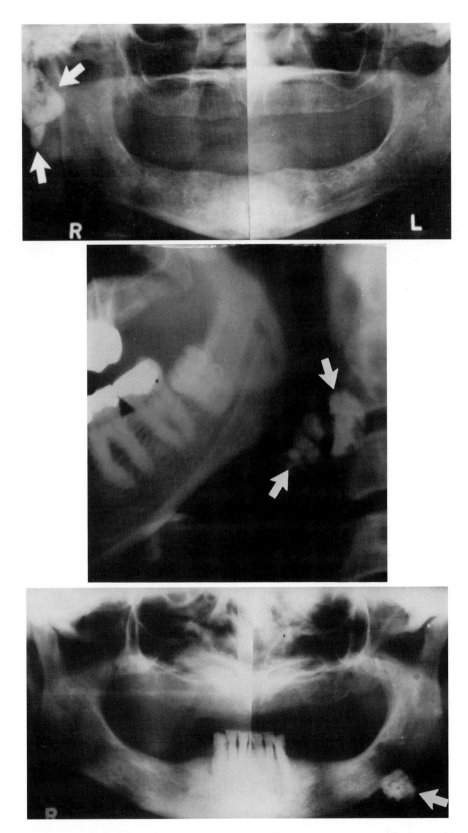

FIG. **26-3** Calcified lymph nodes appear as radiopaque masses, usually located just posterior to the ramus or inferior to the angle of the mandible and occasionally posterior to the ramus.

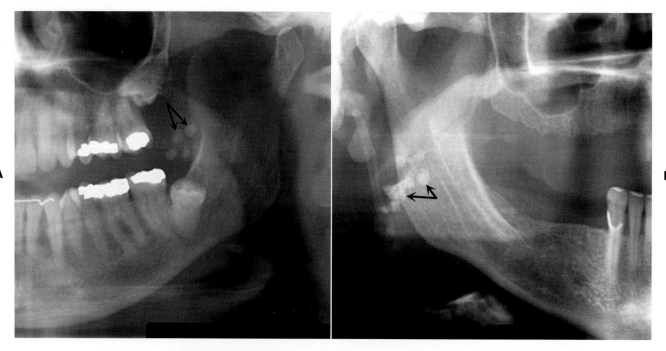

FIG. **26-4** *Dystrophic calcification of the tonsils.* These two examples show positions anterior to the ramus **(A)** and overlapping the posterior aspect of the ramus **(B)** *(arrows).* Note the calcified stylohyoid ligament.

Radiographic Features

Location. In the panoramic film, the image of single or multiple radiopacities overlaps the middle portion of the mandibular ramus in the region where the image of the dorsal surface of the tongue crosses the ramus (Fig. 26-4).

Periphery. The most common appearance is of multiple small, ill-defined radiopacities. However, these calcifications occasionally reach a large size; a range of 0.5 cm^3 to 14.5 cm^3 has been reported.

Internal structure. These calcifications appear slightly more radiopaque than cancellous bone and approximately the same as cortical bone.

Differential Diagnosis

The essential differential diagnosis is a radiopaque lesion within the mandibular ramus, such as a dense bone island. When in doubt, a right-angle view such as a posteroanterior skull view or an open Towne's view may show that the calcification lies to the medial aspect of the ramus.

Treatment

No treatment is required for most tonsillar calcifications. However, large calcifications with associated symptoms are removed surgically.

CYSTICERCOSIS

Definition

When human beings ingest eggs or gravid proglottids from *Taenia solium* (pork tapeworm), the covering of the eggs is digested in the stomach and the larval form *(Cysticercus cellulosae)* of the parasite is hatched. The larvae penetrate the mucosa, enter the blood vessels and lymphatics, and are distributed in the tissues all over the body, including the oral and perioral tissues, especially the muscles of mastication. In body tissues other than the intestinal mucosa, the larvae die and are treated as foreign bodies. After the larvae die, the larval spaces are replaced with fibrous connective tissue that may become calcified after about 3 months. These areas in the tissues are called *cysticerci.*

Clinical Features

Mild cases of cysticercosis are completely asymptomatic. More severe cases have symptoms that range from mild to severe gastrointestinal upset with epigastric pain and severe nausea and vomiting. Invasion of the brain may result in convulsions, irritability, and loss of consciousness. Examination of the head and neck may disclose palpable, firm masses as large as 1 cm in diameter. Multiple small nodules may be felt in the region of the masseter and suprahyoid muscles and in the buccal mucosa and lip.

Radiographic Features

Location. The locations of calcified cysticerci include the muscles of mastication and facial expression, the suprahyoid muscle, and the postcervical musculature.

Periphery and shape. The periphery is well defined, and the shape is elongated, elliptic, or ovoid.

Internal structure. The internal aspect is homogeneous and radiopaque.

Differential Diagnosis

Similarities may exist between a cysticercus and a sialolith in size, form, and density. However, calcified nodules of cysticerci are very likely to be multiple.

Management

Although prevention is the best treatment (proper preparation of pork and avoiding fecal contamination), the symptoms that accompany the initial infestation are best treated by a physician. After the larvae have settled and calcified in the oral tissues, however, they are harmless.

CALCIFIED BLOOD VESSEL

Definition

Arterial walls may calcify in all forms of arteriosclerosis with the deposition of calcium salts within the medial coat of the vessel. Such changes also may represent sequelae of inflammatory processes affecting the vessel walls. Such calcifications occasionally form in the facial, carotid, iliac, femoral, and popliteal arteries.

Clinical Features

Usually no clinical signs or symptoms are present. Although images of calcified arteries of the cheek and oral cavity may appear on oral radiographs of individuals with arteriosclerosis obliterans, their presence does not necessarily indicate occlusive arterial disease. Patients with Sturge-Weber syndrome also develop arterial wall calcification.

Radiographic Features

Location. Calcifications within the carotid artery are located in the soft tissue below the angle of the mandible (Fig. 26-5) and between the hyoid bone and the image of the cervical spine as seen in panoramic images.

Periphery and shape. The calcific deposits in the wall of the artery outline the image of the artery. From the side, the calcified vessel appears as a pair of thin, opaque lines that may have either a straight course or a tortuous path. The calcification also may be less organized and may appear as amorphous or punctate calcifications.

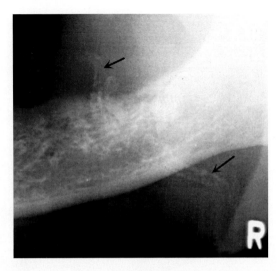

FIG. **26-5** A section of a panoramic image showing calcification of a blood vessel, probably the facial vein *(arrows).*

Internal structure. In a vessel cross-section, the calcified wall appears as a radiopaque circle. Other examples are homogeneously radiopaque.

Differential Diagnosis

Other calcific deposits, phleboliths, miliary osteomas, and sialoliths may be projected over the cheek. Usually the linear nature of the calcified arterial wall indicates the nature of this condition. Calcifications in the carotid artery in the neck must be differentiated from calcified lymph nodes.

Management

Although the calcified vessel in the cheek does not require definitive treatment, the examiner should be alert to the possibility of other lesions in remote locations. Identification of carotid calcifications may indicate the presence of atherosclerotic disease.

Idiopathic Calcification

SIALOLITH

Synonym

Sialolithiasis

Definition

Sialoliths are stones found within the ducts of salivary glands (also see Chapter 29). The flow rate of the saliva and the physiochemical characteristics of the gland secretion may contribute to the formation of a nidus and subsequent precipitation of calcium and phosphate salts. Sialoliths of the minor salivary glands also have been reported.

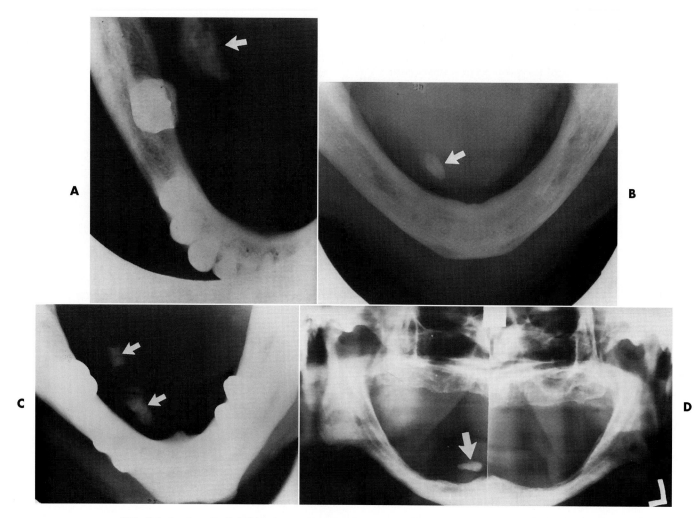

FIG. **26-6** **A** to **C,** Sialoliths *(arrows)* in the duct of a submandibular gland as visualized on standard occlusal projections. Exposure times have been reduced to better demonstrate these calcifications, which are less calcified than the mandible. **D,** Sialoliths also may be visualized on panoramic radiographs, especially in edentulous areas.

Clinical Features

Sialoliths are most common in the submandibular glands of men in their middle and later years. They usually occur singly (70% to 80%) but may occur multiply. Patients with salivary stones may not have any pain, but they usually have a history of pain and swelling in the floor of the mouth and in the involved gland. This discomfort may intensify at mealtimes, when salivary flow is stimulated. Because the stone usually does not block the flow of saliva completely, the pain and swelling gradually subside. Perhaps as many as 9% of patients have recurrent sialolithiasis, and about 10% of patients with sialolithiasis also suffer nephrolithiasis.

Radiographic Features

Location. The submandibular gland is involved more often (83% to 94%) than the parotid gland (4% to 10%) or sublingual gland (1% to 7%), probably because the submandibular gland has a longer duct and more viscous saliva with a higher mineral content. About half of submandibular stones lie in the anterior portion of Wharton's duct, 20% in the posterior portion, and 30% in the gland.

Periphery and shape. Sialoliths located in the duct of the submandibular gland usually are cylindric. Stones that form in the hilus of a submandibular gland tend to be larger and more irregularly shaped (Fig. 26-6).

Internal structure. Some stones are homogeneously radiopaque, and others show evidence of multiple layers of calcification. About 20% or fewer of sialoliths in the submandibular gland and 40% of those in the parotid gland are radiolucent because of the low mineral content of the parotid secretions.

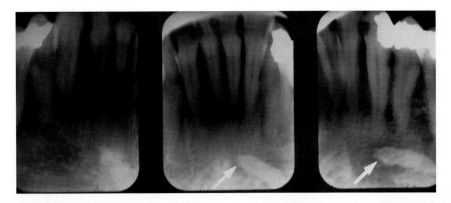

FIG. **26-7** Periapical radiographs showing a sialolith *(arrows)* superimposed on trabecular bone. (Courtesy Dr. L. Hollender, Seattle, Wash.)

Applied Radiology

Salivary stones occasionally are seen on periapical views superimposed over the mandibular premolar and molar apices (Fig. 26-7). The best view for visualizing stones in the anterior portion of Wharton's duct is a standard mandibular occlusal view, which displays the floor of the mouth without overlap from the mandible. Stones in a more posterior location are best visualized on lateral oblique views of the mandible or on a panoramic film. To demonstrate stones in the parotid gland duct, the clinician places a periapical film in the buccal vestibule, and the x-ray beam is oriented through the cheek. Also, stones in the parotid duct can be seen if the patient "blows out" the cheek as an anteroposterior skull view is exposed. An open-mouth lateral skull projection can be used. When producing radiographs to detect sialoliths, the exposure time should be reduced to about half of normal. This helps in detecting stones that are lightly calcified. If a noncalcified stone is suspected, sialography is used (see Chapter 29).

Differential Diagnosis

Sialoliths can be distinguished from other soft tissue calcifications because they usually are associated with pain or swelling of the involved salivary gland. Other calcifications (e.g., lymph nodes) are asymptomatic. If the diagnosis is unclear, the clinician can prescribe a sialogram.

Management

Surgical removal of the stone or gland may be required.

PHLEBOLITHS

Definition

Phleboliths are thought to form in older thrombi in veins or hemangiomas (especially the cavernous type)

with slow blood flow. The thrombus organizes into granulation tissue and occasionally mineralizes, with the deposition of calcium phosphate and calcium carbonate.

Clinical Features

The involved soft tissue may be swollen or discolored by the presence of veins or a soft tissue hemangioma. Applying pressure to the involved tissue should cause a blanching or change in color if the lesion is vascular in nature.

Radiographic Features

Location. Phleboliths most commonly are found in hemangiomas (see Chapter 20).

Periphery and shape. In cross-section the shape is round or oval with a smooth periphery. If the involved blood vessel is viewed from the side, the phlebolith may resemble a straight or slightly curved sausage.

Internal structure. The internal aspect may be homogeneously radiopaque but more commonly has the appearance of laminations. A radiolucent center may be seen, which may represent the remaining patent portion of the vessel (Fig. 26-8).

Differential Diagnosis

A phlebolith may have a shape similar to that of a sialolith. Sialoliths usually occur singly; if more than one is present, they usually are oriented in a single line, whereas phleboliths are commonly multiple and have a more random distribution. The importance of correctly identifying phleboliths lies in the identification of a possible vascular lesion such as a hemangioma. This is important if surgical procedures are contemplated.

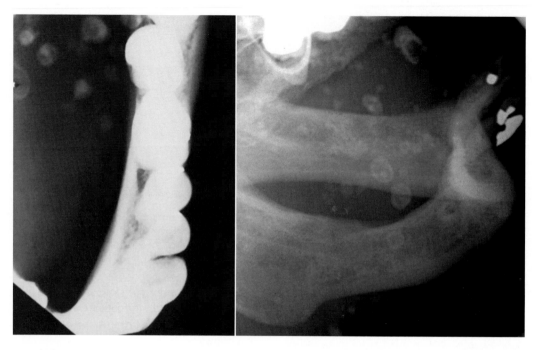

FIG. **26-8** Phleboliths are soft tissue dystrophic calcifications found in veins. They are usually associated with hemangiomas.

Metastatic Calcification

Calcification of the soft tissues in the oral region caused by conditions involving elevated serum calcium and phosphate, such as hyperparathyroidism (see Chapter 23), are extremely rare.

Heterotopic Bone

OSSIFICATION OF THE STYLOHYOID LIGAMENT

Similar and Related Conditions
Conditions similar to ossification of the stylohyoid ligament include Eagle's syndrome, stylohyoid syndrome, and stylohyoid chain ossification.

Definition
Ossification of the stylohyoid ligament usually extends downward from the base of the skull and commonly occurs bilaterally. However, in rare cases the ossification begins at the lesser horn of the hyoid, and in fewer still in a central area of the ligament.

Clinical Features
Even when extensive ossification of one or both stylohyoid ligaments is seen, more than 50% of patients are clinically asymptomatic. The ossified ligament usually can be detected by palpation over the tonsil as a hard, pointed structure. Very little correlation exists between the extent of ossification and the intensity of the accompanying symptoms. One symptom is vague pain on swallowing, turning the head, or opening the mouth. When this entity is associated with discomfort and the patient has a recent history of neck trauma (e.g., tonsillectomy), the condition is called *Eagle's syndrome*. The patient may describe earache, headache, dizziness, or transient syncope. The elongated styloid process probably causes these symptoms by impinging on the glossopharyngeal nerve. Similar clinical findings without a history of neck trauma constitute *stylohyoid syndrome*. These individuals usually are over 40 years of age. This condition is more prevalent than Eagle's syndrome.

Radiographic Features
Ossification of the stylohyoid ligament is detected fairly commonly as an incidental feature on panoramic radiographs. In one study, approximately 18% of a population examined showed ossification of more than 30 mm of the stylohyoid ligament. The ligament shows at least some calcification in individuals of any age.

Location. In a panoramic image the linear ossification extends from the mastoid process and crosses the posteroinferior aspect of the ramus toward the hyoid bone. The hyoid bone is positioned roughly parallel to or su-

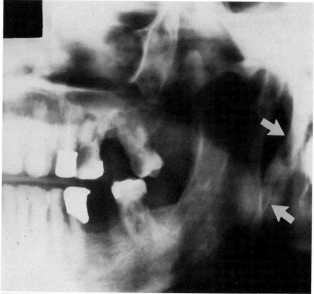

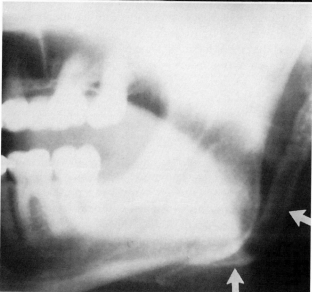

FIG. **26-9** Ossification of the stylohyoid ligament *(arrows)* may be quite prominent, even in individuals with no symptoms.

perimposed on the posterior aspect of the inferior cortex of the mandible.

Shape. The styloid process appears as a long, tapering, thin, radiopaque process that is thicker at its base and projects downward and forward (Fig. 26-9). It normally varies from about 0.5 to 2.5 cm in length. The ossified ligament has roughly a straight outline, but in some cases some irregularity may be seen in the outer surface. The farther the radiopaque ossified ligament extends toward the hyoid bone, the more likely it is that it will be interrupted by radiolucent, jointlike junctions.

Internal structure. Small ossifications of the stylohyoid ligament appear homogeneously radiopaque. As the ossification increases in length and girth, the outer cortex of this bone becomes evident as a radiopaque band at the periphery.

Differential Diagnosis

The symptoms that accompany stylohyoid ligament ossification and Eagle's syndrome generally are vague; however, when they occur with the distinctive radiographic evidence of ligament ossification, little chance exists that the complaint will be confused with another entity. Occasionally, though, the symptoms may be similar to those seen in temporomandibular joint dysfunction.

Management

Most patients with ossification of the stylohyoid ligament are asymptomatic, and no treatment is required. However, the recommended treatment for symptomatic patients with Eagle's syndrome is amputation of the stylohyoid process. For the more common stylohyoid syndrome, however, a more conservative approach of reassurance and steroid injections is recommended first.

OSTEOMA CUTIS

Definition

Osteoma cutis is a rare soft tissue ossification in the skin. The lesions often occur secondary to acne of long duration, developing in a scar or chronic inflammatory dermatosis. Histologically these lesions are areas of dense viable bone in the dermis or subcutaneous tissue. They occasionally are found in diffuse scleroderma, replacing the altered collagen in the dermis and subcutaneous septa.

Clinical Features

Osteoma cutis can occur anywhere, but the face is the most common site. The tongue is the most common intraoral site (osteoma mucosae). Osteoma cutis does not cause any visible change in the overlying skin other than an occasional color change that may appear yellowish white. If the lesion is large, the individual osteoma may be palpated. A needle inserted into one of the papules is met with stonelike resistance.

Radiographic Features

Location. Radiographically, osteoma cutis most commonly appears in the cheek and lip regions (Fig. 26-10). In this location the image can be superimposed over a tooth root or alveolar process, giving the appearance of an area of dense bone. Accurate localization can be achieved by placing an intraoral film between the cheek and alveolar process to image the cheek alone. As an al-

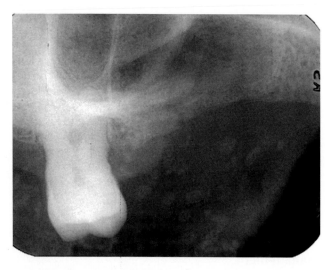

FIG. **26-10** Osteoma cutis is seen here as faint radiopaque calcifications in the cheek.

ternative, a posteroanterior skull view with the cheek blown outward helps localize osteomas in the skin.

Periphery and shape. Osteoma cutis appears as smoothly outlined, radiopaque, washer-shaped images. These single or multiple radiopacities usually are very small, although the size can range from 0.1 to 5 cm.

Internal structure. The internal aspect may be homogeneously radiopaque or may have a radiolucent center that represents normal fatty marrow. Trabeculae occasionally develop in the marrow cavity of larger osteomas.

Differential Diagnosis
The differential diagnosis should include myositis ossificans, calcinosis cutis, and osteoma mucosae. If the blown-out cheek technique is used, the lesions of osteoma cutis appear much more superficial than mucosal lesions. Myositis ossificans is of greater proportions, in some cases causing noticeable deformity of the facial contour.

Management
No treatment is required, but these osteomas occasionally are removed for cosmetic reasons. Although an osteoma cutis usually is quite small, it cannot be removed with a needle and must be excised.

MYOSITIS OSSIFICANS

Definition
Myositis ossificans is a condition in which fibrous tissue and heterotopic bone form within the interstitial tissue of muscle, as well as in associated tendons and liga-

ments. Secondary destruction and atrophy of the muscle occur as this fibrous tissue and bone interdigitate and separate the muscle fibers. Myositis ossificans is divided into two principal forms: localized myositis ossificans and progressive myositis ossificans.

Localized (Traumatic) Myositis Ossificans
Synonyms. *Posttraumatic myositis ossificans* and *solitary myositis*

Definition. Localized myositis ossificans results from acute or chronic trauma or from the heavy muscular strain caused by certain occupations and sports. Muscle injury from multiple injections (occasionally from dental anesthetic) also may be a cause. The injury leads to considerable hemorrhage into the muscle or associated tendons or fascia. This hemorrhage organizes and undergoes progressive scarring. During the healing process, heterotopic bone is formed, and in some cases cartilage is formed as well. The term *myositis* is misleading because no inflammation is involved. The fibrous tissue and bone form within the interstitial tissue of the muscle; no actual ossification of the muscle fibers occurs.

Clinical Features
Localized myositis ossificans can develop at any age in either gender, but it occurs most often in young men who engage in vigorous activity. The site of the precipitating trauma remains swollen, tender, and painful much longer than expected. The overlying skin may be red and inflamed, and when the lesion involves a muscle of mastication, opening the jaws may be difficult. After about 2 or 3 weeks, the area of ossification becomes apparent in the tissues; a firm, intramuscular mass can be palpated. The localized lesion may enlarge slowly, but eventually it stops growing. The lesion may appear fixed, or it may be freely movable on palpation.

Radiographic Features
Location. The most commonly involved muscles of the head and neck are the masseter and sternocleidomastoid. However, other muscles of mastication may be involved, such as the lateral pterygoid muscle. Usually a radiolucent band can be seen between the area of ossification and adjacent bone, and the heterotopic bone may lie along the long axis of the muscle (Fig. 26-11).

Periphery and shape. The periphery commonly is more radiopaque than the internal structure. There is a variation in shape from irregular, oval to linear streaks (pseudotrabeculae) running in the same direction as the normal muscle fibers. These pseudotrabeculae are characteristic of myositis ossificans and strongly imply a diagnosis.

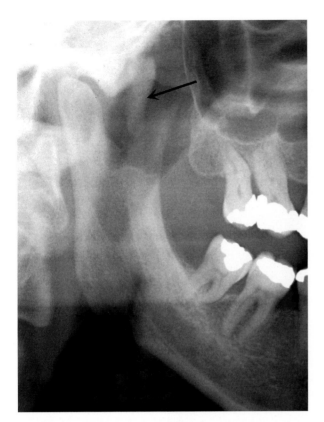

FIG. 26-11 Soft tissue ossification extending from the coronoid process in a superior direction, following the anatomy of the temporalis muscle *(arrow)*. This condition arose after several attempts were made to provide a submandibular nerve block, leaving the patient unable to open the mandible.

Internal structure. The internal structure varies with time. Within the third or fourth week after injury, the radiographic appearance is a faintly homogeneous radiopacity. This organizes further, and within approximately 2 months a delicate lacy or feathery radiopaque internal structure develops, accompanied sometimes by a circumscribed cortical periphery. These changes indicate the formation of bone; however, this bone does not have a normal-appearing trabecular pattern. Gradually the image becomes denser and better defined, maturing fully in about 5 to 6 months. After this period the lesion may shrink.

Differential diagnosis. The differential diagnosis of localized myositis ossificans includes ossification of the stylohyoid ligament and other soft tissue calcifications. However, both the form and location of myositis ossificans often are enough to make the differential diagnosis. Other lesions to consider are bone-forming tumors. Although tumors such as osteogenic sarcoma can form a linear bone pattern (see Chapter 21), the tumor is con-

tiguous with the adjacent bone, and signs of bone destruction often are present.

Management. Rest and limitation of use are recommended to diminish the extent of the calcific deposit. Early surgical removal of the lesion usually stimulates rapid (within 1 month) and extensive recurrence (from origin to insertion of the affected muscle). Recurrence is not likely if removal of the involved area of muscle is postponed until the process has become stationary.

Progressive Myositis Ossificans

Definition. Progressive myositis ossificans is a rare disease of unknown cause that usually affects children before 6 years of age, occasionally as early as infancy. It is more common in males. Progressive formation of heterotopic bone occurs within the interstitial tissue of muscles, tendons, ligaments, and fascia, and the involved muscle atrophies. This condition may be inherited or may be a spontaneous mutation affecting the mesenchyma.

Clinical features. In most cases the heterotopic ossification starts in the muscles of the neck and upper back and moves to the extremities. The disease commences with soft tissue swelling that is tender and painful and may show redness and heat, indicating the presence of inflammation. The acute symptoms subside, and a firm mass remains in the tissues. This condition may affect any of the striated muscles, including the heart and diaphragm. In some cases the spread of ossification is limited; in others it becomes extensive, affecting almost all the large muscles of the body. Stiffness and limitation of motion of the neck, chest, back, and extremities (especially the shoulders) gradually increase. Advanced stages of the disease result in the "petrified man" condition. During the third decade the process sometimes spontaneously arrests; however, most patients die during the third or fourth decade. Premature death usually results from respiratory embarrassment or from inanition through the involvement of the muscles of mastication.

Radiographic features. The radiographic appearance is similar to that described for localized myositis ossificans. The heterotopic bone more commonly is oriented along the long axis of the involved muscle (Fig. 26-12). Osseous malformation of the regions of muscle attachment, such as the mandibular condyles, also may be seen.

Differential diagnosis. In the initial stages of the disease, distinguishing between progressive myositis ossificans and rheumatoid arthritis may be difficult. However, the presence of specific anomalies suggests the diagnosis. In the case of calcinosis, the deposits of amorphous cal-

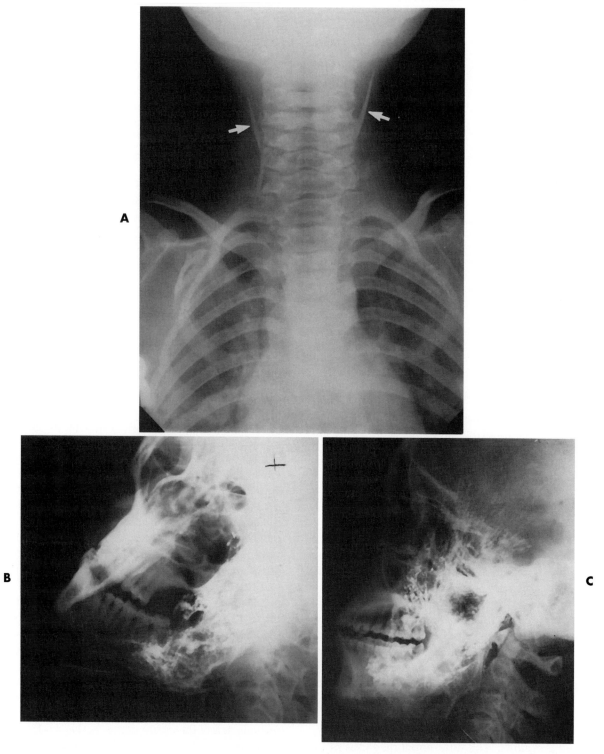

FIG. **26-12   A,** Myositis ossificans, seen as bilateral linear calcifications *(arrows)* of the sternohyoid muscle. **B** and **C,** Extensive ossification of the masseter and temporalis muscles also may be seen. (**A** courtesy Dr. H. Worth, Vancouver, British Columbia; **B** and **C** from Shawkut AH:*Oral Surg* 23:751,1967.)

cium salts frequently resorb, but in progressive myositis ossificans, the bone never disappears.

Management. No effective treatment exists for progressive myositis ossificans. Nodules that are traumatized and that ulcerate frequently should be excised. If interference with respiration or respiratory infection occurs in the later stages of the disease, supportive therapy may be required.

SUGGESTED READINGS

Allen AC: Skin. In Kissane JM, editor: *Anderson's pathology*, ed 8, vol 2, St Louis, 1985, Mosby.

Connor JM: *Soft tissue ossification*, Berlin, 1983, Springer-Verlag.

Monsour PA et al: Soft tissue calcifications in the differential diagnosis of opacities superimposed over the mandible by dental panoramic radiography, *Aust Dent J* 36:94, 1991.

Worth HM: *Principles and practice of oral radiologic interpretation*, St Louis, 1963, Mosby.

DYSTROPHIC CALCIFICATION IN THE TONSILS

Cooper MM et al: Tonsillar calculi: report of a case and review of the literature, *Oral Surg Oral Med Oral Pathol* 55(3):239, 1983.

Pruet CW, Duplan DA: Tonsil concretions and tonsilloliths, *Otolaryngol Clin North Am* 20(2):305, 1987

CYSTICERCOSIS

Rosencrans M, Barack J: Parasitic infection of the mouth: a case report of *Cysticercus cellulosae*, *NY State Dent J* 35:371, 1963.

CALCIFIED BLOOD VESSEL

Allen EV et al: *Peripheral vascular disease*, ed 3, Philadelphia, 1962, WB Saunders.

Carter LC et al: Carotid calcifications on panoramic radiography identify an asymptomatic male patient at risk for stroke: a case report, *Oral Surg Oral Med Oral Pathol Oral Radiol Endod* 85:119, 1998.

Friedlander AH et al: Prevalence of detectable carotid artery calcifications on panoramic radiographs of recent stroke victims, *Oral Surg Oral Med Oral Pathol Oral Radiol Endod* 52:102, 1994.

Hayes JB et al: Calcification of vessels in cheek of patient with medial atherosclerosis, *Oral Surg* 21:299, 1966.

SIALOLITH

Banks P: Nonneoplastic parotid swellings: a review, *Oral Surg* 25:732, 1968.

Ho V et al: Sialolithiasis of minor salivary glands, *Br J Oral Maxillofac Surg* 30:273, 1992.

Iro H et al: Shockwave lithotripsy of salivary duct stones, *Lancet* 339:1333, 1992.

Jensen J et al: Minor salivary gland calculi: a clinicopathologic study of forty-seven new cases, *Oral Surg* 47:44, 1979.

Lustmann J et al: Sialolithiasis: a survey on 245 patients and a review of the literature, *Int J Oral Maxillofac Surg* 19:135, 1990.

Mandel ID, Thompson RH Jr: The chemistry of parotid and submaxillary saliva in heavy calculus formers and nonformers, *J Periodontol* 38:310, 1967.

OSSIFIED STYLOHYOID LIGAMENT

Camarda AJ et al: Stylohyoid chain ossification: a discussion of etiology, *Oral Surg* 67:508, 1989.

Eagle W: Elongated styloid process, symptoms and treatment, *Arch Otolaryngol* 67:172, 1958.

Ettinger RL, Hanson JG: The styloid or "Eagle" syndrome: an unexpected consequence, *Oral Surg* 40:336, 1975.

Grossman JR, Tarsitano JJ: The styloid-stylohyoid syndrome, *J Oral Surg* 35:555, 1977.

Kaufman SM et al: Styloid process variation: radiographic and clinical study, *Arch Otolaryngol* 91:460, 1970.

OSTEOMA CUTIS

Farhood V et al: Osteoma cutis: cutaneous ossification with oral manifestations, *Oral Surg* 45:98, 1978.

Goldstein B et al: Dystrophic calcification in the tongue: a late sequel to radiation therapy, *Oral Surg* 46:12, 1978.

Krolls SO et al: Osseous choristomas of intraoral soft tissue, *Oral Surg* 32:588, 1971.

Peterson WC Jr, Mandel SL: Primary osteomas of the skin, *Arch Dermatol* 87:626, 1963.

Shigehara H et al: Radiographic and morphologic studies of multiple miliary osteomas of cadaver skin, *Oral Surg Oral Med Oral Pathol Oral Radiol Endod* 86:121, 1998.

MYOSITIS OSSIFICANS

Buhain WJ et al: Pulmonary function in myositis ossificans progressiva, *Am Rev Respir Dis* 110:333, 1974.

Cameron JR, Stetzer JJ: Myositis ossificans of the right masseter muscle: report of a case, *J Oral Surg* 3:170, 1945.

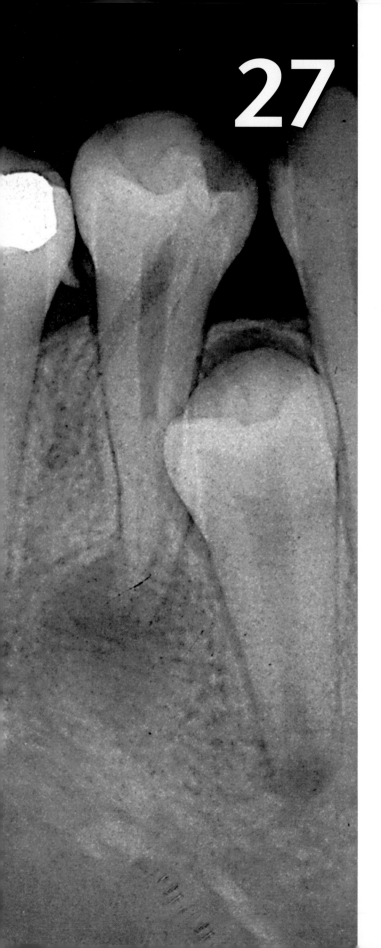

27 Trauma to Teeth and Facial Structures

Radiologic examination is essential for evaluating the sequelae of trauma, including displacement and fracture of teeth and bone, and localizing foreign objects within the soft tissues. Radiology aids in identifying the location and orientation of fractures and indicates the degree of separation or displacement of fracture margins. Follow-up radiographs are useful in evaluating the extent of healing after an injury and the development of long-term changes resulting from the trauma.

Applied Radiology

The prescription of appropriate films can be made only after a careful clinical examination. Multiple projections at differing angles, including at least two views at right angles to each other, are necessary. The application of ideal radiography may be difficult at times because of the nature of the injury and patient discomfort. The most common imaging procedures applied in various forms of trauma follow.

TRAUMA TO TEETH

The investigation of dental trauma always requires intraoral periapical films to obtain adequate image detail. It is important to radiograph not only the involved teeth but also the teeth of the opposing arch. Depending on the severity of the trauma and the ability of the patient to open the mouth, a bisecting-angle technique for intraoral radiography, including occlusal views, may be necessary.

Tooth Fracture

Intraoral periapical films (a minimum of two) should be taken at differing horizontal angulations of the x-ray beam. A panoramic film may serve as a survey film, but it may not have the image detail to reveal a nondisplaced root fracture.

Tooth Avulsion or Fractured Crown

If a tooth or a large fragment of a tooth is missing, a chest film may be considered to rule out aspiration of the tooth. If there are lacerations in the lips or cheek, a soft tissue image may be obtained by placing an intraoral film in the mouth adjacent to the traumatized soft tissue and then exposing it. If the laceration is in the tongue, a standard mandibular occlusal film may be exposed or the tongue can be protruded and then imaged.

Mandibular Fracture

The panoramic film is a good initial survey film for assessing mandibular fracture, but it must not be used alone. The standard occlusal film provides a good right-angle image. Other images that may be used include a posteroanterior skull view and a submentovertex skull view. If panoramic images are not available, lateral oblique views of the mandible are useful.

Trauma to the Mandibular Condyle

The panoramic view should be supplemented with either a transorbital view or a reverse-Towne's skull view in cases of suspected trauma to the mandibular condyle. These anteroposterior views are important to supplement lateral views of the joint, especially in cases of nondisplaced greenstick fractures of the condylar neck. These views may be supplemented with tomographic views and a submentovertex skull view. If the fracture of the condyle is complex, computed tomography (CT) imaging may be required to locate fracture fragments anatomically. Soft tissue injury to the joint capsule or articular disk warrants consideration of arthrography or magnetic resonance imaging (MRI).

Maxillary Fracture

CT is the imaging method of choice to identify the number and location of fractures of the fine structure of the maxilla. Plain radiographs include posteroanterior, Waters', reverse Towne's, and submentovertex skull views.

RADIOGRAPHIC SIGNS OF FRACTURE

The following are general signs that may indicate the presence of a fracture of bone or tooth:

1. *The presence of a radiolucent line (usually sharply defined) within the anatomic boundaries of the structure*—If the line extends beyond the boundaries of the mandible, for instance, it is more likely to represent an overlapping structure.
2. *A change in the normal anatomic outline or shape of the structure*—For instance, a mandible that is noticeably asymmetric between the left and right sides may indicate a fracture. A fracture of the mandible often shows a sharp change in the occlusal plane at the location of the fracture.
3. *A defect in the outer cortical boundary, which may appear as a deviation in the smooth outline, a gap in the outer cortical bone, or a steplike defect.*
4. *An increase in the density of the bone, which may be caused by the overlapping of two fragments of bone.*

A fracture may be missed if the plane of the fracture is not in the same direction as the x-ray beam. For this reason, multiple films at different angulations should be used.

Traumatic Injuries of the Teeth

CONCUSSION

Identifying Characteristics

Definition. The term *concussion* indicates a crushing injury to the vascular structures at the tooth apex and to the periodontal ligament, resulting in inflammatory edema. Only minimal loosening or displacement of the tooth occurs. The injury frequently results in the elevation of the tooth out of the socket so that its occlusal surface makes premature contact on mandibular closing.

Clinical features. The patient usually complains that the traumatized tooth is painful. On examination, the tooth is sensitive to both horizontal and vertical percussion. It may also be sensitive to biting forces, but patients usually modify their bites to remove occlusal stress for the short period that the periodontal ligament is inflamed.

Radiographic features. The radiographic appearance of a dental concussion is widening of the periodontal ligament space. This widening usually occurs only in the apical portion of the periodontal ligament space because the raising of the tooth out of the socket results in an essentially parallel movement of the coronal two thirds of the root surface with the lamina dura (Fig. 27-1). Reduction in the size of the pulp chamber and pulp canals may develop in the months and years after such trau-

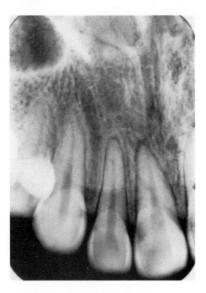

FIG. **27-1** Dental concussion has resulted in widening of the periodontal ligament spaces of the incisors.

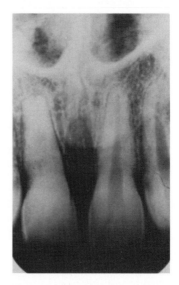

FIG. **27-2** Dental concussion has led to obliteration of the pulp chamber and resorption of the root after an injury.

matic injury (Fig. 27-2). A slow-developing pulp necrosis may result in an increase in the width of the pulp chamber and canals compared with the adjacent teeth because of the death of odontoblasts responsible for laying down secondary dentin. Pulpal necrosis may occur, resulting in the development of a periapical lesion.

Management. Because displacement of the tooth or teeth does not occur, the appropriate treatment is conservative and may include slight adjustment of the opposing teeth (if necessary), repeated vitality tests, and radiographic examination during the period after the injury.

LUXATION

Identifying Characteristics

Definition. Luxation of teeth is dislocation of the articulation (represented by the periodontal attachment) of the tooth. Such teeth are both abnormally mobile and displaced. *Subluxation* of the tooth denotes an injury to the supporting structures of the tooth that results in abnormal loosening of the tooth without frank dislocation.

Traumatic forces, depending on their nature and orientation, can cause *intrusive luxation* (displacement of teeth into the alveolar bone), *extrusive luxation* (partial displacement of teeth out of the sockets), or *lateral displacement* (movement of teeth other than axial displacement). In intrusive and lateral luxation, comminution (crushing) or fracture of the supporting alveolar bone accompanies dislocation of the tooth.

The movement of the apex and disruption of the circulation to the traumatized tooth that accompanies

luxation usually induce temporary or permanent pulpal changes, which may result in complete or partial pulpal necrosis. If the pulp survives, the rate of hard tissue formation by the pulp accelerates and continues until it obliterates the pulp chamber and canal. This may take place in permanent and deciduous teeth.

Clinical features. An adequate history is helpful in identifying luxation and ordering the appropriate radiographs. Subluxated teeth are in their normal location but are abnormally mobile. There may be some blood flowing from the gingival crevice, indicating periodontal ligament damage. Subluxated teeth are extremely sensitive to percussion and masticatory forces. The clinical crowns of intruded teeth may appear shortened. Maxillary incisors may be driven so deeply into the alveolar ridge that they appear to be avulsed (lost). The displaced tooth may cause some damage to adjacent teeth, including any developing succedaneous teeth. Depending on the orientation and magnitude of the force and the shape of the root, the root may be pushed through the buccal or, less commonly, the lingual alveolar plate, where it can be seen and palpated. On repeated vitality testing, the sensitivity of a luxated tooth may be temporarily decreased or nondetectable, especially shortly after the accident. Vitality may return, however, after weeks or even several months.

The teeth most frequently subjected to luxation are the maxillary incisors in both the deciduous and permanent dentitions. The mandibular teeth are seldom involved. The type of luxation varies with age, possibly as an expression of change in the nature of maturing bone.

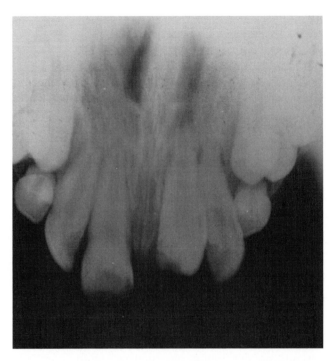

FIG. **27-3** Intruded maxillary central incisor after trauma. Note the obliteration of the apical lamina dura and the fractured incisal edges of both central incisors.

Intrusions and extrusions are the primary dislocations found in the deciduous teeth. In the permanent dentition, the intrusive type of luxation is seen less frequently. When teeth are luxated, in either dentition, usually two or more are involved, and seldom just a single tooth.

Radiographic features. Radiographic examinations of luxated teeth may demonstrate the extent of the injury to the root, periodontal ligament, and alveolar bone. A radiograph made at the time of injury serves as a valuable reference point for comparison with subsequent radiographs. As with dental concussion, the minor damage associated with subluxation may be limited to elevation of the tooth out of the socket. The sole radiographic finding may be a widening of the apical portion of the periodontal ligament space. Slight elevation of the tooth may not be radiographically apparent.

The identification and evaluation of dislocated teeth may require multiple radiographic projections. The depressed position of the crown of an intruded tooth is often apparent on a radiograph (Fig. 27-3), although a minimally intruded tooth may be difficult to demonstrate radiographically. Intrusion may result in partial or total obliteration of the periodontal ligament space. Multiple radiographic projections, including occlusal views, may show the direction of displacement and its relationship to the outer cortical bone and developing teeth.

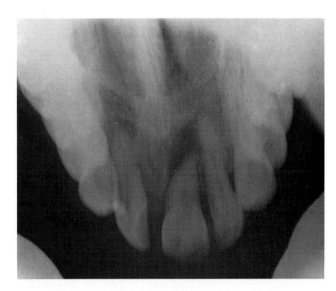

FIG. **27-4** The central incisor has been extruded after trauma. Note the increased radiolucency about the apical portion of the tooth due to an increased width of the periodontal ligament space and an inflammatory lesion.

An extrusively luxated tooth results in increased width of the periodontal ligament space. The widening may be accentuated in the apical region, whereas in a more severely extruded tooth all the periodontal ligament space may be increased. A laterally luxated tooth may show a widened periodontal ligament space, with greater width on the side of impact (Fig. 27-4). Often these teeth are somewhat extruded.

Management. A subluxated permanent tooth may be restored to its normal position by digital pressure shortly after the accident. If swelling precludes repositioning, minimal reduction of antagonists to relieve discomfort may be necessary. Stabilize teeth by splinting to prevent further damage to the pulp and periodontal ligament. However, remove a dislocated tooth if its apex is near its succedaneous tooth. If the alveolar bone over the root of a luxated tooth has been fragmented and displaced, reposition the fragments by digital pressure. Periodically examine a subluxated primary tooth after the injury. If it causes some discomfort as the result of extrusion, it can be removed without undue concern for occlusal problems.

AVULSION

Identifying Characteristics
Definition. *Avulsion* (or *exarticulation*) is the term used to describe the complete displacement of a tooth from the alveolar process. Teeth may be avulsed by direct trauma when the force is applied directly to the tooth, or by indirect trauma (e.g., when indirect force is applied

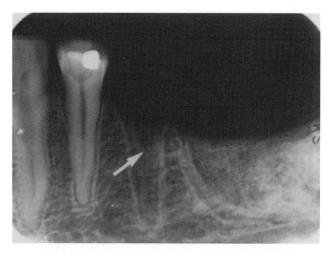

FIG. 27-5 Bone formation in a healing socket develops from the lateral walls and may leave a central radiolucent line *(arrow)* that is suggestive of a pulp canal in a retained tooth fragment.

to teeth as the result of the jaws striking together). Avulsion occurs in about 15% of traumatic injuries to the teeth. Fights are responsible for the avulsion of most permanent teeth, whereas accidental falls account for the traumatic loss of most deciduous teeth.

Clinical features. Maxillary central incisors are the teeth most often avulsed from both dentitions. The appearance of the alveolar process around the missing tooth depends on the time between its loss and the clinical examination. Typically this injury occurs in a relatively young age group, when the permanent central incisors are just erupting and the periodontal ligament is immature. Most often only a single tooth is lost, and fractures of the alveolar wall and lip injuries are frequently seen.

Radiographic features. In a recent avulsion the lamina dura of the empty socket is apparent and usually persists for several months. The replacement of the socket site with new bone requires months and, in some cases, years. As new bone forms, the opposite walls of the healing socket approach each other, reducing the socket width. Time passes, and only a thin vertical radiolucent shadow remains and may have a similar appearance to a pulp canal. In some instances the new bone replacing the socket is very dense and radiopaque and may appear similar to a retained root (Fig. 27-5). The missing tooth may be in adjacent soft tissue, and its image may occasionally project on radiographs near the empty alveolus. To differentiate between an intruded tooth and an avulsed tooth lying within the soft tissues, a radiograph of the lacerated lip or tongue should be produced.

Management. If the avulsed tooth is not found by clinical or radiographic examination, a chest radiograph may be considered to rule out aspiration of the tooth. Reimplanting permanent teeth after avulsion often restores function. If the tooth is intact and without extensive caries or periodontal disease, and the length of time that the tooth is outside the oral cavity has not been extensive, success is possible. The less time that elapses between avulsion and reimplantation, the better the prognosis. Successful reimplantation depends largely on the viability of the residual periodontal ligament fibers. If the apical foramen is open, endodontic therapy may not be required. Endodontic therapy can be delayed until the first signs of apical resorption are radiographically detected (usually 2 or 3 weeks after reimplantation). If the apical foramen is closed, endodontic treatment is required, but it should be delayed 1 or 2 weeks. External root resorption may occur in the months and years after reimplantation, and the resorption may progress to complete the destruction of the root. Reimplanting avulsed deciduous teeth carries the danger of interfering with the developing succedaneous teeth.

FRACTURES OF THE TEETH

Dental Crown Fractures

Definition. Fractures of the dental crown account for about 25% of traumatic injuries to the permanent teeth and 40% of injuries to the deciduous teeth. The most common event responsible for the fracture of permanent teeth is a fall, followed by accidents involving vehicles (e.g., bicycles, automobiles) and blows from foreign bodies striking the teeth. Fractures involving only the crown normally fall into three categories:

1. Fractures that involve only the enamel without the loss of enamel substance (*infraction* of the crown or crack)
2. Fractures that involve enamel or enamel and dentin with loss of tooth substance but without pulpal involvement (*uncomplicated fracture*)
3. Fractures that pass through enamel, dentin, and pulp with loss of tooth substance (*complicated fracture*)

Clinical features. Fracture of the dental crowns most frequently involves anterior teeth. *Infractions,* or cracks in the enamel, are quite common but frequently are not readily detectable. Illuminating crowns with indirect light (directing the beam in the long axis of the tooth) causes cracks to appear distinctly in the enamel. Histologic studies show that they pass through the enamel but not into the dentin. The pattern and distribution of these cracks are unpredictable and apparently relate to the trauma.

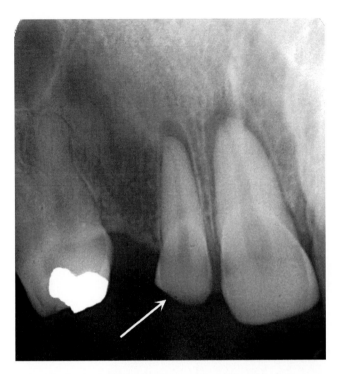

FIG. 27-6 An incisal edge fracture involving the right maxillary lateral incisor *(arrow)* and subluxation of both the central and lateral incisors.

Uncomplicated fractures do not involve the pulp. Uncomplicated crown fractures that do not involve the dentin usually occur at the mesial or distal corner of the maxillary central incisor. Loss of the central portion of the incisal edge is also common. Fractures that involve dentin can be recognized by the contrast in color between dentin and the peripheral layer of enamel. The exposed dentin is usually sensitive to chemical, thermal, and mechanical stimulation. In deep fractures, the pink image of the pulp may shine through the thin remaining dentinal wall.

Uncomplicated fractures that involve both the enamel and the dentin of permanent teeth are more common than complicated fractures. In contrast, the incidence of complicated and uncomplicated fractures is about equal in the deciduous teeth.

Complicated crown fractures are distinguishable by bleeding from the exposed pulp or by droplets of blood forming from pinpoint exposures. The pulp is visible and may extrude from the open pulp chamber if the fracture is old. The exposed pulp is sensitive to most forms of stimulation.

Radiographic features. The radiograph provides information regarding the location and extent of the fracture and the relationship to the pulp chamber, as well as the stage of root development of the involved tooth (Fig.

27-6). This initial film also provides a means of comparison for follow-up studies of the involved teeth.

Management. Although crown infractions do not require treatment, the vitality of the tooth should be questioned and determined. The sharp edges of enamel that result from an uncomplicated fracture may be smoothed by grinding and may require restoration for cosmetic reasons. It is reasonable to delay this procedure for a number of weeks until the pulp has recovered and is starting to lay down secondary dentin. The prognosis for teeth with fractures limited to the enamel is quite good, and pulpal necrosis develops in fewer than 2% of such cases. If a fracture involves both dentin and enamel, the frequency of pulpal necrosis is about 3%. Oblique fractures have a worse prognosis than horizontal fractures because a greater amount of dentin is exposed. The frequency of pulpal necrosis increases greatly with concussion and mobility of the tooth.

Treatment of complicated crown fractures of permanent teeth may involve pulp capping, pulpotomy, or pulpectomy, depending on the stage of root formation. If a coronal fracture of a deciduous tooth involves the pulp, it is usually best treated by extraction.

Dental Root Fractures

Definition. Fractures of tooth roots are uncommon and account for 7% or fewer of traumatic injuries to permanent teeth and for about half that many in deciduous teeth. This difference probably results from the fact that the deciduous teeth are less firmly anchored in the alveolus.

Clinical features. Most root fractures occur in maxillary central incisors. The coronal fragments are usually displaced lingually and slightly extruded. The degree of mobility of the crown relates to the level of the fracture: the closer the fracture is to the apex, the more stable the tooth is. When testing the mobility of a traumatized tooth, place a finger over the alveolar bone. If movement of only the crown can be detected, root fracture is likely. Fractures of the root may occur with fractures of the alveolar bone, which are commonly not detected. This is most often observed in the anterior region of the mandible, where root fractures are infrequent. Although root fracture is usually associated with temporary loss of sensitivity (by all usual criteria), the sensitivity of most teeth returns to normal within about 6 months.

Radiographic features. Fractures of the dental root may occur at any level and involve one (Fig. 27-7) or all the roots of multirooted teeth. Most of the fractures confined to the root occur in the middle third of the root. The ability of the film to reveal the presence of a

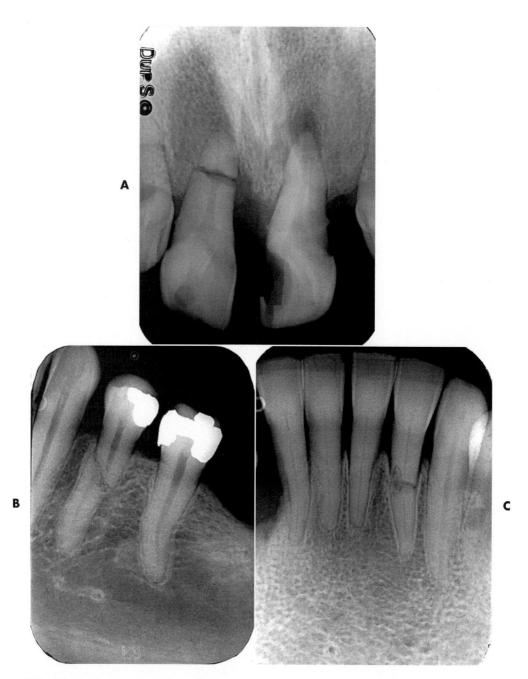

FIG. **27-7**   **A,** A recent horizontal fracture of the right maxillary central incisor and apical rarefying osteitis related to the left central incisor. **B,** A healed fracture with slight displacement of the fragments. **C,** A healed fracture with an increase in the distance between the fracture segments due to root resorption.

root fracture depends on the degree of distraction of the fragments and whether the x-ray beam is in alignment with the plane of the fracture. When visible the fracture appears as a sharply defined radiolucent line confined to the anatomic limits of the root. If, however, the orientation of the beam is not directly through the plane of the fracture, the image of the fracture appears as a more poorly defined gray shadow. Most nondisplaced root fractures are usually difficult to demonstrate radiographically, and several views at differing angles may be necessary. In some instances when the fracture line is not visible, the only evidence of a fracture may be a localized increase in the periodontal ligament space adjacent to the fracture site (Fig. 27-8).

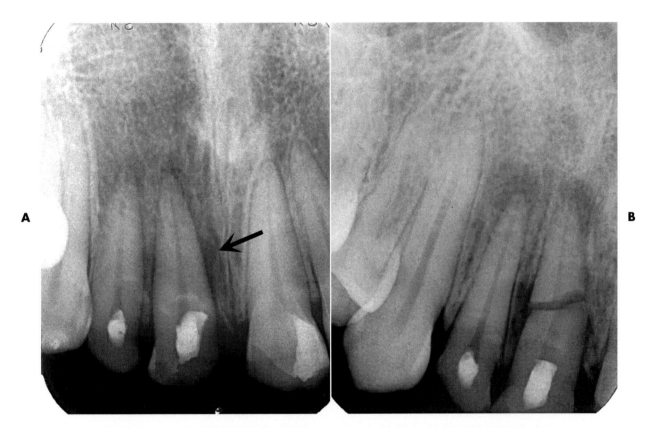

FIG. **27-8**   Incisal fractures involving the maxillary central incisors and the right lateral incisor. In addition, there is subtle evidence of a root fracture involving the distal aspect of the root of the right central incisor **(A).** The fracture line is not apparent on the mesial aspect of the root because the plane of fracture is not in alignment with the x-ray beam. However, there is widening of the periodontal membrane space on the mesial surface *(arrow)* at the site of the fracture. **B,** Dislocation of the root fragments.

Most fractures are transverse and oblique and the shadow of the fracture line at the buccal and lingual surfaces may suggest the presence of more than one (comminuted) fracture (Fig. 27-9). Longitudinal root fractures are relatively uncommon but are most likely in teeth with posts that have been subjected to trauma. The width of fractures tends to increase with time, probably because of resorption of the fractured surfaces. Over time, calcification and obliteration of the pulp chamber and canal may be seen.

Differential diagnosis. The superimposition of soft tissue structures such as the lip, ala of the nose, and nasolabial fold over the image of a root may suggest a root fracture (see Fig. 27-9). To avoid this diagnostic error, note that the soft tissue image of the lip line usually extends beyond the tooth margins. Fractures of the alveolar process may also overlap the root and suggest a root fracture.

Management. Fractures in the middle or apical third of the root of permanent teeth can be manually reduced to

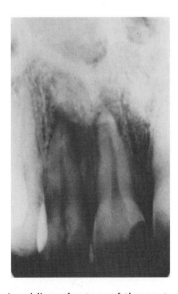

FIG. **27-9**   An oblique fracture of the central incisor root mimics a comminuted fracture. A longitudinal fracture of the lateral incisor also is evident. Note how the soft tissue outline of the nose simulates a fracture of the central incisor root tip.

the proper position and immobilized. Prognosis is generally favorable; the incidence of pulpal necrosis is about 20% to 24%. The more apical the fracture is, the better the prognosis. Perform endodontic therapy only when evidence exists of pulpal necrosis. It is common for bone resorption to occur at the site of the fracture rather than at the apex. When the fracture occurs in the coronal third of the root, the prognosis is poor and extraction is indicated unless the apical portion of the root fragment can be extruded orthodontically and restored. The roots of fractured deciduous teeth that are not badly dislocated may be retained with the expectation that they will be normally resorbed. Attempts at removal may result in damage to the developing succedaneous tooth.

Crown-Root Fractures

Definition. Crown-root fractures involve both the crown and roots. Although uncomplicated fractures may occur, crown-root fractures usually involve the pulp. About twice as many affect the permanent as the deciduous teeth. Most crown-root fractures of the anterior teeth are the result of direct trauma. Many posterior teeth are predisposed to such fractures by large restorations or extensive caries.

Clinical features. The typical crown-root fracture of an anterior tooth has a labial margin in the gingival third of the crown and courses obliquely to exit below the gingival attachment on the lingual surface. Displacement of the fragments is usually minimal. Crown-root fractures occasionally present with bleeding from the pulp. The patient with a crown-root fracture usually complains of pain during mastication. The teeth are sensitive to occlusal forces, which cause separation of the fragments.

Radiographic features. These fractures are often not visible in the radiographic image because the x-ray beam is rarely aligned with the plane of the fracture. Also, distraction of the fragments is usually not present. The vertical fractures of crown and root that are mainly tangential to the direction of the radiographic beam are readily apparent on the radiograph. Unfortunately, this is not common.

Management. Removal of the coronal fragment permits the evaluation of the extent of the fracture. If the coronal fragment includes as much as 3 to 4 mm of clinical root, successful restoration of the tooth is doubtful and removal of the residual root is recommended. Also, if the crown-root fracture is vertical, prognosis is poor regardless of treatment. If the pulp is not exposed and the fracture does not extend more than 3 to 4 mm below the epithelial attachment, conservative treatment is likely to be successful. Uncomplicated crown-root fractures are frequently encountered in posterior teeth, and

with the appropriate crown-lengthening procedures (gingivectomy and ostectomy), the tooth is likely to be amenable to successful restoration. If only a small amount of root is lost with the coronal fragment but the pulp has been compromised, it is likely that the tooth can be restored after endodontic treatment.

Vertical Root Fractures

Definition. Vertical root fractures run lengthwise from the crown toward the apex of the tooth. Usually both sides of a root are involved. The crack is usually oriented in the facial-lingual plane in both anterior and posterior teeth. These fractures usually occur in the posterior teeth in adults, especially in mandibular molars. They are usually iatrogenic, following insertion of retention screws or pins into vital or nonvital teeth. Uncrowned posterior teeth that have been treated endodontically are most at risk. Large occlusal forces are another etiology for vertical root fracture, particularly in restored teeth.

Clinical features. Patients with vertical root fractures complain of persistent dull pain (cracked tooth syndrome), often of long duration. This pain may be elicited by applying pressure to the involved tooth. Pain may be nonexistent or mild. The patient may have a periodontal lesion resembling a chronic abscess or a history of repeated failed endodontic therapy. Occasionally, definitive diagnosis can be made only by inspection after surgical exposure.

Radiographic features. If the central ray of the x-ray beam lies in the plane of the fracture, the fracture may be visible as a radiolucent line on the radiograph. Usually, however, radiographs are not useful in identifying vertical root fractures in their early stages. Later, after the development of an inflammatory lesion, there will be evidence of bone loss. The widening of the periodontal membrane space and this bone loss are usually not centered at the apex but often positioned more coronally towards the alveolar crest. Lesions may also extend apically from the alveolar crest and resemble periodontal lesions.

Management. Single-rooted teeth with vertical root fractures must be extracted. Multirooted teeth may be hemisected and the intact remaining half of the tooth restored with endodontic therapy and a crown.

TRAUMATIC INJURIES TO THE FACIAL BONES

Injury to the facial bones may occur in one or more of the bones. Facial fractures most frequently occur in the zygoma or mandible and, to a lesser extent, in the maxilla. Radiography plays a crucial role in the diagnosis and management of traumatic injuries to the facial bones. The appropriate radiologic investigation is prescribed only after a thorough examination of the teeth and facial bones. Obtaining the history of the trauma also contributes to the selection of the appropriate radiographs. Obtaining multiple views (at least two at right angles) aids in assessing the location, extent, and displacement of fractures. Some fractures are not readily apparent when the x-ray beam is not oriented parallel to the plane of the fracture.

Mandibular Fractures

The most common mandibular fracture sites are the condyle, body, and angle, followed less frequently by the parasymphyseal region, ramus, coronoid process, and alveolus. The most common cause of mandibular fractures is assault, followed by automobile accidents, falls, and sports injuries. About half of all mandibular fractures occur in individuals between 16 and 35 years of age, and fractures are more likely on Fridays and Saturdays than on other days of the week. Males are affected about three times as frequently as females. Trauma to the mandible is often associated with other injuries, most commonly concussion (loss of consciousness) and other fractures, usually of the maxilla, zygoma, and skull.

Mandibular Body Fractures

Definition. The mandible is the most commonly fractured facial bone. It is important to realize that a fracture of the mandibular body on one side is frequently accompanied by a fracture of the condylar process on the opposite side. Trauma to the anterior mandible may result in a unilateral or bilateral fracture of the condylar processes. When a heavy force strikes a small area laterally, fracture of the angle, ramus, or even the coronoid process may result. In children, fractures of the mandibular body usually occur in the anterior region. Mandibular fractures are classified as favorable or unfavorable, depending on their orientation. Unfavorable fractures are those where the action of muscles attached to the mandible are likely to displace the fracture margins. For instance if a fracture site in the body of the mandible slants posteriorly and inferiorly such that the masseter and internal pterygoid muscles pull the ramus segment away from the body of the mandible, the fracture is unfavorable. In favorable fractures, muscle action tends to reduce the fracture.

Clinical features. A history of injury is typical, substantiated by some evidence of the trauma that caused the fracture, such as contusions or wounds in the skin. Frequently the patient experiences swelling and a deformity that is accentuated when the patient opens the mouth. A discrepancy is often present in the occlusal plane, and manipulation may produce crepitus or abnormal mo-

bility. Intraoral examination may reveal ecchymosis in the floor of the mouth. In the case of bilateral fractures to the mandible, a risk exists that the digastric and mylohyoid muscles will pull the mandible against the pharynx and compromise the airway.

Radiographic features. The radiographic examination of a suspected fracture should include a panoramic view; however, it is important to supplement this film with right-angle views. These include occlusal and extraoral views such as the posteroanterior and submentovertex skull views. Frequently such supplemental views disclose fractures not evident on panoramic projections. The margins of fractures usually appear as sharply defined radiolucent (dark) lines of separation that are confined to the structure of the mandible. They are best visualized when the x-ray beam is oriented in the plane of the fracture.

Displacement of the fragments results in a cortical discontinuity or "step" (Fig. 27-10). An irregularity in the occlusal plane is often apparent, indicating the fracture site. Occasionally, the margins of the fracture overlap each other, resulting in an area of increased radiopacity at the fracture site. Nondisplaced mandibular fractures may involve both buccal and lingual cortical plates or only one cortical plate. An incomplete fracture involving only one cortical plate is often called a *greenstick fracture*. Such fractures usually occur in children. An oblique fracture that involves both cortical plates may cause some diagnostic difficulties if the fracture lines in the buccal and lingual plates are not superimposed (Fig. 27-11). In this case, two fracture lines are apparent, suggesting two distinct fractures when in reality only one exists. A right-angle view such as an occlusal view and the fact that the two fracture lines join at the same point on the inferior border of the mandible help with the correct diagnosis.

Differential diagnosis. The superimposition of soft tissue shadows on the image of the mandible may simulate fractures. A narrow air space between the dorsal surface of the tongue and the soft palate superimposed across the angle of the mandible in a panoramic image may appear as a fracture. The air space between the dorsal surface of the tongue and the posterior pharyngeal wall can appear similar to a fracture on lateral views of the mandible. Similar appearances can occur in the region of soft palate superimposition on the ramus.

Management. The management of a fracture of the mandible presents a variety of surgical problems that involve the proper reduction, fixation, and immobilization of the fractured bone. Minimally displaced fractures are managed by closed reduction and intermaxillary fixation, whereas fractures with more severely displaced

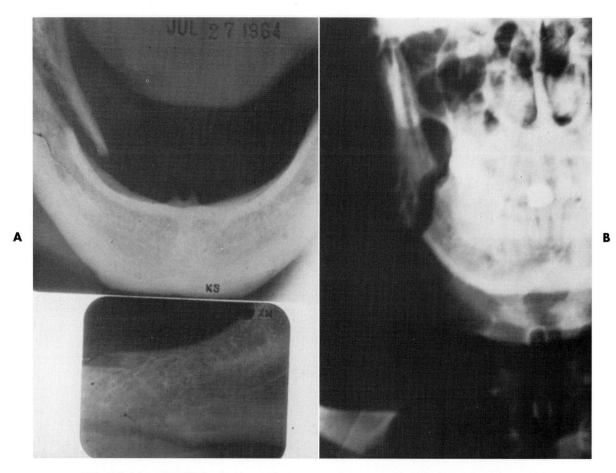

FIG. **27-10** *Mandibular fractures.* **A,** Fracture of the mandibular body, showing medial and superior displacement of the posterior fragment. **B,** Fracture through the angle of the mandible, with lateral displacement of the ramus. (**B** courtesy B. Sanders, DDS, Los Angeles.)

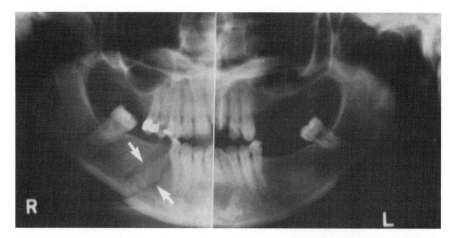

FIG. **27-11** Single fracture of the mandibular body, with separation of the fracture lines on the buccal and lingual plates simulating two fractures *(arrows).* Note how the fracture lines meet at the inferior cortex.

fragments may require open reduction. Treatment for fractures of the body often includes antibiotic therapy because a tooth root may be in the line of the fracture. When the fracture line involves third molars, severely mobile teeth, or teeth with at least half their roots exposed in the fracture line, the involved teeth are often extracted to reduce the risk of infection and problems with fixation.

Mandibular Condyle Fractures

Definition. Fractures in the region of the condyle can be divided into condylar neck fractures and condylar head fractures. Condylar neck fractures are more common and are located below the condylar head. When a condylar neck fracture occurs, the head is usually displaced medially, inferiorly, and anteriorly (as a result of pull from the lateral pterygoid muscle). Severe trauma may displace the condylar head into the skull or sinuses. Fractures of the condylar head are fissure-like, with a vertical cleft dividing the head; they may result in multiple fragments in a compression-like fracture. Almost half the patients with condylar fractures also have fractures in the mandibular body.

Clinical features. The clinical symptoms of a fractured condylar process are not always apparent, so the preauricular area must be carefully examined and palpated. A condylar fracture may be suspected when the clinician cannot palpate the condyle in the external ear canal when the jaw is closed. Movement of the jaw may cause crepitus. The patient may have pain on opening or closing the mouth, but so much swelling and trismus may exist that the patient is unable to move the jaw. Usually an anterior open bite is present, with the last molars in contact. Also, the mandible may be displaced forward or, in the case of a unilateral fracture, deviated toward the side of the fracture, especially on opening. A significant feature is the inability of the patient to bring the jaw forward because the external pterygoid muscle is attached to the condyle.

Radiographic features. Radiographic examination of the condyles should always include lateral and anteroposterior views of each condyle. Appropriate lateral projections include panoramic (Fig. 27-12), Parma (Fig. 27-13), and lateral oblique views of the ramus and condylar regions. Frontal views include reverse-Towne's and transorbital projections. Nondisplaced fractures of the condylar process may be difficult to detect on lateral views and are best demonstrated on anteroposterior views. Careful tracing of the outer cortical plate of the posterior border of the ramus, the condylar head, and the condylar notch on the lateral and posteroanterior projections may reveal the presence of fractures.

Studies of remodeling of fractured condyles show that young persons have much greater remodeling potential than do adults. In children younger than 12 years, most fractured condyles show a radiographic return to normal morphology after healing, whereas in teenagers the remodeling is less complete, and in adults only minor remodeling is observed. The extent of remodeling is also greater with fractures of the condylar head than with condylar neck fractures with displacement of the condylar head. The most common deformities are medial inclination of the condyle, abnormal shape of the condyle, shortening of the neck, erosion, and flattening. Early condylar fractures commonly result in hypoplasia of the ipsilateral side of the mandible.

Management. The technical details of treating condylar fractures vary according to whether one or both condyles are involved, the extent of displacement, and the occurrence and severity of concomitant fractures. The treatment is directed to relieve acute symptoms, restore proper anatomic relationships, and prevent bony ankylosis. If a malocclusion develops, intermaxillary fixation may be provided in an attempt to restore proper occlusion. Often fractures are not reduced because of the morbidity of the procedure and the size and position of the fracture fragments.

Fractures of the Alveolar Process

Definition. Simple fractures of the alveolar process may involve the buccal or lingual cortical plates of the alveolar process of the maxilla or mandible. Commonly these fractures are associated with traumatic injuries to teeth that are luxated with or without dislocation. Several teeth are usually affected, and the fracture line is most often horizontal. The labial plate of the alveolar process is more prone to fracture than the palatal plate.

Some fractures extend through the entire alveolar process (in contrast to the simple fracture that involves only one cortical plate) and may be apical to the teeth or involve the tooth socket. These are also commonly associated with dental injuries and extrusive luxations with or without root fractures.

Clinical features. A common location of alveolar fractures is the anterior aspect of the maxilla. Simple alveolar fractures are relatively rare in the posterior segments of the arches. In this location, fracture of the buccal plate usually occurs during removal of a maxillary posterior tooth. Fractures of the entire alveolar process occur in the anterior and premolar regions and in an older age group.

A characteristic feature of alveolar process fracture is marked malocclusion with displacement and mobility of the fragment. The attached gingiva may have lacerations. When the practitioner tests the mobility of a single tooth, the entire fragment of bone moves. The teeth in the fragment also have a recognizable dull sound when

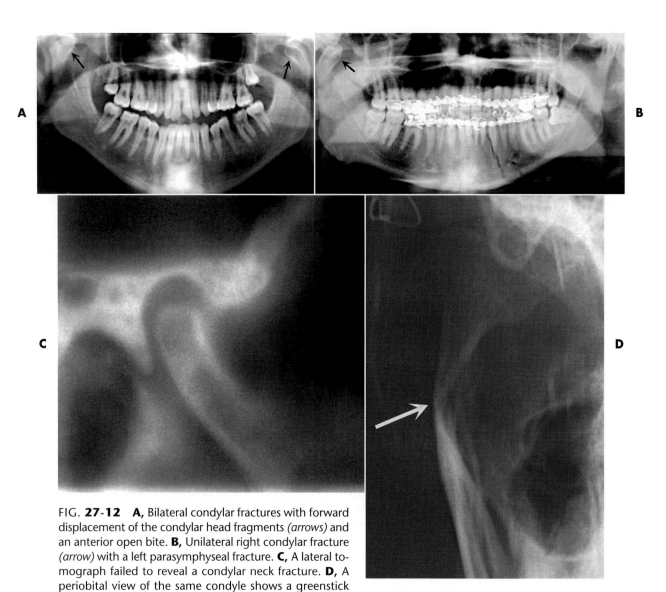

FIG. **27-12 A,** Bilateral condylar fractures with forward displacement of the condylar head fragments *(arrows)* and an anterior open bite. **B,** Unilateral right condylar fracture *(arrow)* with a left parasymphyseal fracture. **C,** A lateral tomograph failed to reveal a condylar neck fracture. **D,** A periobital view of the same condyle shows a greenstick condylar neck fracture.

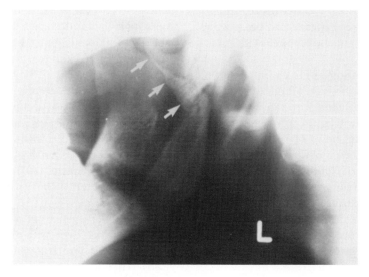

FIG. **27-13** *A Parma view demonstrating a fracture of the left condyle.* Note the increased radiopacity in the ramus near the fracture line due to overlapping fragments *(arrows).*

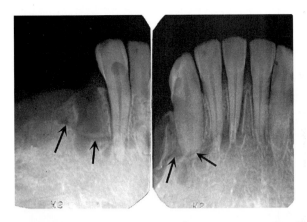

FIG. **27-14** These two images demonstrate an alveolar fracture extending from the distal aspect of the mandibular right cuspid in an anterior direction *(arrows)* and through the tooth socket of the right central incisor.

percussed. The detached bone may include the floor of the maxillary sinus, which may cause bleeding from the nose on the involved side. Ecchymosis of the buccal vestibule is usually evident.

Radiographic features. Intraoral radiographs often do not reveal fractures of a single cortical wall of the alveolar process, although evidence exists that the teeth have been luxated. However, a fracture of the anterior labial cortical plate may be apparent on a lateral extraoral radiograph if some bone displacement occurs and if the direction of the x-ray beam profiles the fracture site. Fractures of both cortical plates of the alveolar process are usually apparent (Fig. 27-14). The closer the fracture is to the alveolar crest, the greater the possibility that root fractures are present. It may be difficult to differentiate a root fracture from an overlapping fracture line of the alveolar bone. Several films produced with different projection angles help with this differentiation. If the fracture line is truly associated with the tooth, the line does not move relative to the tooth structure. Fractures of the posterior alveolar process may involve the floor of the maxillary sinus and result in abnormal thickening of the sinus mucosa.

Management. Fractures of the alveolar process are treated by repositioning the displaced teeth and associated bone fragments with digital pressure. Gingival lacerations are sutured. If the luxated permanent teeth are splinted and stable, intermaxillary fixation is not necessary. Permanent teeth are splinted for about 6 weeks. The faster healing in children permits their removal in about half that time. A soft diet for 10 to 14 days is recommended. Antibiotic coverage is provided because of communication with tooth sockets. Teeth that have lost their vascular supply may eventually require endodontic treatment.

MAXILLARY FRACTURES

Midface Fractures

Definition. Fractures of the midfacial region may be limited to the maxilla alone or may involve other bones, including the frontal, nasal, lacrimal, zygoma, vomer, ethmoid, and sphenoid. Such complex fractures may be quite variable but often follow general patterns classified by Léon Le Fort: zygomatic (complex), horizontal, pyramidal, and craniofacial disjunction fractures. These fractures may be evident clinically or radiographically. They are rare in children.

The radiographic interpretation of fractures of the midface is difficult because of the complex anatomy in this region and the multiple superimpositions of structures. A plain film examination should include posteroanterior, Waters', reverse Towne's, lateral skull, and submentovertex projections. Each film should be searched systematically for fractures in the frontal bone, nasion, orbital walls, zygomatic arches, and maxillary antrum. Fractures may appear as linear radiolucencies that are usually widest at discontinuities in the cortical margins of bone, alterations of normal skeletal contour, displaced fragments of bone, and separated bony sutures. Some fractures are not apparent because of minimal separation of the bony margins, orientation of the fracture at an oblique angle to the x-ray beam, or superimposition of fracture lines over other complex anatomic structures. Abnormal soft tissue densities may both help and hinder the examination of facial trauma. When the fracture tears the antral or nasal mucosa, radiographs reveal densities associated with edema and bleeding in those areas and thus help to identify regions of fracture. However, facial edema detracts from the clarity of the radiographs, and preexisting inflammatory or allergic paranasal sinus disease may be misleading.

CT is the diagnostic imaging method of choice for maxillary fractures. It provides image slices (axial and coronal images using bone algorithm) through the maxilla, allowing for the display of osseous structures without the images of overlapping anatomy. This provides suitable image detail to detect bony fractures and changes in the soft tissues, such as herniation of orbital fat and extraocular muscle and tissue swelling. As an aid in determining the spatial orientation of fractures or bone fragments, the CT images may be reformatted in three-dimensional images.

Horizontal Fracture (Le Fort I)

Definition. The Le Fort I fracture is a relatively horizontal fracture in the body of the maxilla that results in detachment of the alveolar process of the maxilla from the middle face. It is the result of a traumatic force directed to the lower maxillary region. The fracture line passes above the teeth, below the zygomatic process, and through the maxillary sinuses and tuberosities to the in-

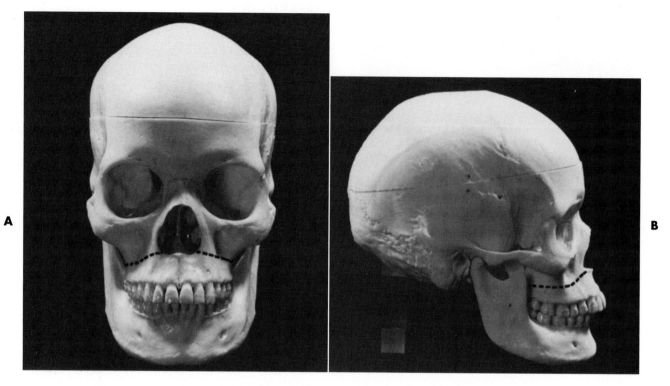

FIG. **27-15** Usual position of the Le Fort I horizontal fracture on a frontal **(A)** and lateral **(B)** view.

ferior portion of the pterygoid processes (Fig. 27-15). It may be unilateral or bilateral. In the unilateral fracture, an auxiliary fracture exists in the midline of the palate. The unilateral fracture must be distinguished from a fracture within the alveolar process (as discussed previously), which does not extend to the midline. Fractures of the mandible (54%) and zygoma (23%) may also be found in these patients.

Clinical features. If the fragment is not distally impacted, it can be manipulated by holding onto the teeth. If the fracture line is at a high level, the fragment may include the pterygoid muscle attachments, which pull the fragment posteriorly and inferiorly. As a result, the posterior maxillary teeth contact the mandibular teeth first, resulting in an anterior open bite, retruded chin, and long face, an appearance characteristic of this type of fracture. If the fracture is at a low level, no displacement may occur. Other symptoms may include an associated swelling and bruising about both eyes, pain over the nose and face, deformity of the nose, and flattening of the middle of the face. Epistaxis is inevitable, and occasionally double vision and varying degrees of paresthesia over the distribution of the infraorbital nerve occur. Manipulation may reveal a mobile maxilla and crepitation.

Radiographic features. This fracture may be difficult to detect. The views to use are the posteroanterior, lateral skull, and Waters' projections and CT scans. Both maxillary sinuses are usually radiopaque and may show air-fluid levels. The lateral view may disclose a slight posterior displacement of the fragment (the inferior portion of the maxilla below the fracture line), and if present the fracture line through the pterygoid bones. The intervertebral spaces of the cervical spine may simulate fracture lines in the posteroanterior skull views. This type of fracture unites rapidly, so if a few days lapse between injury and radiographic examination, the fracture may not be detectable radiographically.

Management. If the fracture is not displaced and is at a relatively low level in the maxilla, it can be treated by intermaxillary fixation. Those that are high, with the fragment displaced posteriorly or with pronounced separation, require craniomaxillary fixation in addition to intermaxillary fixation. A unilateral horizontal fracture is usually immobilized by intermaxillary fixation. However, if it cannot be reduced manually, elastic traction in the required direction (across the palate or between the arches) is employed. Antibiotics are usually administered because the fracture line involves the maxillary sinuses.

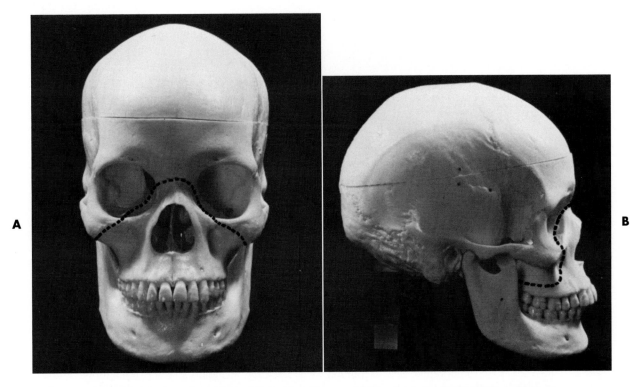

FIG. **27-16** Usual position of the Le Fort II pyramidal fracture on a frontal **(A)** and lateral **(B)** view.

Pyramidal Fracture (Le Fort II)

Definition. The Le Fort II fracture has a pyramidal appearance on the posteroanterior skull radiograph—hence the name. It results from a violent force applied to the central region of the middle third of the facial skeleton. This force separates the maxilla from the base of the skull by causing fractures of the nasal bones and frontal processes of the maxilla (Fig. 27-16). The fractures extend laterally through the lacrimal bones and floors of the orbits and inferiorly through the zygomaticomaxillary sutures (Fig. 27-17). Frequently on one side the fracture passes through the suture or through the zygomic complex and on the other side it passes around and beneath the base of the zygomatic process of the maxilla. From this area, it then passes posteriorly along the lateral wall of the maxilla, across the pterygomaxillary fossa, and through the pterygoid plates. It usually extends through the maxillary sinuses. The frontal and ethmoid sinuses are involved in about 10% of cases, especially in severe comminuted fractures.

Clinical features. In contrast to the Le Fort I (horizontal) fracture, characterized by only slight swelling about the upper lips, the Le Fort II injury results in massive edema and marked swelling of the middle third of the face. Typically, an ecchymosis around the eyes develops

within minutes of the injury. The edema about the eyes is likely to be so severe that it is impossible to see the eyes without prying the lids open. The conjunctivas over the inner quadrants of the eyes are bloodshot, and if the zygomatic bones are involved, this ecchymosis extends to the outer quadrant. The broken nose is displaced; because the face has fallen, the nose and face are lengthened. An anterior open bite occurs (with molars in contact). Epistaxis is inevitable, and a cerebrospinal fluid rhinorrhea may also result. Palpation reveals the discontinuity of the lower borders of the orbits. By applying pressure between the bridge of the nose and the palate, the "pyramid" of bone can be moved. Other common symptoms include double vision and variable degrees of paresthesia over the distribution of the infraorbital nerve.

Radiographic features. The radiographic examination reveals fractures of the nasal bones, both frontal processes of the maxilla (and ethmoid and frontal sinuses, if involved), and the infraorbital rims on both sides (and the floor of both orbits). Fractures in the zygoma or zygomatic process of the maxilla, separation of the zygomaticomaxillary sutures on both sides, deformity and discontinuity of the lateral walls of both maxillary sinuses, thickening of the lining mucosa or

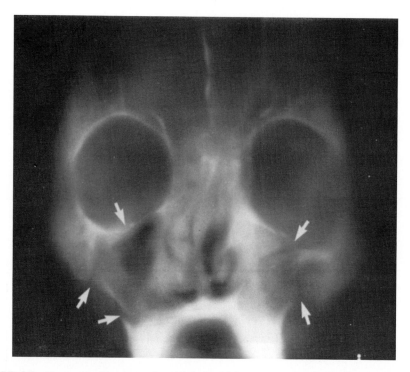

FIG. **27-17** Tomographic view of multiple facial fractures, including a Le Fort II fracture and fractures through the ethmoid bone, infraorbital rims *(arrows)* and lateral wall of the maxilla *(arrows)*. (Courtesy Dr. C. Schow, Galveston, Tex.)

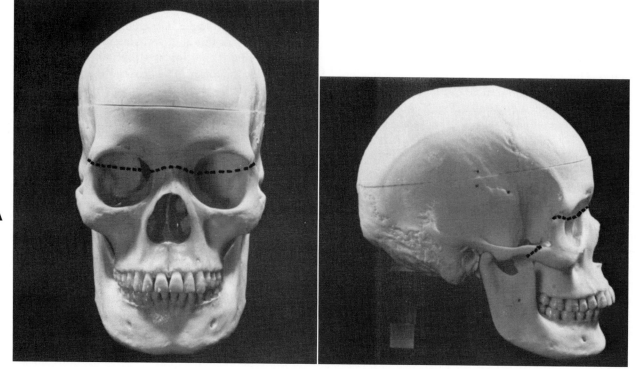

FIG. **27-18** Usual position of the Le Fort III craniofacial disjunction fracture on a frontal **(A)** and lateral **(B)** view.

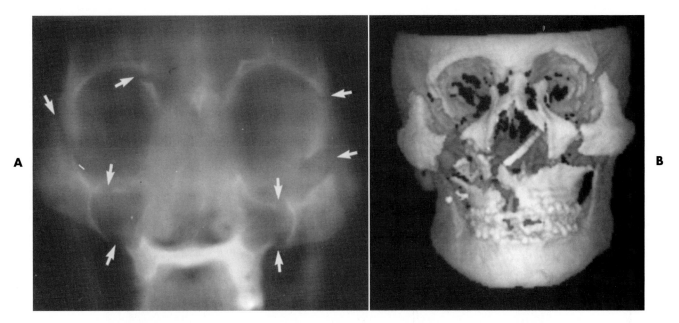

FIG. **27-19** **A,** Tomographic view of multiple facial fractures, including a Le Fort III, through the ethmoid bones, lateral walls of the orbits *(arrows)*, infraorbital rims *(arrows)*, and lateral walls of the maxilla *(arrows)*. **B,** Three-dimensional reformatted CT image of another patient with comparable facial fractures. Note the separation of each zygomaticofrontal suture as well as fractures of the ethmoid bone, each anterior maxilla inferior to the orbit, and the maxillary alveolar ridge from the midface. (**A** courtesy C. Schow, DDS, Galveston, Tex. **B** courtesy M. Alder, DDS, San Antonio, Tex.)

increased radiopacity of the maxillary sinus and sometimes the frontal and ethmoid sinuses, and fractures through both pterygoid plates (Fig. 27-18) also occur. CT examination is required to supplement plain views of the skull because of multiple superimposition of structures.

Examining the floor of the orbit in Waters' projections of the skull may be difficult because two different radiopaque lines often represent the lower limit of the orbit. One is the actual floor of the orbit, which is often thin and difficult to discern. The other is the inferior rim of the orbit, which is usually thicker bone and appears above the floor of the orbit. The presence of a less distinct orbital floor may suggest a blowout fracture of the orbital floor. The presence of herniated orbital contents through the floor and into the maxillary sinus is a useful sign of a blowout fracture. However, orbital floor fractures do not always have associated soft tissue herniation. CT imaging is useful in arriving at an accurate diagnosis.

Management. The treatment of this fracture is accomplished by reduction of the downward displacement of the maxilla. The maxilla is fixed in place by intermaxillary wires or arch bars. Usually treatment includes open reduction and interosseous wiring of the infraorbital rims. The accompanying fractures of the nose, nasal sep-

tum, orbital floor, and detached medial canthal ligaments also require repair. Leakage of cerebrospinal fluid requires the attention of a neurosurgeon. Antibiotics are required because of communication of the fractures with the paranasal sinuses.

Craniofacial Disjunction (Le Fort III)

Definition. A Le Fort III midface fracture results when the traumatic force is of sufficient magnitude to completely separate the middle third of the facial skeleton from the cranium. The fracture line usually extends through the nasal bones and the frontal processes of the maxilla or nasofrontal and maxillofrontal sutures, across the floors of the orbits, and through the ethmoid and sphenoid sinuses and the zygomaticofrontal sutures (Fig. 27-19). It passes across both pterygomaxillary fissures and separates the pterygoid plates where they arise from the sphenoid bone (at their roots). If the maxilla is displaced and freely movable, a fracture must also have occurred in the area of the zygomaticotemporal suture. Because the zygoma or zygomatic arch is involved, these injuries are as a rule associated with multiple other maxillary fractures. Mandibular fractures are also observed in half the cases.

Clinical features. Craniofacial disjunction produces a clinical appearance similar to pyramidal fracture. How-

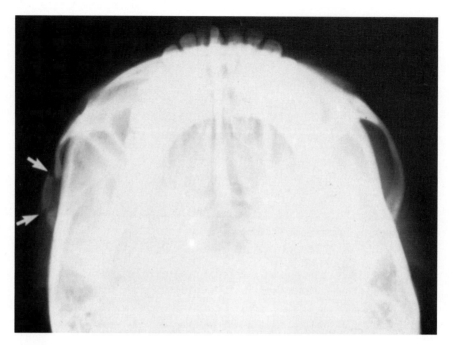

FIG. **27-20** Fractures of the zygomatic arch *(arrows)* are demonstrated on this submentovertex projection with reduced exposure time.

ever, this injury is considerably more extensive. The soft tissue injuries are severe, with massive edema. The nose may be blocked with blood clot, or blood, serum, or cerebrospinal fluid rhinorrhea may be present. Bleeding may occur into the periorbital tissues and all quadrants of the conjunctiva; a number of eye signs of neurologic importance are likely to be present. A "dish face" deformity is characteristic of these fractures, as is an anterior open bite (because of retroposition of the maxillary incisors) with the posterior teeth in occlusion. Although the mandible is wide open, the patient is unable to separate the molars. Intraoral and extraoral palpation reveals irregular contours and step deformities, and crepitation is also apparent when the fragments are moved.

Radiographic features. The radiographic projections of Le Fort III fractures usually are hazy because of extensive soft tissue swelling. The main radiographic findings are separated nasofrontal, maxillofrontal, zygomaticofrontal, and zygomaticotemporal sutures (Fig. 27-20). The nasal bones, frontal processes of the maxilla, both orbital floors, and pterygoid plates are likely to show radiolucent lines and discontinuity in some of these areas. The ethmoid and sphenoid sinuses are radiopaque, indicating the presence of fractures; the frontal sinus is also frequently involved. Associated fractures of the walls of the maxillary sinuses also result in a radiopaque appearance.

It is extremely difficult to document these multiple fractures with plain films alone; therefore CT images in concert with the clinical information is required.

Management. The associated severe soft tissue injury necessitates initial hemorrhage control, airway maintenance, and repair of lacerations. Surgery may be delayed until the edema has sufficiently resolved. The treatment of transverse fractures is complicated because fixation of the loose middle third of the facial skeleton is difficult because of the fact that fractures of the zygomatic arch occur. The only possibilities are external immobilization or immobilization within the tissues. In the former, the loose maxilla is suspended by wires through the cheeks from a metal head frame (halo) or fixed by using external pins anchored in bone. The other possibility is immobilization within the tissues by using internal wiring to the closest solid bone superior to the fracture. A number of complications may develop during or after this treatment.

Zygomatic Fractures

Definition. Unilateral fractures involving the zygoma are of two types: zygomatic arch fractures, in which just the arch is fractured, and zygomatic complex fractures, in which the zygomatic bone is separated from its frontal, maxillary, and temporal connections. Bilateral zygomatic fractures occur in association with Le Fort II and III fractures, described previously. Injuries to the zygomatic arch usually result from a forceful blow to the side of the face. Although the blow may displace the fragment medially, the arch is so well supported superiorly by the temporalis muscle and inferiorly by the masseter muscle that it is rarely displaced upward or downward. The arch may fracture at its center, resulting in a V-shaped medial displacement, or near its articulation with the zygomatic process of the maxilla, resulting in medial displacement of the anterior end of the zygomatic bone.

Clinical features. Flattening of the upper cheek with tenderness and dimpling of the skin over the zygomatic arch and zygomaticofrontal suture and a fullness of the lower cheek may occur after zygomatic complex fracture. Step defects may be palpated in the zygomaticofrontal area and along the infraorbital rim. Some of the clinical characteristics of a zygomatic fracture may not be apparent much longer than an hour after trauma. Subsequently, they are masked by edema for about a week. In most cases, circumorbital ecchymosis and hemorrhage into the sclera (near the outer canthus) occur. Additional symptoms include unilateral epistaxis (for a short time after the accident), anesthesia or paresthesia of the cheek, and an altered level of the eye. The presence of diplopia suggests a significant injury to the floor of the orbit. Mandibular movement may be limited if the displaced zygomatic bone impinges on the coronoid process.

Radiographic features. Because of edema obscuring the clinical features, the radiographic examination may provide the only means of determining the presence and extent of the injury. The occipitomental (Waters') radiograph provides an image of the whole zygoma and maxillary sinus. The submentovertex projection provides a good view of the zygomatic arch. CT images can provide valuable three-dimensional information.

The zygomatic arch may fracture at its weakest point, about 1 cm posterior to the zygomaticotemporal suture. Separation or fracture of the frontozygomatic suture may occur. Fractures do not usually occur through the zygomaticomaxillary suture, but medially within the thin bone comprising the lateral wall of the antrum. As a result of this type of fracture, in some cases the maxillary antrum may become radiopaque and demonstrate a fluid level resulting from bleeding into the sinus.

Panoramic views of the zygomatic arch often reveal the zygomaticotemporal suture as a radiolucent line, which may even have the appearance of a discontinuity in the inferior border. This is a variation of normal anatomy and should not be misinterpreted as a fracture.

Management. When symptoms include minimal displacement of the zygomatic arch and no cosmetic deformity or impairment of eye movement, no treatment may be required. Otherwise, reduction is usually indicated. Fractures of the arch may be reduced through an intraoral or extraoral approach. If a fractured zygoma is treated within 5 days, the bones frequently snap into place and do not require fixation. When treatment has been delayed more than 5 days, the fragments can usually be reduced, but they do not remain in place. In such delayed treatment cases, the zygoma is fixed in place by elastic traction anchored to a headcap. If treatment of the fracture is delayed for several months, it is almost impossible to reduce, and treatment is not generally undertaken. In this instance, the treatment is focused on the associated structures with the objective of restoring function and appearance.

MONITORING THE HEALING OF FRACTURES

Radiographic examination of the facial bones after trauma is usually necessary to measure the degree of reduction from treatment and to monitor the continued immobilization of the fracture site during repair. The monitoring of fracture repair should include examination of both the alignment of the cortical plates of the involved bone and remodeling and remineralization of the fracture site. During normal healing the fracture line increases in width about 2 weeks after reduction of the fracture. This results from the resorption of the fractured ends and small sequestered fragments of bone. Evidence of remineralization usually occurs 5 to 6 weeks after treatment. Unlike the long bones of the skeleton, rarely is a callus formed in healing jaw fractures. The complete remodeling of the fracture site with obliteration of the fracture line may take several months. On rare occasions, fracture lines may persist for years, even when the patient has made a clinically complete recovery. Possible complications of healing include osteomyelitis of the fracture site, malalignment of the fracture segments, inflammatory lesions related to nonvital teeth near or in the line of the fracture, and nonunion of fractured segments.

SUGGESTED READINGS

Brook IW, Wood N: Aetiology and incidence of facial fractures in adults, *Int J Oral Surg* 12:293, 1983.

Daffner RH: Imaging of facial trauma, *Curr Probl Diagn Radiol* 26:153,1997.

Dingman TM, Natvig AC: *Surgery of facial fractures,* Philadelphia, 1967, WB Saunders.

Gerlock AJ Jr, Sinn DP, McBride KL: *Clinical and radiographic interpretation of facial fractures,* Boston, 1981, Little, Brown.

Hunter JG: Pediatric maxillofacial trauma, *Pediatr Clin North Am* 39:1127,1992.

Kaban LB: Diagnosis and treatment of fractures of the facial bones in children 1943-1993, *J Oral Maxillofac Surg* 51:722, 1993.

Koltai PJ, Rabkin D: Management of facial trauma in children, *Pediatr Clin North Am* 43:1253, 1996.

Laine FJ, Conway WF, Laskin DM: Radiology of maxillofacial trauma, *Curr Probl Diagn Radiol* 22:145,1993.

Matteson SR et al: Advanced imaging methods, *Crit Rev Oral Biol Med* 7:346, 1996.

Matteson S, Tyndall D: Pantomographic radiology: II, pantomography of trauma and inflammation of the jaws, *Dent Radiol Photogr* 56:21, 1982.

Newman J: Medical imaging of facial and mandibular fractures, *Radiol Technol* 69(5):417, 1998.

Shumrick KA: Recent advances and trends in the management of maxillofacial and frontal trauma, *Facial Plast Surg* 9(1):16, 1993.

TRAUMA TO TEETH

Andreasen JO: *Traumatic injuries of the teeth,* Philadelphia, 1981, WB Saunders.

Josell SD, Abrams RG: Traumatic injuries to the dentition and its supporting structures, *Pediatr Clin North Am* 29:717, 1982.

LUXATION

Andreasen JO: Luxation of permanent teeth due to trauma: a clinical and radiographic follow-up study of 189 injured teeth, *Scand J Dent Res* 78:273, 1970.

AVULSION

Lenstrup K, Steiller V: A follow-up study of teeth replanted after accidental loss, *Acta Odont Scand* 17:503, 1959.

TOOTH CROWN FRACTURE

Ravn JJ: Follow-up study of permanent incisors with enamel fractures as a result of acute trauma, *Scand J Dent Res* 89:213, 1981.

Ravn JJ: Follow-up study of permanent incisors with enamel-dentin fracture after acute trauma, *Scand J Dent Res* 89:355, 1981.

Stockton LW, Suzuki M: Management of accidental and iatrogenic injuries to the dentition, *J Can Dent Assoc* 64:378, 1998.

CRACKED TOOTH SYNDROME

Fox K, Youngson CC: Diagnosis and treatment of the cracked tooth, *Prim Dent Care* 4:109, 1997.

Turp JC, Gobetti JP: The cracked tooth syndrome: an elusive diagnosis, *J Am Dent Assoc* 127:1502, 1996.

TOOTH ROOT FRACTURE

Andreasen JO, Hjorting-Hansen E: Intra-alveolar root fractures: radiographic and histologic study of 50 cases, *J Oral Surg* 25:414, 1967.

Bender IB, Freedland JB: Clinical considerations in the diagnosis and treatment of intra-alveolar root fractures, *J Am Dent Assoc* 107:595, 1983.

Hovland EJ: Horizontal root fractures. Treatment and repair, *Dent Clin North Am* 36:509, 1992.

Luebke RG: Vertical crown-root fractures in posterior teeth, *Dent Clin North Am* 28:883, 1984.

Schetritt A, Steffensen B: Diagnosis and management of vertical root fractures, *J Can Dent Assoc* 61:607, 1995.

Schmidt BL, Stern M: Diagnosis and management of root fractures and periodontal ligament injury, *J Calif Dent Assoc* 24:51, 1996.

Walton RE, Michelich RJ, Smith GN: The histopathogenesis of vertical root fractures, *J Endodont* 10:48, 1984.

Wright EF: Diagnosis, treatment, and prevention of incomplete tooth fractures, *Gen Dent* 40:390, 1992.

COMPUTED TOMOGRAPHY OF JAW FRACTURES

Creasman CN et al: Computed tomography versus standard radiography in the assessment of fractures of the mandible, *Ann Plast Surg* 29:109, 1992.

Johnson DH: CT of maxillofacial trauma, *Radiol Clin North Am* 22:131, 1984.

Kassel EE, Noyek AM, Cooper PW: CT in facial trauma, *J Otolaryngol* 12:2, 1983.

Marsh JL et al: In vivo delineation of facial fractures: the application of advanced medical imaging technology, *Ann Plast Surg* 17:364, 1986.

Raustia AM et al: Conventional radiographic and computed tomographic findings in cases of fracture of the mandibular condylar process, *J Oral Maxillofac Surg* 48:1258, 1990.

TRAUMA TO THE MANDIBLE

Bailey BJ, Clark WD: Management of mandibular fractures, *Ear Nose Throat J* 62:371, 1983.

Chayra GA, Meador LR, Laskin DM: Comparison of panoramic and standard radiographs for the diagnosis of mandibular fractures, *J Oral Maxillofac Surg* 44:677, 1986.

Clark WD: Management of mandibular fractures, *Am J Otolaryngol* 13:125, 1992.

Ellis E, Moos KF, El-Attar A: Ten years of mandibular fractures: an analysis of 2,137 cases, *Oral Surg* 59:120, 1985.

Olson RA et al: Fractures of the mandible: a review of 580 cases, *J Oral Maxillofac Surg* 40:23, 1982.

Reiner SA et al: Accurate radiographic evaluation of mandibular fractures, *Arch Otolaryngol Head Neck Surg* 115:1083, 1989.

Winstanley RP: The management of fractures of the mandible, *Br J Oral Maxillofac Surg* 22:170, 1984.

CONDYLAR FRACTURES

Consensus Conference on Open or Closed Management of Condylar Fractures. 12th ICOMS. Budapest, 1995, *Int J Oral Maxillofac Surg* 27:243, 1998.

Dahlstrauom L, Kahnberg KE, Lindahl L: 15 year follow-up on condylar fractures, *Int J Oral Maxillofac Surg* 18:18, 1989.

Dimitroulis G: Condylar injuries in growing patients, *Aust Dent J* 42:367, 1997.

Hall MB: Condylar fractures: surgical management, *J Oral Maxillofac Surg* 52:1189, 1994.

Hayward JR, Scott RF: Fractures of the mandibular condyle, *J Oral Maxillofac Surg* 51:57, 1993.

Sahm G, Witt E: Long-term results after childhood condylar fractures: a computer-tomographic study, *Eur J Orthod* 11:154, 1989.

Silvennoinen U et al: Different patterns of condylar fractures: an analysis of 382 patients in a 3-year period, *J Oral Maxillofac Surg* 50:1032, 1992.

Walker RV: Condylar fractures: nonsurgical management, *J Oral Maxillofac Surg* 52:1185, 1994.

FRACTURES OF THE ALVEOLAR PROCESS

Andreasen JO: Fractures of the alveolar process of the jaw: a clinical and radiographic follow-up study, *Scand J Dent Res* 78:263, 1970.

TRAUMA TO THE MAXILLA

Banks P: *Kiley's fractures of the middle third of the facial skeleton*, Bristol, UK, 1981, Wright.

Close LG: Fractures of the maxilla, *Ear Nose Throat J* 62:365, 1983.

Harris JH et al: An approach to mid-facial fractures, *CRC Crit Rev Diagn Imaging* 21:105, 1984.

Luce EA: Developing concepts and treatment of complex maxillary fractures, *Clin Plast Surg* 19:125, 1992.

Marciani RD: Management of midface fractures: fifty years later, *J Oral Maxillofac Surg* 51:960, 1993.

Teichgraeber JF, Rappaport NJ, Harris JH Jr: The radiology of upper airway obstruction in maxillofacial trauma, *Ann Plast Surg* 27:103, 1991.

Tung TC et al: Dislocation of anatomic structures into the maxillary sinus after craniofacial trauma, *Plast Reconstr Surg* 101:1904, 1998.

ZYGOMATIC COMPLEX FRACTURES

Fujii N: Classification of malar complex fractures using computed tomography, *J Oral Maxillofac Surg* 41: 562, 1983.

McLoughlin P, Gilhooly M, Wood G: The management of zygomatic complex fractures—results of a survey, *Br J Oral Maxillofac Surg* 32:284, 1994.

Prendergast ML, Wildes TO: Evaluation of the orbital floor in zygoma fractures, *Arch Otolaryngol Head Neck Surg* 114:446, 1988.

Sands T et al: Fractures of the zygomatic complex: a case report and review, *J Can Dent Assoc* 59:749, 1993.

Winstanley RP: The management of fractures of the zygoma, *Int J Oral Surg* 10(suppl 1):235, 1981.

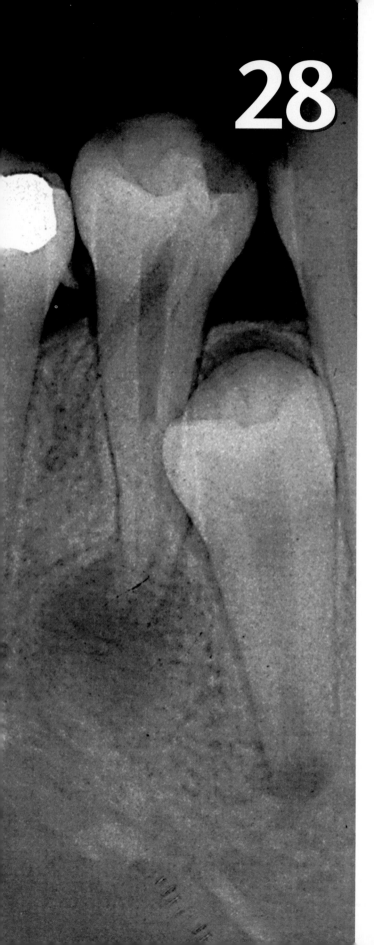

28 Developmental Disturbances of the Face and Jaws

In this chapter the term *"developmental"* indicates the process of growth and differentiation of the craniofacial structures. Disturbances may result in various morphogenic abnormalities, including the following:

- Abnormalities in the structure and shape of hard and soft tissues
- Abnormalities in the quantity and organization of structures and tissues
- Abnormalities in the function of structures (e.g., the temporomandibular joint) and tissues

Often the etiology of these developmental disturbances is poorly understood, but the list of possible agents includes genetic abnormalities, teratogenic agents (e.g., alcohol), and the environmental conditions of the developing embryo. The list of deviations in morphology and related syndromes is extensive. This chapter briefly reviews only the more common developmental abnormalities.

Cleidocranial Dysplasia

SYNONYM

Cleidocranial dysostosis

DEFINITION

Cleidocranial dysplasia is a developmental anomaly of the skeleton and teeth. It can be inherited as an autosomal dominant characteristic in either gender, or it can appear spontaneously.

CLINICAL FEATURES

Cleidocranial dysplasia primarily affects the skull, clavicles, and dentition. The face appears small in contrast to the cranium. This is the result of hypoplasia of the maxilla, a brachycephalic skull (reduced anteroposterior dimension with increased skull width), and the presence of frontal and parietal bossing. The bridge of the nose may be broad and depressed, and hypertelorism (excessive distance between the eyes) is present. The absence of clavicles allows excessive mobility of the shoulder girdle (Fig. 28-1).

Characteristically, patients with cleidocranial dysplasia show prolonged retention of the primary dentition and delayed eruption of the permanent dentition. Extraction of primary teeth does not stimulate eruption of underlying permanent teeth. A study of teeth from patients

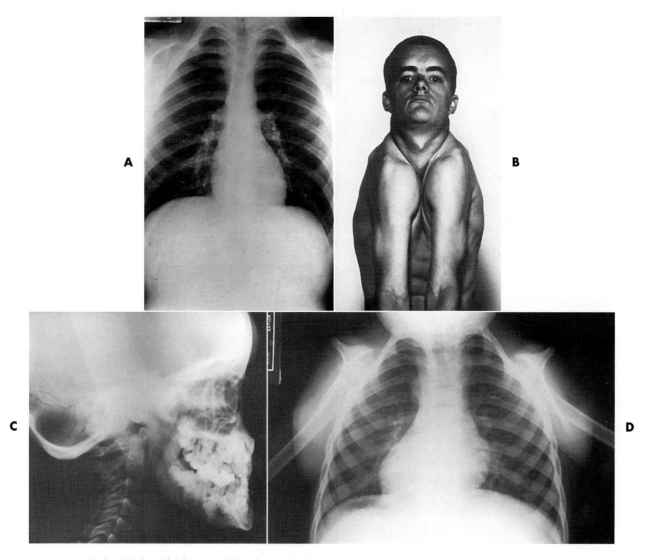

FIG. **28-1** *Cleidocranial dysplasia.* **A,** Chest radiograph; note the absence of clavicles. **B,** The result is excessive mobility of the shoulders. Note also the frontal bossing and underdeveloped maxilla. **C,** On a lateral radiograph, note the wormian (sutural) bones in the occipital region and the supernumerary teeth. **D,** Chest of a 5-year-old boy showing absence of the clavicles. (**D** courtesy Department of Radiology, Baylor University Hospital, Dallas, Tex.)

589

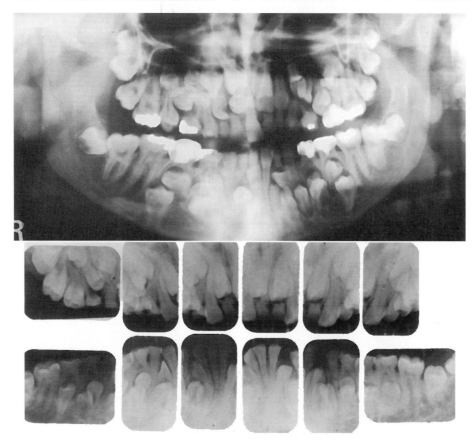

FIG. **28-2** Cleidocranial dysplasia results in prolonged retention of the primary dentition and multiple unerupted supernumerary teeth.

with cleidocranial dysplasia revealed a paucity or complete absence of cellular cementum on both erupted and unerupted teeth. Often unerupted supernumerary teeth are present, and considerable crowding and disorganization of the developing permanent dentition may occur.

RADIOGRAPHIC FEATURES

General Radiographic Features
The characteristic skull findings are brachycephaly, delayed or failed closure of the fontanels, open skull sutures, and multiple wormian bones (small, irregular bones in the sutures of the skull that are formed by secondary centers of ossification in the suture lines). In the most severe cases, very little formation of the parietal and frontal bones may occur. Typically the clavicles are underdeveloped to varying degrees and, in approximately 10% of cases, they are completely absent. Other bones also may be affected, including the long bones, vertebral column, pelvis, and bones of the hands and feet.

Radiographic Features of the Jaws
The maxilla and paranasal sinuses characteristically are underdeveloped, resulting in maxillary micrognathia. The mandible is not involved.

Radiographic Features Associated with the Teeth
Characteristic features include prolonged retention of the primary dentition and multiple unerupted supernumerary teeth (Fig. 28-2). The number of supernumerary teeth varies; as many as 63 have been reported. The unerupted teeth develop most commonly in the anterior maxilla and bicuspid regions of the jaws. Many resemble bicuspids, and these unerupted teeth may develop dentigerous cysts.

DIFFERENTIAL DIAGNOSIS

Cleidocranial dysplasia may be identified by the family history, excessive mobility of the shoulders, clinical examination of the skull, and pathognomonic radiographic findings of prolonged retention of the primary teeth with multiple unerupted supernumerary teeth.

MANAGEMENT

Care in cleidocranial dysplasia is directed toward retention of the erupted primary teeth.

Craniofacial Dysostosis

SYNONYMS

Crouzon syndrome and *Crouzon's disease*

DEFINITION

Craniofacial dysostosis (Crouzon's disease) is a developmental anomaly transmitted as an autosomal dominant condition with variable expression. Of these cases, 33% to 56% may be spontaneous mutations. In patients with Crouzon's disease, all cranial sutures close early (cranial synostosis); this results in various skull malformations caused by increased intracranial pressure.

CLINICAL FEATURES

Patients characteristically have frontal bossing, hypertelorism, and exophthalmos (protruding eyes). They may become blind as a result of early suture closure and increased intracranial pressure. The nose often is prominent and pointed. The maxilla frequently is narrow, has a high vault, and is underdeveloped, resulting in crowding of the dentition.

RADIOGRAPHIC FEATURES

General Radiographic Features

A skull examination reveals the absence of sutures. Prominent cranial markings are noted, the result of increased intracranial pressure from the brain. These markings may be seen as multiple radiolucencies appearing as depressions (digital impressions) of the inner surface of the cranial vault, which results in a beaten metal appearance (Fig. 28-3).

Radiographic Features of the Jaws

The maxilla is hypoplastic; no changes are seen in the mandible.

DIFFERENTIAL DIAGNOSIS

Skull radiographs that show definite and widespread digital impressions and premature synostosis suggest craniofacial dysostosis. However, this condition must be differentiated from others that also involve craniosynostosis.

MANAGEMENT

Although many patients have progressive impairment and some have mental retardation, they have normal life spans. Consequently, maxillofacial surgery may be considered for correction of facial deformity, and neurosurgery may be performed to treat the progressive visual complications and open the sutures.

Mandibulofacial Dysostosis

SYNONYM

Treacher Collins syndrome

DEFINITION

Mandibulofacial dysostosis is a developmental anomaly that can be inherited as an autosomal dominant trait with variable expressivity, although at least half of these cases arise as spontaneous mutations.

CLINICAL FEATURES

Individuals with mandibulofacial dysostosis often show a wide range of anomalies, depending on the severity of the condition. The most common clinical findings are relative underdevelopment of the zygomatic bones, resulting in a narrow face; a downward inclination of the palpebral fissures; underdevelopment of the mandible, resulting in a downturned, wide mouth; malformation of the external ears; absence of the external auditory canal; and occasional facial clefts (Fig. 28-4). The palate develops with a high arch or cleft in 30% of cases. Hypoplasia and a steep mandibular angle may give the patient an anterior open bite. Maldevelopment of the external ear and auditory canal may result in partial or complete deafness.

RADIOGRAPHIC FEATURES

General Radiographic Features

A striking finding is the diminished size of the zygomatic bones. The auditory canal, mastoid air cells, and articular eminence often are smaller than normal or absent.

Radiographic Features of the Jaws

The mandible is hypoplastic, showing accentuation of the antegonial notch and a steep mandibular angle, which gives the impression that the mandible is bending in an inferior and posterior direction (see Fig. 28-4). The condyles are positioned posteriorly and inferiorly. The maxillary sinuses may be underdeveloped or absent.

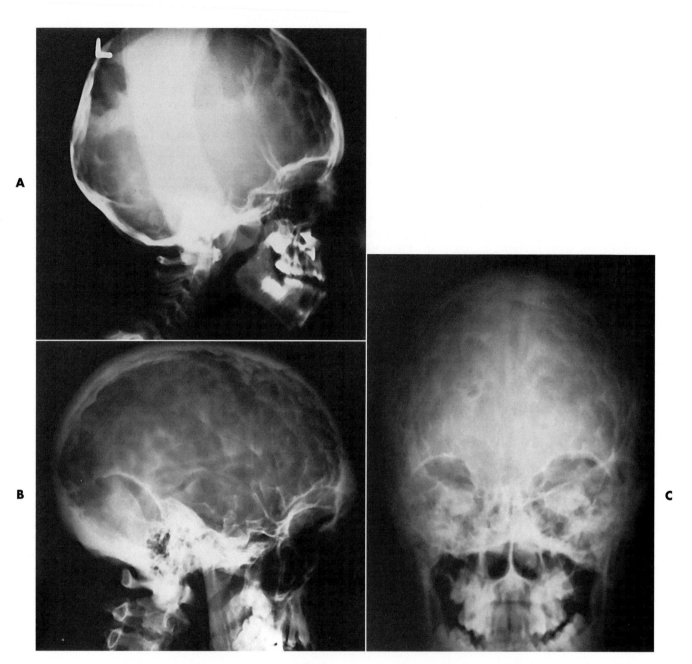

FIG. **28-3**   **A,** Craniofacial dysostosis results in early closure of the cranial sutures and depressions (digital impressions) on the inner surface of the calvarium from growth of the brain. **B** and **C,** Closure of the cranial sutures in another patient. Note also the prominent digital markings. (**B** and **C** courtesy Department of Radiology, Baylor University Hospital, Dallas, Tex.)

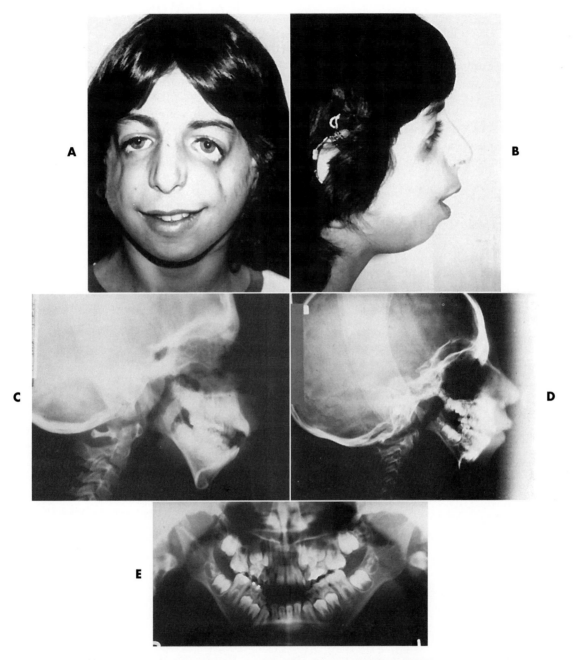

FIG. **28-4** **A** and **B,** Mandibulofacial dysostosis. Note the characteristic facies: downward-sloping palpebral fissures, colobomas of the outer third of the lower lids, depressed cheek-bones, receding chin, little if any nasofrontal angle, and a nose that appears relatively large. **C** to **E,** Correlation of radiographic features with clinical features: short mandibular rami, steep mandibular angle, and an anterior open bite. The zygomas are poorly formed.

DIFFERENTIAL DIAGNOSIS

Other disorders that may result in severe hypoplasia of the entire mandible include Hallermann-Streiff syndrome, Pierre Robin syndrome, and condylar agenesis.

MANAGEMENT

Growth of the facial bones during adolescence results in some cosmetic improvement. Surgical intervention may also be used to improve the osseous and ear defects.

Hemifacial Hypertrophy

DEFINITION

Hemifacial hypertrophy is a condition in which half of the face, including the jaws, alone or in concert with other parts of the body, grows to unusual proportions. The cause of this condition is unknown, but it seems unlikely that heredity plays a part.

CLINICAL FEATURES

Hemifacial hypertrophy begins during youth, sometimes at birth, and usually continues throughout the growing years. It often occurs with other abnormalities, including mental deficiency, skin abnormalities, compensatory scoliosis, genitourinary tract anomalies, and various neoplasms, including Wilms' tumor of the kidney, adrenocortical tumor, and hepatoblastoma. Females and males are affected with approximately equal frequency. The dentition of affected individuals may show unilateral enlargement and accelerated development. Primary teeth usually are shed prematurely. The tongue and alveolar bone enlarge on the involved side.

RADIOGRAPHIC FEATURES

Radiographic examination of the skulls of these patients reveals, on the affected side, enlargement of the bones, including the mandible (Fig. 28-5), maxilla, zygoma, and frontal and temporal bones.

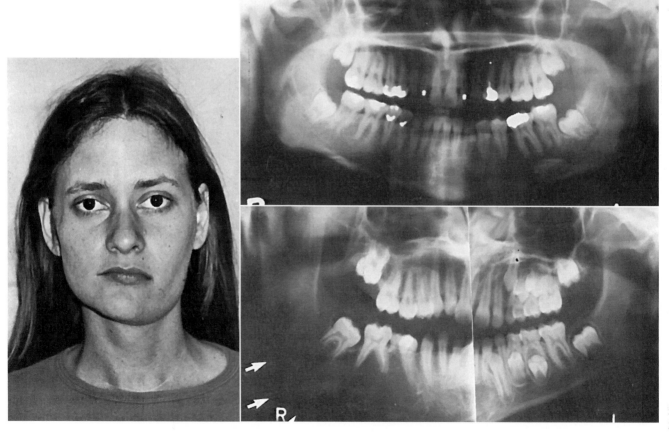

FIG. **28-5 A** and **B,** Hemifacial hypertrophy, revealing enlargement of the left mandible and maxilla. **C,** In a different example, note the marked enlargement of the right maxilla and mandible and the accelerated development of the dentition on that side.

DIFFERENTIAL DIAGNOSIS

The differential diagnosis should consider hemifacial hypoplasia (of the opposite side), arteriovenous aneurysms, hemangioma, and congenital lymphedema. Also, severe condylar hyperplasia that may involve half of the mandible should be considered (see Chapter 24). The presence of enlarged teeth and the rapid eruption of the dentition suggest hemifacial hypertrophy.

Segmental Odontomaxillary Dysplasia

SYNONYM

Hemimaxillofacial dysplasia

DEFINITION

Segmental odontomaxillary dysplasia is a developmental abnormality of unknown etiology that affects the posterior alveolar process of one side of one maxilla, including the teeth and attached gingiva.

CLINICAL FEATURES

The abnormality is always unilateral and results in enlargement of the alveolar process, gingiva, and teeth. Frequently teeth are missing (most commonly the bicuspids), and some of the teeth that remain are unerupted. Unilateral hypertrichosis and facial enlargement have been reported in a few cases.

RADIOGRAPHIC FEATURES

The density of the maxillary alveolar process is increased, with a greater number of thick trabeculae that appear to be aligned in a vertical orientation (Fig. 28-6). The roots of the deciduous teeth are larger than on the unaffected side and usually are splayed in shape. The crowns of the deciduous teeth and sometimes the permanent teeth are enlarged. Enlargement of pulp chambers and irregular resorption of the roots of de-

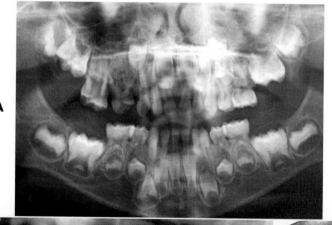

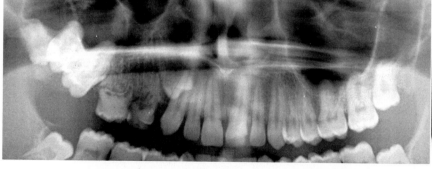

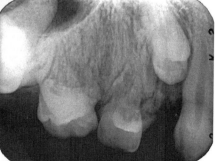

FIG. **28-6** **A,** A panoramic view of segmental odontomaxillary dysplasia. Note the large left maxillary deciduous molars compared with the right side and the lack of formation of the bicuspids, delayed eruption of the first molar, and the dense bone pattern of the left maxillary alveolar process. **B** and **C,** A second case demonstrating the coarse trabecular pattern of the right maxillary alveolar process and delayed eruption of the maxillary right first bicuspid and molars.

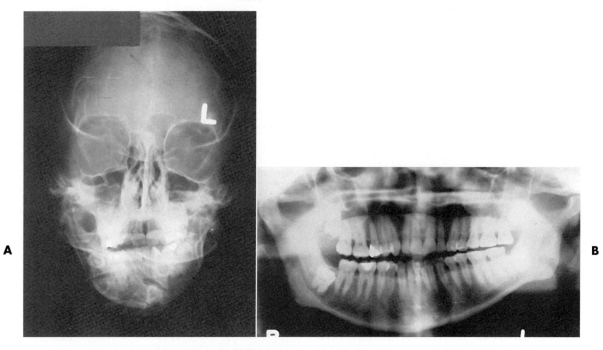

FIG. **28-7**   **A** and **B,** Hemifacial hypoplasia, showing reduced size of the left maxilla and mandible.

ciduous teeth also may be seen. The maxillary sinus does not pneumatize the alveolar process and thus appears smaller than on the contralateral side.

Hemifacial Hypoplasia

SYNONYMS

Hemifacial microsomia, lateral facial dysplasia, and *Goldenhar's syndrome*

DEFINITION

Patients with hemifacial hypoplasia display reduced growth of half of the face. This condition most commonly is unilateral but occasionally may involve both sides. When the whole side of the face is involved, the mandible, maxilla, zygoma, external and middle ear, parotid gland, fifth and seventh cranial nerves, musculature, and other soft tissues are diminished in size. Most cases occur spontaneously, but familial cases have been reported. The disorder does not appear to have a gender predilection.

CLINICAL FEATURES

Hemifacial hypoplasia usually begins early in life. Patients with this condition have a striking appearance caused by progressive failure of the affected side to grow,

which gives the involved side of the face a reduced dimension. In addition, aplasia or hypoplasia of the external ear (crumpled, distorted pinna) is common, and the ear canal often is missing. In some patients the skull is diminished in size. In about 90% of cases, malocclusion is present on the affected side.

RADIOGRAPHIC FEATURES

The primary radiographic finding is a reduction in the size of the bones on the affected side. This change is clearest in the mandible, which may show a reduction in the size of or, in severe cases, lack of any development of the condyle, coronoid process, or ramus. The body is reduced in size, and a portion of the distal aspect may be missing (Fig. 28-7). The dentition on the affected side may show a reduction in the number or size of the teeth. CT examination shows a reduction in the size of the muscles of mastication.

DIFFERENTIAL DIAGNOSIS

The changes of hemifacial hypoplasia are very characteristic. Condylar hypoplasia, especially that caused by a fracture at birth or by juvenile arthrosis (Boering's arthrosis), may be similar, but it does not produce the ear changes (see Chapter 24). Exposure of the face of a child to radiation therapy during growth also may result in underdevelopment of the irradiated tissues.

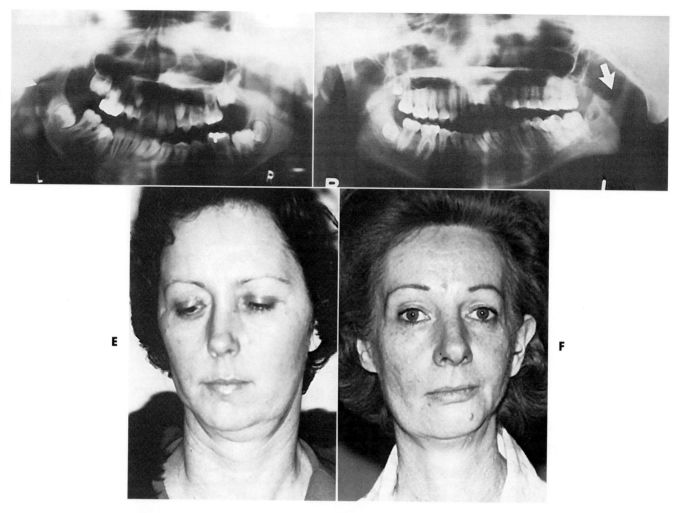

FIG. **28-7, cont'd   C,** Lack of formation of most of the right ramus and all of the condyle and coronoid process. **D,** Severe hypoplasia of the left ramus, condyle, and coronoid process *(arrow).* **E** and **F,** Two women with hemifacial hypoplasia. (**E** and **F** courtesy Department of Oral Diagnosis, Baylor College of Dentistry, Dallas, Tex.)

MANAGEMENT

Orthodontic intervention may correct or prevent malocclusion. Also, the ear and mandibular abnormalities may be repaired by plastic surgery. The hearing loss may be partly corrected by hearing aids or possibly by surgery.

Hyperplasia of the Maxillary Tuberosity

DEFINITION

Hyperplasia of the maxillary tuberosity is a condition in which each maxillary tuberosity is excessively enlarged. The cause of this condition is currently unknown. A genetic influence has not been established.

CLINICAL FEATURES

Hyperplasia of the maxillary tuberosity results in bilateral enlargement of the maxillary tuberosities, a situation easily identified by clinical examination. The condition develops in adults and may result in difficulty with dentures and normal mastication.

RADIOGRAPHIC FEATURES

Radiographs show bilaterally enlarged maxillary tuberosities (Fig. 28-8). Bone density may be increased, but the bone pattern is normal.

DIFFERENTIAL DIAGNOSIS

The differential diagnosis includes bilateral enlargement caused by florid osseous dysplasia (see Chapter 22).

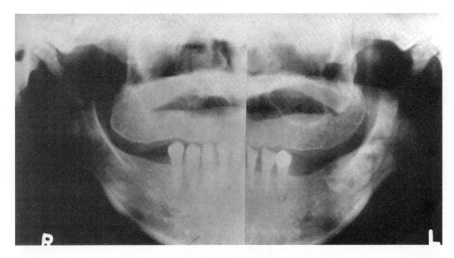

FIG. **28-8** Hyperplasia of the maxillary tuberosities, revealed as opaque bony enlargements of these regions of the maxilla.

MANAGEMENT

When treatment is required, surgical reduction may be considered.

Developmental Salivary Gland Defect

SYNONYMS

Stafne defect, Stafne bone cyst, static bone cavity, and *latent bone cyst*

DEFINITION

A developmental salivary gland defect of the mandible is the development of a deep, well-defined depression in the lingual surface of the posterior body of the mandible. More precisely, the most common location is within the submandibular gland fossa and often close to the inferior border of the mandible. In developmental bone defects investigated surgically, an aberrant lobe of the submandibular gland extends into the bony depression. The etiology remains unknown, but the condition is a developmental anomaly that has been documented to develop in patients as old as 30 years and as young as 11 years.

CLINICAL FEATURES

Developmental salivary gland defects are relatively rare, with an incidence of about 4 in every 1000 adults. They are asymptomatic and next to impossible to palpate, generally discovered only during radiographic exami-nation of the area. More cases have been reported in men than in women.

RADIOGRAPHIC FEATURES

A developmental salivary gland defect is a round, ovoid, or, occasionally, lobulated radiolucency that ranges in diameter from 1 to 3 cm (Fig. 28-9). The defect is located below the inferior alveolar nerve canal and anterior to the angle of mandible, in the region of the antegonial notch. Rare examples are located in the apical region of the mandibular premolars or cuspids and are related to the sublingual gland fossa. The margins of the radiolucent defect are well defined by a dense radiopaque line. This cortical margin usually is thicker on the superior aspect. This appearance is the result of the x-rays passing tangentially through the relatively thick walls of the depression. The lesion may involve the inferior border of the mandible. Computed tomography (CT) images commonly reveal tissue of fat density within the defect (Fig. 28-10).

DIFFERENTIAL DIAGNOSIS

The appearance and location of the radiographic image of this developmental bone defect are characteristic and easily identified. Developmental salivary gland defects can be readily differentiated from odontogenic lesions such as cysts because the epicenter of odontogenic lesions is located above the inferior alveolar canal. However, when the defect is related to the sublingual gland and appears above the canal, odontogenic lesions should be considered in the differential diagnosis.

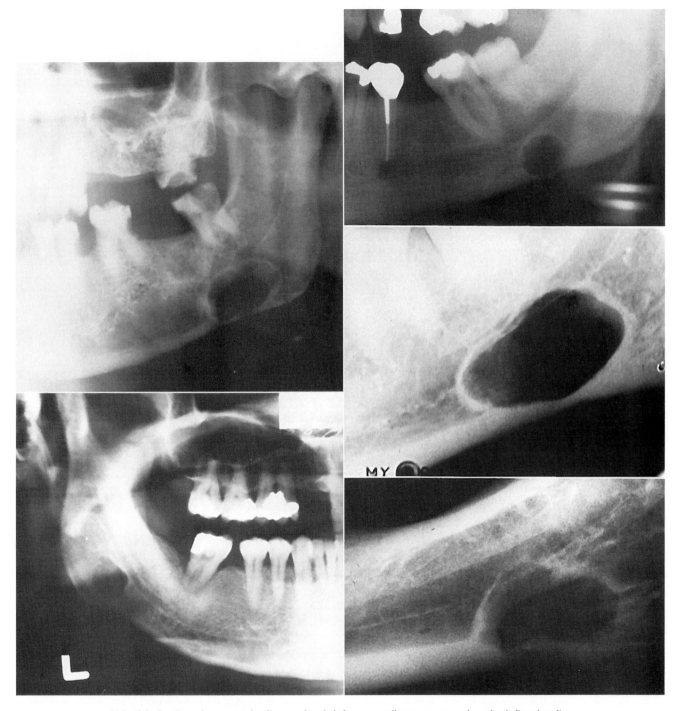

FIG. **28-9** Developmental salivary gland defects usually are seen as sharply defined radiolucencies beneath the mandibular canal in the region of the submandibular gland fossa. These defects can erode the inferior border of the mandible.

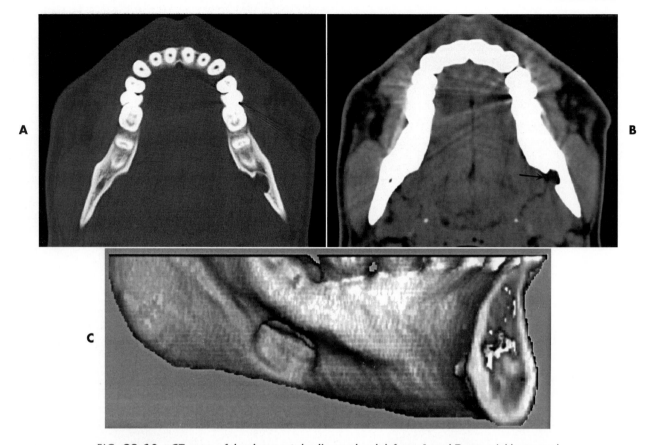

FIG. **28-10** *CT scans of developmental salivary gland defects.* **A** and **B** are axial bone and soft tissue windows of the same case. Note the well-defined defect extending from the medial surface of the mandible and the corresponding soft tissue image, which shows radiolucent tissue within the defect that has the density equivalent of fat tissue *(arrow).* **C,** A three-dimensional, reformatted CT image revealing a defect extending from the medial surface of the mandible.

MANAGEMENT

Recognition of the lesion should preclude any treatment or surgical exploration or the need for advanced imaging such as CT. The defect may increase in size with time. There are rare reports of salivary gland neoplasms developing in the soft tissue within the defect. Destruction of the well-defined cortex of the defect may indicate the presence of a neoplasm.

Cleft Palate

DEFINITION

A failure of fusion of the developmental processes of the face during embryonic life may result in a variety of facial clefts. The most prevalent of these conditions are cleft lip with cleft palate and isolated cleft lip or cleft palate. The overall incidence of cleft lip and cleft palate is about 1 per 1000 live births. The causes of facial clefts are not fully understood, but hereditary factors are considered to be most important. Other factors that have received considerable attention include nutritional disturbances; environmental teratogenic agents; stress, which results in increased secretion of hydrocortisone; defects of vascular supply to the involved region; and mechanical interference with the closure of the embryonic processes. Clefts involving the lower lip and mandible are extremely rare.

CLINICAL FEATURES

The disorder shows gender differences in the frequency of occurrence, but these differences vary among races. Clefts of the lip may be either a unilateral or bilateral condition. Bilateral cleft lip is more prevalent, and when unilateral, the left side is more frequently involved. The

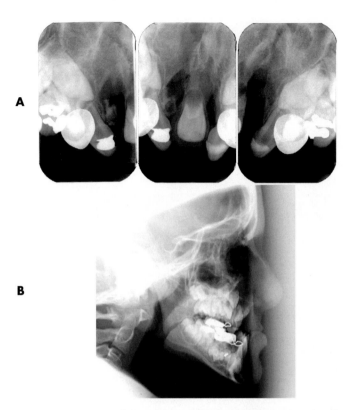

FIG. **28-11** Cleft palate results in defects in the alveolar ridge and abnormalities of the dentition. **A,** Bilateral clefts of the maxilla in the lateral incisor regions and defects of the dentition. **B,** Lateral cephalometric view showing underdevelopment of the maxilla.

cleft may extend just through the lip or may extend up into the nostril. Bilateral cleft lip is more frequently associated with cleft palate. Clefts of the palate may also vary in severity, involving only the uvula or soft palate or extending all the way through the palate and including the alveolar ridge on one or both sides. Defects in the alveolar ridge usually occur near the maxillary lateral incisor. The palatal defect may result in impaired speech.

RADIOGRAPHIC FEATURES

The radiographic appearance of this cleft is a well-defined vertical radiolucent defect in the alveolar bone as well as numerous dental anomalies (Fig. 28-11). These may include the absence of the maxillary lateral incisor and the presence of supernumerary teeth in this region. Often the involved teeth are malformed and poorly positioned. In patients with cleft lip and palate, a mild delay in the development of maxillary and mandibular teeth may occur. Affected children of both genders also have an increased incidence of hypodontia in both arches.

MANAGEMENT

Management of these defects is complex, requiring the coordinated efforts of a surgeon, orthodontist, dentist, speech therapist, and occasionally a psychologist.

Focal Osteoporotic Bone Marrow

SYNONYM

Marrow space

DEFINITION

Focal osteoporotic bone marrow is a radiologic term indicating the presence of radiolucent defects within the cancellous portion of the jaws. Histologic examination reveals normal areas of hematopoietic or fatty marrow. The etiology is unknown but has been postulated to be (1) bone marrow hyperplasia, (2) persistent embryologic marrow remnants, or (3) sites of abnormal healing following extraction, trauma, or local inflammation. This entity is a variation of normal anatomy.

CLINICAL FEATURES

Focal osteoporotic bone marrow defects are usually clinically asymptomatic and are commonly an incidental radiographic finding. These marrow spaces are more common in middle-aged women.

RADIOGRAPHIC FEATURES

A common site for focal osteoporotic bone marrow is the mandibular molar-premolar region. Other sites include the maxillary tuberosity region, mandibular retromolar area, edentulous locations, occasionally the furcation region of mandibular molars, and rarely near the apex of teeth. The radiographic appearance of focal osteoporotic bone marrow space is quite variable. The internal aspect is radiolucent because of the presence of fewer trabeculae in comparison with the surrounding bone. The periphery may be ill-defined and blending or may appear to be corticated. The immediate surrounding bone is normal without any sign of a bone reaction (Fig. 28-12).

DIFFERENTIAL DIAGNOSIS

A small simple bone cyst may have a similar appearance because there is usually no bone reaction at the periphery of a simple bone cyst. When the osteoporotic bone marrow occurs in the furcation region or at the apex of

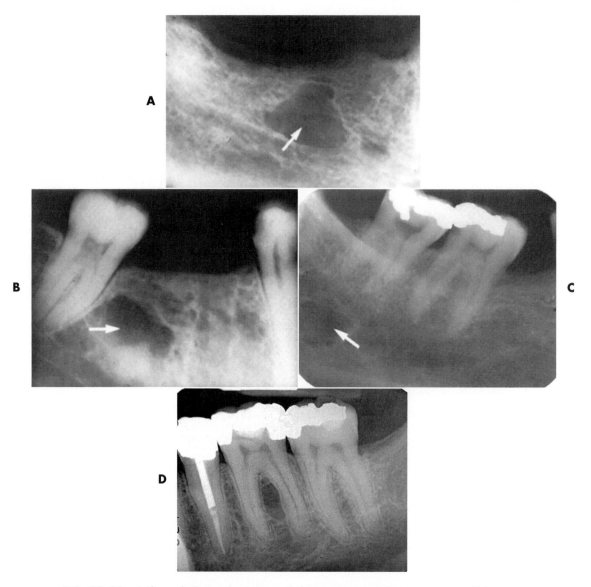

FIG. **28-12** **A** through **C,** Focal osteoporotic bone marrow defect, seen as a radiolucency *(arrow)*. A few internal trabeculae may be present, and the periphery varies from well defined to ill defined. **D,** An example located in the furcation of a mandibular first molar. Note that the periodontal ligament space and lamina dura are intact.

a tooth, the differential diagnosis includes the presence of an inflammatory lesion. If the area is normal bone marrow, the lamina dura should be intact. Very early inflammatory lesions that have not yet stimulated a visible osteoblastic response may appear similar.

MANAGEMENT

No treatment is required for the osteoporotic bone marrow space. When doubt exists about the true nature of the radiolucency, a longitudinal study with films at 3-month intervals may be prescribed. The marrow space should not increase in size.

SUGGESTED READINGS

Elmslie FV, Reardon W: Craniofacial developmental abnormalities, *Curr Opin Neurol* 11:103, 1998.

Friede H: Abnormal craniofacial growth, *Acta Odontol Scand* 53:203, 1995.

Goodman RM, Gorlin RJ: *Atlas of the face in genetic disorders,* ed 2, St Louis, 1977, Mosby.

Gorlin RJ et al: *Syndromes of the head and neck,* ed 3, New York, 1990, Oxford University Press.

Shafer WG et al: *Oral pathology,* ed 4, Philadelphia, 1983, WB Saunders.

Worth HM: *Principles and practice of oral radiologic interpretation,* Chicago, 1963, Year Book.

Zarb GA et al: *Temporomandibular joint and masticatory muscle disorders,* Copenhagen, 1994, Munksgaard.

CLEIDOCRANIAL DYSPLASIA

Ishii K et al: Characteristics of jaw growth in cleidocranial dysplasia, *Cleft Palate Craniofac J* 35:161, 1998.

Jensen BL, Kreiborg S: Craniofacial growth in cleidocranial dysplasia: a roentgencephalometric study, *J Craniofac Genet Dev Biol* 15:35, 1995.

Jensen BL, Kreiborg S: Development of the dentition in cleidocranial dysplasia, *J Oral Pathol Med* 19:89, 1990.

Rushton MA: Anomaly of cementum in cleidocranial dysostosis, *Br Dent J* 100:81, 1956.

Seow WK, Hertzberg J: Dental development and molar root length in children with cleidocranial dysplasia, *Pediatr Dent* 17:101, 1995.

Yamamoto H et al: Cleidocranial dysplasia: a light microscope, electron microscope, and crystallographic study, *Oral Surg Oral Med Oral Pathol* 68:195, 1989.

CRANIOFACIAL DYSOSTOSIS

Bruce DA: Consensus: craniofacial synostoses: Apert and Crouzon syndromes, *Childs Nerv Syst* 12:734, 1996.

MANDIBULOFACIAL DYSOSTOSIS

Dixon MJ: Treacher Collins syndrome, *J Med Genet* 32:806, 1995.

Herman TE, Siegel MJ: Special imaging casebook: Treacher Collins syndrome, *J Perinatol* 16:413, 1996.

Marres HA et al: The Treacher Collins syndrome: a clinical, radiological, and genetic linkage study on two pedigrees, *Arch Otolaryngol Head Neck Surg* 121:509, 1995.

Posnick JC: Treacher Collins syndrome: perspectives in evaluation and treatment, *J Oral Maxillofac Surg* 55:1120, 1997.

HEMIFACIAL HYPERTROPHY

Fraumeni JF et al: Wilms' tumor and congenital hemihypertrophy: report of five new cases and review of the literature, *Pediatrics* 40:886, 1967.

Ringrose RE et al: Hemihypertrophy, *Pediatrics* 36:434, 1965.

Rowe NH: Hemifacial hypertrophy: review of the literature and addition of four cases, *Oral Surg* 15:572, 1962.

SEGMENTAL ODONTOMAXILLARY DYSPLASIA

Danforth RA et al: Segmental odontomaxillary dysplasia: report of eight cases and comparison with hemimaxillofacial dysplasia, *Oral Surg Oral Med Oral Pathol* 70:81, 1990.

DeSalvo MS et al: Segmental odontomaxillary dysplasia (hemimaxillofacial dysplasia): case report, *Pediatr Dent* 18:154, 1996.

Miles DA et al: Hemimaxillofacial dysplasia: a newly recognized disorder of facial asymmetry, hypertrichosis of the facial skin, unilateral enlargement of the maxilla, and hypoplastic teeth in two patients, *Oral Surg Oral Med Oral Pathol* 64:445, 1987.

Packota GV et al: Radiographic features of segmental odontomaxillary dysplasia: a study of 12 cases, *Oral Surg Oral Med Oral Pathol Oral Radiol Endod* 82:577, 1996.

HEMIFACIAL HYPOPLASIA

Figueroa AA, Fields H: Craniovertebral malformation in hemifacial microsomia, *J Cranio Genet Dev Biol* 1(suppl):167, 1985.

Finegold M: Hemifacial microsomia. In Bergsma D, editor: *Birth defects compendium,* ed 2, New York, 1973, Alan R Liss.

Marsh JL et al: Facial musculoskeletal asymmetry in hemifacial microsomia, *Cleft Palate J* 26:292, 1989.

Mazzeo N et al: Progressive hemifacial atrophy (Parry-Romberg syndrome): case report, *Oral Surg Oral Med Oral Pathol Oral Radiol Endod* 79:30, 1995.

DEVELOPMENTAL SALIVARY GLAND DEFECT

Hansson L: Development of a lingual mandibular bone cavity in an 11-year-old boy, *Oral Surg* 49:376, 1980.

Karmiol M, Walsh R: Incidence of static bone defect of the mandible, *Oral Surg* 26:225, 1968.

Parvizi F, Rout PG: An ossifying fibroma presenting as Stafne's idiopathic bone cavity, *Dentomaxillofac Radiol* 26(6):361, 1997.

Tolman DE, Stafne EC: Developmental bone defects of the mandible, *Oral Surg* 24:488, 1967.

CLEFT PALATE

Brouwers HJ, Kuijpers-Jagtman AM: Development of permanent tooth length in patients with unilateral cleft lip and palate, *Am J Orthod Dentofacial Orthop* 99:543, 1991.

Derijcke A et al: The incidence of oral clefts: a review, *Br J Oral Maxillofac Surg* 34:488, 1996.

Habel A et al: Management of cleft lip and palate, *Arch Dis Child* 74:360, 1996.

Harris EF, Hullings JG: Delayed dental development in children with isolated cleft lip and palate, *Arch Oral Biol* 35:469, 1990.

Hibbert SA, Field JK: Molecular basis of familial cleft lip and palate, *Oral Dis* 2:238, 1996.

Koch H et al: Cleft malformation of lip, alveolus, hard and soft palate, and nose (LAHSN): a critical view of the terminology, the diagnosis and gradation as a basis for documentation and therapy, *Br J Oral Maxillofac Surg* 33:51, 1995.

Smahel Z, Mullerova Z: Craniofacial growth and development in unilateral cleft lip and palate: clinical implications (a review), *Acta Chir Plast* 37:29, 1995.

Wyszynski DF et al: Genetics of nonsyndromic oral clefts revisited, *Cleft Palate Craniofac J* 33:406, 1996.

FOCAL OSTEOPOROTIC BONE MARROW

Barker B et al: Focal osteoporotic bone marrow defects of the jaws, *Oral Surg* 38:404, 1974.

Crawford B, Weathers D: Osteoporotic marrow defects of the jaws, *J Oral Surg* 28:600, 1970.

Schneider LC et al: Osteoporotic bone marrow defect: radiographic features and pathogenic factors, *Oral Surg* 65:127, 1988.

Standish S, Shafer W: Focal osteoporotic bone marrow defects of the jaws, *J Oral Surg* 20:123, 1997.

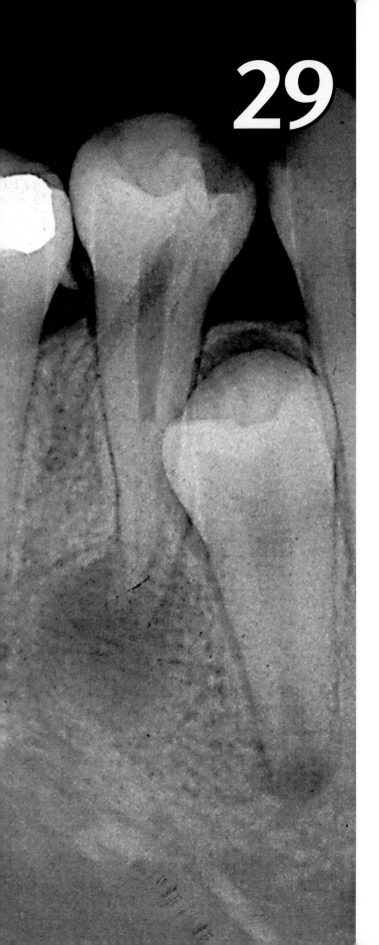

29 Salivary Gland Radiology

BYRON W. BENSON

Definition of Salivary Gland Disease

Dental diagnosticians are responsible for detecting disorders of the salivary glands. A familiarity with salivary gland disorders and applicable current imaging techniques is an essential element of the clinician's armamentarium. Both major and minor salivary glands may be involved pathologically; however, this chapter deals primarily with the major glands. Salivary gland disease processes may be divided into the following clinical categories: inflammatory disorders, non-inflammatory disorders, and space-occupying masses. Inflammatory disorders are acute or chronic and may be secondary to ductal obstruction by sialoliths, trauma, infection, or space-occupying lesions such as neoplasia. Noninflammatory disorders are metabolic and secretory abnormalities associated with diseases of nearly all the endocrine glands, malnutrition, and neurologic disorders. Space-occupying masses are cystic or neoplastic; the neoplasms are benign or malignant.

Clinical Signs and Symptoms

Diseases of the major salivary glands may have single or multiple clinical features. Unilateral or bilateral swellings in the areas of the parotid and submandibular glands should create a clinical suspicion of salivary gland disease. Pain and altered salivary flow may be present. Because the periodicity and longevity of these symptoms are important in the differential diagnosis, a review of the medical histories and physical conditions of patients may provide important information. A history of skin, endocrine, or swallowing abnormalities may suggest a systemic collagen disease or metabolic disorder that may be the cause of the clinical salivary gland disorder.

Differential Diagnosis of Salivary Enlargements

ENLARGEMENTS OF THE PAROTID AREA

Unilateral enlargements of the parotid area are categorized by the presence of a discrete, palpable mass or a diffuse swelling. If no mass is apparent, sialadenitis should be considered. Sialadenitis may be primary or secondary to ductal obstruction (retrograde). A mass superficial to the gland suggests lymphadenitis, an infected preauricular cyst, an infected sebaceous cyst, benign lymphoid hyperplasia, or an extraparotid tumor. A mass intrinsic to the gland suggests a neoplasm (benign or malignant), intraglandular lymph node, or hamartoma. Rapid growth, facial nerve paralysis, rock-hard texture, pain, and older age of occurrence are clinically suggestive of malignant neoplasms.

The differential diagnosis of asymptomatic bilateral enlargements of the parotid area may include benign lymphoepithelial lesion (Mikulicz's syndrome), Sjögren's syndrome, alcoholism, medication (iodine and certain heavy metals), and Warthin's tumor. Painful bilateral enlargement may occur after radiation treatment or secondary to bacterial or viral sialadenitis (including mumps) when accompanied by systemic symptoms.

A differential diagnosis of diffuse facial swelling in the parotid region, but not related to abnormalities of the gland, includes hypertrophy of the masseter muscle, accessory parotid gland, lesions related to the temporomandibular joint, and osteomyelitis of the ramus of the mandible. A palpable mass superficial to the gland suggests lymphadenitis, an infected preauricular cyst or sebaceous cyst, benign lymphoid hyperplasia, or extraparotid tumor (Box 29-1).

ENLARGEMENTS OF THE SUBMANDIBULAR AREA

Unilateral enlargement of the submandibular area associated with tender lymph nodes is suggestive of sialadenitis, which may be primary or secondary to ductal obstruction or decreased salivary flow (retrograde). Unilateral enlargement without tender lymph nodes sug-

---

BOX 29-1
Differential Diagnosis of Enlargements in the Salivary Gland Areas

Parotid Gland Area
UNILATERAL
Bacterial sialadenitis
Sialodochitis
Cyst
Benign neoplasm
Malignant neoplasm
Intraglandular lymph node
Masseter muscle hypertrophy
Lesions of adjacent osseous structures

BILATERAL
Bacterial sialadenitis
Viral sialadenitis (mumps)
Autoimmune sialadenitis
Warthin's tumor
Alcoholic hypertrophy
Medication-induced hypertrophy (iodine, heavy metals)
HIV-associated multicentric cysts
Masseter muscle hypertrophy
Accessory salivary glands
TMJ-related lesions

Submandibular Gland Area
UNILATERAL
Bacterial sialadenitis
Sialodochitis
Fibrosis
Cyst
Benign neoplasm
Malignant neoplasm

BILATERAL
Bacterial sialadenitis
Autoimmune sialadenitis
Lymphadenitis
Branchial cleft cyst
Submandibular space infection

---

gests a neoplasm, cyst, lymphoepithelial lesion, or fibrosis. An intraglandular mass may be neoplastic or cystic. Neoplasms of the submandibular gland have a greater chance of being malignant than do those of the parotid gland. In turn, sublingual gland neoplasms have a still greater chance of being malignant than do those of the submandibular glands. As with parotid neoplasms, rapid growth, rock hard texture, pain, and older age of occurrence are clinically suggestive of malignancy. Masses superficial or adjacent to the submandibular gland are assumed to be lymph nodes or extraglandular neoplasms.

Bilateral enlargement of the submandibular gland area suggests bacterial or viral sialadenitis. Although mumps is primarily a viral infection of the parotid glands, it may also occur in the submandibular glands. Other causes of swelling in the submandibular region include enlarged lymph nodes, submandibular space infection, and branchial cleft cyst (see Box 29-1).

Applied Diagnostic Imaging of the Salivary Glands

Diagnostic imaging of salivary gland disease is undertaken to differentiate inflammatory processes from neoplastic disease, distinguish diffuse disease from focal suppurative disease, identify and localize sialoliths, and demonstrate ductal morphology. In addition, diagnostic imaging attempts to determine the anatomic location of a tumor, differentiate benign from malignant disease, demonstrate the relationship between a mass and adjacent anatomic structures, and aid in the selection of biopsy sites.

ALGORITHM FOR DIAGNOSTIC IMAGING

Plain film radiography is typically the appropriate starting point for imaging the major salivary glands. It can demonstrate dystrophic calcifications and the possible involvement of adjacent osseous structures. Obstructive and inflammatory conditions are ductal system disorders appropriate for evaluation with sialography. Because inflammatory conditions are the most common abnormality, sialography is the next logical step in the investigation. If the patient is allergic to the iodine contrast agent used in sialography, ultrasonography or scintigraphy (nuclear medicine) may be selected as an alternative imaging modality. If sialography eliminates inflammatory disorders or suggests the presence of a space-occupying mass, then computed tomography (CT) or magnetic resonance imaging (MRI) is appropriate for evaluation. Ultrasonography is an alternative technique to differentiate cystic lesions from solid masses. Functional disorders such as xerostomia are appropriately imaged with sialography or scintigraphy. Scintigraphy can provide important physiologic information that may be helpful in forming the differential diagnosis.

PLAIN FILM RADIOGRAPHY

Plain film radiography is a fundamental part of the examination of the salivary glands and may provide suffi-

cient information to preclude the use of more sophisticated and expensive imaging techniques. It has the potential to identify unrelated pathoses in the areas of the salivary glands that may be mistakenly identified as salivary gland disease, such as resorptive or osteoblastic changes in adjacent bone causing periauricular swelling mimicking a parotid tumor. Panoramic and conventional posteroanterior (PA) radiographs may demonstrate bony lesions, thus eliminating salivary pathosis from the differential diagnosis. Unilateral or bilateral functional or congenital hypertrophy of the masseter muscle may clinically mimic a salivary tumor. A plain film extraoral radiograph may demonstrate a deep antegonial notch, overdeveloped mandibular angle, and exostosis on the outer surface of the angle in cases of masseter hypertrophy.

Plain film radiographs are most useful when the clinical impression, supported by a compatible history, suggests the presence of sialoliths (stones or calculi) or phleboliths. Such an examination should include both intraoral and extraoral images to demonstrate the entire region of the gland. Several sialoliths may be present at different locations. It is expedient to use about half the usual exposure to avoid overexposure of the sialoliths. However, this technique must be qualified by the appreciation that 20% of the sialoliths of the submandibular gland and 40% of those of the parotid gland are not well calcified and therefore are radiolucent and not visible in plain films. Radiolucent sialoliths are rarely found in the sublingual glands. Sialography is indicated if clinically suspected sialoliths are not demonstrated by plain film radiography. The radiographic image of a sialolith superimposed over bone must be differentiated from calcified lymph nodes, phleboliths, myositis ossificans, multiple miliary osteomas of the skin, and calcified acne scars.

INTRAORAL RADIOGRAPHY

Sialoliths in the anterior two thirds of the submandibular duct are typically imaged with a topographical mandibular occlusal projection as described in Chapter 8 (Fig. 29-1). The posterior part of the duct is demonstrated with a posterior oblique view, wherein the head of the patient is tilted back and maximally inclined toward the unaffected side. The central ray is directed parallel with the mandible in the area of the submandibular fossa and into the posterior part of the floor of the mouth.

Parotid sialoliths are more difficult to demonstrate than the submandibular variety as a result of the tortuous course of Stensen's duct around the anterior border of the masseter and through the buccinator muscle. As a rule, only sialoliths in the anterior part of the duct, anterior to the masseter muscle, can be imaged on an intraoral film. To demonstrate sialoliths in the

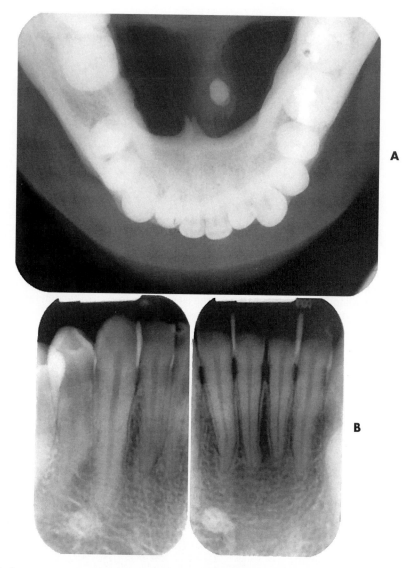

FIG. **29-1** **A,** Underexposed mandibular occlusal radiograph demonstrating radiopaque sialolith in Wharton's duct. Note the classic laminated appearance. **B,** Periapical radiographs of the same case. The radiopaque calculus can be localized lingual to the teeth by applying appropriate object localization rules.

anterior part of the duct, an intraoral film is held with a hemostat against the cheek, as high as possible in the buccal sulcus and over the parotid papilla. The central ray is directed perpendicular to the center of the film.

EXTRAORAL RADIOGRAPHY

A panoramic projection frequently demonstrates sialoliths in the posterior duct or reveals intraglandular sialoliths in the submandibular gland if they are within the image layer (Fig. 29-2). The image of most parotid sialoliths is superimposed over the ramus and body of the mandible, making lateral radiographs of limited value. To demonstrate sialoliths in the submandibular gland,

the lateral projection is modified by opening the mouth, extending the chin, and depressing the tongue with the index finger. This usually moves the image of the sialolith inferior to the mandibular border, where its image is more apparent.

Sialoliths in the distal portion of Stensen's duct or in the parotid gland are difficult to demonstrate by intraoral or lateral extraoral views. However, a PA projection with the cheeks puffed out may move the image of the sialolith free of the bone, rendering it visible on the projected image. This technique may also demonstrate interglandular sialoliths that may be obscured during sialography. Less mineralized sialoliths may also be obscured by heavy soft tissue shadows in the PA view.

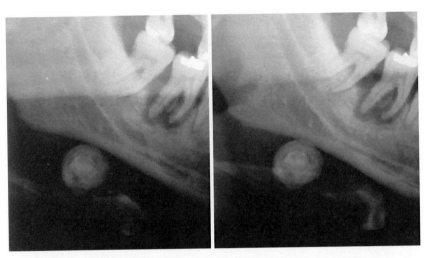

FIG. **29-2** *Stereoscopic panoramic plain film projections.* Note the laminated appearance of this sialolith in the submandibular gland. The image of the sialolith is magnified because of its relatively lingual placement in the image layer. Taken from slightly different horizontal angles, a three-dimensional appearance is presented when viewed with stereobinoculars.

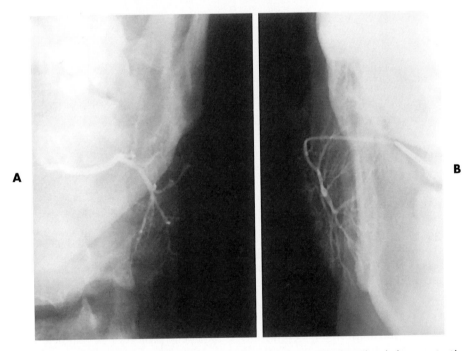

FIG. **29-3** *Sialograms.* **A,** PA projection of the submandibular gland demonstrating prominent superior and posterior extensions of the gland. The peripheral margins of the submandibular gland lie in close proximity to the inferior and anterior margins of the parotid gland. **B,** PA projection of the parotid gland, which was filled using a pressure-regulated pump for optimal parenchymal opacification. Lack of parenchymal blush suggests edema.

SIALOGRAPHY

First performed in 1902, sialography is a radiographic technique wherein a radiopaque contrast agent is infused into the ductal system of a salivary gland before imaging with plain films, fluoroscopy, panoramic radiography, conventional tomography, or CT. Sialography provides a straightforward demonstration of the ductal system (Fig. 29-3). The parotid and submandibular glands are more readily studied with this technique than is the sublingual gland. Although the sublingual gland is difficult to infuse intentionally, it may be fortuitously opacified while infusing Wharton's duct to image the submandibular gland.

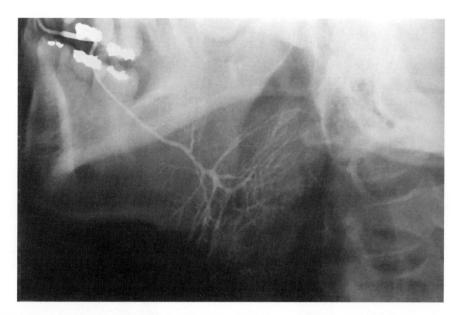

FIG. **29-4** *Sialogram of normal submandibular gland.* This lateral view demonstrates the ductal filling stage before parenchymal opacification.

A survey or "scout" film is usually made before the infusion of the contrast solution into the ductal system as an aid in verifying the optimal exposure factors and patient positioning parameters. Radiopaque sialoliths may also be demonstrated, in addition to extraglandular pathosis and bone disease, which may be responsible for the clinical symptoms.

The closed system technique is frequently recommended for making sialograms. A lacrimal probe is used to dilate the sphincter at the ductal orifice before the passage of a cannula (blunt needle or catheter) connected by extension tubing to a syringe containing contrast agent. Lipid-soluble (e.g., Ethiodol) or non–lipid-soluble (e.g., Sinografin) contrast solution is slowly infused until the patient feels discomfort (usually between 0.2 and 1.5 ml, depending on the gland being studied). Fluoroscopic monitoring of the filling phase is recommended by some; otherwise the procedure is monitored with static films. The intent is to opacify the ductal system all the way to the acini. The image of the ductal system appears as "tree limbs," with no area of the gland devoid of ducts (Fig. 29-4). With acinar filling, the "tree" comes into "bloom," which is the typical appearance of the parenchymal opacification phase (Fig. 29-5). The gland is allowed to empty for 5 minutes without stimulation. If postevacuation images suggest contrast retention, a sialogogue such as lemon juice or 2% citric acid may be administered to augment evacuation by stimulating secretion.

Sialography is indicated for the evaluation of chronic inflammatory diseases and ductal pathoses. However, it is no longer considered the preferred study for space-occupying masses. Contraindications to sialography include acute infection, known sensitivity to iodine-

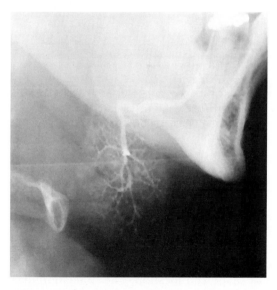

FIG. **29-5** *Sialogram of normal submandibular gland.* This lateral view demonstrates parenchymal filling. Normal fine branching is visible. Lack of parenchymal blush at the anteroinferior margin is caused by radiographic burnout.

containing compounds, and anticipated thyroid function tests.

COMPUTED TOMOGRAPHY

CT is useful in evaluating structures in and adjacent to salivary glands; it distinguishes both soft and hard tissues as well as minute differences in soft tissue densities (Fig. 29-6). (See Chapter 12 for a description of the CT

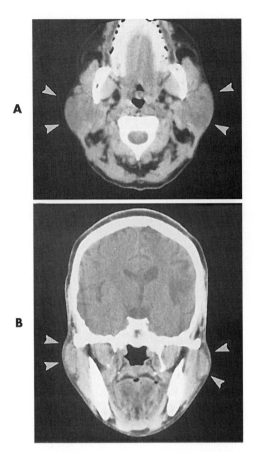

FIG. **29-6** *CT images.* **A,** Axial view demonstrating bilateral enlargement of the parotid glands *(arrows).* **B,** Coronal view of the same patient. The clinical/histopathologic diagnosis was autoimmune parotitis. (Courtesy Department of Radiology, Baylor University Medical Center, Dallas, Tex.)

process.) Glandular tissues are usually easily discernible from surrounding fat and muscle. The parotid glands are more radiopaque than the surrounding fat but less opaque than adjacent muscles. Although the submandibular and sublingual glands are similar in density to adjacent muscles, they are readily identified on the basis of shape and location. The submandibular and sublingual glands are most easily identified on directly acquired contrast-enhanced coronal CT scans. CT is useful in assessing acute inflammatory processes and abscesses as well as cysts, mucoceles, and neoplasias. Some consider CT to be the preferred method for the investigation of masses in or near the salivary glands.

MAGNETIC RESONANCE IMAGING

MRI typically provides better soft tissue images than does CT; it also results in fewer problems with streak artifacts from metallic dental restorative materials (Fig. 29-7). (See Chapter 12 for a description of the basic concepts and principles of nuclear MRI.) Although indica-

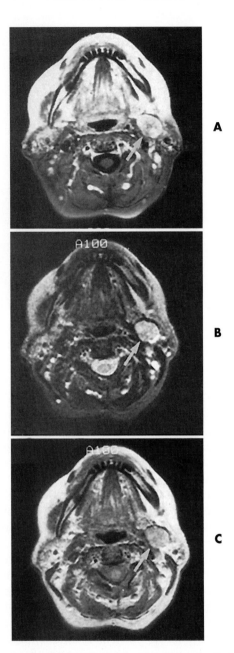

FIG. **29-7** *Gadolinium-enhanced MRIs.* A well-defined mass in the deep lobe of the left parotid gland as imaged with **A,** T1-weighted format; **B,** T2-weighted format; and **C,** proton density–weighted format. The appearance is typical of benign salivary tumors. Histopathologic diagnosis was pleomorphic adenoma. (Courtesy Department of Radiology, Baylor University Medical Center, Dallas, Tex.)

tions for CT and MRI occasionally overlap, MRI demonstrates as well as or better than CT the margins of salivary gland masses, internal structures, and regional extension of the lesions into adjacent tissues or spaces, as occurs with some lesions of the deep lobe of the parotid. MRI also discloses the major vessels, identified as areas of no signal (dark) without the use of contrast medium.

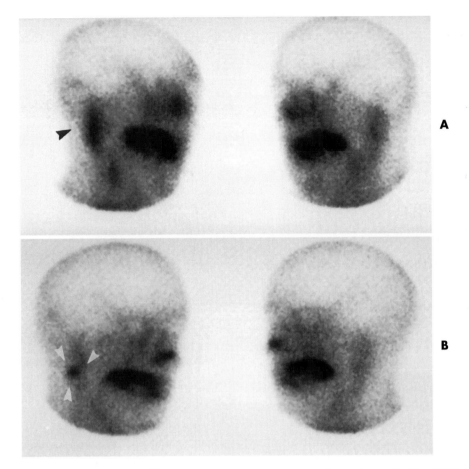

FIG. **29-8** *Scintigraphy.* **A,** ⁹⁹ᵐTc-pertechnetate scan of the salivary glands (right and left anterior oblique views) demonstrates increased uptake of radioisotope in the right parotid gland *(black arrow).* **B,** Scintigram taken after administration of sialogogue (lemon juice) demonstrates retention of isotope in right parotid gland *(white arrows).* This is a typical presentation of salivary stasis, Warthin's tumor, and oncocytoma.

NUCLEAR MEDICINE (SCINTIGRAPHY)

Nuclear medicine, or scintigraphy, provides a functional study of the salivary glands, taking advantage of the selective concentration of specific radiopharmaceuticals in the glands. (See Chapter 12 for a description of the nuclear medicine procedures used to acquire images.) When ⁹⁹ᵐTc-pertechnetate is injected intravenously, it is concentrated in and excreted by glandular structures, including the salivary, thyroid, and mammary glands. The radionuclide appears in the ducts of the salivary glands within minutes and reaches maximal concentration within 30 to 45 minutes. A sialogogue is then administered to evaluate secretory capacity.

All major salivary glands can be studied at once by scintigraphy. It is especially advantageous for conditions in which sialography is contraindicated as well as for patients whose ducts cannot be cannulated.

Although this technique has high diagnostic sensitivity, it lacks specificity and demonstrates little morphology. Pathosis may be demonstrated by an increased, decreased, or absent radionuclide uptake (Fig. 29-8). The diagnosis of salivary gland tumors from nuclear medicine scans is not completely reliable. Current levels of resolution only consistently visualize tumors exceeding 1.0 to 1.5 cm. CT and MRI are preferred for the evaluation of salivary masses.

ULTRASONOGRAPHY

Compared with CT and MRI, ultrasonography has the advantages of being relatively inexpensive, widely available, painless, easy to perform, and noninvasive. (For a full description of ultrasonography, see Chapter 12.) The primary application of ultrasonography is the differentiation of solid masses from cystic ones. Recent

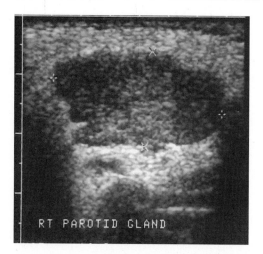

FIG. **29-9** *Ultrasound image of right parotid gland.* A well-delineated, solid mass is suggested by echo returns within the lesion. Ultrasound appearance is typical of a benign salivary tumor. (Courtesy Department of Radiology, Baylor University Medical Center, Dallas, Tex.)

studies suggest that this technique may also be helpful in diagnosing sialoliths (Fig. 29-9).

Image Interpretation of Salivary Gland Disorders

OBSTRUCTIVE AND INFLAMMATORY DISORDERS

Sialolithiasis

Synonyms. *Calculus* and *salivary stone*

Definition. Sialolithiasis is the formation of a calcified obstruction within the salivary duct.

Clinical features. Sialoliths may be calcified to different degrees and can obstruct the secretory ducts. Ductal obstruction may result in chronic retrograde infections because of a decrease in salivary flow. Clinical symptoms include intermittent swelling, pain with eating, and superimposed infection resulting from stasis. Sialoliths may form in any of the major or minor salivary glands or their ducts, but usually only one gland is involved. The submandibular gland and Wharton's duct are by far the most frequently involved (83% of cases). If one stone is found, at least a one in four chance exists that others are present.

Radiographic features. Plain films and ultrasound images are appropriate examinations when a clinical suspi-

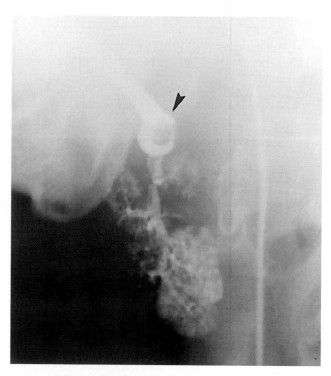

FIG. **29-10** *Sialogram.* Slightly oblique lateral view demonstrating parenchymal opacification of the submandibular gland. *Arrow* points to an obstruction (radiolucent sialolith) within the main duct. Filling of the gland parenchyma is patchy resulting from fibrosis occurring secondary to chronic obstruction.

cion exists of obstructive sialolithiasis (see Fig. 29-1). Depending on their degree of calcification, sialoliths may appear either radiopaque or radiolucent (20% to 40% of cases). Sialography is helpful in locating obstructions that are undetectable with plain radiography, especially if the sialoliths are radiolucent. The contrast agent usually flows around the sialolith, filling the duct proximal to the obstruction. The ductal system is frequently dilated proximal to the obstruction. If the obstruction itself is not recognizable, its presence is inferred by the ductal dilation. The sialolith is typically less radiodense than the adjacent contrast agent that has flowed around it (Fig. 29-10). Small sialoliths distal to the end of the cannula or those that are superimposed with contrast agent may be obscured by the technique. Radiolucent sialoliths appear as ductal filling defects (Fig. 29-11). Sialography should not be performed if a radiopaque stone has been shown by plain radiography to be in the distal portion of the duct, because the procedure may displace it proximally into the ductal system, which might complicate its subsequent removal. CT may also detect minimally calcified sialoliths not noted on plain films.

Ultrasonography is of limited value in the diagnosis of inflammatory and obstructive diseases, but recent

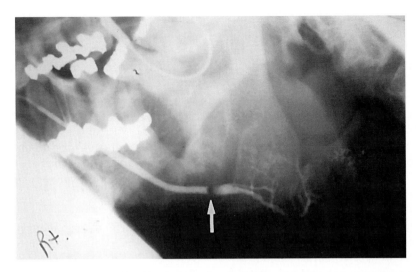

FIG. **29-11** *Sialogram.* Lateral view of submandibular glands demonstrating a radiolucent sialolith in the main duct.

studies indicate it is fairly reliable in demonstrating sialoliths. More than 90% of stones larger than 2 mm are detected as echo-dense spots with a characteristic acoustic shadow.

Treatment. Treatment of sialolithiasis may consist of encouragement of spontaneous discharge through the use of sialogogues to stimulate secretion. Sialography may also stimulate discharge, especially if a oil-based contrast agent is used. If discharge does not occur, local incision or total surgical excision of the involved salivary gland may be indicated.

Bacterial Sialadenitis
Synonyms. *Parotitis* and *submandibulitis*

Definition. Bacterial sialadenitis is an acute or chronic bacterial infection of the terminal acini or parenchyma of the salivary glands.

Clinical features. Acute bacterial infections most commonly affect the parotid gland, but the submandibular gland may also be involved. Most cases are unilateral and may occur at any age. The typical clinical presentation is swelling, redness, tenderness, and malaise. Enlarged regional lymph nodes and suppuration may also be noted. Those most commonly afflicted are elderly persons, postoperative patients, and debilitated patients who have poor hygiene as a result of reduced salivary secretion and retrograde infection by the oral flora (usually *Staphylococcus aureus* and *S. viridans*). Reduced salivary secretion may also be drug related or secondary to occlusion of a major duct. Untreated acute suppurative infections typically form abscesses. Diagnosis is based on clinical observation, systemic symptoms, and the expression of pus from the duct.

Chronic inflammation may affect any of the major salivary glands, causing extensive swelling and culminating in fibrosis. This may be a consequence of an untreated acute sialadenitis or associated with some type of obstruction resulting from sialolithiasis, noncalcified organic debris, or stricture (scar or fibrosis) formation in the excretory ducts. Bacteria or viruses may not be detected in the gland or saliva. The parotid is most often involved. During periods of painful swelling, pus may be expressed from the ductal orifice and salivary stimulation may cause pain. Episodic in nature, signs of generalized sepsis are seldom. The obstruction may be congenital or secondary to sialolithiasis, trauma, infection, or neoplasia. Typical clinical symptoms are intermittent swelling, pain when eating, and superimposed infection resulting from salivary stasis.

Radiographic features. Sialography is contraindicated in acute infections because disrupted ductal epithelium may allow extravasation of contrast agent, resulting in a foreign body reaction and severe pain. This technique is appropriate for use in cases of suspected chronic infections. Epithelial flattening may lead to mildly dilated terminal ducts and saclike acini, which is demonstrable with sialography. The saclike acinar areas are referred to as *sialectasia*. An even distribution throughout the gland is seen in recurrent parotitis and autoimmune disorders. If they are connected to the ductal system, abscess cavities may fill with contrast media during sialography. Abscess cavities appear on CT as areas of decreased density within an enlarged gland. Ultrasound may distinguish between diffuse inflammation (echo-free, light image) and suppuration (less echo-free, darker image) and detect sialoliths greater than 2 mm in diameter. Ultrasound examination may also demonstrate abscess cavities, if present. MRI and scintigraphy are not likely to provide additional useful information unless the clinician suspects some other disorder coincident with the acute infection (Fig. 29-12). However, scintigraphy is an appropriate alternative examination in cases in which sialography is contraindicated or not technically possible (see Fig. 29-8). Advanced sialadenitis may present in combination with sialolithiasis, sialodochitis, abscess formation, and fistulas.

Treatment. Treatment of bacterial sialadenitis typically begins conservatively with attention to oral hygiene, local massage, increased fluid intake, and the use of oral sialogogues (sour citrus fruit wedges or salivary stimulants). An appropriate antibiotic regimen may also be indicated. If symptoms continue, surgical remedies ranging from partial to total excision of the gland may be considered.

Sialodochitis
Synonym. *Ductal sialadenitis*

Definition. Sialodochitis is an inflammation of the ductal system of the salivary glands.

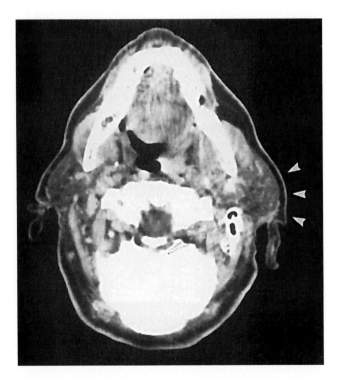

FIG. **29-12** *Contrast-enhanced CT image.* The left submandibular gland *(arrows)* is larger than the right with no suggestion of abscess formation. This appearance is compatible with diffuse parotitis and cellulitis. (Courtesy Department of Radiology, Baylor University Medical Center, Dallas, Tex.)

Clinical features. Dilation of the ductal system is a prominent sialographic presentation of sialodochitis. Although common in the submandibular gland (Fig. 29-13), it is seen almost as often in the parotid gland. If interstitial fibrosis develops, it is apparent in sialograms as a sausage-string appearance of the main duct and its major branches produced by alternate strictures and dilations. CT, MRI, and scintigraphy are not typically indicated in the diagnosis of inflammatory ductal diseases of the salivary glands. They are costly, nonspecific, and probably will not provide any more useful information than sialography.

Treatment. The management of sialodochitis is similar to that described for sialadenitis.

Autoimmune Sialadenitis
Synonyms. *Myoepithelial sialadenitis, Mikulicz's disease, Sjögren's syndrome, benign lymphoepithelial lesion,* and *autoimmune sialosis*

Definition. Autoimmune sialadenitis represents a group of disorders that affect the salivary glands and share an autosensitivity. The range of clinical and histopathologic manifestations suggests that these disorders represent different developmental stages of the same immunologic mechanisms, differing only in the extent and intensity of tissue reaction. Different forms may share a common etiology.

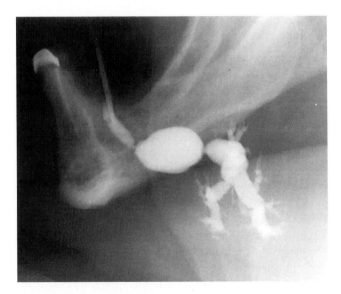

FIG. **29-13** *Sialogram.* Lateral view of the submandibular gland shows intermittent stricture and dilation of the main ducts, which is typical of advanced sialodochitis.

Clinical features. The clinical manifestations range from recurrent painless, unilateral or bilateral swelling of the salivary glands (usually the parotid gland), to a stage that includes enlargement of the lacrimal glands (Mikulicz's disease). Glandular swelling may be accompanied by xerostomia and xerophthalmia (primary Sjögren's syndrome), and subsequently by a connective tissue disease such as rheumatoid arthritis, progressive systemic sclerosis, systemic lupus erythematosus, or polymyositis (secondary Sjögren's syndrome). The process may progress to benign lymphoepithelial lesions that can assume the proportions of a tumor. A presumptive diagnosis can be made on the basis of any two of the following three features: dry mouth, dry eyes, and rheumatoid disease.

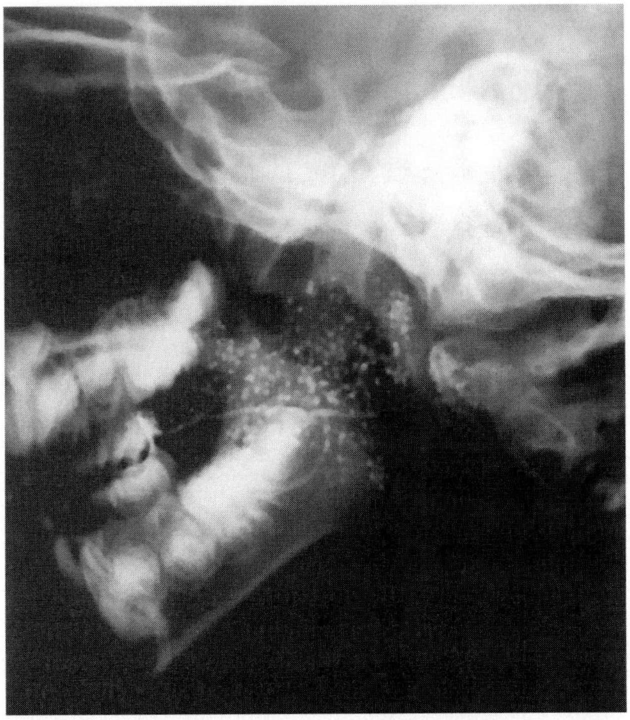

Radiographic features. Sialography is helpful in the diagnosis and staging of autoimmune disorders. The early stages of disease are witness to the initiation of punctate (less than 1 mm) and globular (1 to 2 mm) spherical collections of contrast agent evenly distributed throughout the glands. These collections are referred to as *sialectases* (Fig. 29-14). At this stage, the main duct may appear to be normal but the intraglandular ducts may be narrowed or not even evident. Sialectasia typically remains after the administration of a sialogogue, which is an indication that contrast agent is pooled extraductally and the acini are still functional.

As the disease progresses, the collections of contrast agent increase in size (greater than 2 mm in diameter) and are irregular in shape. These pools of contrast agent are termed *cavitary sialectases*. Cavitary sialectases are fewer in number and less uniformly distributed throughout the glands than are punctate or globular sialectases (Fig. 29-15). Progressively larger cavities of contrast agent and dilation of the main ductal system may also be present. At the endpoint of this disorder, complete destruction of the gland occurs. Cavitation and glandular fibrosis are the result of intercurrent inflammation.

A consensus exists that scintigraphy with ^{99m}Tc-pertechnetate is useful for diagnosing and monitoring the progression of Sjögren's syndrome. Impairment of the parotid and submandibular glands is demonstrated by decreased uptake of the pertechnetate as well as the delay in its stimulated excretion. CT, MRI, and ultrasonography are not particularly diagnostic for autoimmune disorders of the salivary glands (see Fig. 29-6).

FIG. **29-14** *Sialogram of left parotid gland.* Punctate sialectases distributed throughout the gland are suggestive of early autoimmune disease. Clinical/histopathologic diagnosis was Sjögren's syndrome. (Courtesy Department of Radiology, Baylor University Medical Center, Dallas, Tex.)

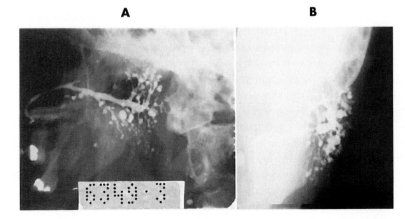

A   **B**

FIG. **29-15** *Sialogram of the left parotid gland.* Punctate (small spherical), globular (larger spherical), and cavitary (largest nonspherical) sialectases with dilation of the main duct are suggestive of advanced autoimmune disease with retrograde infection in **A,** lateral, and **B,** PA, projections. Clinical/histopathologic diagnosis was Sjögren's syndrome. (Courtesy Department of Radiology, Baylor University Medical Center, Dallas, Tex.)

Treatment. The management of autoimmune disorders of the salivary glands is directed toward relief of symptoms. Underlying rheumatoid conditions are systemic and typically treated with antiinflammatory agents, corticosteroids, and immunosuppressive therapeutic agents. Salivary stimulants, increased fluid intake, and artificial saliva and tears are symptomatic treatment regimens for the eyes and mouth. More advanced inflammatory changes may be treated surgically by local or total excision of the symptomatic gland.

NONINFLAMMATORY DISORDERS

Sialadenosis
Synonym. *Sialosis*

Definition. Sialadenosis is a nonneoplastic, noninflammatory enlargement of the salivary glands. It is usually related to metabolic and secretory disorders of the parenchyma associated with diseases of nearly all the endocrine glands (hormonal sialadenoses), protein deficiencies, malnutrition in alcoholics (dystrophic-metabolic sialadenoses), vitamin deficiencies, and neurologic disorders (neurogenic sialadenoses).

Clinical features. Affected glands are typically hypotrophic, although diabetic and alcoholic sialadenosis may result in enlarged parotid glands.

Radiographic features. Sialography may demonstrate atrophy of the affected glands or a normal appearance. CT and MRI provide a more straightforward depiction of the smaller than normal glands. Diminished salivary gland size and a decrease in radioisotope uptake may be apparent on scintigraphic examination.

Treatment. The management of sialadenosis hinges on identifying the etiology of the metabolic or secretory disorder. Conservative treatment, including local massage, increased fluid intake, and the use of oral sialogogues (sour citrus fruit wedges or salivary stimulants), is appropriate.

Cystic Lesions
Definition. Cysts of the salivary glands are rare (less than 5% of all salivary gland masses) and most commonly occur unilaterally in the parotid gland. They may be congenital (branchial), lymphoepithelial, dermoid, or acquired, including mucous retention cysts (obstructions from any etiology). Cystic salivary lesions may be intraglandular or extraglandular in nature and may progress to such proportions that they are clinically palpable and must be distinguished from neoplasia. Cystic neoplasms do occur, but they are discussed separately in

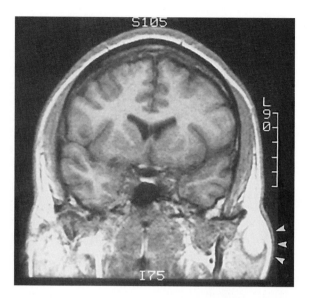

FIG. **29-16**   *Coronal section MRI.* The high-signal mass *(arrows)* in the left parotid gland was diagnosed as a cyst. This patient was found to be HIV positive. (Courtesy Department of Radiology, Baylor University Medical Center, Dallas, Tex.)

this chapter. Mucous extravasation pseudocysts lack an epithelial lining and result from ductal rupture. Ranulas are retention cysts that usually occur secondary to obstruction of the sublingual duct. Benign lymphoepithelial cysts are thought to be sequelae of cystic degeneration of salivary inclusions within lymph nodes. Multicentric parotid cysts associated with human immunodeficiency virus (HIV) have been reported. These lesions are accompanied by cervical lymphadenopathy, occur bilaterally, and are usually in the superficial portion of the parotid gland (Fig. 29-16). A secondary parotitis may develop.

Radiographic features. On sialographic examination, cystic masses are indirectly visualized only by the displacement of the ducts arching around them. Cystic lesions typically appear as well-circumscribed, low-density areas when examined with CT, having CT numbers between 10 and 18 Hounsfield units (HU). The scintigraphic appearance of a salivary gland cyst, like other space-occupying lesions, is that of an area of decreased radioisotope uptake (a "cold spot"). As such, scintigraphy does not contribute to the development of a differential diagnosis because malignant tumors and benign tumors are also almost always "cold" too. When imaged with ultrasound, cysts are sharply marginated and echo-free (represented as a dark area) (Fig. 29-17).

Treatment. Management of cystic lesions is typically surgical, involving local or total excision of the gland.

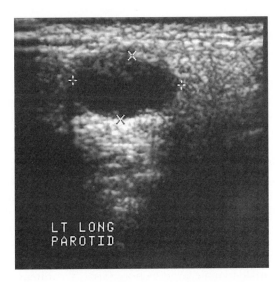

FIG. **29-17** *Ultrasound image of the parotid gland.* Echo-free mass with well-defined margins presents a typical cystic appearance. (Courtesy Department of Radiology, Baylor University Medical Center, Dallas, Tex.)

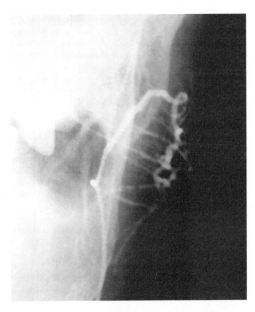

FIG. **29-18** *Sialogram of left parotid gland (PA view).* A mass within the gland is inferred by the appearance of the ducts displaced around the lesion. This is referred to as the "ball-in-hand" appearance, which is typical of a space-occupying mass. (Courtesy Department of Radiology, Baylor University Medical Center, Dallas, Tex.)

Benign Tumors

Salivary gland tumors are relatively uncommon and occur in less than 0.003% of the population. They account for about 3% of all tumors. Some 80% of the salivary tumors arise in the parotid, 5% in the submandibular, 1% in the sublingual, and 10% to 15% in the minor salivary glands. The majority (70% to 80%) of these tumors occur in the superficial lobe of the parotid gland. Most are benign or low-grade malignancies. High-grade malignancies are uncommon. The incidence of benign neoplasms of major salivary glands appears to increase with the size of the gland.

Radiographic features. Benign tumors and low-grade malignancies typically have well-defined margins, which are most apparent on CT or MRI examinations. Because of the higher density of the submandibular gland, which can equal that of the neoplasm and obscure the tumor, the injection of intravenous contrast is required during the CT examination. This causes the tumor to appear more radiopaque because the vascularity of the tumor is greater than the adjacent salivary gland tissue. CT sialography may also be helpful in delineating the tumor. Interrogation of the CT densities of tumors is not predictive except for lipid-containing or vascular tumors. In the ultrasound examination benign masses are typically less echogenic than parenchyma, sharply defined, and of essentially homogeneous echo strength and density. Benign tumors may

present as low-intensity (dark) or high-intensity (light) signals on T1-, T2-, and proton density–weighted images. Their relative intensity on the different MRIs is somewhat predictive of lipid, vascular, or fibrous tissues. Sialography is of limited value, but it may suggest a space-occupying mass when the ducts are compressed or smoothly displaced around the lesion (the "ball-in-hand" appearance) (Fig. 29-18).

Treatment. The management of benign tumors of the major salivary glands is typically surgical. Benign tumors of the parotid gland may be either partially or totally excised. Submandibular and sublingual glands are invariably totally excised.

Benign Mixed Tumor
Synonym. *Pleomorphic adenoma*

Definition. The benign mixed tumor is a neoplasm arising from the ductal epithelium of major and minor salivary glands exhibiting epithelial and mesenchymal components.

Clinical features. Pleomorphic adenomas account for 75% of salivary gland tumors. Of these, 80% are found in the parotid gland, 4% in the submandibular gland, 1% in the sublingual gland, and 10% in the minor salivary glands. This tumor typically occurs in the fifth decade of life as a slow-growing, unilateral, encapsulated, asymptomatic mass. A slight female predilection exists. The benign mixed tumor is characteristically sharply circumscribed, infrequently lobulated, and found within a normal gland. Recurrence occurs in 50% of cases after excision.

Radiographic features. The CT presentation of the benign mixed tumor is a sharply circumscribed and essentially round homogeneous lesion that has a higher density than the adjacent glandular tissue. T1-weighted MRIs present the benign mixed tumor as an area of relatively lower signal intensity (dark area) than adjacent glandular tissue. The tumor has a greater intensity (intermediate brightness) on proton density–weighted MRIs and appears as a homogeneous high-intensity (bright) area on T2-weighted images (see Fig. 29-7). Foci of low signal intensity (dark areas) usually represent areas of fibrosis or dystrophic calcifications. The presence of calcification (signal void) in a parotid neoplasm favors benign mixed tumor as the diagnosis.

Benign mixed tumor does not usually concentrate ^{99m}Tc-pertechnetate. Therefore the tumor appears as a cold spot when examined by scintigraphy. Solid tumors larger than 5 mm are usually well visualized.

Warthin's Tumor
Synonym. *Papillary cystadenoma lymphomatosum*

Definition. Warthin's tumor is a benign tumor arising from proliferating salivary ducts trapped in lymph nodes during embryogenesis of the salivary glands.

Clinical features. Warthin's tumor is the second most common benign neoplasm of the salivary glands, accounting for 2% to 6% of the parotid tumors. In the parotid gland, it is usually found in the inferior lobe of the gland. This unusual type of tumor is slowly growing, painless, and frequently bilateral. Warthin's tumor typically afflicts males over the age of 40.

Radiographic features. CT, MRI, and scintigraphy are the preferred techniques for imaging Warthin's tumor. The CT and MRI appearance of this tumor is not specific and is typical of benign salivary tumors as described for the benign mixed tumor. In general, the detection of this lesion with MRI is as good or better than with CT. Warthin's tumors are characteristically intensely hot on ^{99m}Tc-pertechnetate scans. Oncocytomas (oxyphilic adenoma) may also accumulate the ^{99m}Tc-pertechnetate, but they are less common (less than 1% of all salivary gland tumors) and are less likely to be bilateral (see Fig.

29-8). The ultrasound presentation is that of a solid mass (hypoechoic) (see Fig. 29-9).

Hemangioma
Synonym. *Vascular nevus*

Definition. Hemangioma is a benign neoplasm of proliferating endothelial cells (congenital hemangioma) and vascular malformations, including lesions resulting from abnormal vessel morphogenesis.

Clinical features. Hemangioma is the most frequently occurring nonepithelial salivary neoplasm, accounting for 50% of the cases. As many as 85% arise in the parotid gland. It is the most common salivary gland tumor during infancy and childhood. The average age at diagnosis is 10 years with 65% occurring in the first two decades of life. They are frequently unilateral and asymptomatic. A 2:1 female-to-male predilection exists. Treatment is by local excision for those that do not undergo spontaneous remission.

Radiographic features. Phleboliths are common in this tumor and are well demonstrated on plain films. They appear as calculi with a radiolucent center. Displaced ducts curving about the mass may also be apparent on sialography. Hemangiomas appear as cold spots with scintigraphy. The CT presentation of hemangioma is a soft tissue mass that is well distinguished from surrounding tissue, especially when intravenous contrast enhancement is used. Although ultrasound usually demonstrates well-defined margins in the hemangioma, ill-defined margins may also be noted. Strongly hypoechoic, hemangiomas may have a complex ultrasonographic appearance resulting from the multiple interfaces in the lesion. Phleboliths image as multiple hyperechoic areas within the body of the gland itself.

Lipoma
Definition. Lipoma is a benign neoplasm composed of mature fat cells.

Clinical features. Although lipoma is the most common mesenchymal tumor, it is very rare in the salivary glands. Occurring predominantly in females, the clinical presentation is typical of benign salivary tumors. Most are found in the parotid gland as round or ovoid, moderately firm nodules that are usually painless and mobile. The treatment of choice is local excision, and the prognosis is good.

Radiographic features. CT is particularly helpful in imaging lipomas because of the high lipid content of the tumor, which has a very low CT number (-80 HU). T2-

weighted MRI examinations demonstrate lipoma as a dark mass, which differs from the bright T2 appearance of most salivary tumors. The sialographic, ultrasound, and scintigraphic appearances of lipoma are typical of those previously described for benign salivary tumors.

MALIGNANT TUMORS

About 20% of tumors in the parotid are malignant, compared with 50% to 60% of submandibular tumors, 90% of sublingual tumors, and 60% to 75% of minor salivary gland tumors. Thus the incidence of malignant tumors appears to be inversely proportional to the size of the gland.

Treatment. The management of malignant tumors of the major salivary glands is typically surgical. Low-grade malignant tumors of the parotid gland may be either partially or totally excised. Submandibular and sublingual glands are invariably totally excised. Higher-grade tumors may require radical neck dissection. Combinations of surgery, therapeutic radiation, and chemotherapy may also be used.

Mucoepidermoid Carcinoma

Definition. Mucoepidermoid carcinoma is a malignant tumor of epidermoid, intermediate, and mucous cells of the salivary glands.

Clinical features. This is the most common malignant salivary gland tumor (35%). Just over half occur in the major salivary glands; the rest are found in the minor glands, with the palate being the most frequent location. The aggressiveness of the lesion varies with its histologic grade. A wide age range exists, with the highest prevalence in the fifth decade of life. A slight predilection for females exists. The low-grade variety rarely metastasizes. Clinically, this tumor appears as a movable, slowly growing, painless nodule not unlike a benign mixed tumor. It is usually only 1 to 4 cm in diameter. The prognosis is good; the 5-year survival rate is greater than 95%.

In contrast to low-grade mucoepidermoid carcinomas, high-grade tumors often cause facial pain and paralysis, have ill-defined margins, and are relatively immobile. Metastasis by blood and lymph are common, with recurrence in half the patients after excision. The prognosis is poor and varies with the histologic grade; the 5-year survival rate may be as low as 25%.

Radiographic features. Low-grade mucoepidermoid carcinomas are typically not apparent on plain films unless destructive changes to adjacent osseous structures have occurred. The sialographic, CT, MRI, ultrasonographic, and scintigraphic presentations of this tumor are similar to those previously described for benign salivary tumors.

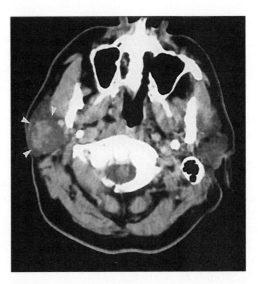

FIG. **29-19** *Contrast-enhanced CT image.* Mass in right parotid gland demonstrates a poorly marginated, heterogeneous, slightly lobulated appearance. Poorly defined margins suggest a low-grade malignancy rather than a benign tumor, even though the CT appearance of both is similar. Histopathologic diagnosis was low-grade mucoepidermoid carcinoma. (Courtesy Department of Radiology, Baylor University Medical Center, Dallas, Tex.)

However, low-grade mucoepidermoid carcinoma may present a lobulated or irregularly sharply circumscribed appearance on CT scans or MRIs (Fig. 29-19).

The radiographic diagnosis of high-grade mucoepidermoid carcinoma typically relies on the appearance of irregular margins and ill-defined form when the mass is examined with CT or MRI. The CT section shows the tumor as an irregular homogeneous mass, not much more dense than the parenchyma. A CT with intravenous contrast shows the tumor as a sharply defined homogeneous mass that is considerably more dense than on the conventional CT. CT is also a reliable technique for the detection of bony invasion.

In contrast to the low-grade malignancies and benign neoplasms, high-grade mucoepidermoid carcinoma, like most high-grade malignancies, has low signal intensity on T1-weighted and T2-weighted MRIs. The T1-weighted images have lower intensity (dark) than the surrounding structures and are relatively homogeneous. T2-weighted images of the tumor are more heterogeneous and intense (brighter) than T1-weighted images and are just slightly darker than the surrounding tissues. Regardless of clinical presentation and margins, low signal intensity is suggestive of a high-grade malignancy.

Cavitary sialectasia and ductal displacement may be noted on sialographic images of this tumor. As with most malignant tumors, the ultrasonographic presentation of high-grade mucoepidermoid carcinoma is a homogeneous echo pattern with low to medium reflectivity (because of the densely packed cells) and attenuation. Diffuse or poorly defined margins are also apparent on ultrasound. Although benign tumors and low-grade malignancies usually have well-defined margins and high-grade malignancies usually have poorly defined margins, an inflammatory response in a benign neoplasm may mimic the appearance of a high-grade malignancy.

Malignant Mixed Tumor

Synonyms. *Carcinoma ex mixed tumor, carcinoma ex pleomorphic adenoma,* and *malignant pleomorphic adenoma*

Definition. Malignant mixed tumor is a malignant tumor arising from the epithelial components of a pre-existing benign mixed tumor (carcinoma ex mixed tumor) or from both epithelial and mesenchymal components (malignant mixed tumor). It may also be detected by unexplained metastasis of a histologically benign mixed tumor.

Clinical features. The benign mixed tumor comprises about 15% of malignant salivary neoplasms. Carcinoma ex mixed tumor is the most common of the three histopathologic variations. The malignant mixed tumor typically begins as a slowly growing mass that suddenly undergoes rapid proliferation, often accompanied by pain and facial paralysis. Metastasis is early and the prognosis is unfavorable.

Radiographic features. The presentation of this tumor is similar to that of the high-grade mucoepidermoid carcinoma previously described.

Other Malignant and Metastatic Tumors

Although the incidence of other malignant tumors of the major salivary glands is low, a significant variety exists in their histogenesis. Of all malignant salivary gland tumors, 23% are adenoid cystic carcinomas; however, the majority of these neoplasms develop in the minor salivary glands.

Adenocarcinoma accounts for 6.4% of all salivary gland malignancies, with acinic cell carcinoma, primary lymphoma, and squamous cell carcinoma occurring with even less frequency. Pain, paresthesia, and even paralysis may be present, especially in high-grade tumors. Interestingly, the pain associated with acinic cell carcinoma is not considered to be as grave a sign as in other malignant salivary tumors. Tumor spread may be by direct invasion or metastasis. Adenoid cystic carcinomas also spread along nerve sheaths. Malignant lymphoma has an incidence 40 times greater in patients with Sjögren's syndrome than in the general population.

Metastasis of tumors of the salivary glands is not un-

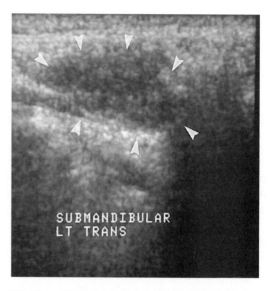

FIG. **29-20** *Ultrasonography.* The mass in the submandibular gland *(arrows)* demonstrates a heterogeneous hypoechoic pattern compared with the adjacent tissue. The histopathologic diagnosis was adenoid cystic carcinoma. (Courtesy Department of Radiology, Baylor University Medical Center, Dallas, Tex.)

usual. Metastatic lesions in the parotid gland are more common than in the other salivary glands because of the extensive lymphatic and circulatory components of the parotid gland. Most metastatic lesions of the parotid gland are via the lymphatic system and include squamous cell carcinoma, lymphoma, and melanoma. Although considerably fewer lesions are the result of hematogenous dissemination, metastasis from the lung, breast, kidney, and gastrointestinal tract has been reported.

Radiographic features. The presentation of these tumors is nonspecific and similar to that of the high-grade mucoepidermoid carcinoma previously described. Ultrasonography may demonstrate echo-free cystic areas in adenoid cystic carcinomas (Fig. 29-20).

SUGGESTED READINGS

Del Balso AM et al: Diagnostic imaging of the salivary glands and periglandular regions. In Del Balso AM, editor: *Maxillofacial imaging,* Philadelphia, 1990, WB Saunders.

Lufkin RB, Hanafee WN: *MRI of the head and neck,* New York, 1992, Raven Press.

Rabinov K, Weber AL: *Radiology of the salivary glands,* Boston, 1985, GK Hall Medical Publishers.

Rankow RM, Polayes IM: *Diseases of the salivary glands,* Philadelphia, 1976, WB Saunders.

Seifert G et al: *Diseases of the salivary glands,* Stuttgart, Germany, 1986, George Thieme Verlag.

Van den Akker HP: Diagnostic imaging in salivary gland disease, *Oral Surg* 66:625, 1988.

Watson MG: Investigation of salivary gland disease, *Ear Nose Throat J* 68:84, 1989.

PLAIN FILM RADIOGRAPHY

Lowman RM, Cheng GK: Diagnostic radiology. In Rankow RM, Polayes IM, editors: *Diseases of the salivary glands*, Philadelphia, 1976, WB Saunders.

Ollerenshaw R, Ross SS: Radiological diagnosis of salivary gland disease, *Br J Radiol* 24:538, 1951.

SIALOGRAPHY

Eisenbud L, Cranin N: The role of sialography in the diagnosis and therapy of chronic obstructive sialadenitis, *Oral Surg* 16:1181, 1961.

Hettwer KJ, Folsum RC: The normal sialogram, *Oral Surg* 26:790, 1968.

Manashil GB: *Clinical sialography*, Springfield, 1978, Charles C Thomas.

Whaley K et al: Sialographic abnormalities in Sjögren's syndrome, rheumatoid arthritis, and other arthritides and connective tissue diseases. A clinical and radiological investigation using hydrostatic sialography, *Clin Radiol* 23:474, 1972.

Yune HY, Klatte EC: Current status of sialography, *Am J Roent Rad Ther Nuc Med* 115:420, 1972.

COMPUTED TOMOGRAPHY OF THE MAJOR SALIVARY GLANDS

Bryan RN et al: Computed tomography of the major salivary glands, *AJR* 139:547, 1982.

Lloyd RE, Ho KH: Combined CT scanning and sialography in the management of parotid tumors, *Oral Surg Oral Med Oral Pathol* 65:142, 1988.

Mooyaart EL, Panders AK, Vermeij A: CT scanning of tumors in or near the parotid or submandibular glands, *Diagn Imag Clin Med* 53:177, 1984.

Saluk PH et al: High resolution computed tomography of the major salivary glands: current status, *J Comput Assist Tomogr* 9:39, 1985.

MAGNETIC RESONANCE IMAGING OF THE MAJOR SALIVARY GLANDS

Kaneda T et al: MR of the submandibular gland: normal and pathologic states, *AJNR* 17:1575, 1996.

Mendelblatt S et al: Parotid masses: MR imaging, *Radiology* 163:411, 1987.

Som PM, Biller HF: High-grade malignancies of the parotid gland; identification with MR imaging, *Radiology* 173:823, 1989.

Swartz et al: MR imaging of parotid mass lesions: attempts at histopathologic differentiation, *J Comput Assist Tomogr* 13:789, 1989.

NUCLEAR MEDICINE (SCINTIGRAPHY) OF THE MAJOR SALIVARY GLANDS

Chaudhuri TK, Stadalnik RC: Salivary gland imaging, *Sem Nucl Med* 10:400, 1980.

Garcia RR: Differential diagnosis of tumors of the salivary glands with radioactive isotopes, *Int J Oral Surg* 3:330, 1974.

Greyson ND, Nikko AM: Radionuclide salivary scanning, *J Otolaryngol* 11:3, 1982.

Mishkin FS: Radionuclide salivary gland imaging, *Sem Nucl Med* 11:258, 1981.

Van den Akker HP, Busemann-Sokole E: Absolute indications for salivary gland scintigraphy with ^{99m}Tc-pertechnetate, *Oral Surg* 60:440, 1985.

ULTRASONOGRAPHY OF THE MAJOR SALIVARY GLANDS

Gooding GAW: Gray scale ultrasound of the parotid gland, *AJR* 134:469, 1980.

Gritzman G: Sonography of the salivary glands, *AJR* 153:161, 1989.

Martinoli C et al: Color doppler sonography of salivary glands, *AJR* 163:933, 1994.

Neiman HL et al: Ultrasound of the parotid gland, *J Clin Ultrasound* 4:11, 1975.

Rothberg R et al: Diagnostic ultrasound imaging of parotid disease—a contemporary clinical perspective, *J Otolaryngol* 13:232, 1984.

OBSTRUCTIVE AND INFLAMMATORY DISORDERS

Dijkstra PF: Classification and differential diagnosis of sialographic characteristics in Sjögren syndrome, *Semin Arthritis Rheum* 190:10, 1980.

Gonzales L, Mackenzie AH, Tarar RA: Parotid sialography in Sjögren's syndrome, *Radiology* 97:91, 1970.

Hughes M et al: Scintigraphic evaluation of sialadenitis, *Brit J Radiol* 67:328, 1994.

Langlais RP, Kasle MJ: Sialolithiasis: the radiolucent stones, *Oral Surg Oral Med Oral Pathol* 40:686, 1975.

Scully C: Sjögren's syndrome: clinical and laboratory features, immunopathogenesis, and management, *Oral Surg* 62:510, 1986.

Som PM et al: Manifestations of parotid gland enlargement: radiographic, pathologic, and clinical correlation—part 1, the autoimmune pseudosialectasias, *Radiology* 141:415, 1981.

NONINFLAMMATORY DISORDERS

Chilla R: Sialadenosis of the salivary glands of the head, *Acta Otorhinolaryngolgica* 26:1, 1981.

CYSTS AND NEOPLASMS

Boles R et al: Malignant tumors of salivary glands: a university experience, *Laryngoscope* 60:729, 1980.

Byrne MN et al: Preoperative assessment of parotid masses: a comparative evaluation of radiographic techniques to histologic diagnosis, *Laryngoscope* 99:284, 1989.

Del Balso AM, Williams E, Tane TT: Parotid masses: current modes of diagnostic imaging, *Oral Surg* 54:360, 1982.

Eneroth CM: Salivary gland tumors in the parotid gland and the palate region, *Cancer* 27:1415, 1971.

Mirich DR, McArdle CB, Kulkarni MV: Benign pleomorphic adenomas of the salivary glands: surface coil MR imaging versus CT, *J Comp Assist Tomogr* 11:620, 1987.

Shugar JMA et al: Multicentric parotid cysts and cervical adenopathy in AIDS patients. A newly recognized entity: CT and MR manifestations, *Laryngoscope* 98:772, 1988.

Thawley SE, Panbje WR: *Comprehensive management of head and neck tumors*, Philadelphia, 1987, WB Saunders.

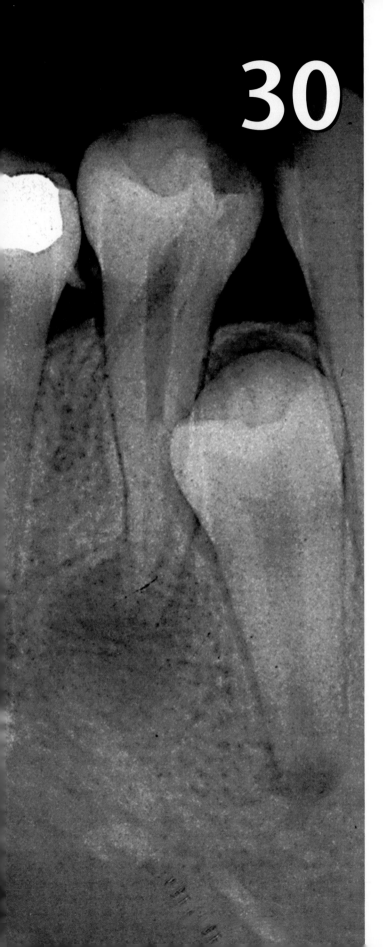

30 Orofacial Implants

VIVEK SHETTY
BYRON W. BENSON

Few advances in dentistry have been as dramatic as the use of prosthetic implants to restore orofacial form and function. Implant technology has enabled the practitioner to help affected patients regain the ability to chew normally and function without embarrassment. With long-term success rates approaching 95% and higher, implant systems are rapidly entering the mainstream of dental practice. These implants typically function as part of a system combining metal fixtures integrated with bone, abutments fastened to fixtures, and a variety of dental appliances attached to the abutments. Because successful implantation depends on close integration of the fixture and the supporting bone, radiographic imaging is an important element of implant therapy. The burgeoning acceptance of these devices has been attributed in part to the increasingly sophisticated imaging techniques used in all phases of implant treatment, including preoperative treatment planning, intraoperative assessment (integration), and postoperative assessment (function) (Fig. 30-1).

Dentists must be knowledgeable about contemporary implant imaging techniques and familiar with the radiographic appearance of various fixtures (Figs. 30-2 and 30-3). Implants encountered on routine dental radiographs may range from fracture fixation devices to alloplastic materials used for augmentation (Figs. 30-4, 30-5, and 30-6). However, most of these devices are dental implants used to restore lost masticatory function by replacing missing teeth. Although subperiosteal and transosteal implant systems are still used occasionally, nearly all dental implants used today are root-form devices placed within bone (endosteal implants). Therefore this chapter focuses on the radiographic aspects of endosteal dental implants.

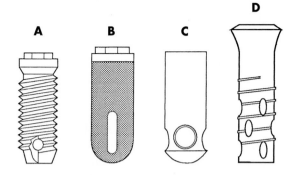

FIG. **30-1** *Four common types of root-form implant fixtures.*
A, Brånemark. **B,** IMZ. **C,** Integral. **D,** ITI.

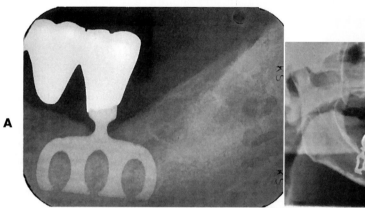
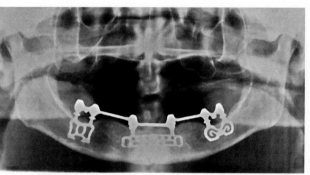

FIG. **30-2** **A,** Blade implant integrated with bone to support a fixed bridge (periapical radiograph of a mandibular molar). **B,** Three blade implants integrated with bone using common abutments to support a mandibular denture region. (**A** courtesy Krishan Kapur, DDS, Los Angeles, Calif.)

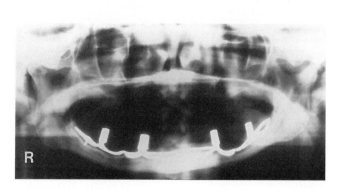

FIG. **30-3** Subperiosteal implant used for aiding denture support.

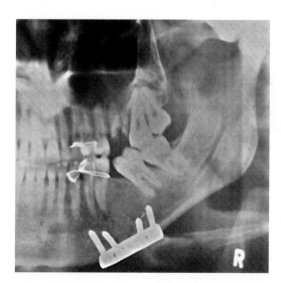

FIG. **30-4** Bone plate (with screws) used to aid the healing of a fractured mandible.

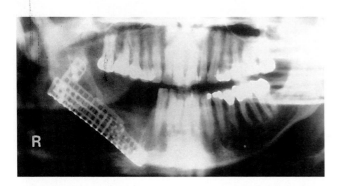

FIG. **30-5** Bone tray used to reconstruct a defect in the body of the mandible.

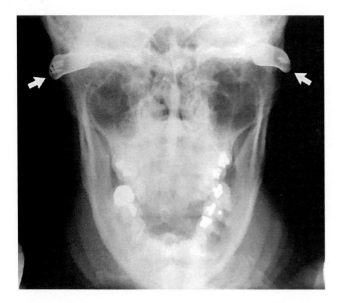

FIG. **30-6** Alloplastic implants substituting for the surgically altered right and left articular fossae (reverse Towne's projection).

Radiographic Assessment of Dental Implants

Although useful and cost-effective, the conventional methods of implant imaging generally are considered inadequate for comprehensive implant evaluation. Newer techniques that permit cross-sectional visualization and interactive image analysis may be considered the standard of care, especially for complex reconstructions. The choice of radiographic techniques often is a function of the various phases of the surgical and restorative procedures (Table 30-1). In every instance the imaging strategy most appropriate for a particular phase of the implant therapy should always be a collective decision of the implant team—the restorative dentist, surgeon, and radiologist (Table 30-2).

Preoperative Planning

Radiographic visualization of potential implant sites is an important extension of clinical examination and assessment. Radiographs help the clinician visualize the alveolar ridges and adjacent structures in all three dimensions and guide the choice of site, number, size, and axial orientation of the implants. Site selection includes consideration of adjacent anatomic structures such as the incisive and mental foramina, inferior alveolar canal, existing teeth, nasal fossae, and maxillary sinuses. Pathologic conditions, such as retained root fragments, impacted teeth, and osteomyelitis, that could compromise the outcome must be identified and located relative to the site of the proposed implant. The variety of radiographic techniques available to assist the clinician includes intraoral radiography (film and digital), cephalometric radiography, panoramic radiography,

---

TABLE **30-1**

Commonly Used Radiographic Procedures with Time Intervals for Treatment Planning and Assessment of Dental Implants

STAGE OF TREATMENT	TIME (MONTHS)	RADIOGRAPHIC PROCEDURES
Treatment planning	−1	Periapical, panoramic radiography; conventional tomography; reformatted computed tomography; cephalometric radiography
Surgery (fixture placement)	0	Imaging only for correction of problems
Healing	0 to 3	Imaging only for correction of problems
Remodeling	4 to 12	Periapical, panoramic radiography; scanography
Maintenance (without problems)	13+	Periapical, panoramic radiography; scanography (follow up approximately every 3 years)
Complications	Anytime	Periapical, panoramic radiography; scanography; conventional tomography (as indicated)

conventional tomography, computed tomography (CT), and stereoscopic (paired) x-ray imaging.

In evaluating a potential implant site, particular attention should be given both to the quality and quantity of bone required for placement of the fixture. The bone must have the necessary dimensions and quality to provide support for the implant fixture. Cortical bone typically is best suited to withstand the functional loading forces of dental implants. The thicker the cortical bone, the greater the likelihood of osseous integration and subsequent success. Bone quantity is assessed by documenting the height and width of available alveolar bone, as well as the morphology of the ridge. The chances of successful implantation increase as more bone is available for anchorage. A cross-sectional image to document the facial-lingual width and height of the ridge, along with the inclination of the bone contours, is especially useful in the preoperative planning phase. Ridge width

measurements aid in maximal engagement of cortical bone, and ridge height measurements aid in the selection of the longest appropriate fixture to maximize anchorage and distribution of masticatory forces. Frequently, morphologic features such as osseous undercuts and ridge concavities that are not immediately apparent on clinical examination become evident with cross-sectional imaging. This information may dictate the choice of implant and its axis of orientation.

Accurate bone measurements are essential for determining the optimal size and length of the proposed implants. The clinician should be aware that the magnification factor of radiographic images may vary with the imaging technique used. Except for reformatted CT, all radiographic images are magnified because the object is never in the same plane as the film. The clinician must consider this magnification factor when calculating the dimensions of the bone at the implant site. To obtain

TABLE 30-2
Summary of Techniques for Implant Imaging

IMAGING TECHNIQUE	APPLICATIONS	ADVANTAGES	DISADVANTAGES
Intraoral periapical radiography	S, M, E, A, R	Readily available High image definition Minimal distortion Least cost and radiation risk	Limited imaging area No facial-lingual dimension Limited reproducibility Image elongation and foreshortening
Intraoral occlusal radiography	S, M, A	Readily available High image definition Gross facial-lingual dimension Relatively large imaging area Least cost and radiation risk	No facial-lingual dimension of ridge Limited reproducibility Not feasible for maxilla Image superimposition
Panoramic radiography	S, M, E, A, R	Readily available Large imaging area Minimal cost and radiation risk	No facial-lingual dimension Moderate image definition Technique errors common Inconsistent magnification Geometric distortion
Conventional tomography	S, M, E	Good image definition Minimal superimposition Facial-lingual dimension Uniform magnification Accurate measurements Moderate cost	Somewhat limited availability Special training needed for interpretation Sensitive to technique errors Higher radiation risk for multiple sites
Reformatted computed tomography	M, E, A, R	Allows evaluation of all possible sites Minimal superimposition Uniform magnification (1:1) Accurate measurements Bone density evaluation Simulates placement with software	Limited availability of reformatting software Sensitive to technique errors Metallic image artifacts Special training needed for interpretation Higher cost and radiation risk

S, Single implant; *M,* multiple implants (2 to 5); *E,* edentulous (6+); *A,* augmentation procedure; *R,* reconstruction procedure.

the actual dimensions of the available bone, the measurements obtained from the radiographs (usually in millimeters) are divided by the magnification factor (usually 1.0 to 1.8) for the particular imaging technique being used. The magnification factor of some techniques may be variable (periapical, panoramic) or fixed (conventional tomography). Reformatted CT images can be corrected to life size. If the magnification factor is constant, clear plastic overlays with 1 mm grids or diagrams of available implant sizes can be produced with the same magnification factor as the image.

Imaging Techniques

The ideal imaging technique for dental implant radiography should have several essential characteristics, including the ability to visualize the implant site in the mesial-distal, facial-lingual, and superior-inferior dimensions; the ability to allow reliable, accurate measurements; a capacity to evaluate the density of trabecular bone and cortical thickness; a capacity to correlate the imaged site with the clinical site; reasonable access and cost to the patient; and minimal radiation risk. Usually a combination of radiographs is used. The following is a review of the imaging techniques applicable to dental implant case management.

INTRAORAL RADIOGRAPHY

Intraoral images may be acquired on film or as direct digital images. Periapical and occlusal radiographic films provide images with superior resolution and sharpness. Maxillary and mandibular periapical radiographs commonly are used to evaluate the status of adjoining teeth and remaining alveolar bone in the mesial-distal dimension. They also have been used for determining vertical height, architecture, and bone quality (bone density, amount of cortical bone, and amount of trabecular bone). Although readily available and relatively inexpensive, periapical radiography has geometric and anatomic limitations. Periapical radiographs, made on a dentate arch, typically are made with the paralleling technique, creating an image with minimal foreshortening and elongation. Because an edentulous alveolar ridge may not have the same "long axis" as a tooth, positioning the film in a consistent and repeatable fashion is difficult, and the image may be foreshortened or elongated (Fig. 30-7). Also, it frequently is difficult to place the film either superior or inferior enough to evaluate the entire maxillary or mandibular ridge all the way to the inferior cortical margin. One study reported that 25% of mandibular periapical radiographs did not demonstrate the mandibular canal. In cases when the

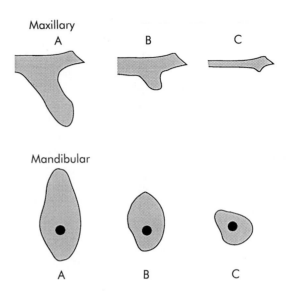

FIG. **30-7** Patterns of bone morphology in the anterior maxilla *(above)* and posterior mandible *(below)* in potential implant therapy patients. Minimal resorption **(A)**, moderate resorption **(B)**, and severe resorption **(C)** of alveolar bone. (Modified from Brånemark P-I et al: *Tissue integrated prostheses,* Chicago, 1985, Quintessence.)

canal was identifiable, only 53% of measurements from the alveolar crest to the superior wall of the mandibular canal were accurate within 1 mm.

Because periapical radiographs are unable to provide any cross-sectional information, occlusal radiographs sometimes are used to determine the facial-lingual dimensions of the mandibular alveolar ridge. Although somewhat useful, the occlusal image records only the widest portion of the mandible, which typically is located inferior to the alveolar ridge. This may give the clinician the impression that more bone is available in the cross-sectional (facial-lingual) dimension than actually exists. The occlusal technique is not useful in imaging the maxillary arch because of anatomic limitations.

LATERAL AND LATERAL-OBLIQUE CEPHALOMETRIC RADIOGRAPHY

Lateral cephalometric radiography provides an image of known magnification (usually 7% to 12%) that documents axial tooth inclinations and the dentoalveolar ridge relationships in the midline of the jaws. The soft tissue profile also is apparent on this film and can be used to evaluate profile alterations after prosthodontic rehabilitation. Although this projection provides a cross-sectional evaluation of the ridges, this dimension is seen only at the midline. The images of structures not in the midline are superimposed on the contralateral side, complicating the evaluation of other implant sites. Oc-

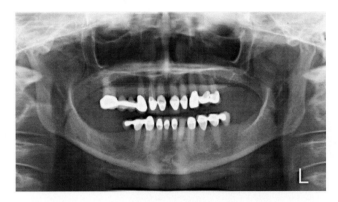

FIG. **30-8** Evaluation of potential implant sites by panoramic radiograph. (Courtesy Oral and Maxillofacial Imaging Center, Baylor College of Dentistry, Dallas, Tex.)

casionally, lateral-oblique cephalometric radiography is used with one side of the body of the mandible positioned parallel to the film cassette. Image magnification on these views is not predictable, because the body of the mandible is not the same distance from the cassette as is the rotation center of the cephalostat. Thus measurements made from these films are not reliable. In general, cephalometric radiographs are of limited use in the selection of implant sites.

PANORAMIC RADIOGRAPHY

Although the resolution and sharpness of panoramic radiographs are less than those of intraoral films, panoramic projections provide a broader visualization of the jaws and adjoining anatomic structures. Panoramic radiography units are widely available, making this imaging technique very popular as a screening and assessment instrument. Panoramic radiographs are useful in making preliminary estimations of crestal alveolar bone and cortical boundaries of the mandibular canal, maxillary sinus, and nasal fossa (Fig. 30-8).

Information acquired from panoramic radiographs must be applied judiciously because this technique has significant limitations as a definitive presurgical planning tool. Angular measurements on panoramic radiographs tend to be accurate, but linear measurements are not. Image size distortion (magnification) varies significantly between films from different panoramic units and even within different areas of the same film. Vertical measurements are unreliable because of foreshortening and elongation of the anatomic structures, since the x-ray beam is perpendicular neither to the long axis of the anatomic structures nor to the film plane. The negative vertical angulation of the x-ray beam also may cause lingually positioned objects such as mandibular tori to be projected superiorly on the film, which may result in

an overestimation of vertical bone height. Furthermore, the anatomic vertical axis varies within the film image, particularly in nonmidline areas. Panoramic radiographs provide a two-dimensional image with no cross-sectional information.

Similarly, dimensional accuracy in the horizontal plane of panoramic radiographs is highly dependent on the position of the structures of interest relative to the central plane of the image layer. The horizontal dimension of images of structures located facial or lingual to the central plane but still within the image layer tends to be minimized or magnified. The degree of horizontal size distortion is difficult to ascertain on panoramic radiographs because the shape of the image layer is configured to a population average. However, the anatomic morphology of few individuals conforms totally to that image layer. In summary, horizontal image magnification with panoramic radiographs varies from 0.70 to 2.2 times actual size, although some manufacturers still claim a 1.25 average magnification (at the central plane of the image layer). Errors in patient positioning can compound further the measurement limitation in the horizontal dimension. Compared with contact radiographs of dissected anatomic specimens, only 17% of panoramic measurements between the alveolar crest and superior wall of the mandibular canal were found to be accurate within 1 mm.

CONVENTIONAL TOMOGRAPHY

Conventional tomography provides reliable dimensional measurements at proposed implant sites, including the cross-sectional (facial-lingual) dimension. It also is reasonably widely available. Used as an adjunct to screening films, cross-sectional tomograms enhance visualization of the available bone. This technique produces a cross-sectional, flat-plane image layer that is perpendicular to the x-ray beam. Images of anatomic structures of interest are relatively sharp, and images of structures outside the image layer are blurred beyond recognition by the motion of the x-ray tube and film. The thickness, orientation, and anatomic location of the image layer can be predetermined and manipulated. It is imperative that the image layer be a true cross-section of the dental arch, rather than oblique. Scout films (usually a submentovertex or panoramic projection) or wax bite registrations commonly are used to determine the appropriate cross-sectional angulation. The complex (multidirectional) tube motion of current conventional tomographic units minimizes image superimposition and provides fixed, uniform image magnification, allowing for accurate measurements. Complex tube motion also permits use of a thicker image layer while retaining diagnostic quality. A thicker image layer is

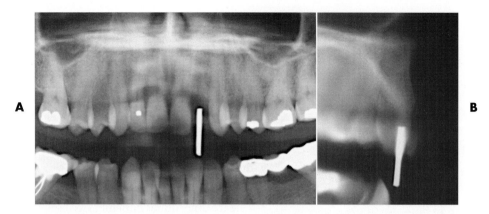

FIG. **30-9** Conventional tomographic series of the maxilla using Scanora integrated imaging system (Orion Corporation/Soredex, Helsinki, Finland). Metal rods retained within an acrylic imaging stent are used to indicate the planned implant sites. **A,** A scout panoramic radiograph used to orient subsequent tomograms. **B,** Cross-sectional tomograms appropriate for measuring the height and width of the alveolar ridge, as well as the axial orientation of the proposed implant. This tomogram suggests that the axial orientation of the proposed implant may need to be altered for optimal placement. (Courtesy Oral and Maxillofacial Imaging Center, Baylor College of Dentistry, Dallas, Tex.)

desirable to maximize image contrast, making the identification of structures such as the mandibular canal more predictable.

The dimensional accuracy of cross-sectional tomograms is particularly useful in measuring the distance between the alveolar crest and adjacent structures, such as the floor of the nasal fossa, maxillary sinus floor, mandibular canal, mental canal, and inferior mandibular cortex. The appropriate axis of insertion of the implant may also be predicted. Measurements are directly acquired from the films and subsequently corrected by the magnification factor used. As an alternative, acetate overlays with appropriately magnified 1 mm grids may be used.

The clinical utility of conventional tomograms can be enhanced by the use of an imaging stent. The stent facilitates correlation of the tomograms to the scout film and provides a practical method of relating the radiographic information to the surgical site. The intended implant sites are identified by radiopaque spheres or rods (metal, composite resin, or gutta-percha) retained within an acrylic stent. The imaging stent subsequently may be used as a surgical guide. For optimal visualization, the width of the markers should be less than the thickness of the tomographic image layer.

Diagnostic dentures coated with barium paste also may be used during imaging. The site markers are visualized in a mesial-distal direction on the scout films and in the facial-lingual dimension on the cross-sectional conventional tomograms. Typically, two to three cross-sectional tomographic slices are required to image each intended implant site adequately. Conventional tomog-

raphy is especially convenient in the planning of single-site implants or those within a quadrant (Figs. 30-9 and 30-10).

COMPUTED TOMOGRAPHY

Patients who are edentulous or who are being considered for multiple implants and augmentation procedures may be best imaged with CT. CT studies are planned on a lateral scout image of the selected jaw with alignment corrections made as needed. Direct axial images are then acquired as thin, overlapping axial scans with approximately 30 axial sections per jaw. These images usually are acquired perpendicular to the occlusal plane. The sequential axial images subsequently are manipulated to produce multiple two-dimensional images in various planes, using a computer-based process called *multiplanar reformatting (MPR).* In general, three basic images are reformatted: axial images with a superimposed curve, cross-sectional images, and panoramic-like curved linear images. An axial scan including the full contour of the mandible (or maxilla) at a level corresponding to the dental roots is selected as a reference for the reformatting process. The computer places a series of sequential dots on the selected scan and connects them to develop a customized arch or curve unique for each jaw. The computer program then generates a series of lines perpendicular to the curve. These lines are made at constant intervals (usually 1 to 2 mm) and numbered sequentially on the axial image to indicate the position at which each cross-sectional slice will be reconstructed. Cross-sectional reconstructions are made

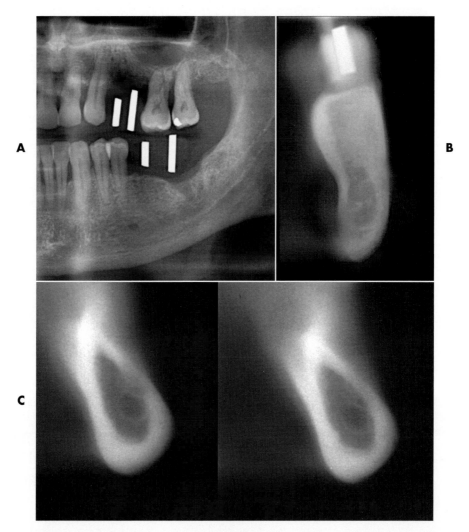

FIG. **30-10** Conventional tomographic series of the mandible using Scanora integrated imaging system (Orion Corporation/Soredex, Helsinki, Finland). Metal rods retained within an acrylic imaging stent have been used to indicate the planned implant sites. **A,** Scout panoramic radiograph used to orient the subsequent tomograms. **B,** Cross-sectional tomograms appropriate for measuring the height and width of the alveolar ridge and the axial orientation of the proposed implant. Note the mental canal and foramen on the buccal aspect of the mandible. **C,** Another case demonstrating a corticated mandibular canal. An imaging stent was not used in this case. (Courtesy Oral and Maxillofacial Imaging Center, Baylor College of Dentistry, Dallas, Tex.)

perpendicular to the curve, and panoramic (curved linear) reconstructions are made parallel with the curve. Three-dimensional representations may also be constructed in various orientations (Figs. 30-11 and 30-12).

These reformatted images provide the clinician with two-dimensional diagnostic information in all three dimensions. Typical studies provide information on the continuity of the cortical bone plates, residual bone in the mandible and maxilla, the relative location of adjoining vital structures, and the contour of soft tissues covering the osseous structures. Studies have reported that 94% of CT measurements between the alveolar

crest and wall of the mandibular canal were accurate within 1 mm. Three-dimensional reformations are particularly useful in the planning of augmentation procedures such as a sinus lift. Unlike conventional tomograms, reformatted CT images provide the radiographic density values of cortical plates and trabecular bone, which may be useful in managing the case. Reformatted CT images also may be used with interactive software to simulate implant orientation and placement on a computer screen before surgery.

Reformatted CT studies provide diagnostic information on all available implant sites with a dental arch. The

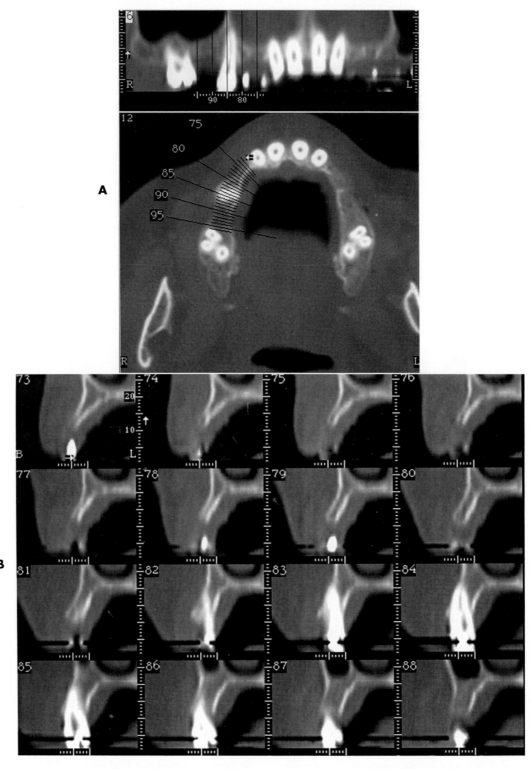

FIG. **30-11**   Reformatted CT study of the maxilla using 3-D Dental software (Columbia Scientific, Inc., Columbia, Md.). **A,** Axial and panoramic-like curved linear reconstructed images using an imaging stent incorporating gutta-percha markers. **B,** Cross-sectional images that correlate with the images in **A.** These images typically are printed life-size for ease of evaluation. (Courtesy Oral and Maxillofacial Imaging Center, Baylor College of Dentistry, Dallas, Tex.)

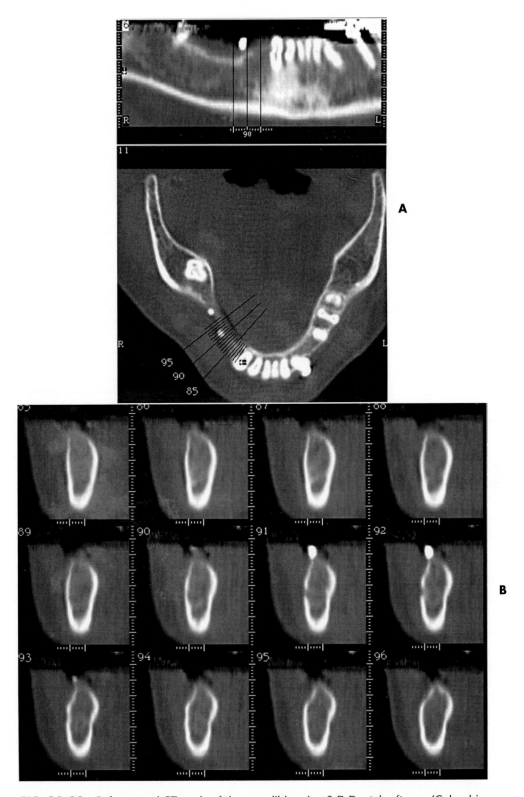

FIG. **30-12** Reformatted CT study of the mandible using 3-D Dental software (Columbia Scientific, Inc., Columbia, Md.). **A,** Axial and panoramic-like curved linear reconstructed images. An imaging stent with gutta-percha markers was used in this case. **B,** Correlating cross-sectional images. These images typically are printed life-size for ease of evaluation. (Courtesy Oral and Maxillofacial Imaging Center, Baylor College of Dentistry, Dallas, Tex.)

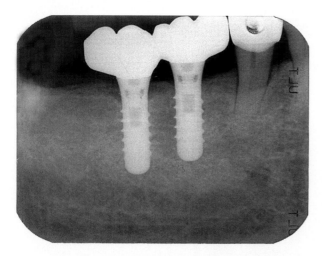

FIG. **30-13**   A periapical radiograph of two successful dental implants. Note the close apposition of the bone to the surface of each implant. A minor amount of saucerization is present at the alveolar crest adjacent to the distal fixture.

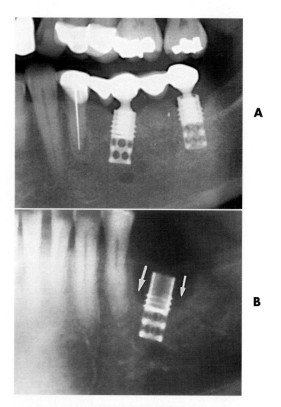

FIG. **30-14**   **A,** Periapical radiograph of marginal bone loss ("saucerization" type) around the cervical region of a root-form dental implant. **B,** Marginal bone loss around the cervical region of a root-form dental implant (portion of a panoramic radiograph).

reformatted images typically are presented life-size on photographic prints or radiographic film. The panoramic (curved linear) images are helpful in identifying mesial-distal relationships and noncorticated mandibular canals. However, the quality of the reformatted CT study depends on the ability of the patient to remain still during image acquisition, because movement may result in subsequent geometric image distortion. Metallic restorations can cause streak image artifacts. However, the streaking is only within the axial plane and does not affect axial slices superior or inferior to it. As with conventional tomography, it is desirable to localize anticipated implant sites with imaging stents incorporating nonmetallic radiopaque markers (gutta-percha, composite resin). Barium-coated diagnostic dentures may also be used to establish the spatial relationships between the anticipated prosthesis and fixtures.

INTRAOPERATIVE AND POSTOPERATIVE ASSESSMENTS

Intraoral and panoramic radiographs usually are adequate for both intraoperative and postoperative assessments. If threaded root-form fixtures have been placed, the optimal radiographic image must separate the threads for best visualization. This may not always be a predictable procedure because the exact angulation of the implant is not known. The angulation of the x-ray beam must be within 9 degrees of the long axis of the fixture to open the threads on the image on most threaded fixtures (Fig. 30-13). Angular deviations of 13 degrees or more result in complete overlap of the threads. In general, periapical radiographs are appropriate for longitu-

dinal assessments. Mesial and distal marginal bone height is measured using known interthread measurements and comparing that with the bone level in previous periapical radiographs. The presence of relatively constant and distinct bone margins suggests successful osseous integration. Resorptive changes, if present, are evidenced by apical migration of the alveolar bone or indistinct osseous margins. These adverse changes are progressive and should be differentiated from the initial circumscribed resorptive osseous changes around the cervical area of the fixture induced by the surgical procedure itself. Studies suggest that the rate of marginal bone loss after successful implantation is approximately 1.2 mm in the first year, subsequently tapering off to about 0.1 mm in succeeding years. Occasionally areas of marginal bone gain also may be noted.

A clinically stable fixture is invariably associated with the radiographic appearance of normal osseous tissue in intimate contact with the implant surface. The development of a thin radiolucent area that closely follows the outline of the implant usually correlates to clinically detectable implant mobility and is an important indicator of failed osseointegration (Figs. 30-14, 30-15, and

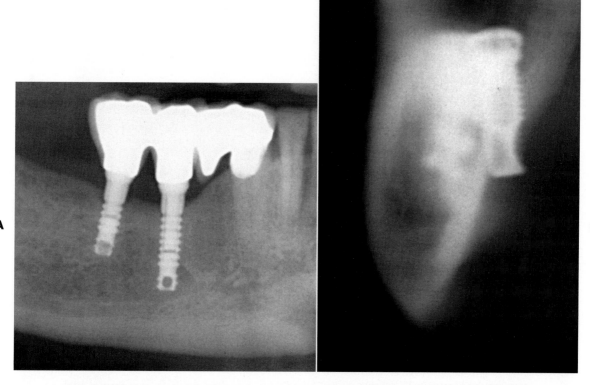

FIG. **30-15** **A,** Panoramic image demonstrating an apparently successful implant placement. **B,** Conventional tomogram of the distal implant reveals perforation of the lingual cortical plate of the mandible and encroachment on the submandibular gland fossa.

TABLE **30-3**
Radiographic Signs Associated with Failing Endosseous Implants

RADIOGRAPHIC APPEARANCE	CLINICAL IMPLICATIONS
Thin radiolucent area that closely follows the entire outline of the implant	Failure of the implant to integrate with adjoining bone
Radiolucent area around the coronal portion of the implant	Periimplantitis resulting from poor plaque control, adverse loading, or both
Apical migration of alveolar bone on one side of the implant	Nonaxial loading resulting from improper angulation of the implant
Widening of the periodontal ligament space of the nearest natural abutment	Poor stress distribution resulting from biomechanically inadequate prosthesis-implant system
Fracture of the fixture	Unfavorable stress distribution during function

30-16). Changes in the periodontal ligament space of associated teeth (natural abutment) also are useful in monitoring the functional competence of the prosthesis-implant system. Any widening of the periodontal ligament space compared with preoperative radiographs indicates poor stress distribution and forecasts implant failure (Table 30-3). After successful implantation, radiographs may be made at regular intervals to assess the success or failure of the implant fixture. Advanced imaging studies may be necessary for adequate assessment in some cases.

Subtle areas of bone resorption adjacent to the fixture may be made evident with intraoral digital images by evaluating a density profile graph of radiographic density values, a feature available on most digital imaging units. If intraoral digital images are acquired at the time of surgery, they may be compared with subsequent digital images either by subjective visualization or digital

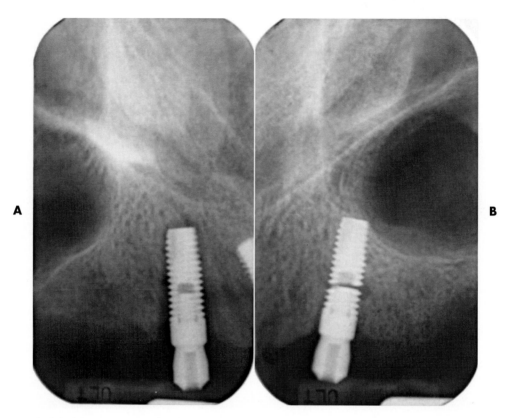

FIG. **30-16** **A,** Periapical radiographs of perifixtural bone loss around a root-form dental implant, indicating failure of osseous integration. **B,** Periapical views of a fractured endosseous implant.

subtraction. Digital subtraction is a computerized process that may reveal areas of bone resorption not apparent visually. Occasionally, stereoscopic plain films or scanograms, which provide the appearance of three dimensions, may be helpful in assessing multiple implant fixtures within a segment of the alveolar ridge. However, measurements may not be reliable on stereoscopic projections.

In summary, imaging is an integral part of dental implant therapy, and a variety of imaging techniques are used for implant assessment. Cross-sectional imaging is increasingly considered integral to optimal implant placement, especially in the case of complex reconstructions. An initial assessment of the feasibility of implant placement may appropriately be made with panoramic radiography. If required, an intraoral radiograph can provide the higher resolution required to evaluate suspected areas of pathosis. Should the initial assessment be favorable and a decision made to proceed with the placement of implants, a cross-sectional image is indicated. Conventional tomography is appropriate for single-implant sites, whereas reformatted CT is preferred for multiple sites or for an edentulous ridge in

which all possible implant sites are to be considered. Assessment of implanted fixtures typically is performed with periapical and panoramic radiography. However, specific cases may require more advanced imaging studies, depending on the nature of the clinical concern.

SUGGESTED READINGS

COMPARATIVE DOSIMETRY

Avendanio B et al: Estimate of radiation detriment: scanography and intraoral radiology, *Oral Surg Oral Med Oral Pathol Oral Radiol Endod* 82:713, 1996.

Frederiksen NL et al: Effective dose and risk assessment from computed tomography of the maxillofacial complex, *Dentomaxillofac Radiol* 24:55, 1995.

Frederiksen NL et al: Risk assessment from film tomography used for dental implant diagnostics, *Dentomaxillofac Radiol* 23:123, 1994.

Scaf G et al: Dosimetry and cost of imaging for osseointegrated implants with film-based and computed tomography, *Oral Surg Oral Med Oral Pathol Oral Radiol Endod* 83:41, 1997.

COMPUTED TOMOGRAPHY

Golec TS: CAD-CAM multiplanar diagnostic imaging for sub-periosteal implants, *Dent Clin North Am* 30:85, 1986.

Kopp CD: Stent-assisted CT in three phases of osseointegration, *Academy Osseointegration* 1:1, 1985.

Kraut RA: Utilization of 3D/DENTAL software for precise implant site selection: clinical reports, *Implant Dent* 1:134, 1992.

McGivney GP et al: A comparison of computer-assisted tomography and data-gathering modalities in prosthodontics, *Int J Oral Maxillofac Implants* 1:55, 1986.

Schwarz MS et al: Computed tomography. I. Preoperative assessment of the mandible for endosseous implant surgery, *Int J Oral Maxillofac Implants* 2:137, 1987.

Schwarz MS et al: Computed tomography. II. Preoperative assessment of the maxilla for endosseous implant surgery, *Int J Oral Maxillofac Implants* 2:143, 1987.

Schwarz MS et al: Computed tomography in dental implantation surgery: osseointegration, *Dent Clin North Am* 33:555, 1989.

Shimura M et al: Presurgical evaluation for dental implants using a reformatting program of computed tomography: maxilla/mandible shape pattern analysis (MSPA), *Int J Oral Maxillofac Implants* 5:175, 1990.

Wishan MS et al: Computed tomography as an adjunct in dental implant surgery, *Int J Oral Maxillofac Implants* 8:31, 1988.

CONVENTIONAL TOMOGRAPHY

Ekestubbe A et al: The use of tomography for dental implant planning, *Dentomaxillofac Radiol* 26:206, 1997.

Fernandes RJ et al: A cephalometric tomographic technique to visualize the buccolingual and vertical dimensions of the mandible, *J Prosthet Dent* 58: 466, 1987.

Gröndahl K et al: Reliability of hypocycloidal tomography for the evaluation of the distance from the alveolar crest to the mandibular canal, *Dentomaxillofac Radiol* 20:200, 1991.

Kassebaum DK et al: Cross-sectional radiography for implant site assessment, *Oral Surg Oral Med Oral Pathol* 70:674, 1990.

Poon C et al: Presurgical tomographic assessment for dental implants. I. A modified imaging technique, *Int J Oral Maxillofac Implants* 7:246, 1992.

Stella JP, Tharanon W: A precise radiographic method to determine the location of the inferior alveolar canal in the posterior edentulous mandible: implications for dental implants. I. Technique, *Int J Oral Maxillofac Implants* 5:15, 1990.

Stella JP, Tharanon W: A precise radiographic method to determine the location of the inferior alveolar canal in the posterior edentulous mandible: implications for dental implants. II. Clinical application, *Int J Oral Maxillofac Implants* 5:23, 1990.

GENERAL IMAGING TECHNIQUES

Benson BW: Diagnostic imaging for dental implant assessment, *Texas Dent J* 112:37, 1995.

Frederiksen NL: Diagnostic imaging in dental implantology, *Oral Surg Oral Med Oral Pathol Oral Radiol Endod* 80:540, 1995.

Hollender L, Rockler B: Radiographic evaluation of osseointegrated implants of the jaws, *Dentomaxillofac Radiol* 9:91, 1980.

Klinge B et al: Location of the mandibular canal: comparison of macroscopic findings, conventional radiography, and computed tomography, *Int J Oral Maxillofac Implants* 4:327, 1989.

Miles DA, Van Dis ML: Implant radiology, *Dent Clin North Am* 37:645, 1993.

Milgrom P, Getz T: Implants: growing concern, *Dental Claims and Insurance News* 8:1, 1994 [newsletter].

Pharoah MJ: Imaging techniques and their clinical significance, *Int J Prosthodont* 6:176, 1993.

Reisken AB: Implant imaging: status, controversies, and new developments, *Dent Clin North Am* 2:47, 1998.

Sewerin I: Identification of dental implants on radiographs, *Quintessence Int* 23:611, 1992.

Strid K-G: Radiographic procedures. In Brånemark P-I, editors: *Tissue-integrated prostheses,* Chicago, 1985, Quintessence.

Strid K-G: Radiographic results. In Brånemark P-I et al, editors: *Tissue-integrated prostheses,* Chicago, 1985, Quintessence.

GENERAL IMPLANTOLOGY

Block MA et al, editors: *Implants in dentistry,* Philadelphia, 1997, WB Saunders.

Brånemark P-I et al, editors: *Tissue integrated prostheses,* Chicago, 1985, Quintessence.

Cranin AM et al: A statistical evaluation of 952 endosteal implants in humans, *J Am Dent Assoc* 94:315, 1977.

Smith RA: New developments and advances in dental implantology, *Oral Maxillofac Surg Infections* 52:42, 1992.

IMAGING TECHNIQUES (IMAGING STENTS)

Israelson H et al: Barium-coated surgical stents and computer-assisted tomography in the preoperative assessment of dental implant patients, *Int J Periodont Restorative Dent* 12:53, 1992.

PANORAMIC RADIOGRAPHY

Lindh C, Petersson AR: Radiologic examination of the mandibular canal: a comparison between panoramic radiography and conventional tomography, *Int J Oral Maxillofac Implants* 4:249, 1989.

Tal H, Moses O: A comparison of panoramic radiography with computed tomography in the planning of implant surgery, *Dentomaxillofac Radiol* 20:40, 1991.

Truhlar RS et al: A review of panoramic radiography and its potential use in implant dentistry, *Implant Dent* 2:122, 1993.

Index

637

ISBN 0-8151-9491-9